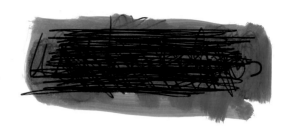

ORBITAL TUMORS

Second Edition

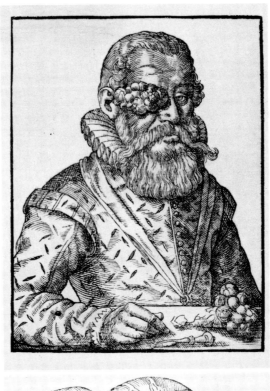

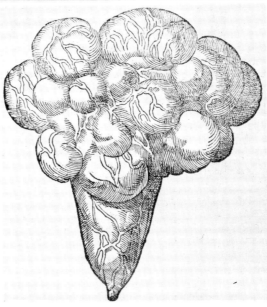

(*Above*) A very early illustration of an orbital tumor in a 56-year-old man. The tumor was removed with the surgical tool lying on the table in front of the patient.

(*Below*) The enucleated pathologic specimen. The patient survived the operation.

(*From Fabricius von Hilden W [Fabricii Hildani G*]: Wund-Artzney, gantzes Werck, und aller Bücher, so viel deren vorhanden. [Auss dem Lateinischen in das Teutsche Sprach übersetzt durch Friderich Greiffen.] Frankfurt am Main, Johann Beyers, 1652, pp 3, 13.)

ORBITAL TUMORS

Second Edition

JOHN W. HENDERSON

M.S. (Ophthalmology), M.A. (Anatomy), D.Sc. (Honorary), M.D.
Former Chairman, Department of Ophthalmology, Mayo Clinic;
Emeritus Professor of Ophthalmology, Mayo Medical School;
Rochester, Minnesota

in collaboration with

GEORGE M. FARROW, M.D., M.S. (Pathology)

Head of Section, Department of Surgical Pathology, Mayo Clinic;
Associate Professor in Pathology, Mayo Medical School;
Rochester, Minnesota

1980

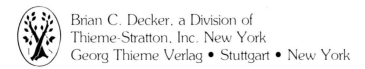
Brian C. Decker, a Division of
Thieme-Stratton, Inc. New York
Georg Thieme Verlag • Stuttgart • New York

Publisher: Brian C. Decker, a Division of
Thieme-Stratton Inc.
381 Park Avenue South
New York, New York 10016

ORBITAL TUMORS

ISBN 0-913258-77-6

Last digit is print number 9 8 7 6 5 4 3 2 1

Affectionately dedicated to
Nadine, Sally, and Holly

Preface

Eight years have passed since the manuscript was finalized for the first printing of *Orbital Tumors*. In this interval, several major advances have occurred in this field. Foremost in overall importance has been the burgeoning application of computed tomography to orbital diagnostics. In this short interval, the technology of computed tomography has passed from its infancy to a sophisticated family of fourth generation scanners. This has provided a window to the orbital deep by which soft tissue masses are now visualized; a wonderment beyond imagination at the time I started clinical practice.

Also noteworthy have been the changing concepts in the terminology, diagnosis, and treatment of some of the individual tumors. Malignant lymphomas, for one, have undergone such changes in their histopathologic classification that new names have made passé such old and familiar terms as *reticulum cell sarcoma* and *lymphosarcoma*. In addition, the use of immunochemistry in the entire spectrum of lymphoproliferative diseases may, in the future, provide a supplementary means for differentiating the malignant from the nonmalignant tumors as well as the individual lymphomas from each other. The scourge of orbital rhabdomyosarcoma has been definitely mitigated by the use of adjuvant chemotherapy and radiotherapy, and the treatment protocols of cooperative treatment centers have made possible a controlled judgment of prognosis. In addition, newer orbital lesions, such as Wegener's granulomatosis, have been sufficiently documented to warrant inclusion in the classification of orbital tumors. Electron microscopy has become a most useful supplement to light microscopy in determining the tissue genesis of some tumors of equivocal origin. All of this and more has made parts of the first edition woefully out-of-date.

Finally, in the eight-year interval, there has been a priceless opportunity to extend further the follow-up observation of the original consecutive series of 465 patients and to enlarge the scope of our study to a total of 764 consecutive cases. This has permitted an observation of some patients for 27 years or longer and has revealed new information concerning the long-term (30 to 40 years) or natural history of some tumors. Such data have revealed the minatory behavior of many benign recurrent mixed tumors and orbital meningiomas, and the lethal course of orbital hemangiopericytomas; features heretofore suspected but not well documented. Our concept of the clinical course of these as well as other tumors has been revised accordingly by the lengthened period of study.

All this has made a major revision of *Orbital Tumors* desirable, but such an endeavor could not be undertaken without consideration of the economic realities of such a publication. Simply stated, the spiraling costs of printing must be weighed against the still narrow readership appeal of the subject relative to the more populated subspecialty groups. Our publisher, Brian C. Decker, believed such a project feasible and W.B. Saunders, publisher of the first edition, graciously released the various copyright restrictions.

In keeping with budgetary guidelines, all copy of the first edition was carefully revised and re-edited so as to make room for all new subject material without increasing the original size of the text. Also, in the interests of conserving space, we have followed the custom of the former edition in listing only key references at the conclusion of each chapter rather than duplicating in-depth bibliographies that can be found elsewhere in the literature. We believe these alterations will still provide an attractive updating of the text for the benefit of the faithful readers of the first edition and provide a stimulating overview of the subject to a newer generation of ophthalmologists.

In preparing this revision I have again relied heavily for advice and counsel on my close collaborater, Dr. George Farrow, and his associates in the Department of Surgical Pathology of the Mayo Clinic. Dr. Peter Banks and Dr. Edward Soule, also of this department, generously provided data important to the updating of the chapters on malignant lymphoma and rhabdomyosarcoma. Other standbys from the staff of the Mayo Clinic who helped in the preparation of this as well as the first edition were Dr. Omer Burgert, Jr. (Pediatrics), Dr. Martin Van Herik (Radiophysics), Dr. Colin Holman (Radiology), and Dr. Kenneth Devine (Surgical Oncology of the Head and Neck). Dr. Thomas McDonald (Otorhinolaryngology) shared with me his viewpoint on some of the tumors secondarily invading the orbit from sources in the nose, nasopharynx, and paranasal sinuses. Other sources of information and new figures are carefully acknowledged in the text. Mr. John Prickman of the Department of Publications, Mayo Clinic, and Mary Donchez of New York shared in editing and assembling the revised manuscript. Dolores Sexton willingly typed the many addenda so necessary to a revised manuscript. Most important, during the two-year period of preparation, was the steadfast backing of the publisher, Brian C. Decker.

Now back, once again, to the cushioned chaise lounge for rest and recuperation, but ever curious about the progress of orbital tumor patients.

John Warren Henderson, M.D.

Contents

III / SURGICAL APPROACHES TO ORBITAL TUMORS

SECTION I

Applied Anatomy
of the Orbit

Diagnosis of
Orbital Tumors

1

Applied Anatomy of the Orbit

Although the orbit is defined by some in terms of its bony components and contours, others regard it as a cavity or space in which are housed those tissues and organs contributing to the function of the eye. The former is properly termed the *bony orbit* and the latter, the *orbital cavity*. In medical parlance the word *orbit* frequently includes both the space and its surrounding bone, that is, the *bony socket*. Throughout this text the word orbit will be used with its broadest denotation, and the reader may judge from the context whether the reference is to orbital bone or socket cavity, or both. The eye, of course, is the principal resident of this compartment, the bones and adnexal structures being carefully adapted for its protection and support. Nature has designed this orbit so nicely that the eye, particularly anteriorly, fits as smoothly as a hand in a glove and almost as snugly as a cork in a bottle.

It follows, then, that when something goes amiss with this contact arrangement — such as the edema of inflammation, the swelling of an expanding tumor, or the dilatation of vascular channels — direct pressure is exerted on the eye. The result is forward expulsion of the eye from the protective environs of its orbit.

GENERAL ORBITAL TOPOGRAPHY

Among the various descriptions of the orbit, Whitnall's (1932) is one of the most graphic. He compared the orbit to a pear, the anterior orbital aperture corresponding to the base of the pear and the optic canal, to its stalk. The volume of this orbital spaced is only 29 ml. The *measurements* of the principal meridians of the orbital cavity are noted by all texts of anatomy and, as these values are so nearly alike, it is convenient to consider its size (in adults) by taking a standard of 40 mm for each meridian: that is, for height, width, and depth.For practical purposes the anterior aperture of the orbit in diameter is about the size of a half-dollar; in children and infants these values are correspondingly less.

Just as the body of the pear has a greater circumference than its base, so too the roomiest portion of the orbit is about 15 mm inside the orbital rim. This space would be quite adequate for the exploring finger were it not for the protective overhang of the circumference of the orbital rim. Access to the orbital cavity through this narrow space is easier on the nasal and inferior sides of the orbit. The width of these avenues of approach is about a finger's breadth. To facilitate palpation of orbital structures through these narrow apertures, some

3

physicians use the little finger, but the proprioceptive sense of this digit is not nearly as acute as that of the index finger.

The *anterior portion* of the orbit, wherein are lodged the eye and lacrimal gland, is roughly quadrangular. Posterior to these structures there seems less need for support, and the bony floor merges into the other three walls of the compartment, which now becomes triangular. Although the volume of the orbit is reduced, adnexal tissues are not as crowded in this area as they are more anteriorly. The transfrontal and lateral surgical approaches, by circumventing the eyeball and lacrimal gland, have proved more useful in reaching this retrobular space than the older route of anterior orbitotomy.

At the *apex*, where the three remaining walls merge, are located the posterior outlets of the orbit: the *optic foramen* and *superior orbital fissure.* The former, with its prolongation posteriorly making the optic canal, is frequently unroofed by the neurosurgeon either during his dissection for meningioma or during the excision of a glioma extending along the optic nerve. This remote area is approximately 5 cm from the nearest skin surface. The ophthalmic surgeon also must be well acquainted with this apical area in order to facilitate removal of "intra-orbital" meningiomas, which are encountered rarely in the course of lateral orbitotomy, and resection of long sections of the optic nerve in cases such as intraocular retinoblastoma and optic nerve glioma. However, neither neurosurgeon nor ophthalmologist is anxious to disturb structures adjacent to the superior orbital fissure, for through it pass at least eight nerves of assorted diameters and several blood vessels. This is a veritable "no man's land."

The student or the young surgeon rummaging around the rear of the orbit for the first time usually has some misconceptions as to the exact location of these orifices. Figure 1 shows their position as viewed from the front, but the photographer or medical illustrator often positions the skull at an angle to reveal best all the major bony structures and foramina of the orbit (Fig. 2). In such illustrations, the optic foramen appears to be located close to the intersection of lines drawn through the vertical transverse diameters, and the illusion is given that the orbit is cone-shaped in a direct anteroposterior axis, the apex of the cavity being nearly equidistant from the four sides. The observer may not realize, however, that such views do not represent a true front view of the orbit. Instead, the line of visual regard is actually parallel to the axis of the optic canal and, when such a line is projected forward, it passes through the anterotemporal portion of the orbit, not the true anteroposterior meridian of the skull. Actually, the position of the optic foramen is more medial and superior to that represented in such photographs. If one aligns the orbital cavities of a skull with the observer's eye level, an imaginary line running through the sagittal plane of the observer's nose and the nasal bone of the cadaver, the optic foramina will be directly posterior along the medial walls of the orbit (Figs. 1 and 2). If the observer's head is kept steady and not moved laterally, the right optic foramen of the skull will almost be concealed from the view of the observer's left eye by a slight lateral bulge of the medial wall as it passes along the ethmoid sinus; the situation is similar when the observer tries to locate the position of the left optic foramen with the right eye. This knowledge of the true versus the false location of the apex of the orbit is pertinent to those surgical situations wherein the orbit is approached from the anterior or lateral aspect; the optic foramen is further from the surgeon and, surprisingly, more inaccessible than

Figure 1. True anterior view of orbits. Camera has been positioned along midline axis of skull. Right optic foramen is concealed by slight lateral bulge of medial wall of orbit as it passes along ethmoid sinus. Left optic foramen is only slightly visible as a small dimple (*small arrow*). *Large arrow* superior orbital fissure.

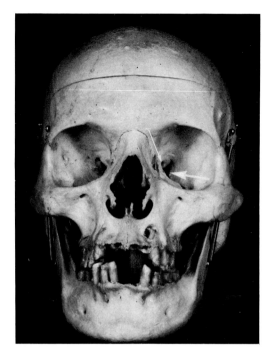

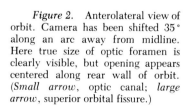

Figure 2. Anterolateral view of orbit. Camera has been shifted 35° along an arc away from midline. Here true size of optic foramen is clearly visible, but opening appears centered along rear wall of orbit. (*Small arrow*, optic canal; *large arrow*, superior orbital fissure.)

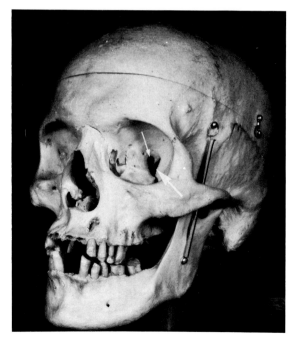

expected. Although the visual axis of the eye is on a saggital plane, the antero-posterior axis of the orbit is offset laterally.

ORBITAL WALLS

The makeup and configuration of the bony walls and rim of the orbit and the application of this knowledge to the problem of orbital tumors are chiefly the concern of the roentgenologist and the surgeon. The superior, nasal, and inferior walls are of greater interest to the former, for it is through study of these barriers that roentgenographic evidence of invasion of the orbit by tumors in adjacent cavities is usually found, and primary tumors may erode these walls in their effort to escape the orbit. (Further comment on the nature of these changes will be found in Chapter 2.) From a surgeon's standpoint the orbit may be entered from any direction, but those anatomic features relating to the superior and lateral rims and walls are more pertinent to the modern surgical approaches.

Superior Wall. The superior wall, or roof, is rather thin throughout its extent, and the periorbita easily peels away from its undersurface. On the intracranial side the dura can be lifted almost as easily. Because the roof is perforated neither by major nerves nor by blood vessels, it is easy to nibble away this bony partition with rongeurs without serious consequences, a fact that is utilized in the transfrontal approach to the orbit. Except when eroded by mucoceles or epidermoid cysts, the roof is an effective barrier that prevents accidental contact with dura underneath the frontal lobes during anterior and lateral orbitotomy.

Lateral Wall. Because the lateral orbital surgical approach is popular, the lateral wall concerns the ophthalmic surgeon more than other bony partitions. In practice, it has some similarities to the roof: it is almost as devoid of foramina, and its anterior portion can be broached without serious hemorrhage; the zygomaticotemporal vessels and nerves piercing the bone just posterior to the midportion of the lateral rim usually do not pose a problem; and the periorbita is reasonably easy to separate from the bone, even in the area of the orbital tubercle where several fascial bands and tendons insert. However, at this point any similarity to the roof of the orbit ceases.

Any exterior approach to the lateral side of the orbit must take into account the tough and thick *lateral rim*, which is but the forward extension of the lateral wall (Fig. 2). This rim is the strongest portion of the orbit, and even the suture line between the zygoma and the frontal bone is not easily jimmied except by the heaviest chisels, saws, and drills. Even so, malignant tumors of the lacrimal gland seem to erode this tough bone as easily as they exert pressure on the eye. That portion of the zygomatic bone constituting the lateral rim and the anterior one-third of the lateral wall protects the posterior half of the eye; the anterior half of the eye thus has an unencumbered vista laterally (Fig. 3). Palpation of retrobulbar tumors, therefore, should be easier from the lateral rather than from the nasal side of the eyeball, but the lacrimal gland, which fills the anterior portion of the superotemporal quadrant, largely nullifies this anatomic advantage. The lateral wall, which is thick along its front surface, becomes thinner as it passes posteriorly to its junction with the forward and lateral extension of the greater wing of the sphenoid bone.

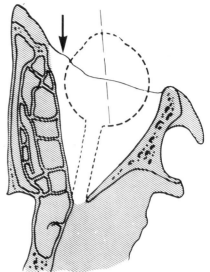

Figure 3. Transverse section of right orbit with diagrammatic representation of eye in relation to nasal and lateral bony walls. Anterior half of eye on lateral surface is not protected by bone. (*Arrow* indicates approximate line of superior bony rim of orbit superimposed on drawing.)

This portion of the sphenoid bone, comprising the posterior two-thirds of the lateral wall, is also wedge-shaped but in a direction inverse to the wedge of the adjacent zygomatic bone. This configuration of the sphenoid makes it difficult to dissect or remove bone posterior to the suture line; biting forceps or drills encounter thicker and thicker bone with but little additional exposure of the orbital contents. Another hindrance to extensive removal of bone beyond this point is the possibility of encountering orbital branches of the middle meningeal artery and vein that penetrate the sphenoid bone posterior to the zygomatic-sphenoid suture; bleeding from this source in the depth of the orbit can unexpectedly complicate manipulations and can be difficult to stem. The zygomatic-sphenoid suture is an important landmark because along this line, bone invariably fractures when one is creating the flap common to all modifications of the Krönlein operation (Fig. 4.) Once the bone flap has been turned, the

Figure 4. Mid-horizontal section through orbits (superior halves): note triangular shapes of bony orbits, broad expanse of orbital roofs, parallel position of medial walls, and thin portion of lateral walls (*arrow*) corresponding to suture line between left sphenoid and zygomatic bones. Dehiscence is present in roof of right orbit. (From Berke RN: A modified Krönlein operation. Trans Am Ophthalmol Soc 51:193–227, 1953. By permission of the American Ophthalmological Society.)

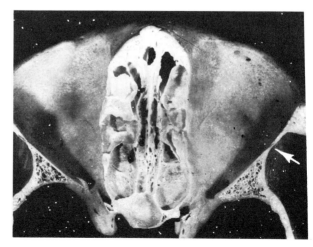

surgeon has direct access to the superolateral and inferolateral quadrants of the orbit posterior to the eye. Since these quadrants are the favorite lurking places of orbital tumors, the surgical anatomy of this area is germane.

Inferior Wall.   The inferior wall, although entered least often during surgery for tumor, is a most important partition to those who specialize in repair of orbital fractures. Almost bisecting this wall from a posterior to anterior direction is the infraorbital groove (part sulcus, part canal) housing the infraorbital nerve and artery. Probably the presence of these structures in the middle of the surgical field is one factor discouraging the antral approach to tumors located in the inferior quadrants of the orbit. On their orbital surfaces the infraorbital nerve and vessel are covered with periorbita. Since orbital tumors rarely originate beneath the periorbita in this area, there is no need to elevate the periorbita during orbitotomy, as so frequently is done in the superior and lateral zones of the orbit. Thus, the surgeon has little reason to disturb the nerves and vessels within the bony groove. If the vessels are accidentally torn, hematoma of the inferior orbit and ecchymosis of the lower eyelid may complicate the immediate postoperative period. The thin inferior wall is easily eroded by upward extension of antral carcinomas.

In practice, upward displacement of the eye sometimes is the initial clue to an otherwise silent neoplasm in the maxillary sinus. When erosion of bone occurs in this area, reactive fibrosis of the covering periorbita may then effectively prevent infiltration of tumor into the orbital soft tissue structures. In the case of primary tumors, the space between periorbita and the eye is more significant: "that is where the action is." This space, although confined by the nearness of the eye to its floor, is not difficult to examine, and palpation of orbital tumors is easier here than in other orbital spaces because the orbital septum is thinner and less of a barrier. Instruments also pass easily beneath the suspensory ligament. This hammock, cradling its rotund occupant, can be elevated to provide more space for surgical maneuver. Visibility is usually direct, and tumors on the floor of the orbit usually are not located too far from the surface, nor do large vessels harass the operator. On the nasal side, the bony origin of the inferior oblique muscle is such that it does not usually interfere with inferior orbitotomy. However, more posteriorly, one must take care to note the presence of the ciliary ganglion. This will not be permanently damaged as long as dissection is blunt and spreading rather than sharp and cutting. Considering the ease of access along the inferior wall, it is regrettable that a greater proportion of tumors are not found in this area.

Medial Wall.   The thinnest of the four walls is the medial. It is frequently eroded by chronic inflammatory lesions, cysts, and neoplasms that originate in the adjacent air sinuses and seek egress via the orbit. Also it is easily fractured by the surgeon's instruments if elevation or removal of the covering periorbita becomes necessary during orbitotomy. This area usually is approached through an incision along the superior nasal bony rim because the wide, thick, medial palpable tendon and the underlying lacrimal drainage apparatus discourage an approach along the midportion of the medial orbital rim. Furthermore, most diagnostic problems originate superior rather than inferior to the medial palpebral tendon. It is along this wall also that hemorrhage is most troublesome. Two foramina in the ethmoid bone transmit arteries, and unless these vessels can be identified and ligated, hemorrhage can so obscure the field of exploration as to seriously hinder careful dissection. In addition, the medial palpebral, the frontal, and the dorsal nasal arteries all pass forward near the medial wall to supply structures outside the orbit. That portion of the lacrimal drainage apparatus consisting of the lacrimal sac and its bony walls lies along the most forward extension of the medial wall but, for the purposes of discussion, will be considered as lying outside the bony orbit proper.

The *superior rim* of the bony orbit is most important because it is encountered more frequently during orbitotomy than are either the inferior or the nasal margins. Also, the diagnostician must learn to palpate along its edge in searching for tumor. For surgical purposes, the superior rim is not considered a part of, nor is it removed with, its adjacent wall as is the lateral margin, except when it is necessary to uncover an epidermoid cyst deeply placed in the frontal bone (see Chapter 4). Its curvature, overhang and thickness are admirable suited to the protection of the eye, and these features also discourage casual prying and snooping into the attic of the orbit. The *supraorbital notch* (sometimes an actual foramen), located at the junction of the medial one-third and lateral two-thirds, is its most important landmark. The supraorbital vessels and nerve curve almost at a right angle along the surface of this notch as they leave the orbit. The vessels may bleed vigorously during orbitotomy with this approach, but the surgeon may carefully dissect inferior to their course, leaving them intact, or may ligate them before entering the orbit proper. The accompanying nerve — the more important of the two major structures passing through the notch — is another matter. Those of us who are able to enjoy the normal function of this nerve and its branches as they pass over our scalps have difficulty understanding the depression and discomfort of those whose nerve supply in this area after a superior orbitotomy is no longer intact. The lack of sensation seems to be a constant and nagging annoyance. The unwary surgeon may sever or tear the nerve during manipulations, and the duration of nerve dysfunction seems proportional to the degree of trauma. If the nerve is severely damaged, regeneration may never be complete; if nerve transmission is permanently impaired, the loss can be a source of recrimination for the patient in an otherwise successful convalescence; and if the injury is only partial, the zone of anesthesia will persist for several months and then be succeeded by bizarre sensations (akin to those of herpes zoster) along the course of the nerve as regeneration slowly occurs.

Just medial to the notch and hanging from the undersurface of the rim is the *trochlea*, its ribbon-like tendon of the superior oblique muscle fanning downward to the eye. Another important structure to the palpating finger is the palpebral lobe of the *lacrimal gland*, which is located beneath the other side (temporal) of the superior rim. When mischief occurs either in the gland proper or adjacent to it, the ensuing swelling pushes the palpebral lobe forward, and the examiner uninitiated to the lobular feel of this structure can easily mistake it for an orbital tumor. It is therefore important to be familiar with the normal feel of these structures as sensed by the tip of an index finger; otherwise, palpating them in a patient with a protruding eye may erroneously lead to the diagnosis of an orbital tumor.

Along the entire circumference of the forward lip of the orbital rim is the fibrous roll of tissue representing the junction of the periosteum, the periorbita, and the orbital septum. This fibrous band is thicker at, and more adherent to, the superior rim than at and to, other areas of the bony margin. The extension of the orbital septum from this fibrous-bony junction into the structures of the eyelids represents the anterior boundary of the orbital cavity. The fusion of these fibrous connective sheaths along the superior rim is also important to the surgeon, who must dissect either through or adjacent to the junction arc in approaching tumors nestling in the upper quadrants. Once this fibrous roll of tissue is peeled away from its tight attachment to the bony rim, the peripheral space between periorbita and bone usually is entered easily with a periosteal elevator.

RETICULAR TISSUE AND ORBITAL SPACES

The spaces and closets in the orbital household not occupied by eye, optic nerve, extraocular muscles and their sheaths, levator palpebrae superioris, lacrimal gland, and assorted smaller vessels and nerves are clinically important, as it is here that most orbital tumors reside. Some have favorite hiding places in the various spaces. Furthermore, most tumors, once established, will not stray beyond the anatomic boundaries of a space unless they are either large or malignant or unless they represent an infiltrative process such as pseudotumor. For the clinician making a preoperative differential diagnosis, this behavior is pertinent, and knowledge of the main compartments and their boundaries permits a choice of the most direct approach to the tumor. These spaces and planes are usually classified on the basis of their circumferential position in relation to the eye. Normally, the bulk of this area is occupied by tissue commonly referred to as the *orbital fat*. The surgeon casually encountering normal fat in the course of either enucleation or operation for blepharoptosis will note its pretty yellow color and the ease with which individual lobules, bulging into the surgical field, can be plucked away with forceps without apparent harm to other structures. The surgeon soon learns, however, not to disturb or trifle unnecessarily with this tissue, because blood persistently oozes from the torn edges of the connective tissue septa separating the lobules of fat.

The fat lobules lie in the interstices of a web of modified connective tissue called either the *reticular tissue* or the *orbital reticulum*. This tissue is the supporting framework of the orbital fat, anchoring it to other modified fascial structures of the orbit, such as Tenon's capsule, orbital septum, check ligaments, intermuscular septa, and the fascial covering of the extraocular muscles. It also is reflected around the optic nerve, the lacrimal gland, the blood vessels, and the nerves; it provides all structures of the orbit with a snug scaffold of support.

Benign encapsulated tumors do not alter the normal structure of reticular tissue and fat, except that these structures are under greater pressure and, when the periorbita has been opened, bulge more persistently into the operative field. However, when the marauder is a malignant neoplasm or when the tumor is inflammatory (pseudotumor or endocrine exophthalmos), this basic matrix may alter, depending on the nature and duration of the invader. The reticular septa become tougher and vascular, bleed readily and persistently, and are more difficult to dissect. The fat turns a tan or dirty yellow, is less soft, and seems to heal with much scarring. In the type of reaction associated with endocrine exophthalmos, the fat may undergo such swelling and hypertrophy that it mimics the form and feel of a firm neoplasm. In other words, the orbital fat and its reticular framework may be very reactive tissues and are not as inert as is commonly assumed. Therefore, the less disturbance of these structures during orbitotomy, the better the functional and cosmetic results.

The attachments, septal divisions, and boundaries of the orbital reticulum also are pertinent to the surgical attack on the tumor that usurps this space. The surgical anatomy of this tissue may be considered in relation to either the anteroposterior axis of the orbit or the circumferential position relative to the eye.

Peripheral (Subperiosteal) Space. The space between periorbita and bone usually is called the *periosteal* or *subperiosteal space.* The term "subperiosteal" with its prefix may be confusing when used as a reference to tumors growing along the roof of the orbit. The reader may not be sure whether the prefix, meaning beneath or under, indicates that the tumor is between periorbita and bone or between periorbita and the eye. As this plane is the most distant of the several spaces from the eye, the term *peripheral* seems more useful and appropriate. Normally this is only a potential space. It is delimited anteriorly by the fusion of periorbita with the periosteum and orbital septum along the rim of the orbit. The other boundaries are formed by attachment of the periorbita to various fissures and foramina in the rear of the orbit and by its junction with the dural sheath along the optic nerve. Elsewhere, the periorbita is reasonably easy to separate from the adjacent bone. Along the roof, tumors originating in bone tend to insinuate themselves along the peripheral space and to separate periorbita from bone. The periorbita then becomes thicker and tougher (unless subject to extreme pressure for a long duration), forming an effective floor barrier against the spread of tumor toward the eye. This space is a favorite lurking place for meningiomas, dermoid cysts, epidermoid cysts, mucoceles, myelomas, osteomatous tumors, hematomas, and forms of fibrous dysplasia. The neoplasms and cysts of this group seldom occur along the inferior and temporal walls of the orbit. Tumors occurring in the upper part of this space usually push the eye straight temporally and somewhat forward. It is with tumors occurring in the peripheral space that roentgenograms are most helpful.

Anterior Space. This space surrounds the eyeball in the way a doughnut encircles its hole. In a frontal plane, the space is delimited internally by the extraocular muscles and intermuscular membrane and peripherally by periorbita. In a sagittal view, its anterior boundary is formed by the orbital septum, but its posterior limit roughly corresponds to the plane of the posterior wall of the eye. In the latter area, the anterior space merges imperceptibly with the posterior retrobulbar space. Tumors in the anterior space tend to push the eye toward one quadrant of the orbit (for example, downward and inward, upward and outward) as well as forward and usually can be palpated. Malignant lymphomas, capillary hemangiomas of childhood, intrinsic neoplasms of the lacrimal gland, and pseudotumors often are found in this space. The fat hypertrophy of a progressive endocrine orbitopathic condition often extends into this zone and, on palpation, mimics the consistency and contour of an inflammatory pseudotumor. Tumors residing in this space usually are explored by the anterior orbitotomy approach.

Posterior (Retrobulbar) Space. This space extends from the back surface of the eye to the orbital apex and is bounded peripherally by the periorbita. It encompasses an area often referred to as the "muscle cone," surgeons or clinicians noting that a tumor is either within or outside the muscle cone. This statement implies that a membrane or sheath passes circumferentially between the extraocular muscles in this area of the orbit and presumes that such a sheath may be more theoretic than real. Some connective tissue septa resembling a sheath are present in the upper nasal quadrant of Figure 5, passing clockwise between the conjoined superior rectus-levator palpebrae muscle bundle and the superior oblique and between the latter and the medial rectus, but no circumferential intermuscular septum is evident between (clockwise) medial rectus and inferior rectus, inferior rectus and lateral rectus, and lateral rectus and superior rectus-levator palpebrae muscle bundle. Our own experience, based on numerous sallies into the temporal quadrants of the orbit through a lateral orbitotomy, does not support the concept of a circumferential intermuscular septum posterior to the eye. Once the periorbita has been broached, the interior of the orbital cavity is easily entered without passage through any definite septum, either above or below the lateral rectus muscle, that would justify the designation of an intermuscular sheath. Furthermore, in this retro-ocular area (Fig. 5), no significiant space exists outside the alleged muscle cone except in the lower nasal-posterior quadrant (peripheral and inferior to the medial rectus) of the orbit. Therefore, on a practical anatomic basis, surgeons might well abandon the concept of positioning tumors in relation to a muscle cone and, instead, simply refer to this area as the retrobulbar space. Many of the circumscribed orbital tumors, such as the cavernous hemangioma of adults, the solitary neurofibroma, neurilemomas, nodular orbital meningiomas, and optic gliomas, find this space convenient for their slow expansion. Such tumors usually are removed by the ophthalmic surgeon through a lateral orbitotomy.

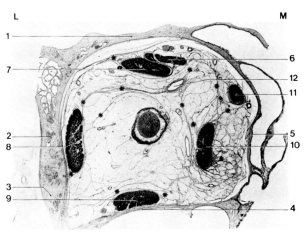

Figure 5. Frontal section of right orbit in retrobulbar area, 2.1 mm from back of eyeball. L = lateral; M = medial; 1 = frontal bone; 2 = greater wing of sphenoid; 3 = zygomatic bone; 4 = maxilla; 5 = ethmoid; 6 = superior levator palpebrae muscle; 7 = superior rectus muscle; 8 = lateral rectus muscle; 9 = inferior rectus muscle; 10 = medial rectus muscle; 11 = superior oblique muscle; 12 = superior ophthalmic vein. Asterisks indicate connective tissue septa. (× 3) (From Koornneef L: New insights in the human orbital connective tissue. Arch Ophthalmol 95: 1269–73, 1977. By permission of the American Medical Association.)

LEVATOR PALPEBRAE SUPERIORIS

The levator palpebrae superioris, which spreads as a broad, thin canopy across the anterior space beneath the roof of the orbit in its forward extension toward the eyelid, deserves special mention. Because of its position, the muscle usually is manipulated during orbitotomy either through the brow or by a transfrontal approach. Its thin structure makes it particularly liable to injury by either tumor or surgeon, and some degree of permanent blepharoptosis often results. This muscle, therefore, after the eye and the optic nerve, is the most important surgical structure in the orbit. Tumors originating in the peripheral space along the roof of the orbit, particularly large cysts, press downward, and the pressure of the expanding mass often fuses the periorbita with the surface of the levator muscle. In such a situation the surgeon can scarcely differentiate the muscle from the capsule forming the floor of the cyst, and the unwary surgeon may unknowingly remove some of this muscle while performing a neat and complete excision of the cyst, thereby causing a traumatic or cicatricial blepharoptosis that defies satisfactory repair. Blepharoptosis not only is a cosmetic blemish but also may so cover the eye that it is useless for vision. Such complications may well make patients believe that they would have been better off without the operation.

The levator palpebrae superioris also is easily infiltrated by malignant neoplasms and inflammatory pseudotumors. The surgeon may not realize that the levator as well as tumor has been removed until the frozen tissue report identifies striate muscle bundles. During the preoperative assessment, it is well to be wary of the patient who already has the symptom of blepharoptosis. This symptom can only mean that the disease is close to, or has actually involved, the levator muscle, and the surgeon must consider how much worse any well-intentioned operative manipulations may make the situation. As a general rule, the competence and skill of a surgeon working in the upper quadrants of the orbit can be judged by the degree and permanence of the postoperative blepharoptosis.

LACRIMAL GLAND

Another important structure, not only because of its size but also because it harbors some of the most vicious of the orbital neoplasms, is the lacrimal gland. In size, it is the second largest organ in the orbit; in position, it fills the entire forward portion of the superotemporal quadrant. The student on first observing this gland in the living subject during lateral orbitotomy often comments that it is much larger than he had imagined. Posteriorly, the tip of the gland extends almost to the zygomatic-sphenoid suture, so that a surgeon entering the superior quadrant from a lateral approach must either push it forward or retract it to one side to gain better access and visibililty into the posterior orbit. Some surgical texts suggest that the posterior one-third of the gland can easily be amputated — for better exposure or for decompression of the orbital contents — without affecting function. Overlooked is the fact that the blood supply from the lacrimal branch of the ophthalmic artery enters the gland in this area and that this vessel, if there is only one, is something to reckon with when severed.

Anteriorly, the gland is divided into superior and inferior lobes by the lateral sweep of the aponeurosis of the levator palpebrae superioris. The smaller, inferior lobe really lies outside the orbit, but it is connected to the main and larger lobe by an isthmus of tissue, so that both lobes are a functional continuum. The need to become familiar with the feel of the forward, inferior lobe has already been noted. It is also wise to become acquainted with the lobular appearance of the main gland in conscious persons to avoid partial excision in the mistaken belief that the gland represents the suspected tumor. This instance of mistaken identity is particularly prevalent in cases of pseudotumor.

Bibliography

Beard C, Quickert MH: Anatomy of the Orbit (A Dissection Manual). Birmingham, AL: Aesculapius Publishing Company, 1969

Hollinshead WH: Textbook of Anatomy. Third edition. Hagerstown, MD: Medical Department, Harper & Row, Publishers, 1974, pp. 881-927

Koornneef L: New insights in the human orbital connective tissue. Arch Ophthalmol 95:1269-73, 1977

Warwick R: Eugene Wolff's Anatomy of the Eye and Orbit: Including the Central Connexions, Development, and Comparative Anatomy of the Visual Apparatus. Seventh edition. Philadelphia: WB Saunders Company, 1976

Whitnall SE: Anatomy of the Human Orbit and Accessory Organs of Vision. Second edition. London: Oxford University Press, 1932

2

Diagnosis of Orbital Tumors

The many important factors in the clinical evaluation and diagnosis of orbital tumors will be noted in this chapter. Here we will first meet the patients: we will measure the proptosis, palpate the orbit, perform the routine ocular examination, analyze the subjective symptoms in relation to objective findings, and decide which ancillary or special studies are necessary. These varied facets of the initial study often are minimized by many ophthalmologists in their hurry to proceed to surgical biopsy. Of course, biopsy is important, but it assumes that precise pathologic evaluation is always possible from a smidgen of tissue, and it implies that surgical tampering with the tumor is harmless. Furthermore, many clinicians, so bamboozled by the reputed diagnostic accuracy of computed tomography and ultrasonography in the past decade, believe all these preliminaries unnecessary. A broad approach to this problem is necessary in an effort to find a rightful balance between surgical and nonsurgical evaluation. Here, we want to emphasize the foresight rather than the hindsight of diagnosis.

CLINICAL APPROACH TO ORBITAL DISORDERS

Assessment of Proptosis

The tissues within the orbit are arranged so snugly and utilize so efficiently the space within their small compartment that any increase in their bulk or the lodgement of any additional components must cause displacement of some of the structures already present. By reason of its suspension in the middle orbital hollow and its lack of firm anchorage, the eye is easily displaced and usually is the first structure to reflect some increase in orbital bulk by its protrusion. Protrusion or measurable displacement is almost pathognomonic of orbital tumor and was present in 84% of the primary tumors listed in Chapter 3, Table 2.

There are, however, some infrequent exceptions to the rule that protrusion of the eye is invariably a sign of orbital tumor. For example, the eye, by reason of either an increase in size (high myopia) or retraction of its eyelids (endocrine dysfunction), may only appear to be protruding. Also, relative protrusion may occur in an infant or child whose orbital growth has been retarded by previous x-ray irradiation. In other situations, the eye may actually protrude, but the disturbance may be outside the orbit (passive congestion of orbital contents secondary to intracranial vascular malformations, fistulas in the area of the cavernous sinus, or midbrain tumor) or the tumor might be located so far anteriorly in the orbit (psuedotumor, malignant lymphoma, and infantile hemangi-

oma) that a palpable mass or blepharoptosis would precede actual displacement
of the eye. In contrast, tumors (for example, meningioma and optic nerve
glioma) in the rear of the orbit might become manifest by papilledema and
visual loss before significant pro rusion develops. Finally, in some types of carcinoma metastatic to the orbit, ,he eye may actually become enophthalmic (for
example, scirrhous carcinoma metastatic from the breast). These and other
exceptions to the common rule will be noted below.

The protrusion of the eye that so commonly occurs in primary orbital tumors is now called either exophthalmos or proptosis. Both terms are very old in
medical usage but had different meanings relevant to the eye up to the latter
half of the 19th century. Today, the two terms have become synonomous in
their reference to the eye, but *exophthalmos* almost exclusively denotes the
orbital manifestations of endocrine dysfunction, and this usage will continue in
this text. *Proptosis,* instead, will be used chiefly in reference to orbital tumors,
as the verbal element *ptosis* is more in keeping with the downward displacement that occurs more commonly in this type of orbital problem than in endocrine exopthalmos.

One of the first steps in our diagnostic observation is to measure the
amount of proptosis of the affected eye and to compare it either to a predetermined standard norm or to the position of the unaffected fellow eye. Several
instruments (for example, the exophthalmometer) have been developed to help
furnish this information. Most of these devices measure, in an anteroposterior
plane, the distance between the apex of the cornea and some point on the bony
margin of the orbit.

In our tumor study, the Hertel exophthalmometer or the Krahn modification of this device was used to measure most cases of proptosis. With these ex-
ophthalmometers the forward distance of the front surface of the eye in relation
to the lateral rim of the orbit averages 16 to 17 mm in adults and slightly less
in children, with a range of 14 to 21 mm. Anything less than 14 mm can usually
be considered an enophthalmos, and values this low are occasionally encountered in some types of metastatic disease (see Section II). The upper limits of
normal are less easy to define. Values higher than 21 mm occasionally are
encountered among patients who have either a familial tendency for prominent
eyes or a moderate degree of myopia.

However, with orbital tumors we are concerned not only with maximum
values but also with the difference in the relative position of one (affected) eye
to the other (normal) eye. In our text, a difference of 3 mm or more is considered significant. All values are subject to latitude because asymmetry of the
patient's face, tilting of the bridge of the exophthalmometer, or exotropia of one
eye may easily exaggerate an otherwise normal difference.

Displacement of Eye

Next in the scheme of study is an inspection of the position of the eye
other than in its forward (proptosis) protrusion. Many orbital tumors push the
eye away from its normal visual axis in a sagittal or vertical plane. The term
displacement will be used to designate this deviation along a plane other than
the anteroposterior axis. Displacement should not be confused with rotation or

deviation of the eye around a vertical axis, as in strabismus. The latter is seldom a sign of orbital tumor except in infants and, ordinarily, is not accompanied by proptosis. In contrast, displacement of the eye is a common diagnostic feature of orbital tumors and almost always is associated with some amount of proptosis. Almost without exception, the direction of displacement is opposite to the position of the growing tumor. Rarely, a benign cyst, such as mucocele, may insinuate itself among the structures in the rear of the orbit so slowly and in such a fashion that the final position of the eye may actually be in the same direction as the origin of the cyst.

Displacement is most commonly *downward*, because the majority of orbital tumors, particularly the cysts and benign neoplasms, occur somewhere in the two upper quadrants of the orbit. Forward proptosis and downward displacement of the eye, so commonly associated with cysts and benign neoplasms located beneath the roof of the orbit, are illustrated in Figures 6 and 7. Further shift of the eye in a temporal or nasal direction simply indicates that the orbital mass is in the upper nasal or upper temporal quadrant of the orbit, respectively. *Lateral* displacement of the eye without significant downward or upward shift and with only minimal proptosis usually results from tumors originating in the area of the ethmoid sinus (for example, mucoceles, chondrosarcomas, carcin-

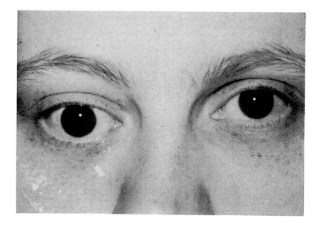

Figure 6. Epidermoid cyst located along roof of right orbit has pushed right eye downward and forward. In spite of marked displacement, right eye has maintained straight-forward visual axis parallel to left eye. No diplopia is present except in extreme upward gaze. Adnexal structures also have adapted to slow growth of tumor, maintaining normal anatomic relationship to displaced eye. Superior palpebral folds are symmetric, and widths of palpebral fissures are nearly equal. There is no edema or redness of eye and adnexa.

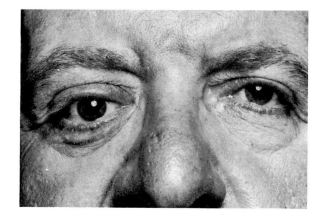

Figure 7. Forward proptosis and downward displacement of right eye due to benign mixed tumor of lacrimal gland. Clinical features are similar to those illustrated in Figure 6.

omas, and even some malignant tumors of the nasopharynx). Figure 8 illustrates such a case; the lateral displacement of the affected eye is easily determined by measuring the distances between the pupils of the eyes and the midline of the bridge of the nose. *Upward* displacement of the eye is observed with tumors frequently found in the inferior quadrants of the orbit, such as malignant lymphoma and carcinoma invading the orbit from a source in the maxillary sinus. Displacement of the eye solely in a *medial* direction is quite rare, because the more shallow bony coverage of the eye laterally permits egress of the expanding tumor before the eye is pushed against the unyielding nasal wall.

An evaluation of the amount of proptosis and displacement of the eye relative to each other also is helpful in determining the position of the tumor. The more forward the tumor in the orbit, the greater the displacement relative to the amount of proptosis. Thus, if there is forward proptosis of 2 mm but downward displacement of 4 mm, the tumor must occupy a more forward position in the orbit than a tumor with forward proptosis of 4 mm but only 2 mm of downward displacement. In general, the more anterior the orbital tumor, the greater the displacement of the eye; the more posterior the tumor, the greater the proptosis. An exception to this rule is often observed among the orbital hemangiomas of infancy. Unless their origin is deep, these tumors tend to push themselves, rather than the eye, out of the orbital space. In such situations, the eye may be displaced to one side while its forward protrusion is relatively slight. A straightforward protrusion of the eye with little displacement in any other direction is a characteristic of tumors near the apex of the orbit. Meningiomas, optic nerve gliomas, and cavernous hemangiomas are the more frequent growths exhibiting this type of proptosis.

ORBITAL COVER TEST.   The position of the visual axis of the displaced eye may also provide diagnostic information. The ability of some eyes, even though markedly displaced to maintain a forward visual axis parallel to that of the fellow normal eye is a remarkable example of adaptation and may pose the challenge of "which orbit contains the tumor?" For example, when both eyes of either Figure 6 or Figure 7 are viewed simultaneously from front-face position, their gross misalignment is obvious. However, if right and left orbits are alternately covered (*orbital cover test*) on either side of the midline of the face (use red bookmark to cover one side of face at a time), the uncovered eye and

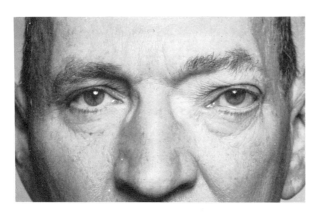

Figure. 8. Mucocele of left ethmoid sinus. Patient had noted variable displacement of left eye and fluctuant mass in nasal portion of left orbit for 21 years. Note wide lateral shift of left eye from midline of face (right eye is in normal position); forward proptosis of left eye is minimal. As in Figures 6 and 7, width of palpebral fissures and position of superior palpebral folds are nearly symmetric, an indication that adnexal structures have adapted to pressure of slowly growing orbital tumor.

adnexal structures appear normal. This gross clinical pattern is quite diagnostic of benign neoplasms and cysts of the orbit. Patients with this appearance usually have an orbital tumor amenable to surgical removal, because slow expansion, unassociated with invasion, permits the extraocular muscles to maintain binocular fixation in spite of increased orbital pressure. In contrast, the more malignant neoplasm primary in the orbit may quickly infiltrate the nearest extraocular muscle, resulting in paresis and consequent strabismus of the affected eye.

Pulsation of Eye

The proptosed eye should also be inspected for any sign of pulsation. Rhythmic movement of the eye, synchronous with the arterial pulse, occurs infrequently in unilateral proptosis. But it is an important clinical sign, because it limits differential diagnosis to a few specific entities. Usually it is caused by an arteriovenous intercommunication located within or behind the orbit. In general, the larger the arteriovenous fistula, the greater the excursion of the pulsating eye, but pulsation may in some cases be so slight as to be easily overlooked. Such a situation is illustrated in Figure 106 (page 163).

The most practical way of detecting pulsation of a small degree is to observe the patient's eye from a direct lateral view. The association of a pulsating, proptosed eye and an arteriovenous shunt is so frequent and striking that the term *pulsating exophthalmos* has become almost synonomous with this clinical entity. However, the examiner should remember that an arteriovenous communication is not the sole cause of a pulsating, proptosed eye. Any disorder that creates an abnormal intercommunication between the orbital space and intracranial cavity also may produce this clinical entity. In children and infants, such pulsation may be the result of a meningoencephalocele. In adults, it may result from large mucoceles that have eroded the bony walls of both the orbit and the intracranial vault. In any age group, bony dysplasias of the orbit associated with neurofibromatosis may produce a similar clinical picture.

The term "pulsating exophthalmos" is valid in describing a diagnostic feature of arteriovenous fistula only if the pulsation and proptosis are accompanied by the characteristic venous engorgement on the surface of the eye, which is described later in the chapter. Also, pulsating exophthalmos should be distinguished from the postural type of pulsation. Supplementary diagnostic features, such as thrill, bruit, and effects of digital compression over the carotid vessels, are also noted later.

Inspection of Adnexal Structures

Observation may now turn from the protruding eye to those supporting structures whose function and appearance also may be altered by an expanding orbital mass. The eyelids and epibulbar tissues of the eye should be inspected for any change in their color, texture, or structure. The eyelids, in particular, should be scrutinized for any anatomic alterations affecting their role in protect-

ing the protruding eye. The width of the palpebral fissure and the space between the margin of the upper eyelid and the superior palbebral fold should be
measured on the side of the proptosis and compared with those of the fellow
eye. These features deserve emphasis because of their role in the differential
diagnosis of orbital tumors from other orbital disorders. Scanning of the adnexal
structures does not need special instruments nor does it involve any complicated techniques; it does require visual attention and clinical acumen on the
part of the examiner.

Changes in the texture and color of the soft tissues of the eyelid occasionally may be helpful in differential diagnosis. *Swelling, edema,* and *redness* of
these tissues are infrequent in the primary neoplasm-cyst group of tumors, although there are four common exceptions to this dictum. First, with malignant
epithelial tumors of the lacrimal gland, early, slight edema of the adjacent soft
tissues of the eyelid is the rule. Second, boggy edema of the nasal portion of
the upper eyelid often is associated with mucoceles pushing downward into the
superior nasal quadrant of the orbit from the frontal sinus. Third, some puffiness of the lower lid accompanies malignant lymphoma growing in the inferior
quadrants of the orbit. In all these instances the tumors are located well forward, and tissue swelling probably represents passive edema owing to pressure
of the tumor on the nearby eyelid and interference with lymph drainage.
Fourth, and more puzzling, boggy edema, greater in the lower than in the
upper eyelid, is sometimes associated with a meningioma that either has been
partially removed or has existed undetected in the rear of the orbit for several
years (Fig. 9; see also Fig. 294, page 481). Here it might be postulated that a
large meningioma has gradually reduced the normal venous flow through the
posterior orbital outlets and that the result is a subtle rise of pressure through
the more anterior venous channels of the face. But in none of these four exceptions is there redness of the overlying skin such as would appear with an inflammatory disorder.

Soft tissue swelling more commonly is associated with the proptosis and lid
retraction of the endocrine exophthalmos type of orbital disorder. Both eyelids
usually are affected, and the edema is more firm and the tissues are more
tense with these disorders than with most neoplasms and cysts. Commonly, the

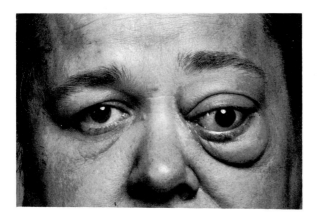

Figure 9. Pronounced downward displacement (9 mm) and
forward proptosis (14 mm) of left
eye associated with boggy edema
of eyelids. Patient has intraorbital
meningioma of 8 years' duration.

soft tissues in the orbital portion of the eyelid are affected more than are tissues in the pretarsal zone. This edema does not pit on pressure.

Rubor of the eyelids (with or without edema) must be regarded with caution in any patient suspected of harboring an orbital tumor. It suggests inflammation, and surgical exploration of such cases should be deferred or even avoided. The most intense rubor and edema affect infants with orbital cellulitis; in these cases, the eyelids may be so swollen as to cover the proptosed eye. An increase in heat locally and a systemic rise in temperature should make possible a differentiation of these acute inflammatory lesions from disorders like orbital cysts, neoplasms, vascular malformations, and endocrine exophthalmos. Rubor, less intense but equally diffuse, may be observed in adults who have malignant lymphoma of the eyelids, but lack of proptosis rules out orbital involvement in these cases. Redness of the eyelids also frequently accompanies fast-growing neoplasms located in the more anterior areas of the orbit; these are rhabdomyosarcoma in children and adolescents and metastatic carcinoma in adults. In these conditions, the short duration of symptoms and the rapid day-to-day changes in the patient's appearance should suggest their malignant character. Less well known are the rubor and minimal edema affecting the eyelids of some patients with pseudotumor of the more acute types (See Fig. 329, page 521). Rubor alone should make the ophthalmologist carefully consider whether surgical biopsy or a conservative trial of steroid therapy is the wisest approach to management. Lastly, these varying types of degrees of rubor should not be confused with the ecchymosis of the eyelids associated with orbital hematomas, neuroblastomas, amyloid deposits, and leukemia infiltrates.

As illustrated in Figures 6, 7, and 8, the widths of the palpebral fissures of the displaced eyes are the same as, or are within a millimeter of, similar measurements on the normal side. In these illustrations the margins of the lower eyelids are parallel to the inferior limbus of the eyes, and the arch of each upper eyelid is symmetric in relationship to the upper margin of the corneas. The curves and positions of the superior palpebral folds of the eyelids of the displaced and normal eyes also are symmetric. This pattern — *proptosis without alteration in the anatomic relationship of the overlying eyelids* — is particularly characteristic of benign neoplasms and cysts. A simple and useful way of bringing out this striking diagnostic feature is alternate coverage of the eyes and face while facing the patient at a distance of several feet (*orbital cover test*). The explanation for this phenomenon probably is the slowness of growth of the benign cyst of neoplasm.Equal pressure is exerted on all structures by the expanding tumor, so that the eye and adnexal structures maintain a reasonably normal anatomic relationship to each other as they are pushed out of the orbit together. An exception is observed in cases of long-standing benign tumor wherein increasing orbital pressure pushes the eye beyond the limits of elasticity of the protective eyelids (Fig. 10; see also Fig. 75, page 118). Protrusion of this extent usually is noted when the tumor has been present for more than 4 or 5 years. Although the eyeball then protrudes well beyond the normal protective mantle of the eyelids, exposure keratitis seldom develops. Some malignant neoplasms primary in the orbit may produce a similar clinical picture, but their growth is so rapid that the eye is pushed out of its socket before the eyelids have time to adapt to the increased orbital bulk; this phenomenon is more com-

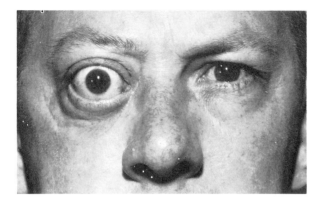

Figure 10. Extreme proptosis of right eye due to cavernous
hemangioma that slowly enlarged
for 12 years. Eye has been pushed
beyond protective elasticity of
eyelids.

monly observed among the malignant tumors of children than those of adults
Fig. 11). The protruding and displaced eye of malignant vis-á-vis benign and
long-standing disease may be distinguished, of course, by the duration of
symptoms.

In endocrine exophthalmos, different factors prevail — even though, to a
casual observer, the overall appearance of protrusion may be similar to the
proptosis of orbital neoplasms and cysts. As noted in Chapter 3, an exposition on
the subject of endocrine exophthalmos will not be attempted: a textbook could
be written on this subject alone. However, some of the orbital effects of this
hormonal disorder must be noted here because the *tumefaction of tissue* due to
endocrine exophthalmos may predominantly affect one orbit and thus easily be
confused with the clinical signs of other orbital tumors. Actually, a true unilateral form of the disease probably is quite rare, and the more common bilateral and symmetric form of endocrine exophthalmos seldom offers any problem in the differential diagnosis of orbital tumors. Sometimes, months to a year
may elapse between the onset of symptoms in one orbit and their appearance
in the other. Until the bilateral form of the disease becomes manifest, such
occurrences pose a challenge in the differential diagnosis of this unilateral
orbital disorder. Fortunately, such cases are quite uncommon. More often,
subtle and early manifestations of endocrine exophthalmos are overlooked in the
less affected eye, such cases being asymmetric forms of endocrine exophthalmos rather than unilateral examples of the disease.

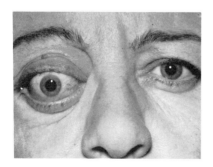

Figure 11. Proptosis and displacement of right
eye from rapidly growing cellular hemangiopericytoma of only 10 months' duration. Increase in intraorbital pressure was so rapid that adnexal structures could
not maintain their usual protective relationship.

Figure 12 illustrates some of the problems in the differential diagnosis of exophthalmos. The diagnosis of malignant neoplasm of one orbit was made but was not confirmed pathologically. Orbitotomy twice was unsuccessful in locating the neoplasm. The problems were similar in another case (see Fig. 16 on Color Plate I, p. 26). Because no laboratory tests can provide an unequivocal diagnosis of endocrine exophthalmos during the euthyroid stage of this hormonal dysfunction, the ophthalmologist's familiarity with the orbital signs and symptoms of the disease becomes ever more important.

In the diagnosis of this endocrine dysfunction, *the most common and important clue is retraction of the eyelids.* This so-called retraction may affect both eyelids but most frequently affects only the upper. The width of the palpebral fissure is always increased with lid retraction, but this change alone is not diagnostic. As already noted, the width of the palpebral fissure may also be altered by some types of neoplasm that push the eyelids apart during their egress from the orbit. In both conditions, there is baring of the sclera either below or above the limbus of the eye or, sometimes, in both locations. It is sometimes stated that differentiation between the unilateral, wide palpebral aperture of the endocrine type and the stretching of the palpebral space from the bulging eye of neoplasm is impossible without the use of an exophthalmometer. But since both endocrine ophthalmology and neoplasm may produce proptosis, exophthalmometry by itself is not diagnostic. Similarly, it is sometimes held that endocrine exophthalmos and proptosis secondary to neoplasm may be differentiated on the basis that the relationship of the lower eyelid to the protruding eye is not altered in endocrine exophthalmos; thus, baring of the sclera superiorly would favor a diagnosis of endocrine exophthalmos. But again, this rule is unreliable because retraction of the lower eyelid occurs more frequently in association with endocrine disorders than is generally suspected. Figures 13 and 14 illustrate some of the asymmetric features of lid retraction and emphasize the unreliability of diagnosis based solely on the position of the lower eyelid.

A diagnosis of lid retraction also cannot depend entirely on the classic concept that the arch of the upper eyelid crosses the cornea at a fixed distance below the superior ocular limbus, because this anatomic relationship may be altered by the age of the patient and the bone makeup of the face: in children,

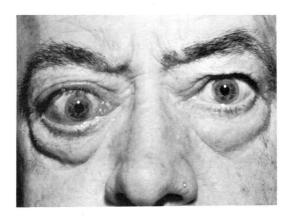

Figure 12. Progressive ophthalmoplegia, proptosis (6 mm), and displacement of right eye over an 11-month period had been associated with two anterior orbitotomies in fruitless search for orbital neoplasm; a third operation (lateral orbitotomy) had been proposed at time of this photograph to permit exploration of posterior orbit. Concern of both patient and physician was so focused on right eye that retraction of left upper eyelid associated with deepening of superior palpebral sulcus remained unnoticed. This case again illustrates asymmetric features of some instances of endocrine exophthalmos. Surgical intervention in such cases only makes the situation worse.

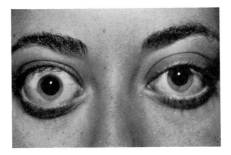

Figure 13. Bilateral exophthalmos (exophthalmometry, 26 mm, each eye) 4 years after thyroidectomy is associated with asymmetric retraction of eyelids of only 2 months' duration. Marked retraction of right upper eyelid and moderate retraction of each lower eyelid are evident, but position of left upper eyelid is within limits of normal.

the arch of the upper eyelid rides higher in relation to the superior ocular limbus than in adults. What constitutes lid retraction in adults would not apply in children if judged only on the basis of bared sclera. Also, in some patients prominence of the eyes, with the sclera visible above the superior ocular limbus, may be a natural familial trait.

More accurate detection of lid retraction follows measurement of the distance or space between the margin of the eyelid and the superior palpebral sulcus. In adults, this distance is reasonably constant; it measures approximately 3 mm. In children, this interval is less. The superior palpebral sulcus is formed by the main cutaneous insertion of the levator palpebrae superioris, and when endocrine factors cause stimulation or contracture of the elevator muscles of the upper eyelid, the superior palpebral sulcus deepens and those tissues overlying the tarsus are pulled upward. The tissue space between the superior palpebral fold and the margin of the eyelid then appears to shorten. In extreme cases, the eyelashes may be positioned directly beneath the exaggerated palpebral fold. and the superior palbebral fold and eyelid margin appear almost merged. In some cases, the upward pull on the margin of the eyelid may be so marked as to cause a slight inversion of the eyelashes (see Fig. 17 on Color Plate I, p 26). Even though the palpebral fissure is widened to accommodate the protruding eye of neoplasm or cyst, *the distance between the eyelashes and superior palpebral fold remains unaltered,* and in many cases, this distance is the same on both the affected and the unaffected sides. In some conditions simulating unilateral orbital disease, this space is wider because of the stretching effect exerted by an enlarging eye on the soft tissues of the overlying eyelid (Fig. 15).

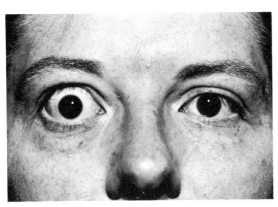

Figure 14. Asymmetric retraction of eyelids (first noticed at onset of thyrotoxicosis 10 years previously) without significant exophthalmos. Note extensive retraction of right upper eyelid and slight retraction of right lower eyelid. Eyelids on left side are normal.

Figure 15. Slowly progressive prominence of left eye simulating unilateral proptosis associated with orbital cysts and benign neoplasms. Apparent proptosis, however, is due to enlarging eye rather than orbital tumor. Left eye had been amblyopic since childhood (with myopia, approximately 20 D). On left, interval between eyelid margin and superior palpebral sulcus is wider than comparable, normal area on right side because soft tissues have gradually stretched to accommodate enlarging left eye.

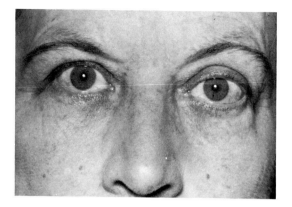

Lid retraction associated with endocrine exophthalmos frequently is described and defined in terms of lid lag. In lid lag, downward excursion of the retracted upper eyelid is limited during inferior rotation of the eye. This test, as an evaluation of lid retraction, seems less dependable and more difficult to measure than an assessment of the lid margin — superior palpebral fold ratio.

Inspection of the Surface of the Eye

In a study of the surface of the eye, much diagnostic information comes from careful attention to the color and distribution of the epibulbar vascular plexus. Vascular dilatation and congestion are seldom associated with the unilateral proptosis of benign neoplasms and cysts. However, in the other groups of orbital disorders — endocrine exophthalmos, vascular malformation, and inflammatory disease — the pattern of dilated vessels on the proptosed eye may be so characteristic as to make possible a specific diagnosis at this point. Dilated, tortuous vessels extending across the surface of the eye in an almost corkscrew-like configuration are particularly diagnostic of some vascular malformations (see Fig. 18 on Color Plate I, p. 26; see also Figs. 105 and 106, page 163). In these cases, the epibulbar veins are dilated to several times their normal caliber and assume a more reddish purple hue than normal. However, the tissue spaces between the engorged vessels retain their normal, nonvascularized color, and furthermore, the vascular arcades seem to terminate at the limbus, a feature rarely observed in other types of orbital disorders unless they are severe and long-standing or unless the proptosed eye is subject to exposure.

The pattern of vascular dilatation in endocrine exophthalmos is different. At each lateral canthus is one, or sometimes two, dilated vascular channel having a more purplish hue than the average epibulbar vessel. Overlying this dilated vessel is a puff of chemotic conjunctiva (see Fig. 17 on Color Plate I, p. 26). In less severe cases of short duration, these changes may not be visible unless the eye is rotated medially or the eyelids are gently pulled apart. As the disease progresses, the purplish discoloration of the dilated vessel becomes more evident, and the area of chemotic conjunctiva enlarges. Branching from the main vessel are several smaller vessels of more nearly normal color that meander along the surface of the eye toward the ocular limbus. In severe endocrine exophthalmos, wherein either the eye is under great pressure from the increased orbital bulk or its surface has

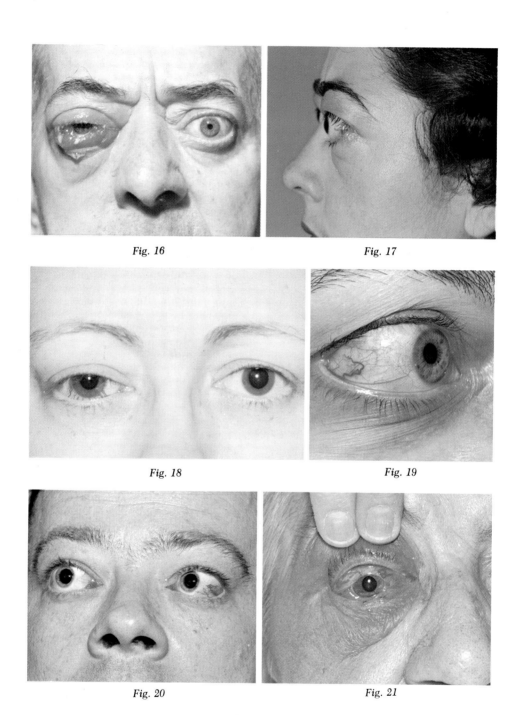

Fig. 16

Fig. 17

Fig. 18

Fig. 19

Fig. 20

Fig. 21

Figures 16 through 21. See opposite page for legends.

been unduly exposed by marked lid retraction, these dilated vessels may actually reach the ocular limbus. However, most often these smaller terminal vessels seem to fade away about midway between their source and the corneoscleral junction (see Figs. 19 and 20 on Color Plate I, p. 26). The degree of ecchymosis accompanying this vascular engorgement seems roughly proportional to the degree of congestion. There may be similar changes at the nasal canthus, but usually these are much less intense. Even in the absence of lid retraction, this distinctive vascular pattern may be considered diagnostic of endocrine exophthalmos and thus may eliminate the need for biopsy or exploratory orbital surgery.

Still other distinctive changes may be noted in the vascular arcades in cases of orbital inflammatory disease. The dilated epibulbar vessels have a brighter hue and a more diffuse distribution; all indicate active rather than passive congestion of the eye. Surgical management of such cases should always be cautious, for surgical manipulation may aggravate both proptosis and orbital disease. Rarely, a mixture of these vascular patterns may suggest a more specific orbital diagnosis. Figure 21 (see Color Plate I, p. 26) illustrates such a case, wherein the reddish purple color and the corkscrew tortuosity of epubulbar vessels superimposed on a background of diffuse, bright-red congestion signify some orbital process that may combine the features of both vascular obstruction and orbital inflammation (for example, orbital thrombophlebitis).

Palpation of the Eye

Next in diagnostic importance to visual inspection of the protruding eye and adnexal structures is the information acquired by touch. Palpation of orbital contents, however, is limited because of the snug approximation of the eye and surrounding orbital bones. Access to the orbital cavity is the width of a fingerbreadth (see Chapter 1). Whether we use the tip of the index finger or distal phalanx of the little finger, it is unlikely (unless the patient is under general anesthesia) that we

---

Figure 16. Asymmetric endocrine exophthalmos. Appearance of right eye suggested acute orbital inflammation or possible malignant neoplasm, and orbitotomy had been suggested to exclude the latter. Preoccupation with right eye made it easy to overlook slight but definite retraction of both upper and lower eyelids on left side. This case illustrates the marked asymmetry that many exist in orbital and adnexal signs of bilateral endocrine exophthalmos.

Figure 17. Marked retraction of upper eyelid with endocrine exophthalmos. Upward pull on eyelid has inverted its margin, so that eyelashes rub against surface of eye and normal tissue interval between margin of eyelid and superior palpebral sulcus is narrowed. Note puff of chemotic conjunctiva overlying engorged epibulbar vessels at lateral canthus, a frequent finding in endocrine exophthalmos that helps to differentiate endocrine exophthalmos from proptosis associated with other orbital disorders.

Figure 18. Dilated vessels extend, corkscrew-like, across surface of right eye to limbus in case of vascular malformation in posterior orbit. This feature differentiates the case from similar unilateral proptosis and ocular displacement associated with benign neoplasms and cysts.

Figure 19. Reddish purple vascular loop at lateral canthus of eye is associated with over-lying chemosis typical of early endocrine exophthalmos.

Figure 20. Prominent vascular pattern at lateral canthus is characteristic of endocrine exophthalmos; dilated vessels fade away midway between their source and limbus. At medial canthus, vascular changes are less marked.

Figure 21. Unilateral proptosis of right eye, diffuse congestion and chemosis of ocular surface, and prominent corkscrew-like vascular pattern adjacent to upper nasal limbus. This combination of patterns of active and passive congestion suggests an orbital process marked by elements of both inflammation and vascular obstruction. It was accompanied by much pain.

can palpate beyond half the depth of the orbit in the temporal quadrants and one-third its depth in the nasal quadrants. Although some structures of the orbit are thus beyond the perimeter of the prying finger, the information that can be gained is important. Interestingly, an abnormal mass could be palpated in approximately 63% of the 764 orbital tumors of the Mayo Clinic series (see Section II). This proportion is surprisingly high when one considers the limitations of palpation and the space in the rear of the eye, beyond the reach of an exploring finger, for potential growth of a tumor. If the palpable masses of hypertrophied fat (frequently mistaken for neoplasm) that are associated with severer forms of endocrine exophthalmos had been included in this survey, the percentage of cases in which palpation was positive would be even higher. On the other hand, this incidence reflects the compact arrangement of orbital structures and the ease with which an intruding mass soon makes its presence known by forward displacement of the eye and adnexal structures.

Some ophthalmologists have advocated small incisions through the conjunctival cul-de-sac to facilitate palpation of the retrobulbar space and localize more precisely a suspected tumor before surgical exploration. The tumor-localizing features of orbital ultrasonography and computed tomography have made such transconjunctival probings unnecessary.

The most fertile field of palpation is across the anterior plane of the two upper orbital quadrants, for this is the more frequent homestead of tumors. In the upper nasal quadrant the *hemangiomas* of infancy frequently are encountered. With a light touch, the finger will feel the definite, smoothly contoured, front surface of this tumor. When more forceful pressure is applied, however, the presenting surface seems to disappear and the fingertip sinks easily into the inner portion of the tumor, as though no wall or barrier existed. Compressibility is characteristic of these soft cystic masses in infants. In adults, the hemangioma is firmer, the feel of this tumor resembles that of some orbital cysts, such as the dermoids, arising from congenital rests. Here, there is less difference between various intensities of pressure than is noted with hemangiomas of infancy. Although the distinct, smooth, anterior surface of the mass can still be identified by light touch, this wall remains as a palpable barrier when the pressure is increased. It is as though one were pushing aside the entire tumor rather than easily invaginating its wall.

Another tumor often palpated in the upper nasal quadrant is the *mucocele*. Its presenting surface does not have quite the rounded contour of other cysts. As the finger pushed deeper, the tumor feels boggy and doughy like a medicine ball in a gymnasium.

In the upper temporal quadrant, the *neoplasms of the lacrimal gland* and the *dermoid cysts* may be palpated. The characteristics of the dermoid have been mentioned. The features of neoplasms, in their early stages, are not such that the benign can be differentiated from the malignant by palpation. The examiner may even by fooled by portions of the gland pushed forward by the neoplasm, mistaking the lobular structure of the gland for the tumor. As the neoplasm breaks out of its confines within the gland and becomes invasive, it usually attaches to the periorbita somewhere along the bony margin from the juncture of the middle and outer thirds (superiorly) to the area of the lateral palpebral raphe (inferiorly). By this stage, the anterior lobe of the lacrimal gland is pushed into the superior conjunctival cul-de-sac and the tactile difference between the hard, fixed neoplasm and the softer, movable, lobulated glandular structure becomes evident. The adenocarcinoma has the characteristics of hardness and immobility to a greater degree than does adenoid cystic carcinoma, although these factors may be influenced by the duration of growth. However, when tumors of comparable size are examined adenoid cystic carcinoma more often seems to be tender than does adenocarcinoma.

Palpation of the space between the nasal and the temporal extremes (the upper-middle two-thirds of the anterior orbital space) is more perplexing. The presenting edge of many tumors can be felt, but something about the local anatomy, combined with either the thickness of the orbital septum or the course of the levator palpebrae superioris, makes tactile identification of tumors less specific. The *hypertrophy of fat* that develops in more advanced endocrine exophthalmos seems more prominent in this area than in other zones of the orbit. Palpation of this fat may dupe the unwary observer into fruitless surgical search for neoplasm. One such example is illustrated in Figure 12. This edematous hypertrophied tissue, although firm or even hard to palpation, still retains its basic lobulated structure. The lobules are large compared to other lobulated structures within the orbit, and the septal dividers can be recognized by light palpation along the anterior surface of the masses. Another important point is that fat hypertrophy develops as a diffuse response to the basic endocrine disease; similar, but usually less distinct, masses can be palpated in the lower quadrants of the orbital cavity. This is a differential point, inasmuch as primary neoplasms rarely appear both above and below the eye.

Inflammatory pseudotumor is another disorder favoring this particular orbital area, and it offers an additional challenge to discerning palpation. Lobulated and similar in appearance to fat hypertrophy, it tends to conform to the contour of structures that offer resistance to its growth, except in the area of the lacrimal gland. Therefore, it becomes flat and dome-shaped as it insinuates itself between the eye and the bony roof of the orbit. The lobulated structure also is lost where it abuts against the back side of the orbital septum. The smooth front surface of this tumor feels like the edge of a very tough pancake.

Primary *malignant lymphomas*, similarly, are frequent residents in the more forward portions of the orbit, and the frequency of identification by palpation in them is higher than in any other primary orbital tumor. These tumors are quite soft. In the upper orbital quadrants, limitations of space and the pressure from surrounding structures tend to compress the neoplasm and conceal its natural contour. In these areas, no distinctive features permit a specific diagnosis by touch alone. The tumors are more easily identified by their color as they expand and push forward into the superior conjunctival cul-de-sac (see Fig. 220, page 352). In the lower quadrants, these factors do not help, and the neoplasm almost may be diagnosed by its "feel." As the lobules of lymphoid tissue expand, they give the main mass a somewhat knobby, nodular contour (see Fig. 219, p. 351). These small lumps, all connected to one another, are about the size of large shotgun pellets. The masses are not tender to touch.

Secondary malignant neoplasms arising from adjacent areas of the face and nose usually can be palpated either in the inferior or in the medial orbital quadrants. The tumors always feel firm and often are surrounded by reactive edema of the adjacent soft tissues. They are more easily diagnosed by roentgen-ray examination than by palpation. The hardest tumors are the *metastatic carcinomas* (usually adenocarcinomas), excepting osteomas and fibrous dysplasia. The metastatic carcinomas are diffuse and indistinctly outlined, and the surrounding soft tissues

rapidly become immobilized by the infiltrative character of the growths. Carcinomas lodge more frequently in the posterior orbit than in the more anterior areas
and therefore will not be palpated as often as the secondary malignant neoplasms that favor a more forward location. The frequency of secondary malignant
neoplasms also is greater than that of the metastatic neoplasms.

Palpation of the orbital contents also should include elicitation of any signs of
tenderness. Antibiotic therapy has eliminated most of the orbital inflammatory conditions that, years ago, caused tenderness and pain. Occasionally, tenderness may
be elicited by palpation of the orbital floor or the nasal quadrants in some cases
of mild proptosis. This may herald an inflammatory lesion or a neoplasm invading
the orbit from an adjacent sinus. Mention already has been made of the tenderness characterizing some adenoid cystic carcinomas; this is due to their early invasion of periorbita in the course of their growth.

Another part of the digital examination is the determination of the pressure
required to push the protruding eye back into its cavity. Resistance to retrodisplacement often is noted as a helpful diagnostic sign in the differentiation of other
conditions, including benign from malignant neoplasms and neoplasms from non-
neoplastic disorders. In general, the more malignant the neoplasm, the more will
retrodisplacement be resisted. However, the size of the tumor may so influence
the degree of retrodisplacement as to invalidate this statement. Thus, benign
tumors, such as osteomas and large cavernous hemangiomas in adults, may resist
retrodisplacement as much as small retrobulbar malignant neoplasms. Similarly,
many cases of progressive, malignant endocrine exophthalmos create greater intraorbital pressure than some neoplasms. Therefore, this test of retrodisplacement
probably is of less value than many of the simple clinical observations already
discussed.

The History

Up to this point in the diagnostic workup, and while the examiner is listening
to the patient, visual inspection and palpation of the proptosed eye and adnexa
have provided much information. Now pertinent information must be sought by
evaluating the patient's history.

Several symptomatic sequences have diagnostic value. For example, in a child,
loss of vision followed by proptosis suggests a tumor in, or adjacent to, the optic
nerve. Also a parent who described an intermittent bluish or purple *discoloration
of the adnexal soft tissues aggravated by crying* is telling the listener that a likely
diagnosis in the infant patient is hemangioma. Then there is the sequence in a
child of *ecchymosis of eyelids followed by proptosis* attributed to some trivial
trauma; this suggests one of the malignant orbital neoplasms of childhood. And any
patient, either adult or child, with sudden onset of *proptosis and soft tissue swelling
accompanied by fever, malaise, and upper respiratory infection* more likely has an
inflammatory orbital disease than a neoplasm. But if this same process waxes and
wanes or extends over a period of many months, a possible mucocele should be kept
in mind. Unexplained *epiphora and proptosis* some weeks later may be a good clue
to an unsuspected malignancy secondarily invading the orbit. Finally, the story of a
persistent and annoying *extrusion of an orbital prosthesis,* placed after enucleation of the eye, is familiar in recurrent malignant melanoma in an adult and in

orbital retinoblastoma in a child. The duration and sequence of symptoms associated with individual tumors will be discussed in more detail in Section II.

As a symptom of orbital neoplasms, moderate or severe *pain is uncommon* and, if mentioned, may indicate a less common orbital problem. When pain is associated with sudden proptosis and orbital swelling in an adult, an inflammatory orbital process is more likely than a neoplasm. Less intense pain associated with sudden proptosis and adnexal swelling suggests metastatic carcinoma. If the onset of pain is late, a malignant neoplasm or vascular disorder in the orbit is a more likely possibility. Vague orbital discomfort also is noted by patients who have had many consultations because of mild but unsolved proptosis of long duration. Such pain probably has a functional rather than an organic basis. Discomfort associated with a swishing sound or a peculiar noise in the vicinity of the orbit is a clue that a vascular intercommunication probably exists. A gritty ocular sensation associated with increased lacrimation in the presence of proptosis differentiates endocrine exophthalmos from other orbital tumors.

In the patient's medical history, some earlier events may have a bearing on the current orbital problem. In particular, the patient should be questioned about any previous operations. Thyroidectomy in women should alert the ophthalmologist to the possible orbital sequelae of endocrine exophthalmos. Although the orbital disorder may have been present for several months, the correct diagnosis may remain unsuspected because of the asymmetic features of the orbital involvement. However, if the orbital disease is unilateral, its onset sudden, and its progress rapid, the excised thyroid tissue might be reexamined for occult carcinoma. Female patients should also be questioned concerning any previous breast surgery, because years may elapse before the first evidence of metastasis. The orbit may be one of the areas to be affected first by such recurrence (see Chapter 17). In elderly men, a history of operations on the prostate gland or stomach also raises the possibility of orbital metastasis. Also, nasal surgery, for example, sinusotomy or polypectomy, in either sex might be the forerunner of an unsuspected mucocele or neoplasm that first becomes manifest by secondary invasion of the orbit. Obscure histopathologic evaluation in previous biopsies of small nodes or lumps might be compatible with early malignant lymphoma of the orbit.

Ocular Examination

Although alteration in the normal position of the eyeball is the most common sign of orbital disease, the eye is only a passive participant in most derangements resulting from orbital tumor. Therefore, there are no sudden or profound changes in visual acuity, the visual field, or intraocular dynamics (as frequently occur with intrinsic eye disease). For these reasons, ocular examination may not give much positive information about the nature of the disorders exterior to the ocular walls, and the routine assessment of the eye, to which the skilled opthalmologist is most accustomed, will be less important in diagnosis than those aspects already mentioned. Those alterations of ocular function that may have some diagnostic value usually result from either the eye's malposition secondary to increased orbital pressure or the direct effect of the orbital mass on the eye itself.

Visual Acuity. Visual acuity is tested first because it usually is considered the most important mirror of ocular efficiency. Benign orbital neoplasms situated in the more anterior portions of the orbit may only minimally disturb central visual acuity, in spite of marked displacement, because the eye seems able to adapt to the slow progression of the orbital disorder without loss of vision. However, if the tumor (either benign or malignant) is located in the posterior orbit, the mass may push directly on the eyeball and alter its curvature. Such pressure makes the eye more hyperopic or less myopic. Unless pressure is of long standing, this reduction of visual acuity is seldom more than two or three lines on the Snellen test chart at 20 feet (6.0 m). A convex spherical lens or cylinder of low power will easily bring the vision to about 20/25 in such cases without a refined refraction. Conversely, a proptosis associated with a decrease in hyperopia or an increase in myopia is more likely due to a progressive myopia than to an orbital tumor (Fig. 15). These eyes may have such high myopia as to be partially amblyopic (the 20/400 level of central acuity).

Patients with moderately severe endocrine exophthalmos also show some change in their ability to read the test types. At distance range, the test letters seem blurred but tend to clear, or the acuity may improve a line or two if the patient blinks or closes the eyes a few moments. This alteration of visual acuity is more often due to corneal drying than to a profound change in refractive error, except in severe cases. At near range, acuity seems more embarrassed than at distance range because of the difficulty in maintaining convergence. More than other orbital problems, the average case of endocrine exophthalmos tends to aggravate an existing presbyopia or make manifest a latent presbyopia. In endocrine exophthalmos, the addition of convex lenses of low dioptric power brings the reading of test types to a normal range. For patients with other orbital tumors that grow near the optic nerve, convex lenses provide less improvement in the reading of test types at close range. Loss of sight not remedied by corrective lenses and associated with slowly progressive proptosis may indicate some tumor directly affecting the optic nerve, such as glioma of the optic nerve or a meningioma, and irremedial visual loss associated with more progressive proptosis of sudden onset is likely to indicate a malignant neoplasm, possibly metastatic.

Visual Fields. Additional information about visual status may be obtained by examination of the visual fields. However, the defects in the visual fields associated with orbital lesions are not nearly as informative or distinctive as those alterations resulting from intracranial disturbances. All orbital neoplasms, if large enough, may produce irregular quadrantic contractions or relative central scotomas because of direct pressure on the eye. Those tumors or orbital conditions that are intrinsic in the optic nerve or affect its sheaths produce central scotomas disproportionately greater than the amount of proptosis. Unfortunately, refined perimetry is not always possible in younger children, in whom these tumors are most common (Fig. 22). Adults with endocrine exophthalmos associated with an optic neuropathy in one eye also may show central defects in the visual field. Defects in the earlier stages of optic nerve involvement in this disorder usually are dense arcuate scotomas running beneath the fixation area. As the disease becomes more fulminant or of longer duration, the defect enlarges and becomes a huge, dense central scotoma (Fig. 23). The defects of meningioma are more irregular in both contour and density and usually affect the peripheral field much sooner than the central field. However, in the advanced stages of meningioma, the visual fields closely resemble those plotted with optic nerve gliomas. The possibility of obtaining useful information in

Figure 22. Complete loss of central and inferior portions of right visual field in 13-year-old girl as a result of grade 1 fibrous astrocytoma involving right optic nerve from near junction with eyeball to approximately 4 mm anterior to the chiasm. Only 2.5 mm of proptosis was present on right side. (From Dodge HW Jr, Love JG, Craig W McK, et al: Gliomas of the optic nerves. Arch Neurol 79:607–621, 1958. By permission of the American Medical Association.)

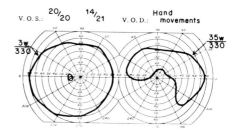

children by the confrontation testing method should not be forgotten. In this age group, perimetry is not feasible and confrontation testing may reveal gross defects in the peripheral field that were neither realized by the parents nor suspected by the ophthalmologist.

Rotation of the Eye. An assessment of the rotation and movement of the affected eye is important because many orbital tumors, as they increase in size, produce some disturbance of ocular motility. The benign cysts and neoplasms, as a group, seem to affect ocular rotation the least. These tumors are usually confined to one quadrant of the orbit, and, in such cases, ocular rotation is normally free except when the eye rotates toward the affected sector. In the restricted sector, the limitation of rotation seldom exceeds 50% of the normal excursion. Furthermore, the weakness of rotation will be most obvious in the last phase of the ocular excursion rather than at the beginning of the muscular contraction. This pattern suggests that mechanical factors acting on the muscle, secondary to the size and position of the orbital mass, are responsible for the limitation of ocular excursion. In contrast, when the muscle or its nerve is compromised by an invasive or infiltrative process, the ocular excursion is impaired at the beginning of the muscular contraction. Also, the rotations of the eye are likely to be impaired in directions of gaze other than toward the orbital quadrant occupied by the tumor.

The most severe impairment of ocular rotation is caused by metastatic carcinomas, some of the pseudotumors, and the acute inflammatory processes of sudden onset. In these, an eye may almost be held, seemingly "frozen," in its primary position of gaze and be able to move in any direction. Among metastatic neoplasms, the scirrhous adenocarcinomas (usually from the breast) show this effect most frequently. These vicious carcinomas cause so much tissue contracture that retraction rather than protrusion of the eye results. The ensuing enophthalmos differentiates the ophthalmoplegia associated with metastatic, scirrhous carcinoma from the

Figure 23. Bilateral optic neuropathy of endocrine exophthalmos in 50-year-old woman. Tangent screen field of right eye shows dense central scotoma, but on left side dense arcuate defect is present. (From Henderson JW: Optic neuropathy of Graves's disease. Trans Am Ophthalmol Soc 55:353–365, 1957. By permission of the American Ophthalmological Society.)

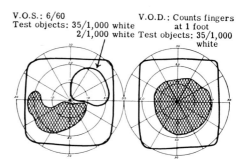

paralysis secondary to other orbital disorders (see Figs. 281 and 282, page 456). Pseudotumor, unless it is exceptionally fulminant, does not produce the so-called frozen eye until a surgical attempt to remove or explore the lesion has been made. Surgical manipulation of some of these lesions may trigger a gross inflammatory reaction that may suggest some very malignant process (Fig. 24) to the ophthalmologist who happens to see such a patient for the first time in this stage of the orbital disease. The ophthalmoplegia that accompanies acute inflammatory disorders of the orbit (cellulitis and thrombophlebitis) of sudden onset may also be quite severe, but movement of the eye is more painful than with other orbital disturbances.

The ophthalmoplegia associated with endocrine exophthalmos also has several characteristic clinical features. Ocular muscle palsy may precede exophthalmos (particularly in those cases of endocrine exophthalmos wherein a definite thyrotoxicosis exists), whereas in other orbital disorders, ophthalmoplegia usually appears after the onset of proptosis; occasionally, proptosis and motility disturbances are nearly simultaneous in onset. In cases of thyrotoxicosis or hyperthyroidism, diplopia usually is first noted in the field of upward gaze, owing to paresis of the superior rectus muscle. This ocular muscle palsy, which initially is rather mild, also is often associated with a retraction of the upper eyelid. This combination of ocular signs in only one eye may not be remembered as a clinical sign of thyroid dysfunction; instead, an orbital tumor may be suspected (Fig. 25). The absence of proptosis rules out orbital neoplasms and cysts. If the endocrine disorder persists, true exophthalmos appears and the motility disturbance becomes more generalized. At this stage, ocular rotations are restricted in a given plane or direction of gaze rather than in the field of action of any one muscle. Further progression of the basic endocrine disorder finally causes the most severe degree of ophthalmoplegia, the protruding eye becoming fixed in the abnormal position of upward or downward gaze. Such eyes can no longer move back to the primary position, owing to contracture of the extraocular muscle in the direction of the deviation rather than a paresis of the opposing muscle such as would be present in the average case of strabismus (Fig. 26).

All cases of ophthalmoplegia associated with proptosis also should have an evaluation of the sensory innervation of the external eye or adnexa. Should anesthesia of the cornea, conjunctiva, eyelids, forehead, or upper face be found, some disturbance of the fifth cranial nerve should be suspected in that area where it enters the orbit in association with the cranial nerves concerned with the innerva-

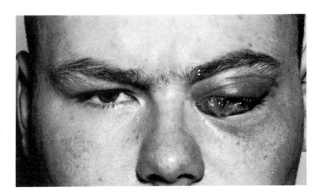

Figure 24. Progressive edema of eyelids, chemosis, ophthalmoplegia, pain, and proptosis of left eye after biopsy of pseudotumor 2 months earlier. Scar of previous orbitotomy is visible along superolateral aspect of left upper eyelid. Additional tumor appeared in lower temporal quadrant of left orbit after the surgical manipulation; this finding, combined with acute, progressive post-operative course, suggested malignant neoplasm.

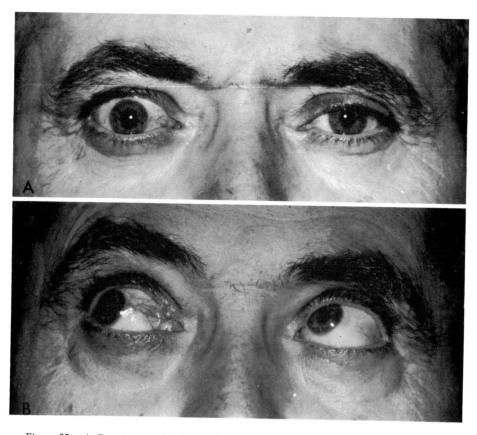

Figure 25. A, Prominence of right eye due to retraction of right upper eyelid. Exophthalmo-meter measurements were within limits of normal. *B*, In right upward gaze, right eye noticeably lags because of mild paresis of right superior rectus. Weakness of superior rectus muscle and retraction of upper eyelid are frequently associated in early endocrine exophthalmos.

Figure 26. Moderate proptosis, marked retraction of upper eyelid, and moderate downward rotation of right eye in endocrine exophthalmos of several months' duration (lateral view). Ophthalmoplegia is so severe that eye cannot be elevated to normal horizontal plane; this defect and eyelid retraction made exposure keratitis likely.

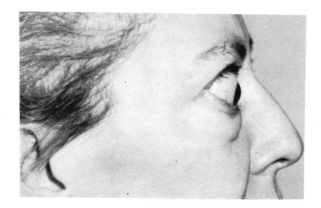

tion of the paretic extraocular muscles. This *superior orbital fisure syndrome* or *syndrome of the sphenoidal fissure* is not specific for orbital tumor but may also be observed in inflammatory processes and after trauma affecting this anatomic area. Its importance lies in pinpointing the probable location of the tumor should other ocular and orbital signs support this as a possible diagnosis.

Ophthalmoscopy. The routine ocular examination continues with a search of the interior of the eye for any change that may support a diagnosis of orbital tumor. *Indentation of the posterior wall* of the eye or any change in its contour reflects the pressure of an expanding orbital tumor. The retina overlying these areas of pressure will show radial lines of stress resembling fine wrinkles. Several authors emphasize the importance of this ocular sign as an aid to the diagnosis of orbital tumor. However, this clinical sign occurs in only a small minority of cases, and by the time indentation of the globe develops, the tumor probably has been present for some time and diagnosis will be more obvious by other means. The sign is more important in localizing the position of the tumor with greater accuracy than would be possible if a change in the curvature of the posterior wall were not present.

Attention is next given to the appearance of the optic disk. *Papilledema* is rare with orbital tumors. Most often it is observed in cases of malignant neoplasms expanding in the retrobulbar space at the apex of the orbit (particularly in children). Papilledema is then an indication of the severity or the rapid progression of the orbital disorder; it is a bad omen. If papilledema occurs in the course of an endocrine exophthalmos, it should be considered an indication for orbital decompression. If papilledema develops after operation for any orbital tumor that has been incompletely removed, permanent loss of vision will likely follow.

As a manifestation of orbital tumor, *pallor of the optic disk* is more common than papilledema. This pallor, as a rule, is not associated with either loss of nerve substance or increase in the size and contour of the optic cup, such as occurs with primary optic atrophy or glaucoma. Pallor and proptosis in an adult suggest meningioma, but in a child an optic nerve glioma is the more likely tumor. More rare than the preceding is the association of pallor with *optico-ciliary* (retinochoroidal) *shunt veins* of the optic disk. If slowly progressive visual loss and indentation of the posterior pole of the eye are also present, a diagnosis of primary, orbital, optic nerve sheath meningioma is virtually certain (Fig. 27).

Finally, the *color and configuration of the retinal venous tree* should be noted. Dilatation, tortuosity, and a deeper bluish hue of these vessels may be seen, particularly with the orbital vascular malformations and occasionally with hemangiomas. When these changes are seen, the orbital disorder may be of great extent or of long duration, and such orbits should be approached surgically, with some caution.

Tonometry. As part of the ocular examination, the intraocular pressure should be measured. In some cases of arteriovenous intercommunication, passive orbital congestion can be so great as to impede the normal outflow of the intraocular fluid. The intraocular pressure in one eye is high and the eye shows the corkscrew pattern of tortuous vessels on its surface, as noted earlier. Figure 107 (page 166) illustrates a case wherein corneoscleral trephination was performed after an erroneous diagnosis of primary glaucoma had been made. Claims also

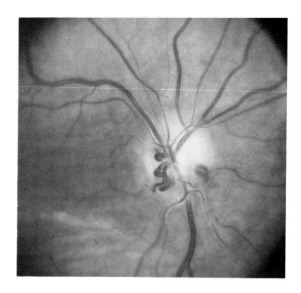

Figure 27. Pallor, grade 4, of right optic disk and shunt veins at the 5 and 8 o'clock positions. (From Hollenhorst RW jr, Hollenhorst RW Sr, MacCarty CS: Visual prognosis of optic nerve sheath meningiomas producing shunt vessels on the optic disk: the Hoyt-Spencer syndrome. Trans Am Ophthalmol Soc 75:141-160, 1977. By permission of the American Ophthalmological Society.)

have been made that an increase in intraorbital pressure associated with endocrine exophthalmos will frequently cause secondary glaucoma. Such observations usually are based on the measurement of the intraocular pressure with the Schiotz tonometer while the patient is supine. In this position, the ophthalmoplegia so frequently present in the disease results in falsely high values. Measurement of intraocular pressure by applanation tonometry gives more nearly correct values. The incidence of glaucoma among patients with endocrine exophthalmos probably is not significantly greater than that in the general population and age groups unaffected by this endocrine disorder. In children or infants, a rise in the intraocular pressure of a proptosed eye may indicate an associated neurofibromatosis.

Auscultation. Auscultation of the orbit is neither a part of the ophthalmologist's routine examination nor, technically, an evaluation of ocular function. However, as part of the overall diagnostic approach, it should be mentioned. It is useful in cases of suspected vascular anomaly or arteriovenous intercommunication. It may also aid the differential diagnosis of cases of pulsating exophthalmos, for not all of these cases have a vascular basis. A bruit is an indication of a vascular disorder either in the orbit or in the retro-orbital portion of the intracranial vault. In general, a bruit is heard best when the stethoscope is placed over the temple on the affected side. Its pitch and volume vary — the softer the bruit, the smaller the vascular lesion, while harsh, high-pitched tones more often accompany widespread tumors — and it is synchronous in most cases with the radial pulse. A thrill also may be detected but not as easily, unless the vascular abnormality is quite large.

Systemic Survey

Most patients in whom orbital tumor is suspected undergo a general physical survey, but this seldom reveals information that aids diagnosis. The primary neoplasms in the orbit, in particular, may remain so localized as to pose no threat nor create any alarm in the overall body economy. Even some of the metastatic neoplasms that stop first in the orbit during their spread may progress so stealthily that much sleuthing is required to discover their source. The neoplasms that invade the orbit by direct extension from neighboring structures may be quite advanced before showing manifestations other than local destructive changes, which are so obvious on roentgenography (see Chapter 16). Many cases of endocrine exophthalmos show no laborabory evidence of dysthyroidism, the diagnosis being made only from the orbital and ocular manifestations.

The patient (or both the parents and the patient, if the latter is a child) should first be surveyed for any changes in the color of the skin (caf áu lait spots) or any masses (molluscum fibrosum) that might suggest a slow-growing neurofibroma. Angiomas around the head and neck and inside the mouth may, in an infant, be a clue to a hemangioma in the nearby orbit. Soft and hard lumps beneath the skin of the eyelids and that of the submaxillary, cervical, or axillary areas may indicate an orbital disorder of lymphomatous type. Extensive surgical scars – in a woman, around the breast, axilla, or neck, and in a man, on the abdomen – may bring out on questioning the almost forgotten information that a "growth" or "cancer" had been "completely removed" some years previously. Stippled and depigmented patches of skin around the face and eyelids, such as occur after irradiation, might suggest a malignant transformation of tissue secondary to excessive irradiation or the orbital spread of a previous surface epithelioma that was once "cured."

Erythrocyte, white blood cell, and differential counts are seldom altered significantly in association with primary orbital lesions except, rarely, in conditions such as leukemia, plasma cell myeloma, and multiple myeloma. The results of routine urinalysis in cases of localized orbital disease are similarly devoid of significance. Special studies of the urine, such as those for amyloid, Bence Jones protein, melanin, vanillylmandelic acid, and homovanillic acid, usually are done after the diagnosis has been established by orbital exploration. These and other special tests pertinent to either diagnosis or prognosis of the individual tumors will be noted among the chapters of Section II.

Roentgenographic Examination

Roentgenographic study of cases of unilateral proptosis has become such an established procedure that it can be considered a routine part of the diagnostic survey. The skull views most commonly ordered are the posteroanterior projections (Caldwell and Waters positions) and lateral orbital views. Optic canal projections usually are not required unless the clinical picture suggests an optic nerve tumor. In recent years, computed tomography and ultrasonography have become almost routine supplements to standard roentgenography as noninvasive refinements for the study of orbital soft tissues. More complex radiographic techniques, such as linear tomography, axial tomography of the optic canals, and basilar skull projections are reserved for the more detailed study of any bone pathology discovered on routine, plain film roentgenography. Invasive procedures requiring the injection of radiopaque material, such as arteriography and phlebography, have a very limited, but necessary, application in the study of certain vascular abnormalities. Other invasive procedures, such as positive and negative contrast orbitography and radioisotope scanning, have largely been replaced by noninvasive procedures in the study of orbital tumors.

Main Features of Roentgenographic Diagnosis.   During the initial study of routine head films, the observer compares the configuration of one orbit with the other. If the size and shape of one orbit are different from the other, the tumor more often is present in the larger orbit. The orbital walls and margins are then more closely scrutinized for irregularities, erosions, and destructive changes such as occur with invasive and malignant lesions. Any abnormal hiatus or dehiscence should be noted; occasionally, an actual absence (dysplasia) of bone is found. Also sought is evidence of atrophy, fossa formation, or hyperostosis due to steady pressure or irritation by the tumor on the adjacent bone. The shadow of the sphenoid bone, in particular, is inspected for evidence of hyperostosis. Less subtle changes indicative of mischief along or adjacent to the optic nerve usually can be observed readily in the special views of the optic canals. Finally, an overall scan of the adjacent sinuses is important to detect those cysts and neoplasms that first must pass through a bony wall before occupying the orbit. Further details of each of these principal features follow.

ENLARGEMENT OF THE ORBIT.   Most readily visualized by the Caldwell projection, expansion of the bony orbit results from increased intraorbital pressure and seems to occur more often with hemangiomas (both adult and infantile types) and neurofibromas (see Fig. 167, page 268). Lymphangiomas, meningiomas, meningoencephaloceles, hemangiopericytomas, and orbital retinoblastomas are less frequent causes of this change. To accommodate the enlarging orbital mass, the walls become more concave. The thinnest wall, the nasal wall, is affected first, but in most cases the distribution of pressure soon creates a symmetric expansion in all meridians. Since the source of the incident ray from the x-ray apparatus is equidistant from each orbit, the comparison of one orbit to the other is valid. The contours of the bony orbit are strikingly symmetric, and a difference of 1 or 2 mm in diameter should be regarded as abnormal. If there is any question about the presence of an orbital enlargement, the diameters of the two orbital entrances may be measured with a millimeter rule, preferably in the vertical meridian.

In our Mayo Clinic series of tumors (Chapter 3), this bony change was noted in approximately 11% of all positive orbital films. Just why this alteration is observed more often with some soft tissue tumors than with others is not known. Similarly, it is not clear why enlargement of the bony orbit occurs with some cases of hemangioma and neurofibroma and not with others. It is natural to assume that the duration of the tumor and the age of the patient contribute to this orbital enlargement; the greater the longevity of the tumor or the younger the patient, the greater the tendency for the bony walls to give way to the relentless pressure. However, in some adult patients with huge hemangiomas of long duration (more than 5 years) associated with extreme proptosis, enlargement of the orbit has not occured; and yet in other adults who have smaller tumors, some enlargement has been noted. In infants, the orbit may expand well beyond its normal diameter during a period of several months, but this change is not necessarily associated with all tumors in this age group. The position of the tumor within the orbital cavity may be more important than hitherto assumed; those in the retrobulbar space seem more capable of exerting the required pressure than tumors in other positions.

Enlargement of the superior orbital fissure also should be mentioned at this point. Some degree of asymmetry in the superior orbital fissures is common, but caution should be exercised in attaching pathologic significance to this finding. Figure 28 illustrates an enlarged, irregular superior orbital fissure that proved

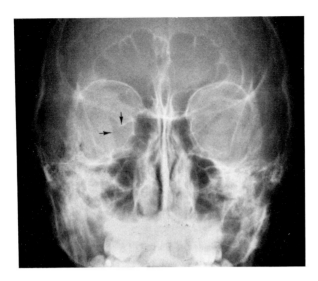

Figure 28. Enlarged, irregular superior orbital fissure (*arrows*) in 15-year-old patient. Its configuration did not change over period of repeated observations.

not to be secondary to an intracranial-orbital tumor. If erosion of the margin of an enlarged fissure occurs, a possible intracavernous carotid aneurysm should be considered. Widening of the fissure also may develop secondary to the pressure of long-standing primary orbital tumors (cavernous hemangioma, meningioma, and hemangiopericytoma) and caroticocavernous fistulas.

BONE DESTRUCTION. Roentgenographically, the most frequent lesions — particularly if secondary neoplasms and cysts from adjacent sinuses are included — are varying degrees of bone destruction. It was present in 18% of the entire series of tumors classified in Chapter 3 and in 45% of those cases having positive orbital films. Bone destruction may take the form of simple surface erosion; interlamellar erosion from, for example, the relentless pressure of an expanding cyst; localized osteolysis due to an irritative or inflammatory lesion; or a diffuse, destructive osteolysis. The last-named condition is usually a bad omen, because it often indicates malignancy. In these cases, the margins of the bony defect are poorly defined and the area of bone destruction is irregular in contour. Bone destruction of this type is most often associated with secondary malignancies from the paranasal sinuses or neoplasms metastatic to the orbit. If such osteolysis is noted in the area of the lacrimal fossa, the likely source is a malignant tumor of the lacrimal gland. Less serious is the more localized bone destruction of mucoceles, hematic cysts, cholesteatomas, or histiocytosis X, wherein the margins of the circumscribed defect show the irregular erosion and fragmentation secondary to irritation and inflammation (see Figs. 67 and 236, pages 102 and 384). Most benign of all types are the sharply outlined defects of dermoid and epidermoid cysts (see Figs. 54 and 54, pages 79 and 80). The smooth borders of these defects may have an almost polished appearance from the long-term effects of pressure.

HYPEROSTOSIS. Next to bone destruction, hyperostosis was the most frequent bony lesion, occurring in about 24% of the positive orbital roentgenograms of the Mayo Clinic series. The three principal orbital lesions producing hyperostosis are meningioma, osteoma, and fibrous dysplasia. Hyperostosis is so frequently associated with one particular orbital condition — meningioma — that it is almost a diagnostic cliché. This roentgenographic alteration most often is noted along the orbital surface of the greater wing of the sphenoid bone (see Fig. 296, page 483). The roentgenographic shadow of such hyperostosis may vary somewhat in density. With long-standing irritation, the shadow may be so dense as to suggest osteoma, the latter being an actual tumor rather than a thickening of bone. However, the shadow of orbital osteomas (see Fig. 119 and 120, pages 201 and 202) usually is well delineated (or even pedunculated) rather than flat and diffuse like the hyperostosis of meningioma.

The hyperostosis of fibrous dysplasia results from a replacement of bone by a more fibrous-like tissue. This replacement sclerosis may be so diffuse and so exuberant as to cause expansion and bulging of the affected bone (see Fig. 137, page 228). The volume of such an orbit is thereby reduced and on plain films appears smaller in overall size than the normal orbit. Hyperostosis and an enlarged lacrimal fossa, singly or together, may occur with lacrimal gland tumors. These changes seem more frequent with benign tumors. The malignant neoplasms in this area more often cause bone destruction, but the incidence of all these bony alterations may depend on the duration of the tumor rather than its type.

BONY DYSPLASIA.   Occasionally seen in orbital roentgenograms, bony dysplasia creates a defect in or an absence of an orbital wall that results in a wide hiatus between orbital cavity and intracranial vault. Most defects of this type that occur around the orbit are large enough to be seen easily in routine roentgenograms. When the defect is present, a diagnosis of neurofibromatosis should be seriously considered (see Figs. 165 and 166, page 267).

CALCIFICATION.   Radiopaque shadows of diagnostic significance also may be seen rarely in the soft tissues of the orbit. Small flakes or clumps of calcium may in younger patients indicate the orbital spread of an unsuspected intraocular retinoblastoma. Larger and more rounded shadows may suggest the concretions associated with vascular abnormalities in the rear of the orbit or a cavernous hemangioma of long duration. Neurofibromas, dermoid cysts, and meningiomas also may show varying degrees of calcification.

OPTIC CANALS.   These projections need not be routinely ordered, because first, it may be a needless expense and, second, findings are positive in only a small percentage of cases. The indications for optic canal studies are more definite but rather limited. As a rule, if an orbital mass is palpable, optic canal views will be negative. However, optic canal views are essential for the following: visual loss (unaccounted for by the change in the refraction of the eye secondary to proptosis), change in the appearance of the optic disk (pallor or papilledema), alteration in the contour of the posterior wall of the eyeball (as viewed by ophthalmoscopy), demonstrable defects on examination of the visual fields, straightforward proptosis, and, particularly, the examination of children. In such instances, the roentgenographic findings may be so diagnostic as to exceed in importance the reliance usually placed on inspection and palpation of the orbit. Although the technique of optic canal projection may vary, the important feature is to orient the ray parallel to the axis of the optic canal and the plane of the film perpendicular to the ray. The optic canal lies at an angle of approximately 37° from the midline. In studying orbital tumors, we are concerned with the difference in size and configuration of the optic canal between the side of the proptosis and the unaffected side. The optic nerve glioma is the most important tumor producing a deformity of the optic foramen. This deformity, of course, is an enlargement of the optic foramen (see Fig. 185, page 295). The diameter of the normal optic canal is about 4.5 mm up to age 1 year. Thereafter, the diameter gradually increases, reaching the adult dimensions of 5.5 to 6 mm by the age of 5 years. We are always suspicious of any diameter greater than 6 mm, and such a finding is an indication for axial tomography of the optic canal (Fig. 29). In addition, axial tomography should be performed in any child with the symptoms noted above, even though the diameter of the optic foramen is normal on plain films. Tomograms may show distortion of the intracranial portion of the canal by a tumor that has not yet advanced anteriorly to the orbital end of the canal.

Supplementary diagnostic procedures utilizing more specialized radiographic techniques now will be noted. All are of more recent origin than the routine roentgenographic examinations just discussed; and, as a group, they represent an attempt to improve the diagnosis among cases that otherwise would appear radiographically negative.

Carotid Angiography. This medium was but one of several procedures devised in the past few decades to visualize orbital soft tissue disease that could not be detected by plain film roentgenography and was beyond the limits of orbital palpation by the diagnostician. Many of these procedures are invasive in that an injection of some medium is required to produce enough contrast between the normal and abnormal soft tissue structures of the orbit to make the pathologic tissue visible on roentgenograms. The introduction of newer noninvasive techniques, such as ultrasonography and computed tomography, have made most of these contrast methods less necessary for the diagnostic evaluation of unilateral proptosis. Positive and negative contrast orbitography, for example, has become almost obsolete, and the once-promising diagnostic procedures of venography and radioisotope scanning have been sharply restricted. Carotid angiography, however, in our opinion, remains a most useful and important adjunct to orbital diagnosis.

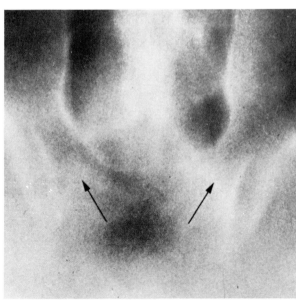

Figure 29. Axial hypocycloidal tomography of optic canals *(arrows).* Excellent view — as if observer were looking at unroofed optic canals in their entire length from above. Accurate comparison of contours of two canals can be made. (From Lloyd GAS: Radiology of the Orbit. London, W. B. Saunders Company, 1975. By permission.)

In the years before the refinements of the noninvasive diagnostic procedures noted above, it was often necessary to use angiography as an exploratory medium when a pathologic condition in the region of the orbital-intracranial partition was only suspected. The patients were subjected to the morbidity and risk inherent in all carotid injections without any assurance that the unknown lesion was in its assumed position or would be visualized if actually present. Now the indications for angiography have become more nearly precise and the risks of angiography are more likely to be justified because the procedure is used only after a noninvasive preliminary procedure, particularly computed tomography, has already discovered the location of the lesion. These more narrow, but important, indications for carotid angiography are the probability, on the basis of clinical assessment or computed tomography, of either a vascular abnormality along the carotid-ophthalmic artery trunk or a meningioma along the orbital surface of the sphenoid bone.

Continuing efforts have been made to improve the quality and diagnostic usefulness of this procedure. Catheter techniques have been developed to permit selective injection of the external and internal carotid system. The x-ray plate changer has been modified to achieve more rapid exposures with good screen contact. Also, the final display has been improved by the use of magnification and subtraction techniques.

The principal role of carotid angiography in orbital diagnosis is to identify the location and extent of ophthalmic artery aneurysms and the pathologic circulation associated with various arteriovenous communications along the ophthalmic artery-cavernous sinus complex that produce unilateral proptosis. In general, angiography should be performed in all cases of pulsating exophthalmos alone and in cases associated with bruit or thrill. In any of these situations, angiography may, surprisingly, uncover a dual blood supply to the orbital mass or reveal an unsuspected locus of a vascular malformation on the side opposite to the affected orbit. All such information is absolutely essential to any surgical approach, whether it be an attempted excision, a trapping or clipping procedure, or selective embolization.

In meningiomas or other vascular tumors adjacent to or involving the sphenoid bone, angiography may be a diagnostic refinement to computed tomography. Such vascular lesions may show such enhancement with contrast on the computed tomographic display that an exact diagnosis is in some doubt. Here, the angiogram may well show whether the lesion is localized or diffuse and, thereby, provide the information for a proper surgical approach. In contrast to the en plaque meningioma secondarily affecting the orbital contents, nodular intraorbital meningioma may show only a faint tumor blush.

VENOGRAPHY (PHLEBOGRAPHY). As orbital angiography developed, it became apparent that concentration of the contrast material in the late phase of an arteriogram was insufficient for visualization of the venous arcades. The next logical step was to devise a method of direct injection of dye into the venous system, and this accomplishment followed by a few years the work on orbital angiography. At present, the frontal vein, preferably on the side of the proptosis, is favored for the introduction of the dye. A 23-gauge scalp needle (a 21-gauge needle may be used to introduce the dye at a more rapid rate if the veins are large enough) is used for the injection of 10 to 12 ml of a suitable contrast medium. The needle must carefully positioned within the lumen of the vein, because extravasation of dye can be irritating. Flow of dye into each orbit is facilitated by a tourniquet (headband) around the forehead and digital pressure over the facial veins. Thus, the venous pattern of the uninvolved orbit may be used as a control in the interpretation of the venogram. Anteroposterior views provide more information than lateral orbital views, and the quality of the final film is enhanced by the use of magnification and subtraction techniques.

Several problems may be encountered in obtaining the ideal venogram. Anatomic difficulties attendant on the introduction of the dye into a suitable vein may make it necessary to cancel the procedure. This flow of dye may not completely fill the venous system of each orbit. More frustrating are cases in which the vein of the affected orbit will not fill at all because of high intra-orbital pressure secondary to a suspected acute pseudotumor, a rapidly progressing asymmetric endocrine orbitopathy, or a rapidly growing neoplasm. Last are those orbital situations in children and some adults when venography cannot be fully accomplished without anesthesia.

In the interpretation of completed films, most attention is directed toward the course of the superior ophthalmic vein, which is visualized best in the anteroposterior projections. This vein arches upward and outward as it enters the orbit near the trochlea. After passage through the anterior one-third of the orbit, the vein angulates in a concave arc downward, outward, and posteriorly. Finally, it levels out, parallel to the lateral orbital wall, until it reaches the superior orbital fissue, where the lumen is slightly constricted before the vein enters the cavernous sinus. Important diagnostic features include unusual displacements of the vein, irregularities or duplications in its caliber, and any increase in the size of the vessel. Because normally its couse is variable and the vein is easily displaced, small deviations in its orbital pattern are not significant and a large deviation is required for diagnostic value (Fig. 30). However, by the time an orbital mass becomes large enough to cause meaningful displacement of the superior orbital vein, the type and position of the orbital tumor likely can be surmised either by observing the direction of proptosis and displacement of the eye or by palplation of the mass.

The greatest value of venography is the demonstration of an orbital varix. Although this condition may be suspected clinically, venography is indispensable not only to confirm the diagnosis but also, more important, to outline the size and extent of the anomaly to facilitate proper surgical planning. If the venogram shows that the varix is fairly well localized to the orbit, it is likely that the venous supply proximal and distal to the mass can be ligated to relieve the proptosis to some extent (Fig. 31). If, instead, venography shows venous ramifications into the pterygoid fossa and intracranial vault, the problem is probably beyond surgical control.

Tomography. Essentially, tomography is a type of body-section roentgenography permitting a study of tissue shadows in one plane of focus of the x-ray machine. It is technically accomplished by moving the x-ray apparatus around a point calculated to lie in the plane of the structure to be studied. Here, we will discuss the bony imaging in the coronal, lateral, and axial positions of the apparatus. The newer (since the first edition of this text) and exciting use of tomography for the imaging of soft tissue (computed tomography) will be noted in the following subchapter.

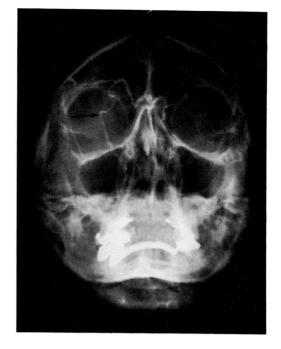

Figure 30. Venogram showing medial displacement (at and below *arrow*) of posterior portion of right superior orbital vein (compare with course of similar vein on left) due to large (4 by 2 by 1.4 cm) cavernous hemangioma in midtemporal portion of right orbit; proptosis on right, 6 mm.

Bony tomography is a most useful refinement of roentgenography because it permits better resolution of the bony defects that usually are apparent on the initial plain film study. Only those tissues at the focal point of the x-ray beam are clearly delineated, because all adjacent structures move in relation to the film plate and their shadows are blurred.

Of the several methods available for moving the x-ray tube to accomplish the objectives of tomography, the linear movement pattern is the most widely employed for orbital studies, because it blurs out the many bony shadows that overlap the orbital contours. Occasionally, a surprisingly large disproportion becomes evident between the abnormality suspected on the plain films and the defect actually present on tomography.

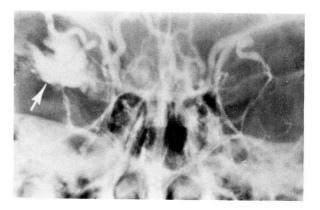

Figure 31. Orbital varix (*arrow*) in 16-year-old girl was confined to orbit and was successfully excised. Varix contained two phleboliths (3 mm and 2 mm). This lesion did not opacify on carotid angiography.

In the coronal plane, tomography shows in more detail the bone destruction associated with dermoid and epidermoid cysts, mucoceles, cholesteatomas, meningoencephaloceles, neoplasms arising in the maxillary antrum, and some malignant neoplasms of the lacrimal gland. Expanding lesions such as aneurysmal bone cysts (see Fig. 146, page 238) also are well defined in these projections.

Lateral tomograms outline the posterior extent of some of these destructive lesions and help determine whether there is any extension into the intracranial vault. We also have found an occasional case in which the destruction of the lateral orbital rim by a malignant tumor of the lacrimal gland is not easily seen on the usual coronal projection but is quite evident on a lateral tomogram.

The axial projections are very important in patients with proptosis who may have either some tumor in the area of the optic canals (Fig. 29) or a destructive process secondarily invading the orbit from the intracranial vault (meningioma, olfactory neuroblastoma) or from the ethmoid-sphenoid sinus area (mucoepidermoid and squamous cell carcinomas) (Fig. 32). In some of these situations, axial tomograms may well determine whether the tumor is operable or inoperable. We also utilize axial tomograms in the staging of tumors in children with suspected rhabdomyosarcoma; particular attention is given to the bony partition between the ethmoid sinus and the orbital cavity.

Computed Tomography

This is a new refinement in body section tomography permitting, for the first time, a clearer imagery of soft tissue structure without the introduction of contrast media. It has been hailed by some as the most important addition to x-ray diagnosis since the discovery of the roentgen ray nearly a century ago. Clinically, computed tomography was first used in neuroradiology of the brain. Subsequently, the scanning apparatus was modified to include the soft tissues of the orbit. Truly, computed tomography has been the most important advance in orbital diagnosis of the past several decades.

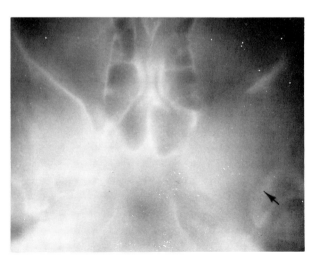

Figure 32. Trispiral basal tomogram of metastatic mucoepidermoid carcinoma that has destroyed floor of middle fossa (*arrow*), foramen ovale, walls of optic canal, and part of greater wing of sphenoid bone. Neoplasm has invaded posterior orbit and produced proptosis. This is an inoperable situation.

The seed for computed tomography was planted by an American neurologist, W. H. Oldendorf, in a nearly forgotten publication in 1961. Here, he described a method for passing a beam of high-energy photons repeatedly from different positions through a given plane in a head phantom. The distribution of the resulting radiodensities was defined by a "simple, on-line" electronic manipulation. He called this technique "spin migration" scanning. A patent was secured, and Oldendorf approached several medical x-ray manufacturers in the hope that a clinically useful apparatus could be developed. For several reasons, his idea was rejected. Furthermore, the more sophisticated ramifications of computed technology had not yet been developed. In other words, the time was not quite appropriate for this new twist in radiographic imaging.

It remained for Mr. Godfrey Hounsfield and his bioengineering associates of EMI Limited, Middlesex, England, to develop the basic head scanner-computer analyzer of present-day techniques. This apparatus was first used clinically in 1972 at the Atkinson Morley Hospital in Wimbledom, England, under the guidance of James Ambrose, M.D. Later, Hounsfield received the MacRoberts Award, a high honor in engineering circles, for the ingenuity and engineering excellence of an apparatus that was to have such a profound, beneficial impact on neuroradiologic diagnosis and patient care. The basic technical features of Hounsfield's invention are illustrated in Figure 33.

The repositioning of the head to permit orbital scanning is illustrated in Figure 34. Additional technical factors in relation to orbital scanning will be found in the bibliography at the end of this chapter. A cross-sectional scan through the midportion of a normal orbit showing ocular detail is illustrated in Figure 35.

In the short span of about 5 years, several dozen articles have described the radiodense imagery of various tumors and lesions of the orbit that heretofore have been unseen in the living patient except by the exploring surgeon. Recent technical modifications utilizing a finer matrix (160 × 160), a narrower collimation of the x-ray beam, thinner tissue sections (4 mm instead of 8 mm), and wider window widths for viewing orbital display have improved the diagnostic capabilities of the instrument to a probable recognition level of more than 90% in instances of abnormal soft tissue lesions. During the scanning procedure, intravenous injection of a contrast substance having a relatively higher density

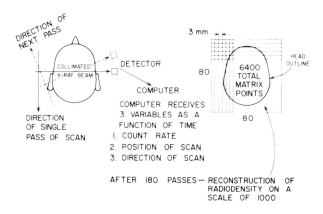

Figure 33. Simplified description of the Hounsfield-EMI scanner. Narrow beam of x-rays is passed through head in horizontal plane. This beam scans at right angles to its own axis, sweeping out entire plane in a little over 1 second. Head occupies center of 80 × 80 matrix. More recent machines have 160 × 160 matrix, which provides better resolution. (From Oldendorf WH: Spin-migration: an early attempt at radiographic transmission section scanning. Bull Los Angeles Neurol Soc 39:138–143, 1974. By permission.)

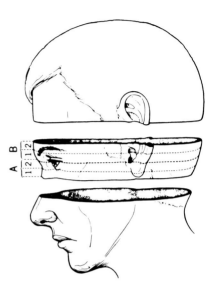

Figure 34. Line diagram illustrates two scans, A and B, parallel to Reid's base line (connects inferior orbital rim with auditory meatus), producing four contiguous slices of orbits from above as though cranial vault were removed. (From Alper MG, David DO, Pressman BD: Use of computerized axial tomography [EMI scanner] in diagnosis of exophthalmos. Trans Am Acad Ophthalmol Otolaryngol 79:OP150–OP165, 1975. By permission of the American Academy of Ophthalmology and Otolaryngology.)

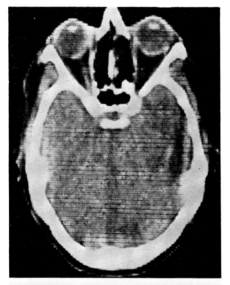

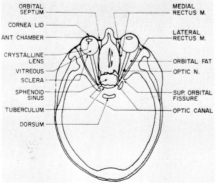

Figure 35. *Top*, Section through midorbit shows ocular detail. *Bottom*, Schematic drawing of section and identification of soft tissue structures within orbit. (From Hilal SK, Trokel SL, Coleman DJ: High resolution computerized tomography and B-scan ultrasonography of the orbits. Trans Am Acad Ophthalmol Otolaryngol 81:OP607–OP617, 1976. By permission of the American Academy of Ophthalmology and Otolaryngology.)

than orbital soft tissue may further enhance the radiographic shadow of some orbital tumors. In addition, the imaging of the optic nerves in their course from the globe to the orbital apex can be improved by changing the plane of scan so that it intersects Reid's base line at an angle of 10°. extending below the line anteriorly and above the line posteriorly.

The computed tomographic appearance of some of the orbital tumors and related lesions pertinent to this text are summarized in the following subsections and supplemented, whenever possible, by photographic reproductions either from our files or from illustrations published by others.*

Hemangioma. The cavernous hemangioma of adults has been the neoplasm most frequently studied by computed tomography. Most of these tumors appear as well-circumscribed, oval, or rounder masses, usually in the more superior cross sections of the orbital scan (Fig. 36). Usually they have a homogeneous appearance and are more dense than other soft tissue tumors (except meningioma). They appear solid because their cystic spaces are not so well delineated by computed tomography as by ultrasonography. Occasionally the tumor has a somewhat speckled appearance that may reflect the image disparity between cystic and solid portions of a longer-standing growth. The dense homogeneity of the tumor may show variable degrees of enhancement with the intravenous injection of a contrast substance. When the hemangioma is confined to the retrobulbar space, differentiating it from the less common intraorbital meningioma may be impossible, because features of contour and density are so similar.

Meningioma. This is a well-delineated mass that has a radiodensity similar to cavernous hemangioma and optic nerve glioma. A frequent diagnostic feature is intraorbital projection from, and attachment to, the sphenoid bone along the posterior partition of the orbit. If the tumor arises from the greater wing of the sphenoid, the lateral rectus muscle shadow will be displaced medially. The sphenoid bone will show variable degrees of increased thickness and sclerosis. The tumor shadow is not always enhanced with contrast media. A meningioma appearing as a thickening of the optic nerve at the extreme apex of

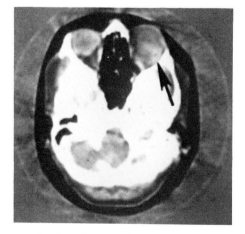

Figure 36. Cavernous hemangioma. Huge (35 by 25 by 20 mm), well-delineated mass (*arrow*) fills retrobular space and lies above optic nerve. Forward extension of tumor partially obscures shadow of eyeball.

---

*It has been difficult to achieve clarity in the reproduction of computed tomographic Polaroid photographs. Therefore, most photographic reproductions appear to be smudged.

the orbit cannot be definitely differentiated by computed tomography from a small optic nerve glioma in the same locality (Fig. 37).

Optic Nerve Glioma.   Many of these tumors along the intraorbital portion of the nerve become quite large — a feature not common with meningioma Fig. (38).

Pleomorphic Adenoma.   Similar in appearance to hemangioma and meningioma, the benign mixed tumor of the lacrimal gland is well circumscribed, fairly radiodense, and homogeneous appearing. The tumor usually is smaller than a cavernous hemangioma. Its anterior position above and lateral to the eyeball and the persistence of its shadow in the more dorsal scanning sections differentiate it from other neoplasms of similar density (meningioma and neurofibroma). If bone erosion is present (usually more visible on linear tomography), the tumor is likely to be one of the malignant epithelial neoplasms intrinsic in the lacrimal gland.

Neurofibroma.   The solitary neurofibroma may arise anywhere in the orbit and may look very similar to any of the previously noted tumors. With high-resolution scanning, slight variations in the homogeneity of its shadow may be visible, corresponding to the lobular form of the tumor (Fig. 39).

Malignant Lymphoma.   This is one of several soft tissue tumors that have a less dense shadow, a more speckled appearance, and a less definite contour than the orbital lesions in the foregoing group. When located in the posterior orbit, the lymphoma does not have scanning features that differentiate it from many other soft tissue disorders. However, when this tumor arises in the more anterior portions of the orbit, it tends to push forward into the eyelid. This feature, combined with a tumor shadow that may extend ventrally or dorsally along the anterior third of the eyeball and may have an indefinite border, suggests lymphoma, particularly if the main mass of the lesion is more pronounced in the inferior cross sections of the orbital scan. Enhancement with injections of contrast media is variable.

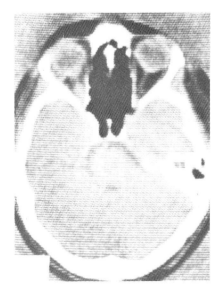

Figure 37. Perioptic meningioma producing slight proptosis and thickening of left optic nerve. Differential diagnosis was between optic nerve glioma and meningioma. (From David DO, Alper MG: Computerized tomography of the orbit and orbital lesions. *In* Orbit Roentgenology. Edited by PH Arger. New York, John Wiley & Sons, 1977, p 206. By permission.)

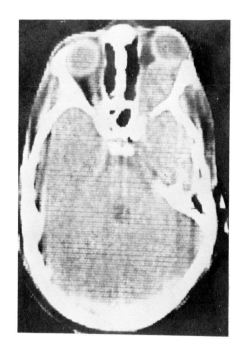

Figure 38. Very large optic nerve glioma. Note marked proptosis of right eye and enlargement of optic canal. (From Hilal SK, Trokel SL, Coleman DJ: High resolution computerized tomography and B-scan ultrasonography of the orbits. Trans Am Acad Ophthalmol Otolaryngol 81: OP607–OP617, 1976. By permission of the American Academy of Ophthalmology and Otolaryngology.)

Metastatic Carcinoma. These lesions have a mottled appearance not unlike some lymphomas, but their distribution in the orbit usually is more extensive and diffuse. Their tendency to infiltrate the extraocular muscles, particularly the levator muscle of the upper eyelid to cause paralytic ptosis (Fig. 40), is a feature that differentiates them from lymphoma. Also, they have a more pronounced enhancement after injection of contrast substances than other soft tissue tumors with similar configurations or contours. In women, the breast is the most likely source of the metastasis, but in men, the orbital masses more likely are metastatic from the kidney, lung, stomach, or prostate. The scirrhous variants of metastatic seedings usually produce enophthalmos rather than proptosis of the eye in the affected orbit.

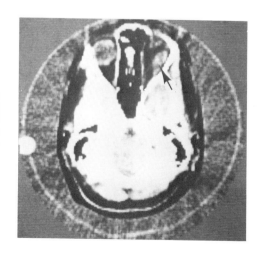

Figure 39. Solitary neurofibroma. This ellipsoid, dense, circumscribed, lobulated tumor (*arrow*) appearing in a dorsal orbital scan is located superior and posterior to eye and above lateral rectus muscle. It is not attached to bone.

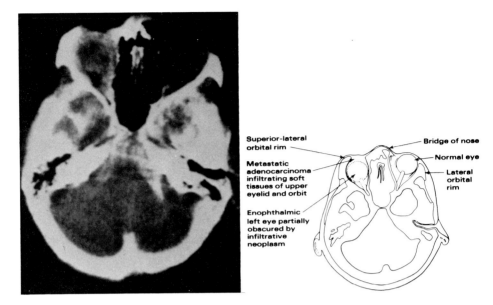

Figure 40. *A*, Metastatic carcinoma in 73-year-old woman with complete left ophthalmoplegia and bilateral carcinoma of breasts. Diffuse infiltration of soft tissues of left orbit, extraocular muscles, and eyelid by metastatic carcinoma, which partially obscures shadow of enophthalmic left eye. *B*, Schematic drawing shows principal features of orbital scan.

Vascular Lesions. Arteriovenous malformations of the orbit and orbital involvement secondary to carotid-cavernous fistulas are visible by computed tomography techniques. Because the scans are noninvasive, they are useful for preliminary assessment of a suspected problem. However, if surgical treatment is contemplated, angiography is needed to provide a more definite outline of the extent and size of the vascular malformation.

Inflammatory Pseudotumor. In our experience, this orbital disorder is the most difficult of the soft tissue abnormalities to assess by computed tomography. In some patients, the scans may be negative except for unexplained unilateral proptosis. In other patients, the tumor shadow may vary from a focal, well-delineated mass to a diffuse, mottled process that may even involve the extra-ocular muscles (Fig. 41). These capricious disorders may be found anywhere in the orbit but do not invade or attach to bone. Rarely, a pseudotumor may be suspected on preoperative scanning when the inflammatory process is so acute, infiltrative, or close to the eye as to produce some scleral thickening on the scanning display (Fig. 42).

Endocrine Orbitopathy. This is another nonneoplastic disorder that has presented problems in diagnosis by computed tomographic methods. In all cases, there is an increase of varying degree in the density and bulk of the orbital reticulum. The increase is often associated with hypertrophy of two or more of the extraocular muscles. The increased density and bulk might suggest the shadow of an infiltrating, low-density, soft tissue neoplasm in the retrobulbar space. The spindle-like shadows of the hypertrophic muscles have easily been interpreted as elliptic, high density, solid neoplasms. False-positive indications for surgical exploration also have resulted from misinterpretation of the com-

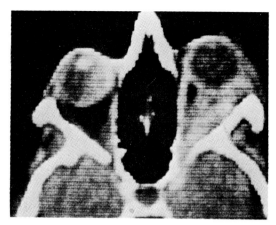

Figure 41. Pseudotumor. Diffuse inflammatory process involves retrobulbar area of right orbit and blends with shadow of lateral rectus muscle. (From Hilal SK, Trokel SL: Computerized tomography of the orbit using thin sections. Semin Roentgenol. 12:137–147, 1977. By permission of Grune & Stratton.)

bined shadows of hypertrophied muscle bundles at the apex of the orbit, particularly when proptosis was marked on one side but of only borderline degree on the less affected side. It is now realized that the anatomic position of the swollen muscle bundles, particularly the superior and inferior recti, does not remain in the horizontal plane of the scanning cross section. Instead, the incidence rays of the scanner section the muscle annulus at an oblique angle. The resulting shadow then appears as a solid tumor with a feathered anterior border (Fig. 43). When a more isolated swelling of a lateral or medial rectus muscle has been surgically explored for probable neoplasm, either the examiner has overlooked hypertrophy of at least one other muscle or the head has been tilted in the scanning apparatus so that the horizontal recti muscles do not lie in the same focal plane. These diagnostic guesses may be resolved by the use of coronally positioned scans, a recent innovation. Here, the shadows of the hypertrophied superior and inferior rectus muscles are more clearly delineated than in horizontal cross sections and help differentiate this orbitopathy from all other soft tissue lesions that cause proptosis. The superior and inferior rectus muscles are involved more often and more extensively by the edema, hypertrophy, and eventual fibrosis of the disease than the medial and lateral recti.

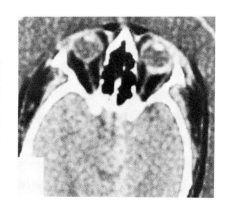

Figure 42. Scan shows definite thickening of sclera along temporal surface of right eye and some thickening of right lateral rectus muscle. These changes usually are enhanced by injection of contrast medium. (From Bernardino ME, Zimmerman RD, Citrin CM, et al: Scleral thickening: a CT sign of orbital pseudotumor. AJR 129:703–706, 1977. By permission of the American Roentgen Ray Society.)

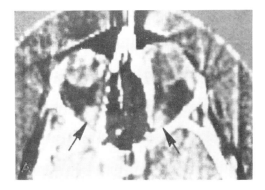

Figure 43. Severe endocrine orbito-pathy. Large orbital apex masses (*arrows*) on both sides are due to enlarged extra-ocular muscles. (From Momose KJ: The place of computerized tomography in oph-thalmology. *In* Controversy in Ophthal-mology. Edited by RJ Brockhurst, SA Boruchoff, BT Hutchinson, et al. Philadel-phia, W. B. Saunders Company, 1977, p 369. By permission.)

There are several other, less common, neoplasms, cysts, or metabolic prob-lems involving the orbit that have been noted one time or another in the litera-ture (Fig. 44). Also, there are a number of tumors that involve bone or break through the bony barriers separating the orbit from adjacent sinuses. Here, computed tomography is but a supplement to more specific data obtained by linear, hypocycloidal, or baso-orbital tomography.

Ultrasonography

The application of the principles of ultrasound to the study of soft tissue dis-orders of the orbit has been one of the major advances in orbital diagnostics of the past 20 years. The principal investigators who have contributed so much to the refinements necessary for the present widespread clinical use of ultra-sonography are Baum, Bronson, Coleman, Oksala, Ossoinig, and Purnell. Ultra-sonography and the more recently discovered computed tomography have made possible a graphic mapping or a picture display of many soft tissue abnormalities that were considered well beyond the realm of discovery not so many years ago.

Briefly, the basic components of an ultrasonic instrument are these: a piezoelectric element that converts an electric source into pulsed waves of ultra-

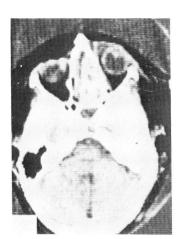

Figure 44. Olfactory neuroblastoma. Nasoethmoidal mass, with destructive bone lesions, encroaching on medial right orbit and producing proptosis. (From Davis DO, Alper MG: Computerized tomography of the orbit and orbital lesions. *In* Orbit Roentgenology. Edited by PH Arger. New York, John Wiley & Sons, 1977, p 200. By permission.)

frequency sound, an acoustic lens that provides direction and form to the incident wave, a collecting unit that reconverts the reflected sound into electric units, and a recorder, such as an oscilloscope. The sound-generating source and sound-receiving device are compactly combined into one unit, the transducer. The principle of ultrasonography is that the sound wave emanating from the transducer is reflected back from tissue interfaces, which have different acoustic impedance properties. This reflected sound is called an echo. The echoes recorded on the oscilloscope can be photographed as a permanent echogram, or ultrasonogram. The two echo displays most commonly used in ophthalmology are A-mode and B-mode.

A-Mode. This method is a time-amplitude, unidirectional system wherein the horizontal axis of the tracing represents the time and distance factor of the sound as it traverses the orbital tissues, and the vertical component represents the intensity of the reflected impulse (Fig. 45). The position of various echoes along the horizontal axis of the tracing corresponds to their relative tissue depth and distance from the source of the sound. A study of the height (amplitude), number, and width of the vertical components of the tracing provides informa-

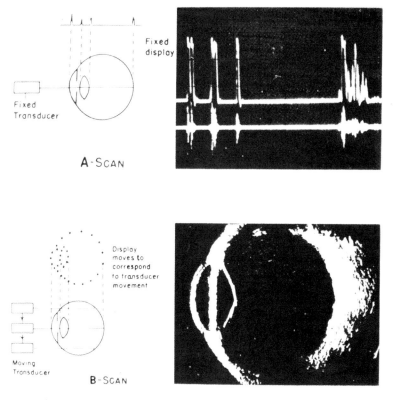

Figure 45. Schematic and photographic representation of A-mode (*Top*) and B-mode (*Bottom*) ultrasonography. *Left,* Orientation of transducer and diagrammatic form of echo display. *Right,* Actual ultrasonogram obtained from normal eye. (From Coleman DJ, Dallow RL: Introduction to ophthalmic ultrasonography. *In* Clinical Ophthalmology. Edited by TD Duane. Hagerstown, MD, Harper & Row, Publishers, 1978, vol. 2, chapter 25, p 2. By permission.)

tion about the cellular characteristics of the tissue through which the sound wave travels. Deductions based on these factors have reached a high degree of sophistication in differentiating abnormal from normal echo patterns. The reflected waves of this scanning mode are better delineated and more correctly recorded if the transducer is held at right angles to the tissues under study. Abnormalities in the apex of the orbit are more difficult to assess with A-mode display than more anterior lesions, because tissues such as the optic nerve and the annulus of the extraocular muscles produce a less sharp, more confluent echo. Also, there is some attenuation of the sound wave by the time it reaches this area of the orbit due to some absorption of the sound energy by the intervening tissues. For the same reason, tumors arising from, or adjacent to, the orbital roof or sphenoid bone are relatively inaccessible ultrasonically.

B-Mode. This is called intensity-modulated ultrasound. Because it utilizes a moving transducer, it is often referred to as a B-scan. It provides a two-dimensional cross section display of the orbital structure under study (Fig. 45). In this system, the reflected echo is modulated to produce a spot of light on the oscilloscope display instead of the vertical wave of the A-mode method. The brightness of each of these light points is proportional to the intensity of the reflected sound wave. B-scan instruments are helpful in providing a two-dimensional view of the size, shape, and position of the soft tissue orbital lesion, but, as with the A-mode method, abnormalities of the bony orbital walls are not well visualized.

In clinical diagnostics, the two methods complement one another. The orbit may be scanned first with the B-mode system to localize the tumor and then its particular tissue component studied in more detail by the A-mode display. Differential diagnosis usually is based on the patterns of sound reflectivity at the surfaces of the mass and the transmission characteristics of the sound wave as it passes through the lesion. From these, the surface of the mass can be classified as smooth or irregular, and the character of the mass can be subclassified as smooth or irregular, and the character of the mass can be subclassified as solid, cystic, vascular, or infiltrative. The ultrasonic patterns of some of the common orbital tumors are as follows.

Hemangioma. These tumors have smooth, well-demarcated borders that appear on the echogram as sharply defined, highly reflective interfaces (Fig. 46A and B). However, the ultrasonic pattern from the interior of these tumors varies according to the type of hemangioma. The fibrous-walled septa between the vascular arcades of the adult cavernous hemangioma reflect the sound in a pattern of irregular, high-amplitude echoes. The more compact, cellular structure of the capillary and infantile hemangioma results in a more regular, low-amplitude echo.

Mucocele. The rounded, well-delimited, smooth surfaces of these tumors show sharply outlined acoustic borders like those of hemangiomas, but the sound wave easily penetrates their cystic interiors (Fig. 46C). A few low-amplitude echoes may be reflected from debris within the interior of the cyst. Dermoid cysts have a similar ultrasonographic display.

Solid Neoplasms. The benign mixed tumor of the lacrimal gland, the solitary orbital neurofibroma, the encapsulated neurilemmoma, the optic nerve glioma, and the nodular meningioma primary in the orbit have similar ultrasonic features. Usually, they have smooth, demarcated contours that produce echoes from their anterior and posterior surfaces of less amplitude than those from hemangiomas, mucoceles, and dermoid cysts. Sound absorption by these tumors is moderately high because of their solid structure (Fig. 46D and E). Tissue discontinuities within these tumors produce irregular echoes of medium amplitude. Ultrasonically, it is difficult to differentiate tumors in this class from one another, particularly those that often grow in the area of the orbital apex. In these situations, B-mode scans may provide helpful supplementary information (Fig. 47).

Infiltrative Lesions. The infiltrative tumors include lymphangioma, metastatic carcinoma, malignant lymphoma, and inflammatory pseudotumor. They are the most difficult group to differentiate by ultrasound. Because the tumors are infiltrative, ultrasonic surface signals may be irregular, indistinct, or of low amplitude. Echograms from the interior of these lesions may vary, showing the good sound transmission and high-amplitude echoes of lymphangioma, the poor sound transmission and low-amplitude echoes of lymphoma, or various combinations of sound transmission and amplitude in metastatic carcinoma and pseudotumor (Fig. 46F).

Endocrine Orbitopathy. Here, the involvement of the orbit is usually more diffuse than with any of the aforementioned lesions and will be more easily visualized by the topographic potentials of the B-mode scan. Enlargement of the extraocular muscles is the most nearly constant ultrasonic clue to this disorder (Fig. 48). The superior and inferior rectus muscles are more frequently involved than the medial and lateral rectus muscles. Such changes are more evident in a B-mode scan taken in a vertical plane.

Vascular Malformations. When the clinical findings suggest a possible orbital vascular abnormality, arteriography may be deferred until the problem has been assessed by a noninvasive, less serious procedure such as ultrasonography. Such ultrasonic surveys are often inconclusive, but one positive example is illustrated in Figure 49. In this case, the signals from the surface of the arteriovenous fistula show a moderate reflectivity like that previously noted with cystic orbital tumors. However, the low-amplitude echoes from the fast-moving blood columns are so rapid that they have a blurred, almost smudged outline, a feature not seen with any other orbital tumors.

Recapitulation

From the foregoing discussion or the numerous laudatory reports in the literature, the reader may assume that either ultrasonography or computed tomography is the only technique needed, nowadays, for complete diagnosis of orbital tumors. Not so! The reader should keep in mind that photographic reproductions of positive orbital displays and the accuracy of the final diagnosis detailed in the literature have almost always been based on retrospective analysis. In other words, the sophisticated diagnostic machines have confirmed the presence of an orbital mass already suspected on the basis of history or clinical data or revealed by successful orbitotomy. With experience, one can accurately diagnose an occasional tumor preoperatively by either method, but, in general, neither technique can accurately differentiated malignant from benign lesions that have similar display patterns. In our opinion, neither test replaces the value of a careful history and an accurate preoperative clinical assessment of the prop-

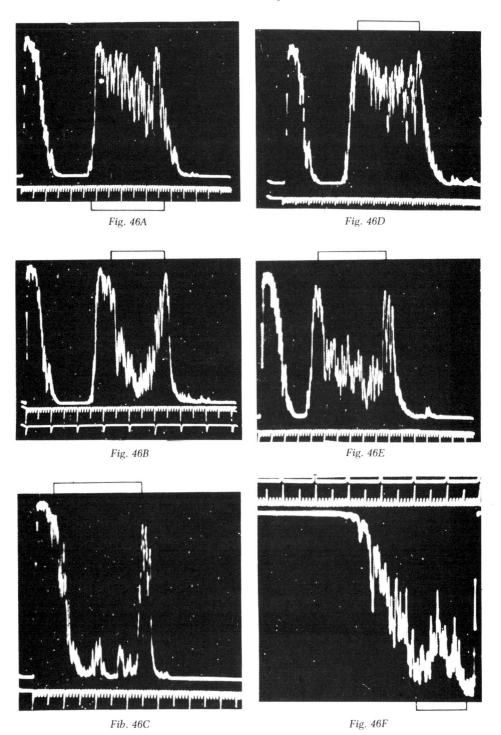

Figure 46. A-mode ultrasonograms. *A*, Cavernous hemangioma. *B*, Capillary hemangioma. *C*, Mucocele. *D*, Benign mixed tumor. *E*, Optic nerve glioma. *F*, Metastatic carcinoma. (From Ossoinig KC, Blodi FC: Diagnosis of orbital tumors. *In* Current Concepts in Ophthalmology. Edited by FC Blodi. St. Louis, C. V. Mosby Company, 1974, vol 4, pp 313–343. By permission.)

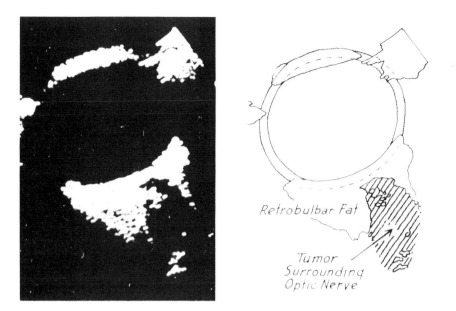

Figure 47. B-scan ultrasonogram of glioma of optic nerve. Tumor produces marked widening of normal nerve shadow. (From Coleman DJ, Lizzi FL, Jack RL: Ultrasonography of the Eye and Orbit. Philadelphia, Lea & Febiger, 1977, p 315. By permission.)

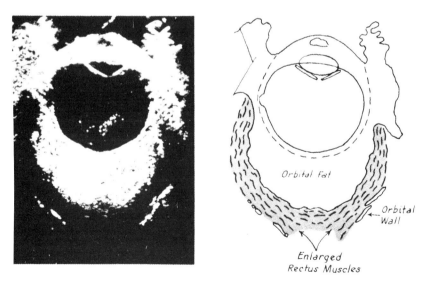

Figure 48. Endocrine orbitopathy. B-scan ultrasonogram shows shadows of enlarged medial and lateral rectus muscles. (From Coleman DJ, Lizzi FL, Jack RL: Ultrasonography of the Eye and Orbit. Philadelphia, Lea & Febiger, 1977, p 328. By permission.)

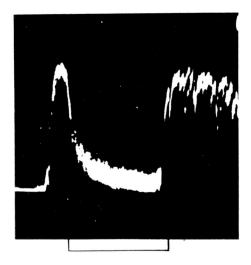

Figure 49. A-scan ultrasonogram of arteriovenous fistula. Note low-amplitude, blurred echoes produced by fast-moving blood flow. (From Ossoinig KC, Blodi FC: Diagnosis of orbital tumors. *In* Current Concepts in Ophthalmology. Edited by FC Blodi. St. Louis, C. V. Mosby Company, 1974, vol 4, p 334. By permission.)

tosis. To us, the value of these special diagnostic techniques is the information they provide about the size, contour, extent, and position of the suspected orbital mass — features sometimes beyond the scope of external ocular evaluation and orbital palpation. Knowledge of these dimensions has helped immensely in planning the surgical approach that most efficiently exposes the lesion.

Because of the high cost of this equipment, some persons have asked which system — ultrasonography or computed tomography — is the best buy when financing is possible for one but not both. If a purchasing budget is the only factor, a fully equipped ultrasonography laboratory would be our choice. If clinical usefulness is a major factor, we would choose the computed tomography apparatus. The latter choice is based on an often overlooked factor, that is, the value to the patient. Whereas in the precomputer period patients often were hesitant to proceed with orbitotomy when orbital roentgenographic findings were negative, now they, too, can see the abnormal shadow on the computer Polaroid print and realize the need for surgical therapy. In addition, they can foresee some of the surgeon's problem in removing a tumor from the cramped confines of the orbit. Also, they can see how close the orbital abnormality is to the eyeball or the optic nerve and, thereby, be tolerant of dissection difficulties that result in postoperative diplopia or reduced vision. On the other hand, few patients can accurately comprehend the interpretive complexities of an orbital ultrasonogram.

Radioisotope Scanning

The use of radionuclides for orbital diagnosis was an offshoot of the radioisotope scans once widely used for the differential diagnosis of brain disease. In this respect, radioisotope scanning was similar in genesis to the earlier development of orbital angiography. In contrast, orbital angiography found a special niche in orbital diagnosis, as we have already noted, but radioisotope scanning was curtailed in its developmental prime by use of the more efficient, noninvasive diagnostic modalities of computed tomography and ultrasonography. At present, we are not aware of any radioisotope center that is relying on this medium for the differential diagnosis of unilateral proptosis to the exclusion of one of the more practical diagnostic adjuncts noted above.

Thermography

Orbital thermography is another diagnostic supplement in the study of orbital disease that has been so overshadowed by the diagnostic reliability of either computed tomography or ultrasonography that publications on it have almost disappeared.

Surgical Biopsy

A discussion of orbital diagnosis would not be complete without consideration of surgical biopsy. Even though we assiduously pursue all the clinical ramifications of unilateral proptosis described in this chapter and correctly analyze the positive clues provided by all the mechanical aids noted above, the histologic verification of the tumor is the goal of all our efforts. Biopsy is the climax of the patient's evaluation; it is the revelation that all concerned, including the patient, are awaiting. Probably more reliance is placed on this diagnostic procedure than on any other.

The objective of biopsy is to remove a portion of the orbital mass and, by either inspection or histopathologic study, to establish the diagnosis. *Incisional biopsy* is the term almost universally applied to this pursuit. *Excisional biopsy*, which requires total or almost complete removal of the tumor, is primarily a method of treatment and only secondarily a procedure for diagnosis. *Frozen tissue study*, a term for a rapid means, now available in most hospitals, for determining the nature of an orbital mass, has become almost synonymous with incisional biopsy in its diagnostic implications, whereas *fixed tissue study* has, more or less, replaced the older connotation of the latter. In our haste to perform frozen tissue study, we may wrongly assume that it will always establish the correct diagnosis. In reality, its accuracy is only in the range of 95%. Also we overlook the possibility that biopsy may deleteriously affect either the course of the tumor or the symptoms of the patient. What, then, is the scope of biopsy in the overall scheme of diagnostic search?

In orbital lesions associated with evidence of inflammation (that is, redness and edema of ocular adnexal structures), incisional biopsy must be done carefully. However, to satisfy the pathologist and to assure that no neoplastic changes are overlooked, resection of a fairly large portion of the mass may be necessary. But such surgical meddling, even though well intentioned, frequently exacerbates the orbital disorder; postoperative hemorrhage or reactive edema increases proptosis. Patients with endocrine exophthalmos and many with pseudotumor are particularly prone to this reaction; many have extensive loss of vision due to increased orbital pressure.

The patient's attitude and response to biopsy also should be considered. Whereas the ophthalmologist's concern is the identity of the orbital disease, the patient may be more alarmed about the progressive protrusion of one eye or the cosmetic liability of such a unilateral flaw. The ophthalmologist looks upon the biopsy principally as a means for information, but the patient, even though understanding the need for diagnosis, also assumes such a surgical undertaking will improve the proptosis or promote resolution of the orbital mass. If biopsy is not soon followed by arrest of the proptosis or improvement in the symptoms, the surgical manipulation has little practical value from the patient's viewpoint. This embarrassing circumstance may be further compounded if the results of incisional biopsy are inconclusive. Among the orbital tumors, lymphomas, pseudotumors, rhabdomyosarcomas, and undifferentiated metastatic carcinomas are prone to this problem when subjected to frozen tissue study.

Other drawbacks to incisional biopsy concern its possible effect on the neoplasm. Biopsy of malignant lacrimal gland tumors is particularly dangerous, because it permits an earlier dissemination and, hence, wider extension of the tumor than would likely have happened had the mass been excised rather than incised. Even the biopsy of benign mixed tumors in this area is hazardous, because it permits escape of tumor cells that have a strong penchant for growing again on some distant day. In cases of carcinoma of adnexal structures such as the eyelids, incisional biopsy may promote fatal dissemination of the neoplasm (meibomian gland carcinoma) or create so much postoperative edema that the borders of the tumor become indefinite, so that the ultimate excision is less precise.

The salient attribute of incisional biopsy combined with frozen tissue study is the rapid assistance it provides the surgeon in making a therapeutic decision. So often, what the surgeon wants to know is whether the orbital mass is benign or malignant. In most cases, neoplastic disease can be quickly differentiated from inflammatory lesions, and a skilled pathologist may further classify the neoplasms as to whether they are amenable to irradiation, should be excised, or are best left alone. Also, if the surgeon can give a definite diagnosis when the patient recovers from anesthesia, the confidence of the patient and relatives is bolstered.

The proper interpretation of fixed-tissue sections of some orbital lesions also is important. It is desirable that the pathologist have training or experience in orbital pathology, because the response of the host reticular tissue (orbital fat) to some orbital invaders may be unique. Thus, the pathologist should know the varied tissue responses to orbital pseudotumors and not misinterpret the profuse lymphocytic collections in some of these specimens as evidence of malignant lymphoma. Conversely, true lymphomatous neoplasm may be considered innocent hyperplasia because the pattern of this neoplasm in the orbit may differ from its customary picture in lymph nodes. The morphologic changes of most orbital tumors have a closer kinship to systemic surgical pathologic findings than to those of the eye lesions. Therefore, a surgical pathologist working routinely with specimens of metastatic carcinomas, particularly the large family of fibrous tissue tumors, is in a better position to recognize the altered nuances of these lesions when they occur in the orbit than an ophthalmic pathologist, who works with a more limited and specialized number of neoplasms.

Fixed-tissue study of an incisional biopsy also is more accurate if the surgeon furnishes the pathologist with a representative section of the lesion. Time and again we have seen the bravado of the surgeon's biopsy nullified by a smidgen of tissue too small to interpret properly. This pitfall is particularly serious when a biopsy is performed on noncircumscribed or infiltrative soft tissue tumors. A proper biopsy specimen should be at least 5 to 10 mm in length in at least one diameter and, preferably, should include material from the periphery as well as the interior of the lesion. There seems to be no need to biopsy most encapsulated tumors, and, in our opinion, circumscribed orbital masses probably can be studied as well after their removal as by preliminary biopsy. Incisional biopsy of encapsulated or circumscribed tumors in the lacrimal gland fossa, in particular, is dangerous because of frequent seeding of potentially malignant cells that serve as a nidus for a future inoperable recurrence. Orbital manifestations of endocrine exophthalmos and pseudotumor should not be subjected to incisional biopsy unless the process is aggressive and has not responded to medical therapy such as administration of the steroid drugs. If biopsy is necessary in a case of pseudotumor, a large and representative specimen should be submitted for histopathologic study to assure adequate analysis of the response within the various tissue strata. Some pseudotumors become partially circumscribed and can be partially excised almost as easily as they can be biopsied. *Whatever the enthusiasm of the ophthalmologist for incisional biopsy, it should be tempered by the understanding that removal of an orbital tumor, not biopsy, is the main objective, for it is the orbital mass that brought the patient to the clinician and the feature for which the patient seeks relief.*

Needle biopsy of an orbital mass is occasionally advocated, but most ophthalmologists oppose such exploratory punctures on grounds of possible harm. Even so, many of these physicians think nothing of thrusting a long needle into the area of the ciliary ganglion adjacent to the optic nerve to secure anesthesia suitable for intraocular surgical procedures. Such retrobulbar blocks are widely used for cataract surgery and occasionally result in some degree of optic atrophy (although such cases are seldom reported). There is, indeed some risk to the insertion of a needle into the orbital contents whether it be for biopsy or for the administration of an anesthetic solution.

A more practical application of the diagnostic potential of needle biopsy is to insert the needle after the tumor has been surgically uncovered. A cystic lesion in infants, for example, may represent an orbital extension of an unsuspected meningocele. Incisional biopsy of such tumors causes unnecessary loss of spinal fluid and opens an avenue to the intracranial cavity. The more cautious insertion of a small-gauge needle will reveal the characteristic clear fluid of such tumors and should prevent the surgeon from bumbling into a situation that he may not be able to handle. If there is any doubt whether the clear content of such a cyst is spinal fluid, the sample can be quickly analyzed for sugar. If sugar cannot be identified, the surgeon may feel more free to proceed with the surgical removal of the cyst. If the specimen is positive for sugar, the case may be turned over to a neurosurgeon. Exploratory needle puncture of a clear tumor in adults may be the means for identifying echinococcus cysts. Actually, exploratory needle puncture may be used on any orbital cyst, regardless of color, if the surgeon has doubts whether incision or excision of the tumor offers the best means for eradication.

Bibliography

A complete bibliography of all facets of diagnosis covered in Chapter 2 has not been attempted. Instead, key references are listed that should provide an interested reader good coverage of specific aspects of orbital diagnosis as well as access to many other publications on the subject.

Clinical Evaluation and Proptosis

Alper MG: Endocrine orbital disease. *In* Orbit Roentgenology. Edited by PH Arger. New York: John Wiley & Sons, 1977, pp 69–92

Grove AS Jr: Evaluation of exophthalmos. N Engl J Med 292:1005–13, 1975

Hepler RS: Clinical diagnosis of orbital tumors. Radiol Clin North Am 10:3–10, 1972

Wright JE, Fells P, Jones BR: The investigation of proptosis. Trans Ophthalmol Soc UK 90:221–39, 1970

Roentgenography

Hanafee WN: Plain views of the orbit. Radiol Clin North Am 10:167–79, 1972

Kirkpatrick JA, Capitanio MA: Radiology of the orbit in infancy and childhood. Radiol Clin North Am 10:143–66, 1972

Lloyd GAS: Radiology of the Orbit. London: W. B. Saunders Company, 1975

Angiography and Venography

Dayton GO: Orbital venography: anatomy, technique, and diagnostic use. Trans Am Ophthalmol Soc 75:459–504, 1977

Dilenge D: Arteriography in tumors of the orbit. CRC Crit Rev Clin Radiol Nucl Med 5:213–50, 1974

Hanafee W: Orbital venography. Radiol Clin North Am 10:63–81, 1972

Vignaud J, Clay C, Aubin ML: Orbital arteriography. Radiol Clin North Am 10:39–61, 1972

Zimmerman RA, Vignaud J: Ophthalmic arteriography. *In* Orbit Roentgenology. Edited by PH Arger. New York: John Wiley & Sons, 1977, pp 135–69

Tomography

Ambrose JAE, Lloyd GAS, Wright JE: A preliminary evaluation of fine matrix computerized axial tomography (Emiscan) in the diagnosis of orbital space-occupying lesions. Br J Radiol 47:747–51, 1974

Hilal SK, Trokel SL: Computerized tomography of the orbit using thin sections. Semin Roentgenol 12:137–47, 1977

Lloyd GAS: Axial hypocycloidal tomography of the orbits. Br J Radiol 48:460–64, 1975

Momose KJ: The place of computerized tomography in ophthalmology. *In* Controversy in Ophthalmology. Edited by RJ Brockhurst, SA Boruchoff, BT Hutchinson, et al. Philadelphia: W. B. Saunders Company, 1977, pp 361–76

Ultrasonography

Baum G: A reappraisal of orbital ultrasonography. Series II. Trans Am Acad Ophthalmol Otolaryngol 69:943–57, 1965

Bronson NR: Development of a simple B-scan ultrasonoscope. Trans Am Ophthalmol Soc 70:365–408, 1972

Coleman DJ: Orbital ultrasonic tomography (B-scan). Trans Am Acad Ophthalmol Otolaryngol 78: OP577–OP580, 1974

Oksala A: Ten years' experiences in clinical ultrasound investigation. Acta Ophthalmol (Copenh) 45: 489–509, 1967

Ossoinig K: Echography of the eye, orbit, and periorbital region. *In* Orbit Roentgenology. Edited by PH Arger. New York: John Wiley & Sons, 1977, pp 223–69

Purnell EW: Ultrasonic interpretation of orbital disease. *In* Ophthalmic Ultrasound. Edited by KA Gitter et al. St. Louis: C. V. Mosby Company, 1969, pp 249–55

Surgical Biopsy

Dehner LP, Rosai J: Frozen section examination in surgical pathology: a retrospective study of one year experience, comprising 778 cases. Minn Med 60:83–94, 1977

Nakazawa H, Rosen P, Lane N, et al: Frozen section experience in 3000 cases: accuracy, limitations, and value in residency training. Am J Clin Pathol 49:41–51, 1968

SECTION II

The Individual Tumors: Clinical Features, Pathology, and Management

WITH THE COLLABORATION OF
GEORGE M. FARROW, M.D.

3

The Tumor Survey

NOMENCLATURE

Because the title of this text signifies our principal interest *in tumors*, it is germane to clarify the context of this term. In the particular fields of pathology, histology, and oncology, the word *tumor*, through common usage, has become almost synonymous with *neoplasm*. Even so, we prefer to use *tumor* in the meaning of its etymologic genesis, that is, a term indicating swelling or abnormal enlargement. In a sense, the true nature of most orbital masses and swellings (tumors) that cause proptosis is unknown until the surgical exploration or histologic examination classifies the lesion as neoplastic or nonneoplastic. The word *tumor* can cover all these presurgical unknowns. Although we will rely heavily on this word throughout the text, we will exclude from our tumor survey most of the conditions associated with infectious agents, collagen disease, and metabolic disorders. The last-named exclusion will eliminate a discussion of a very common cause of proptosis, namely, endocrine orbitopathy (the ophthalmopathy of Graves' disease). However, we will include several inflammatory metabolic, or granulomatous processes that may simulate neoplasms in their progressive growth (Table 1). Also, such lesions as cysts and soft tissue malformations will be considered to be in the domain of our discussion.

Neoplasms, thus, become a subclass of tumors, and we will use the former within its customary meaning of an abnormal, progressively enlarging mass (new growth) that exceeds and is uncoordinated with the function of the surrounding normal tissues. Also, the modifying designations *malignant* and *benign* will be used within the context of their accepted usage, but we would caution the reader not to accept the full literal sense of the word *benign* as it often is applied to several members of the orbital tumor family. For example, as will be noted in Chapter 15, some recurrent benign mixed tumors are not so benign as their cellular classification may seem, because they possess the capabilities of becoming malignant, in the full sense of that term, at some later time. Recurrent meningiomas, although repeatedly designated benign, possess strong inherent tendencies to remain cellularly aggressive and may eventually cause death by their unchecked spread to vital centers. In the realm of pathology, there has been no satisfactory term to designate separately those so-called benign neoplasms with malignant or malaggressive traits.

CLASSIFICATION

Throughout our many years of interest in orbital tumors, the variety of tumors that can originate in, grow in, invade, lodge in, or otherwise usurp

67

TABLE 1. Classification of Orbital Tumors

Cysts
    Developmental (dermoid cyst, epidermoid cyst, teratoma,
        cephaloceles, congenital cystic eye, microphthalmos
        with cyst, perioptic hygroma)
    Mucocele
    Parasitic
    Hematic
    Simple (serous, retention, and implantation cysts)
    Dentigerous
Vascular neoplasms
    Hemangiomas (capillary, cavernous)
    Hemangioendothelioma
    Hemangiopericytoma
    Vascular leiomyoma
    Lymphangioma
Vascular malformations
    Aneurysm
    Varix
    Arteriovenous fistula
    Arteriovenous aneurysm
Tumors of fibrous connective tissue
    Fibroma
    Fibromatoses
    Proliferative nodular fasciitis
    Fibrous histiocytoma
    Fibrosarcoma
    Fibrosarcoma after irradiation
Tumors of osseous and cartilaginous tissue
    Osteoma
    Osteoblastoma
    Giant cell tumor
    Osteogenic sarcoma
    Osteogenic sarcoma after irradiation
    Chondroma
    Mesenchymal chondrosarcoma
    Fibrous dysplasia of bone
    Infantile cortical hyperplasia
    Progressive diaphyseal dysplasia
    Aneurysmal bone cyst
    Chordoma
    Ewing's tumor
Tumors of mesenchymal and adipose tissue
    Myxoma
    Mesenchymoma
    Lipoma
    Liposarcoma
Tumors of nerve sheath origin
    Neurofibroma
    Neurofibromatosis
    Neurilemmoma
    Malignant schwannoma
    Neurofibrosarcoma
Neurocytic and neurogliogenic tumors
    Retinoblastoma
    Medulloepithelioma
    Optic nerve glioma
    Neuroepithelioma
    Ganglioneuroma
    Neuroblastoma
    Chemodectoma
    Olfactory neuroblastoma (esthesioneuroblastoma)
Malignant melanoma

(Continued)

TABLE 1. CLASSIFICATION OF ORBITAL TUMORS (CONTINUED)

Lymphocytic, plasmacytic, and granulocytic neoplasms
    Malignant lymphoma
        Hodgkin's disease
        Well-differentiated lymphocytic lymphoma, diffuse
        Poorly differentiated lymphocytic lymphoma, diffuse
        Nodular lymphoma
        Mixed cell lymphoma
        Large cell (reticulum cell, histiocytic) lymphoma
        Burkitt's lymphoma
    Plasma cell myeloma
    Waldenström's macroglobulinemia
    Granulocytic sarcoma
    Leukemias
Histiocytoses
    Histiocytosis X
    Infantile xanthogranuloma
    Sinus histiocytosis
Intrinsic neoplasms of the lacrimal gland
    Benign mixed tumor
    Malignant mixed tumor
    Adenoid cystic carcinoma
    Adenocarcinoma
    Squamous cell carcinoma
    Mucoepidermoid carcinoma
    Oncocytoma
Secondary epithelial neoplasms
    Squamous cell carcinoma
    Adenoid cystic carcinoma
    Adenocarcinoma
    Malignant mixed tumor
    Mucoepidermoid carcinoma
    Basal cell carcinoma
    Sebaceous carcinoma
    Sweat gland carcinoma
Metastatic carcinoma
Meningioma
Neoplasms of muscle
    Rhabdomyosarcoma
    Rhabdomyoma
    Leiomyoma
    Leiomyosarcoma
Miscellaneous tumors
    Lymphoid inflammatory pseudotumor
    Sarcoid
    Orbital vasculitis
    Wegener's granulomatosis
    Amyloid tumor
    Ectopic lacrimal gland
    Mikulicz's disease
    Wilms' tumor
    Nasal-Orbital polyposis
Tumors of uncertain origin
    Alveolar soft part sarcoma
    Granular cell tumor

space in the relatively small orbital cavity has continued to amaze us. This assortment of trespassers also has piqued the interest of many others, because a small but consistent number of reports are found in yearly summaries of the literature. Some of these reports are based on observations in distant countries where the published material is not easily available for perusal. In still other reports, linguistic nuances and differences in terminology may indicate either a larger variety or a greater number of tumors than would be the case if the report had originated in another country or had been written in another language. The World Health Organization has recognized this lack of uniformity and, in recent years, has published a series of monographs on the histologic typing of tumors of various organs and tissues in an effort to provide a more nearly standard international classification. Such a monograph on the grouping of tumors of the eye and adnexa is pending but has not been published at the time of this writing.

The classification given in Table 1 is a conglomerate of several that have appeared in texts and journals. It is subject to many of the variables already noted. We hope that it includes enough divisions based on histopathologic features to satisfy the purist but at the same time offers a sufficient nexus of tumor behavior and location to be helpful to the clinician. Most of all, this classification has provided a convenient grouping for the subsequent discussion.

INCIDENCE

The nucleus of this study is a series of reports on 764 consecutive orbital tumors obtained from the files of the Mayo Clinic for the 27-year period 1948 through 1974. This series, one of the largest recent compilations of tumors collected from one institution, is a logical source for important clinical and pathologic data relating to orbital tumors. In addition, particular attention has been given to the long-term course of some groups of tumors, since many patients have continued under observation of the Mayo Clinic for many years. This follow-up has provided valuable data on the natural history of some of our tumor family. In this respect, the survey differs from many others wherein large collections of pathologic material have been assembled but protocols have been either incomplete or based on short periods of observation. This long-term study of patients has confirmed the expected course of some tumors but has suggested revision in the prognosis of others. The duration of the study roughly corresponds to the period in which one of us participated in the clinical management of 38% of the patients in the total group.

Much of our incidence data will be based on the Mayo Clinic series, but whenever feasible in the subsequent chapters, we will compare our findings with similar data from other large collections of orbital tumors published in the literature. Our consecutive series of orbital tumors is listed in Table 2. It covers

TABLE 2. SUMMARY OF 764 CONSECUTIVE ORTIBAL TUMORS, MAYO CLINIC, 1948-1974

Histologic type	Primary	Secondary	Metastatic	Generalized	Total
Cyst					93
Dermoid	10				10
Epidermoid	7				7
Simple	1	1			2
Cephalocele		2			2
Hematic	6				6
Teratoma	1				1
Mucocele		65			65

CONTINUED

TABLE 2. CONTINUED

Histologic type	Primary	Secondary	Metastatic	Generalized	Total
Vascular					74
Hemangioma	55				55
Hemangiopericytoma	11	1	1		13
Lymphangioma	5				5
Vascular leiomyoma	1				1
Vascular malformations					43
Aneurysm	2	1			3
Arteriovenous aneurysm	1	4			5
Arteriovenous fistula		35			35
Fibrous connective tissue					10
Fibrosarcoma	3	4			7
Fibrosarcoma after irradiation		1			1
Fibromatosis	1				1
Fibrous histiocytoma		1			1
Osseous and cartilaginous					27
Osteoma	3	6			9
Osteogenic sarcoma		4			4
Osteogenic sarcoma after irradiation		1			1
Chondroma	1				1
Chondrosarcoma		5			5
Fibrous dysplasia	5				5
Aneurysmal bone cyst	2				2
Mesenchymal and adipose tissue					6
Lipoma	2				2
Liposarcoma	3	1			4
Nerve sheath origin					28
Neurofibroma	5				5
Neurofibromatosis	12	1			13
Neurilemmoma	7	1			8
Neurofibrosarcoma				2	2
Neurocytic and neurogliogenic					40
Retinoblastoma		6			6
Optic nerve glioma	19				19
Neuroblastoma			11		11
Olfactory neuroblastoma		4			4
Malignant melanoma	3	27	1		31
Lymphocytic, plasmacytic, granulocytic					63
Malignant lymphoma	38	3		16	57
Plasma cell myeloma	1			3	4
Granulocytic sarcoma	2				2
Histiocytosis X		4		4	8
Mixed					28
Benign	13				13
Malignant	10	5			15
Rhabdomyosarcoma	9	9			18
Carcinoma					163
Squamous cell	1	58	4		63
Adenocarcinoma	4	9	39		52
Adenoid cystic	12	13			25
Basal cell		18			18
Mucoepidermoid	1	1			2
Sebaceous		3			3
Meningioma	23	45			68
Lymphocytic inflammatory pseudotumor	35				35
Sarcoid	5				5
Vasculitis	13				13
Wegener's granulomatosis	4	1			5
Amyloid	1	1			2
Unclassified granuloma	2	1			3
Epithelial papilloma		1			1
Total	340 (45%)	343 (45%)	56 (7%)	25 (3%)	764

tumors primary in the orbit, those that secondarily involve the orbit by direct spread from an adjacent area of the face or head, those that metastasize to the orbit, and those that are but one focus of a multifocal, generalized disease (chiefly, tumors of the hematopoietic system). The number of tumors in each of these categories was as follows:

Primary Tumors	340
Secondary tumors	343
Metastatic tumors	56
Generalized (part of a multifocal process)	25

It will be quite a surprise to many ophthalmologists to note that nearly equal percentage of primary and secondary tumors in the overall total (we were aware of this statistical trend from the survey of a smaller number of tumors published in the first edition). No other large published series (more than 200 cases) of orbital tumors emanating from a department of ophthalmology contains such a large number of secondary tumors. In practice, the ophthalmologist customarily observes or manages most primary tumors and assumes that they are, by far, the most common in the domain of orbital tumors. Therefore, this physician may contend that our incidence of secondary tumors is skewed by a referral of greater numbers of these more difficult cases to a large treatment center than would be seen in an average community practice. In reply, we can say that many of these patients with secondary orbital tumors were first seen in either the department of otorhinolaryngology or the section of maxillofacial surgery as primary care patients rather than as referred patients. Our belief is that physicians in these two surgical specialties manage many patients with secondary orbital tumors, but ophthalmologists will not see these patients unless the physicians are part of an interdependent association of physicians or participate in an active hospital consultation practice.

The five most common primary orbital tumors in our series were as follows:

Hemangiomas	55
Malignant lymphoma	38
Lymphocytic inflammatory pseudotumors	35
Meningioma	23
Optic nerve glioma	19

The five most common secondary tumors were:

Mucocele	65
Squamous cell carcinoma	58
Meningioma	45
Vascular malformations	40
Malignant melanoma	27

The numbers of primary and secondary neoplasms were 246 and 228, respectively.

Age and Sex

The prevalence of certain tumors in children or adults is well known. The age distribution of our patients by type of tumor is listed in Table 3. We note in Table 3 that about 14% (106 cases) of all the tumors are concentrated in the

TABLE 3. AGE AND SEX DISTRIBUTION OF PATIENTS IN ORBITAL TUMOR SURVEY

Male	Female		Age in years at time of orbital diagnosis							
			0-10	11-20	21-30	31-40	41-50	51-60	61-70	70+
11	2	Adenocarcinoma (primary & secondary)				3	3	6	1	
11	28	Adenocarcinoma (metastatic)				5	9	15	8	2
13	12	Adenoid cystic carcinoma (primary & secondary)			4	5	5	7	2	2
1	1	Amyloid						1	1	
	2	Aneurysmal bone cyst	1	1						
15	3	Basal cell carcinoma				1	1	4	5	7
1	1	Cephalocele	2							
1		Chondroma						1		
2	3	Chondrosarcoma					1	2	2	
4	6	Dermoid cyst	4	3	1	2				
1	6	Epidermoid cyst	1	2	1	1	1	1		
1		Epithelial papilloma							1	
1	3	Olfactory neuroblastoma			1	1	1		1	
1		Fibromatosis	1							
5	3	Fibrosarcoma				1	1	2	3	1
2	3	Fibrous dysplasia	2	2	1					
1		Fibrous histiocytoma								1
1	1	Granulocytic sarcoma	2							
26	29	Hemangioma	25	3	3	5	10	6	2	1
5	8	Hemangiopericytoma		1	2	2	6		1	1
6		Hematic cyst			1	2	2	1		
5	3	Histiocytosis X	7	1						
17	18	Lymphocytic inflammatory pseudotumor	1	1	4	4	9	5	6	5
2		Lipoma				1		1		
3	1	Liposarcoma		1		1			2	
2	3	Lymphangioma	3		1		1			
32	25	Malignant lymphoma	2	1	1	1	5	22	19	6
18	13	Malignant melanoma		2	1		7	3	14	4
17	51	Meningioma	2	3	3	19	14	13	11	3
8	5	Mixed tumor (benign)		3	2	2	4	1	1	
10	5	Mixed tumor (malignant)		1	3	1	4	3	1	2
32	33	Mucocele	1	4	7	3	19	12	14	5
	2	Mucoepidermoid carcinoma						1	1	
4	4	Neurilemmoma		1	1	1	2		2	1
8	3	Neuroblastoma	11							
3	2	Neurofibroma			1			3	1	
6	7	Neurofibromatosis	7	4	1	1				
2		Neurofibrosarcoma					1			1
7	12	Optic nerve glioma	11	6	1		1			
3	2	Osteogenic sarcoma		1		1	1	2		
6	3	Osteoma	1	3	1		3		1	
2	2	Plasma cell myeloma							3	1
4	2	Retinoblastoma	6							
13	5	Rhabdomyosarcoma	13	1	2	2				
1	4	Sarcoid					1	2		2
3		Sebaceous carcinoma					1	1		1
2		Simple cyst			1			1		
45	18	Squamous cell carcinoma			5	4	8	15	23	8
1		Teratoma	1							
	3	Unclassified granuloma				1	1			1
	1	Vascular leiomyoma	1							
17	26	Vascular malformation	1	6	7	3	7	11	5	3
4	1	Vasculitis		4	4	1			2	2
7	6	Wegener's granulomatosis				1	2		2	
393	371	Total	106	55	62	76	130	144	130	61

first decade of life but that the fewest tumors are found in the second decade. After age 20, the frequency of tumors gradually increases until age 71, when a fairly sharp decrease occurs. About 53% (404 cases) of all our tumors occurred in the age interval 41 to 70 years. The common tumors of childhood are hypertrophic (juvenile) hemangiomas, capillary hemangiomas, rhabdomyosarcomas, neuroblastomas, and optic nerve gliomas, as has been noted in many pediatric surveys. Not one of the serious carcinomas occurred before the third decade.

Our series shows a distribution of 371 female and 393 male patients, or an approximate ratio of 12:13. Tumors such as metastatic adenocarcinoma and meningioma predominantly affect women and girls, but this preference is offset by the predominance among men of basal cell carcinomas and squamous cell carcinomas secondarily invading the orbit.

Bibliography

Hou PK, Garg, MP; Tumors of the orbit: a report of 193 consecutive cases, In Current Concepts in Ophthalmology. Vol. 3. Edited by FC Blodi. St. Louis: C. V. Mosby Company, 1972, pp 176—85

Jones IS, Jakobiec FA, Nolan BT: Patient examination and introduction to orbital disease. *In* Clinical Ophthalmology. Vol 2. Edited by TD Duane. Hagerstown, MD: Medical Department, Harper & Row, Publishers, 1978, chapter 21, p 17–24

Reese AB: Expanding lesions of the orbit. Trans Ophthalmol Soc UK 91:85–104, 1971

Silva D: Orbital tumors. Am J Ophthalmol 65:318–39, 1968

4

Orbital Cysts

DEVELOPMENTAL CYSTS

DERMOID AND EPIDERMOID CYST

The most frequent and important of the so-called developmental cysts involving the orbit are the dermoid and epidermoid cysts. Although benign, they relentlessly expand and may produce considerable displacement of the eye before they are obliterated.

The term *choristoma* frequently is applied to tumors of this type. The term refers to their origin from an aberrant anlage: in this case, dermal elements that get pinched off along suture lines or diploe in the course of embryonic development. The skull is a common site of origin for these cysts, owing to the number and complicated relationships of its component bones.

Designation of these cysts as *dermoid* (the "oil cyst" of the older literature) or *epidermoid* is based largely on detailed histologic study. Because their source of origin is similar and because transitional types occur, many observers believe a differentiation between the two types is artificial and academic. In much of the literature therefore, the older and more common term, *dermoid* designates both types of cysts. We accept this tendency among writers to lump them together, but we will point out several features in their clinical course and management wherein they differ. Those solid tumors, also of dermal origin, found on the surface of children's eyes now are designated dermoid *tumors*. *Epidermoid* is a newer term rightly replacing the older and familiar designation *cholesteatoma*. The latter implies that cholesterol or its derivates influence formation of the tumor, whereas the cholesterol content of many cysts is but a late manifestation of their growth and degeneration. *Epidermoid cyst* is the more nearly factual and proper term.

INCIDENCE

As recorded in Table 2 (pages 71 and 72) 17 (2.2% of the total tumors) of the cysts are included in our study. In other tumor surveys, dermoid and epidermoid cysts usually approximate 4 to 6% of the total but such series, although comparable to our own in size, contain a higher percentage of primary tumors relative to the total than our survey (Reese 1971, Silva 1968. See Bibliography, Chapter 3). Also, many surveys, particularly those limited to the pediatric age group, include cysts along the upper temporal margin of the orbital rim that are found to be anterior to the orbital septum at the time of excision. This type of cyst is quite common, easily seen and palpated early in life, and accounts for the frequent statement that dermoid cysts are the most common orbital tumors of childhood. We have excluded these anterior cysts from our study because we do not believe they are in the orbital cavity proper (Fig. 50). Cysts arising along the superior rim of the orbit anterior to the orbital septum are more likely to expand forward along the path of the least tissue resistance than to push posteriorly through the tough fibrous tissue of this fascial structure. Lastly, the counts in some surveys are inflated by the unknowing inclusion of lesions that look like orbital dermoid cysts and occur in the upper eyelid but contain a lining of nonkeratizing cells (cuboidal epithelium). These, more properly, should be designated "conjunctival dermoid cysts" (Jakobiec et al, 1978).

In most surveys sex incidence is about equal, but in our series females were affected twice as often (12:5) as males. As for age, these cysts usually are manifest in the first two decades but occasionally are encountered up to the age of 50. Epidermoid cysts generally affect an older age group than dermoid cysts, probably because they are located deeper in the orbit, more often grow in the diploe of bone, and remain latent for longer periods.

CLINICAL FEATURES

That these cysts grow slowly is often implied by the literature. This is true to a degree, but their growth behavior might better be characterized as intermittent. In children and young adults, the cysts may enlarge for several months and then remain dormant or unchanged for an interval. In adults, the cysts must have a long period of latency, for it is difficult to understand how a cyst continuously enlarging since infancy would become manifest only at the age of 40 with clinical symptoms of about a year's duration. Just what triggers the growth of these embryonic anlages at such a late age is not known.

The fact that most cysts (15 of 17 in the Mayo Clinic series) were palpable attests to the size of some of them as well as to their favored site of origin, the anterior portion of the orbit. Statistics tending to support their prevalence in one orbit rather than the other may not be significant, although in our series, there was a definite preponderance in the right orbit (14 of 17 cases). Reports in the literature agree, however, that the cysts favor the upper portion rather than the lower quadrants of the orbit for their growth. Occasionally, instances of a

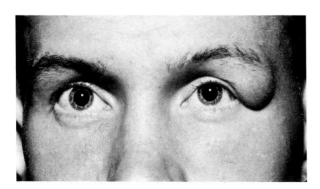

Figure 50. Dermoid cyst entirely confined to adnexal tissues of left upper eyelid anterior to orbital septum; no displacement or proptosis of left eye.

cyst in the inferior portion of the orbit are reported; almost always, the cyst shadow is visible by routine roentgenographic examination, and the cause of the patient's exophthalmos is not diagnostically puzzling. For some years, our impression was that dermoid cysts were more common in the upper temporal quadrants of the orbit, an impression influenced by frequent encounters with cysts in the eyelids and other adnexal structures of this general area. When our series is analyzed, however, the cysts seem nearly equally distributed between upper nasal and upper temporal quadrants, an occasional cyst extending across the midline and occupying both upper quadrants. The epidermoid cyst usually is found deeper in the orbit than the dermoid type and more often erodes bone.

In children, particularly, the cyst soon protrudes forward beneath the upper rim of the orbit. By the time the parents bring the child in for consultation, the "lump" is usually more or less the size of a hazelnut. The mass is smooth, painless, and more often oval than round. It is not attached to skin, as would be the case if it were a sebaceous gland tumor. The mass could almost be rolled between thumb and forefinger were it not still attached to bone along its upper or posterior side. There is little or no displacement of the eye, and the x-ray findings are negative.

In adults, the cyst may not be so easily palpated, probably owing to its more posterior location. Nor does it emerge from the orbit so easily as in children. Under the relentless pushing of the cyst, the eye and adnexal structures gradually are displaced downward, with scarcely any interference of ocular function except for occasional diplopia due to restricted motility of the eye when it moves toward the affected orbital quadrant (see Fig. 6, page 17). The cysts also may find an outlet by growing through bone into the intracranial cavity, an adjacent sinus, or the temporal fossa. Whatever its route of expansion, the cyst may not be palpated until it is large and it is not unknown for a cyst to reach the surface and intermittently evacuate its contents through a fistulous tract (Pollard and Calhoun, Dayal and Hameed, and many others), particularly in the inhabitants of underprivileged countries. In such patients, pressure on the proptosed eye produces a malodorous discharge from the sinus tract. Some cysts in their travel through bone become hourglass-shaped, the bony dehiscence forming just a tiny aperture between the expanded chambers of the bilobed cyst. It was a cyst of this type that Krönlein (1888) first removed by the lateral surgical approach (Fig. 51). The tip of a probing finger will feel the tumor to be smooth and firm but its extent and outline to be vague. Tenderness or pain may be elicited when the finger pushes against the mass. Ballottement of the extraorbital lobe of the cyst also may cause movement of the eye if the bony aperture is large.

ROENTGENOGRAPHIC CHANGES

The most telltale clues are seen on roentgenography (Figs. 52, 53, and 54). The defects are radiolucent and are large in proportion to the overall size of the orbit, and the margins of the fossa or hiatus are distinct. Bone adjacent to the cyst wall becomes polished from pressure, and the terms *sclerotic border* and *well-corticated margins* are used to describe this typical feature. Radiolucency is caused by a high content of fatty material within the cyst. Occasionally, inflammation complicates the cyst and exerts a lytic effect on bone, and in such cases,

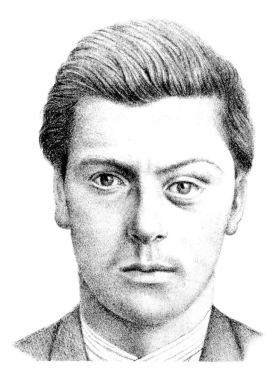

Figure. 51. Preoperative appearance of Krönlein's patient, who had orbital dermoid cyst removed from rear of left orbit by osteoplastic resection of lateral orbital wall. Note fullness of left temporal fossa resulting from expansion of cyst outside orbit. (From Krönlein RU: Zur Pathologie und operativen Behandlung der Dermoidcysten der Orbita. Beitr Klin Chir 4:149-163, 1888.)

the margins of the bony defect are less dense or even irregular but not to the degree seen in malignant lesions.

PATHOLOGY

Differentiation between dermoid and epidermoid types most easily is made by histopathologic study. Each type has a fibrous tissue capsule of various degrees of thickness and toughness. Within its capsule, the simpler of the two cysts, the epidermoid, has a lining of epithelial cells that usually are stratified and capable of producing keratin (Fig. 55). A middle layer containing blood vessels, fat lobules, collagen bundles, sebaceous glands, and hair follicles characterizes the dermoid type (Fig. 56). The epithelial lining may vary in thickness; when it is thin or even absent, cellular collections appear, an indication of an inflammatory component. Somewhere along the circumference of the mass will be a fibrovascular connection to adjacent periorbita. The contents of the cysts may vary from an oily, tan liquid, through a cheesy, yellow or white material, to an inspissated mass with a high content of cholesterol (Fig. 57). In some of the larger and older cysts with stretched and thin walls, bleeding into the lumen gives the contents a chocolate hue. When exposed, cysts that are deeper and larger have a whitish or bluish color, whereas cysts that are smaller and more anterior look yellow.

It is important to do a histologic study on all these cysts at the time of surgery even though they may rupture during the procedure and their lining is eradicated by some means other than excision. There are at least two known instances (Jones, Wright and Morgan) of a probable epidermoid cyst undergoing

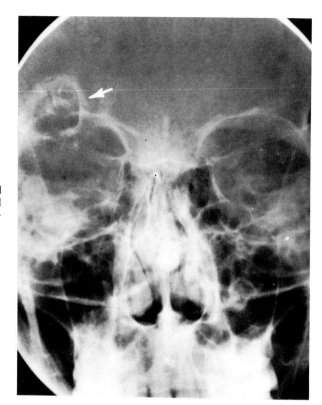

Figure 52. Sharply outlined bony margins (*arrow*) of small epidermoid cyst in superotemporal portion of right orbit.

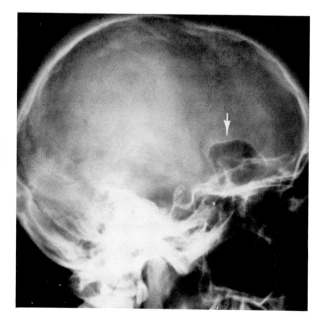

Figure 53. Larger epidermoid cyst (*arrow*) involving roof of orbit (lateral view). Note radiolucency of cyst.

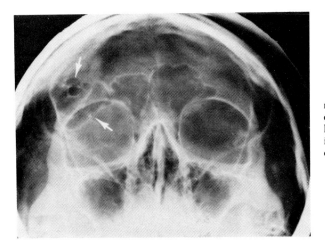

Figure 54. Large epidermoid cyst eroding roof of right
orbit (*lower arrow*) with smaller
hiatus (*upper arrow*) through
inner table of bone into intracranial vault (Waters' view).

malignant transformation into a squamous cell carcinoma. Both patients were
53 years of age, and the carcinoma was eventually fatal. It would be easy to
miss something as serious as this if the cyst were simply evacuated and its wall
not studied histologically.

TREATMENT

Anterior Cysts. The surgical approach to the more forward cysts is by a
slightly curved transverse incision through the skin of the upper eyelid overlying the mass and parallel and adjacent to the superior rim of the orbit. The
capsule of the cyst usually is thick enough to permit relatively easy dissection
along a cleavage plane around the surface of the mass. The goal of surgery is to
remove the mass intact. If dissection is too meticulous in removing all the shreds
of tissue adherent to the capsule, the wall of the cyst will be nicked and the

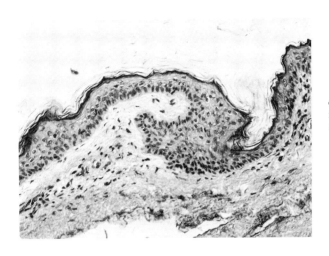

Figure 55. Section of epidermoid cyst. Lining is keratinizing squamous epithelium. (Hematoxylin and eosin, × 160.)

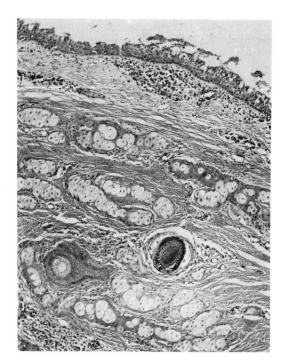

Figure 56. Section of dermoid cyst; squamous epithelial lining, hair, and sebaceous glands in wall. (Hematoxylin and eosin; × 70.)

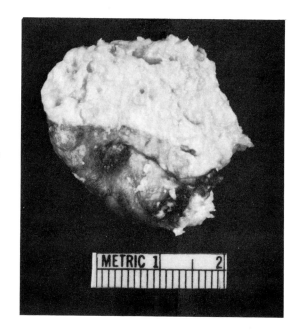

Figure 57. Dermoid cyst (opened) showing sebaceous contents.

contents will extrude. Extrusion of the contents does no harm as long as most of the material is carefully removed. The problem is that the wall of the cyst is less easily identified after the mass has collapsed. A neat and clean removal of the tumor thus becomes more difficult. Somewhere along the surface of the mass, in what always seems the most inaccessible area of dissection, the scissors will cut the main blood supply. A sharp spurt of blood, obscuring the field and halting the careful dissection, may surprise or alarm the surgeon who operates on one of these cysts for the first time, but an appropriately placed hemostat enables easy completion of the excision.

Deeper Cysts. The approach to larger, more deeply placed cysts may require more planning. The outlines and extent of the cyst determined by roentgenograms are helpful. The cysts may be approached through the anterior brow incision, the transcranial route, or the lateral orbit route (see Section III). If roentgenograms locate the cyst near the optic foramen or superior orbital fissure, the transcranial approach is recommended. Similarly, this approach seems wisest for cysts of hourglass and dumbbell shape found along the roof of the orbit when the cystic space on the intracranial side appears larger than the cavity on the orbital side. Proptosis is minimal in such cases. The lateral surgical route is favored for cysts located behind the lacrimal gland and for those extending hourglass-fashion through a tiny dehiscence in the suture line between the zygomatic and sphenoid bones. The anterior route is useful for those lying behind the superior orbital rim and involving the frontal sinus or occupying the deeper portion of the upper nasal quadrant of the orbit.

If the anterior approach is chosen, either the classical cleavage plane between periorbita and roof of the orbit (peripheral space) can be utilized or the cyst can be exposed directly through the frontal bone just above the superior rim of the orbit. With the former method, the cavernous spaces of the cyst lie above and posterior to the lip of the bony orbital rim once the anteroinferior wall of the cyst has been removed. Because the attic compartments of the cyst are poorly illuminated with this approach, the surgeon's maneuvers are hindered. An approach to the anterior surface and main compartment of the cyst by direct passage through the frontal bone may then be helpful. With a Stryker saw or chisel, a small rectangle of bone can be removed from the superior orbital rim directly anterior to the cystic cavity (Fig. 58). The surgical field will then lie in direct view of the surgeon, and brighter illumination of the cavity will be possible.

Whatever the route, intact removal of a cyst in the posterior orbit is seldom accomplished. Some cysts are so stretched and their walls so thin that a good resection of tissue is not easy to obtain. Anterior and inferior walls usually are thickest where the cyst abuts against the resistance of orbital structures. If the cyst erodes bone, the lining may be stripped away with tissue forceps or curette. Sometimes this stripping is difficult to accomplish because of small outpouchings from the main chamber. Also the color of the cyst lining may be so similar to that of underlying bone that the cyst may be overlooked in scattered areas Frequently the intracranial vault and its tough dura are exposed because thin chips of bone break away as the cyst lining is stripped. Such exposure does not seem to pose any problem in the postoperative period as long as dura is not unduly traumatized. A tiny nick in the dura can be closed with a fine silk suture.

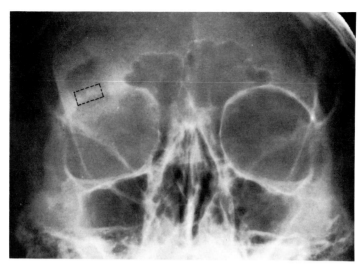

Figure 58. Rectangle (*black dots*) outlining bone to be removed from superior orbital rim to facilitate direct access to large epidermoid cyst in roof of right orbit.

Remnants of the cyst wall that cannot be stripped may be lightly touched with mild desiccating diathermy. This destroys any tags of epithelium that have been overlooked and helps to discourage recurrence. Diathermy desiccation is preferable to chemical cautery (phenol, silver nitrate, and trichloroacetic acid) and coagulation diathermy.

The inferior wall of the cyst may require special handling. This wall, by reason of long-continued counter pressure from orbital structures, becomes fused with the fascial covering of the levator palpebrae superioris. Formerly, we tried to dissect this wall meticulously lest the remnants encourage recurrence. Such dissection probably does more harm than good to the underlying levator muscle and may result in partial, permanent blepharoptosis. Instead of knife or scissors manipulation, light surface diathermy desiccation seems sufficient and minimizes the problem of blepharoptosis.

Meticulous removal of cyst remnants by these methods is no assurance there will be no recurrence. Neither does incomplete resection of a ruptured cyst necessarily mean the operation is in vain, as illustrated by the following experience.

Superior-nasal orbitotomy was performed in a 15-year-old girl because of a 3-year displacement and proptosis of one eye due to a mass in the upper nasal quadrant of the orbit. A large, thin-walled, multiloculated dermoid cyst was found midway back in the orbit. It ruptured quickly on dissection. Its anterior and nasal walls were easily removed, but the medial face of the cyst was fused to the posterior surface of the eye and adjacent portion of the optic nerve. In this junctional area, the cyst wall was lightly electrodesiccated. Proptosis recurred in 4 years. A second orbitotomy was performed, and a smaller dermoid cyst was found in the identical area of the initial cyst. Again, all the cyst wall was excised except that portion that was fused to the optic nerve. This area was again electrodesiccated. No recurrence of the cyst was found 5 years after the second orbitotomy.

After successful eradication of the cyst, the residual bony defect gradually becomes smaller as the years pass. However, if the eye has been greatly displaced for a long time, it may never regain perfect alignment with the other eye.

TERATOMA

Among the several developmental cysts occurring in the orbit, teratomas arouse the most interest, principally because in this area they are pathologic curiousities. Their common sites of growth are the gonads, retroperitoneum, and mediastinum.

TERMINOLOGY AND ORIGIN

Teratoma is derived from the word *teratoid* ("resembling a monster"), but a tumor of such literal denotation occurring in the orbit is of no practical importance. More often, teratoma is defined broadly to indicate a true neoplasm that contains one or more types of tissue, none of which is indigenous to the area in which it grows. On this basis, dermoid and epidermoid cysts, or even cancer, might be considered as examples of teratoma. For correct identification, it seems preferable to use *teratoma* more specifically. The crux of the problem is a matter of embryogenesis: specifically, whether the tumor contains anlage of one, two, or three germinal layers. Dermoid and epidermoid cysts are derived from only one germinal layer. The term *true teratoma* frequently appears in the literature in reference to tumors whose origin seems based on all three germinal anlages. Identification of tissue with an arrangement characteristic of gut is considered diagnostic of such tumors. However, the terms *teratoid cyst* and *teratoid tumor* sometimes are applied to tumors originating from two germinal layers.

A classification into four groups based on various gradations in the complexity of the tumors also has been proposed. Such detailed classifications, technically, are most proper but have less application to tumors as infrequent in the orbit as these. Identification of tissue derived from endoderm often is difficult when these tumors occur in the orbit. Not only is anlage from such a germinal layer most infrequent but also the entire pathologic specimen requires detailed search before presence or absence of such tissue is established. Therefore, one term encompassing tumors with anlage from two or more germinal layers would seem as useful as separate designations for either. The choice seems to lie between the words *teratoid* and *teratoma*. *Teratoma* seems suitable for the brief discussion that follows. Other terms — *embryoma, teratoblastoma,* and *tridermoma* — seldom are used in modern literature.

INCIDENCE

Teratomas of the orbit occur at any age. The oldest age reported in the literature was 63 years. The majority, perhaps 75%, either are present at birth or appear within the first 6 months of life. In our survey, one example was noted in a 30-year-old man. Other large surveys of orbital tumors usually contain one case of teratoma. However, such single-case notations are not too useful for statistical purposes, because age, sex, and other clinical details of the patient are not always stated. Thus, we found 28 reports wherein the age was stated but the sex of the patient was not always included. The tumor seems a little more common in females, by a ratio of 4:3. Barber and associates (1974) at the time of their report had counted 54 cases in the literature, including one patient with bilateral involvement. Ferry (1965) counted 21 cases wherein the tumor (true teratoma) was derived from three germ layers, and he estimated about the same number of tumors derived from only two germ layers. In summary, a lifetime of ophthalmic practice might pass without observation of the tumor, so infrequent is its occurrence.

CLINICAL FEATURES

No other orbital tumor, except possibly rhabdomyosarcoma, manifests such a dramatic unilateral proptosis at or near time of birth as teratoma. If not already present, it blossoms within a few days or months after birth and reaches large size. The tumor of Hoyt and Joe (1962) was 8 by 6 by 4 cm (Fig. 59) and that of Casanovas (1967) was an enormous mass covering the upper face and weighing 83 g with eye attached. The size and the red, angry appearance make an unforgettable visual experience; in description, the tumor has been eloquently compared to large fruit, such as a ripe tomato, an orange, or an apple. Perched on the anterior convexity of the mass, the eyeball appears to be

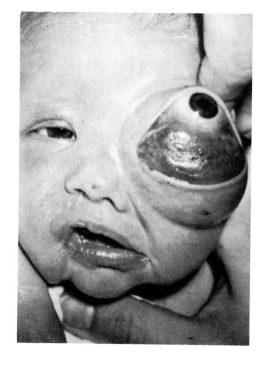

Figure 59. Congenital cystic teratoma of left orbit in 3-day-old infant. Tumor was removed, but eye was preserved. (From Hoyt WF, Joe S: Congenital teratoid cyst of the orbit: a case report and review of the literature. Arch Ophthalmol 68:196–201, 1962. By permission of the American Medical Association.)

squashed, showing the effects of pressure and the signs of destruction. The use-less appendage adds to the picture of overall alarm. Although neither the eye nor the optic nerve is an intrinsic part of the tumor, both usually are removed with it. In recent years, several teratomas have been removed with preservation of the eye, but the cosmetic and functional ocular results of such heroics over a long period of observation have been disappointing. Exenteration usually is per-formed to effect a complete cure. This operation is a formidable challenge to a newborn infant, and in years past some infants did not survive. Barber and associates suggest reducing the size of the mass by aspiration and biopsy until the child is older and can better withstand surgery. If, either on aspiration or subsequent surgery, the mass must be differentiated from other congenital cystic tumors that may communicate with the intracranial space (cephaloceles), the fluid can be chemically analyzed for protein content. The analysis usually shows that protein levels are much higher than normal spinal fluid values. Incomplete excision of the cyst leads to recurrence or continued growth. Roentgenograms may show marked enlargement of the orbit, and this is additional evidence of the pressure exerted by these rapidly expanding tumors.

Teratomas in older patients do not enlarge as rapidly as, and do not attain the size of, those in the newborn. Their clinical pattern is similar to other benign neoplasms and cysts of the orbit. Usually well encapsulated, they are al-most exclusively derived from two germinal layers. The tumor observed in our 30-year-old patient was of this type. For several years, the patient had noted proptosis. The tumor was located in the lateral portion of the orbital cavity. It was a thin-walled, blue-tan cystic mass resembling an epidermoid cyst. The cyst contained an oily liquid like that in dermoid cysts. Teratomas in older persons can be removed without removal of the eye. Roentgenography is not helpful in making a specific diagnosis.

PATHOLOGY

Teratomas may be solid, cystic, or a mixture of these types. The cystic form is most prevalent. Most also are benign, but some solid tumors in newborns are malignant. Because of their origin from multiple germ layers, the tumors may contain a variety of tissues and their histologic patterns may be very complex. The cysts slowly enlarge because of mucus-secreting components. Photomicro-graphs of several interesting cases from the literature are illustrated (one in color) in the Duke-Elder text. The teratoma illustrated in color contained 14 different types of tissue. Such a case is aptly referred to as a "histologist's dream" (Fig. 60).

CEPHALOCELE

Sac-like herniations of brain or its membranes may protrude into the orbit and by their bulk push upon the eye. They must therefore be differentiated from other orbital tumors. They are neither neoplasms nor, strictly, cysts. Yet they may contain fluid or, infrequently, may undergo a secondary cystic degen-eration to resemble a cyst, and they may be appropriately discussed here.

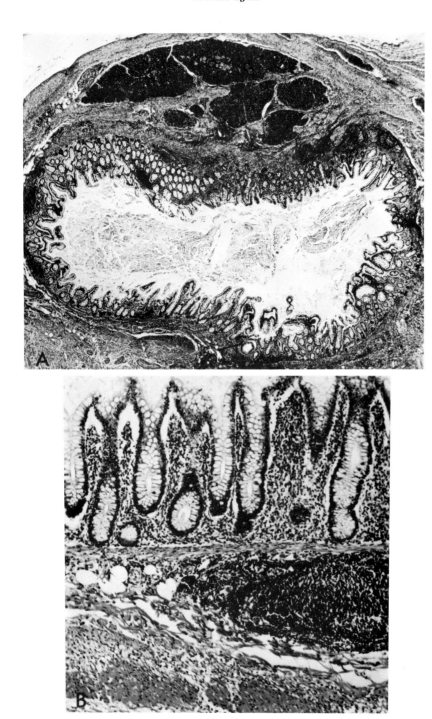

Figure 60. Teratoma of orbit. *A*, Lower power: view shows gut-like structure (×26). *B*, Higher power: view shows colonic-like epithelium (×100). (From Ferry AP: Teratoma of the orbit: a report of two cases. Survey Ophthalmol *10*:434–442, 1965. By permission of the Williams & Wilkins Company.)

TERMINOLOGY AND ORIGIN

Frequently, these herniations are classified according to position (anterior, posterior, frontal, ethmoidal, or sphenoidal) or contents (for example, meningocele, encephalocele, meningoencephalocele). Technically, the latter terms are more specific. Clinically, however, all are so similar that specific diagnosis usually is not possible until they are uncovered either by orbitotomy or by histologic examination. Even histologic examination may not give an entirely accurate diagnosis, because the herniated contents may atrophy from continued pressure; thus, the identity of the original tissue structures may be masked. Moreover, treatment of the herniations is similar. Therefore, the less specific term, *cephalocele*, which encompasses herniations of all types of intracranial contents, seems sufficient. Lesions caused by trauma or secondary to erosion of bone from inflammatory disorders are excluded from this discussion. Pulsating proptosis first appearing in adult life but secondary to a congenital bony dysplasia of the orbit also may be considered an example of cephalocele, but it more properly belongs with neurofibromatosis.

The nidus of the usual cephalocele usually develops during embryonic growth. In a sense, all cephaloceles are congenital, but they may not cause symptoms until later life. It seems plausible that some cephaloceles should commence very early in embryonic life, owing to a failure in normal separation of surface ectoderm from neuroectoderm. Cleavage is faulty, and some portion of brain substance is pinched off from the main mass of neuroectoderm by subsequent bone development. The resulting cephalocele may remain attached to brain by a cord or stalk of tissue. This characteristic might explain many anterior orbital cephaloceles that retain connection with brain in the sutures between the frontal, ethmoid, lacrimal, and maxillary bones. Or, developing bone may succeed in completely isolating the cephalocele within the orbit or adjacent sinus. This seems to be a reasonable explanation for the unusual orbital-ethmoid encephalocele reported by Leone and Marlowe (1970). In this patient, orbital symptoms did not appear until the age of 62 years; surgical exploration did not demonstrate any communication with the cranial cavity.

Other cephaloceles may result from defects in osseous development rather than neural dysgenesis. Here, some quirk prevents proper ossification of bones, such as the ethmoid and sphenoid, so that bony fusion around various orbital foramina and fissures is incomplete. True herniations of intracranial contents, then, may develop through deformed or enlarge bony apertures such as the optic canal and superior orbital fissure. Such cephaloceles develop later in embryonic life than the other type and more often occur in the area of ethmoid and sphenoid bones.

INCIDENCE

At the time of his review, Duke-Elder (1963) noted fewer than 100 cases on record, with a slightly higher prevalence in females. Thus, encephaloceles are not common tumors but occur more frequently than teratomas. Most are found in the young, but nontraumatic cephaloceles have been found in adults and reported as curiosities. Our two cases were in infants, one male and one female.

Anterior cephaloceles are commoner than those in the posterior orbit. Also, because of their position and easier recognition, anterior cephaloceles usually are observed at an earlier age than are those of the posterior orbit.

CLINICAL FEATURES

Anterior cephaloceles are most common in the superior-anterior-medial aspect of the orbit, with the outpouching along suture lines occurring between frontal, maxillary, ethmoid, and lacrimal bones. They protrude either anteriorly onto the face at the junction of nose and eyebrow (Fig. 61) or laterally into the orbital cavity. In the case of lateral protrusion, there is greater displacement of the eye temporally and downward. Almost all anterior cephaloceles are palpable and painless; the herniation feels elastic and is not as firm as other developmental cysts. As to size, the mass may enlarge slowly during a period of months. This feature, as well as possible pulsation, seems more dependent on size of the bony defect between orbital cavity and anterior fossa. The greater the defect, the more prominent the pulsation and more rapid the progression. The skin overlying the more anteriorly placed cephaloceles may become quite thin and vascularized.

Posterior cephaloceles are less obvious, less palpable, and seemingly slower in onset than those in the anterior orbit. However, as they develop, pulsation of the displaced eye may become more evident than is the case with anterior cephaloceles. Motility of the eye also is more affected; the eye is pushed forward and usually downward rather than sideways (Fig. 62).

Congenital defects of the eye, face, and adnexa, are not uncommon with both types of cephaloceles. Acrocephaly, cryptophthalmos, microphthalmos,

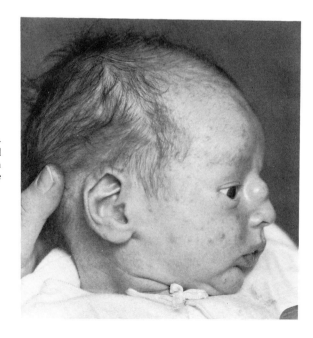

Figure 61. Cephalocele; defect in anterior cranial bones, and globular mass protruding beneath skin of glabella. (See also Figure 65.)

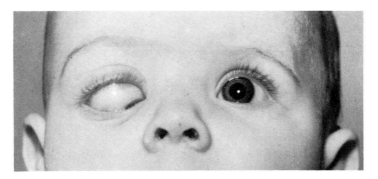

Figure 62. Posterior cephalocele in right orbit, with downward displacement and inward rotation of right eye. Cornea is almost covered by lower eyelid.

buphthalmos, hypertelorism, broad nasal root, and congenital colobomas of the optic nerve and optic disk have been recorded.

Because the encephalocele may arise along the suture line between any of the several bones, because its configuration may be determined by the embryonic stage of the cleavage fault, and because it may differ according to the tissue element incarcerated in the cyst, the bony defects vary considerably in size, position, and configuration. The larger defects are visible on standard views and, for the planned surgical attack, can be outlined in further detail by linear tomography. Smaller defects, however, may not be recognized on the usual orbital roentgenograms because of the overlapping of midline bone shadows. Nonrecognition can lead to an unfortunate experience at orbital exploration for the suspected tumor: The surgeon biopsies the mass only to blunder into a communication with the ventricular system and be confronted with leakage of cerebrospinal fluid. Meningitis, sepsis, and death are known to have resulted from such a surgical misfortune.

A misadventure of an opposite type, based on the roentgenograms in Figure 63, bedeviled one of us. Here, the bony defect was large, was easily visible on standard views, and showed many of the features of a slowly enlarging epidermoid cyst. The 11-year-old female patient did not have any protruding soft tissue mass or any congenital deformity of the face such as might have been associated with an encephalocele. Furthermore, her age was more compatible with the diagnosis of epidermoid cyst. A palpable, hard tumor in the superior nasal quadrant of the orbit was then explored, but when the cystic mass protruding downward into the orbital cavity was amputated, the tumor proved to be an unsuspected meningomyocele.

PATHOLOGY

If surgical exploration has not already made the diagnosis evident, histopathologic study will reveal brain tissue in the specimen submitted for examination. Neural tissue, with its covering pia and arachnoid, is identified more easily in specimens from young patients. When the cephalocele has been long-standing, as in adults, the meningeal layers may be fused and fibrosed and the neural tissue edematous and degenerate; psammoma bodies may even be noted. The

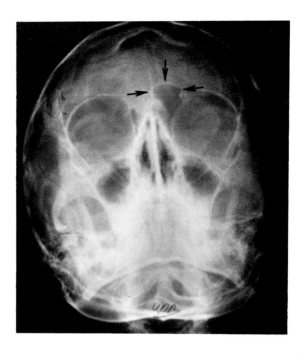

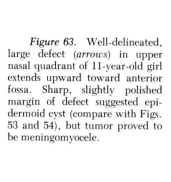

Figure 63. Well-delineated, large defect (*arrows*) in upper nasal quadrant of 11-year-old girl extends upward toward anterior fossa. Sharp, slightly polished margin of defect suggested epidermoid cyst (compare with Figs. 53 and 54), but tumor proved to be meningomyocele.

dura tends to fuse with or incorporate with bony or soft tissue structures adjacent to the herniation (Figs. 64 and 65).

TREATMENT

Careful thought should be given to management of any cystic lesion uncovered at orbitotomy in an infant or child, particularly posterior cephaloceles, for the true nature of the cyst-like mass may be unsuspected. The diagnosis of anterior cephalocele may be more evident before operation. Because latent cephaloceles lurk in the orbits of patients in this age group, needle aspiration of any unexplained cyst is recommended at the time of orbitotomy. The needle should be of very small diameter, and if aseptic technique is strict, there should be no danger. If the fluid is clear, it is given emergency analysis for sugar and protein content before anything further is done.

Antibiotics have made it possible to correct many orbital cephaloceles that would formerly have been surgically fatal. An anterior approach is suitable for some anterior cephaloceles when the preoperative diagnosis is evident and the communication between orbit and intracranial space is small or narrow. The fibrous or membranous pedicle is exposed and ligated, and the herniation into the orbit is excised. A small bony hiatus may be plugged with a piece of muscle, a portion of Silastic sponge, or gel sponge. After careful hemostasis, the plugged defect is covered with periorbita.

For cephaloceles in which the bony dehiscence is large or the diagnosis is established during orbitotomy, definitive treatment is best handled by neurosurgeons through a transcranial approach. After removal of the herniated pouch or restoration of its contents into the proper intracranial fossa, the soft tissues are

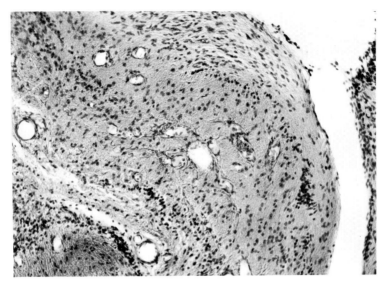

Figure 64. Cephalocele. Clear space to right is lined by flattened ependymal cells and communicates with ventricular system. Surrounding brain tissue consists mainly of glial elements (Hematoxylin and eosin; × 120.)

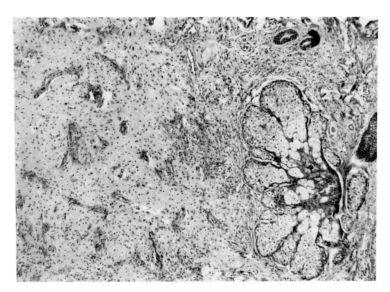

Figure 65. Cephalocele. Brain tissue has developed in intimate association with adnexal skin structures such as sebaceous glands seen to right of sections. (Section from case illustrated in Figure 61; hematoxylin and eosin; × 60.)

carefully closed in layers. Bony defects are sealed by dural substitutes, bone grafts, or acrylic materials. Larger cephaloceles often are adherent to either ocular surfaces or optic nerve. Therefore, dissection must proceed with more than ordinary caution.

CONGENITAL CYSTIC EYE

Another tumor filling an orbit of a newborn should be noted here, if for no other reason than to differentiate it from the other congenital tumor (teratoma) of similar appearance. This tumor, once known as anophthalmos with cyst, is now called *congenital cystic eye* or eyeball (Fig. 65A). It is usually smaller than, and is encountered less frequently in the newborn than, a teratoma. Nor does the cystic eye tumor have quite the frightening appearance of a teratoma, because the protruding mass of the former is not capped by the useless, staring eye of the latter. Indeed, there is no formed eye, because ocular embryogenesis is arrested at about the stage of the primary optic vesicle. Another differentiating feature is the tendency of the enlarged cystic eye to be partially covered by a markedly stretched upper lid; in this age group a teratoma, in contrast, tends to expand through the palpebral fissure beyond the shelter of the eyelids. Also, the congenital cystic eye is covered by normal conjunctiva. Its color is less vivid than that of a teratoma, ranging from blue to rose.

Congenital cystic eye is a benign tumor. Pathologically, it contains tissue elements that would be expected in a primary optic vesicle except in a dysplastic form. Actually, the tumor may be more solid than cystic because of abnormal proliferation of neuroglial tissue. This glial proliferation may be so profuse as almost to mask the primitive retinal rosettes. In the less solid portion of the tumor, a sinusoidal network of dilated capillaries may be found. The cyst

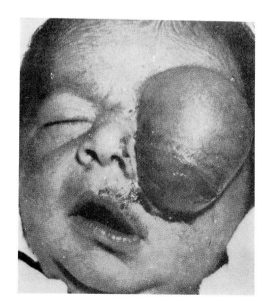

Figure 65A. Congenital cystic eye in 10-day-old infant. Note extreme stretching of upper eyelid. (From: Baghdassarian SA, Tabbara KF, Matta CS: Congenital cystic eye. Am J Ophthalmol 67:269–275, 1973 by permission.)

is self-contained and does not communicate with the intracranial ventricular system but is connected to the brain by a stalk corresponding to the primitive optic nerve. However, this stalk is filled with astrocytes rather than the axons of ganglion cells.

Because the cyst slowly enlarges, it must be removed. Complete excision of the cyst is possible because of its circumscribed, self-contained, and rather solid structure. The normal conjunctiva covering the cyst may be incised, the cyst separated from surrounding orbital tissue, and the optic stalk sectioned, similar to enucleation of an eye. The surgical defect may be partially covered by the conjunctival flaps. The excised tumor usually measures from 20 to 40 mm in its longest diameter.

MICROPHTHALMOS WITH CYST

This developmental cyst usually is classified among congenital anomalies of the eye and is closely allied to the congenital cystic eye discussed above. What may begin as a small hiatus in closure of the embryonic ocular cleft at about the fourth week of embryonic life may, by continued expansion, become large enough to resemble a tumor originating in the orbit; hence, the consideration of this ocular abnormality here. It occurs much more often than other congenital cystlike tumors, such as teratoma and congenital cystic eye.

Three features usually are common to all cases of this condition: eyes that are deformed, defective, and smaller than normal; a cystic mass, of almost any size, that is attached to the eye; and the presence of the cystic mass at birth. The condition may be bilateral or associated with a congenitally cystic eye in the other orbit.

These cysts might best be described as bizarre. Their appearance at birth or in infancy depends on such factors as size of intercommunication between cyst and eye and rate of expansion of the cyst. Thus, a miniature but recognizable eye with a small cystic appendage attached to its inferior surface may be palpated in the rear of the orbit. At the other extreme may be a cystic tumor so large that an eye can neither be seen nor palpated. All variations between these extremes may be observed. Because the cyst continues to expand, it becomes the larger of the two structures. When it pushes against the eyelids and begins to protrude from the orbit, differentiation from other orbital tumors in infancy is pertinent.

Seldom will this condition be confused with teratoma, which is more vivid in color, enlarges more rapidly, and occurs with a formed eye. However, congenital cystic eye and the cystic protruberance of microphthalmos are look-alikes in several ways. The cysts are similar in color, may transilluminate, and expand at the same rate. As a rule, the cyst of microphthalmos first appears as a bulging mass behind the lower lid, whereas the tumor of congenital cystic eye almost always exerts its initial pressure on the upper eyelid. In microphthalmos with cyst, ultrasonography may locate the concealed nubbins of the microphthalmic eye. This condition also may resemble an orbital cephalocele, but the degree of ocular malformation is not as great with the cephalocele as with the cyst. In addition, linear tomography shows bony orbital defects associated with cephaloceles but not with microphthalmos. Routine roentgenography may show orbital enlargement in cases of cephalocele but a smaller orbit than average in cases of microphthalmos with cyst.

The histopathology of microphthalmos with cyst is similar to that already noted in congenital cystic eye, but in the former condition, the dysplastic retina and proliferating neuroglial elements do not cover the entire inner surface of the cyst wall, whereas in the latter, the lining of the primary optic vesicle is more nearly uniform. Cellular components of an astrocytoma were found in the pathologic specimen reported by Bonner and Ide (1974).

Surgical removal of the expanding cyst and its attached eye is the treatment usually recommended. Waring and associates (1976) found that repeated aspiration of the cyst effected a permanent cure in one of their cases.

PERIOPTIC HYGROMA

When preparation of the previous edition of this text was nearly complete, two reports (Smith and associates 1969, Spencer 1972) describing the clinical and histologic features of a cystlike tumor of the sheath of the intraorbital portion of the optic nerve appeared in the ophthalmic literature. Later, two more publications (Miller and Green 1975, Harris et al 1976) reported on three additional patients with similar cystic masses. In a report earlier than any of the above, Holt (1966) recorded two instances of a cystic tumor involving the intracranial portion of the optic nerve but not associated with proptosis. This total of seven well-documented cases is reason to discuss these tumors at this point, particularly those along the intraorbital portion of the nerve associated with proptosis.

These new members of the orbital tumors in this text have been called *perioptic subdural hygroma, arachnoid cyst of the optic nerve* and *cyst of the optic nerve sheath.* Some aberration occurs along the arachnoid of the optic nerve; the result is a collection of clear fluid in the subdural space. Whether the tumors are true cysts, because of possessing a lining layer of cells, or a localized collection of fluid is not known, because the tumors were not excised intact in all cases. In some, an incision through the tumor wall decompressed the mass and relieved some of the visual problems complicating the growth. All but one of these intraorbital *perioptic hygromas* occurred in women between the ages of 33 and 56. The one male patient was 3 years old. A variety of clinical features other than proptosis were noted in the five cases, such as papilledema, empty sellae, enlargement of optic canal, neurofibromatosis, visual field defects, visual loss, optociliary shunt vessels, porencephalic cyst, optic atrophy, and pallor of the optic disk.

In adults, these tumors resemble a meningioma of the intraorbital portion of the optic nerve. In children, of course, perioptic hygroma probably cannot be differentiated from an optic nerve astrocytoma without surgical exploration. Reports of more cases will no doubt be published in the future.

MUCOCELE

A cystic tumor covered by mucous membrane, the mucocele is filled with thick mucous secretion, hence its name. It is primary in one or more paranasal sinuses; persistently expanding, it may erode surrounding bone, often exiting into the adjacent orbit. If the cyst continues to expand within the orbital cavity, the mass may mimic the behavior of many benign growths primary in the orbit. In these circumstances, the tumor is of concern to ophthalmologists, because displacement of the eye may be the initial symptom of an otherwise insidious tumor.

ORIGIN

The cause is debatable. Most rhinologists believe mucoceles to be secondary to obstruction of the ostium of the sinus: for example, obstruction from recurrent bouts of inflammation, trauma, or repeated surgery in and around the nasal cavity and adjacent sinuses. Whatever the origin, continued secretion of mucus gradually fills the obstructed sinus and presses on the bony walls. A minority holds that mucoceles arise as small cysts within the mucous membrane and by continued growth finally obstruct the ostium of the sinus. Similarly, inflammation, trauma, and surgery may contribute to the initial cyst, or it may arise de novo. All these theories differ only about whether the cyst is primarily the cause or the effect of obstruction. It is likely that both circumstances prevail and arguments about causation are academic.

The contents of the cyst may vary widely both in color and in viscosity. Most common is a white or tan mucoid or watery material. If the cyst contains a green or yellow, thick viscid material, it may be called a *pyocele*. The term *hydrops* is now seldom used. *Pyocele* may denote a collection of pus resulting from an inflammatory process primary in the sinus or a mucocele that has become secondarily infected. *Mucocele* implies a more benign process characterized by retention of secretion. Differentiation into pyoceles and mucoceles is not as important as it once was. The use of antibiotics for recurrent sinusitis may so alter the contents of pyoceles that by the time of surgical exploration the exudate has become aseptic or so modified as to no longer warrant the designation "pus." Furthermore, whether the cysts be mucoceles or pyoceles, surgical management, technically, is the same. For this discussion, all these cysts will be treated as a type of mucocele.

HISTORICAL ASPECTS

Mucoceles were among the first orbital disorders to be described. Von Leden (1966) credited Henri Nicolai of Strasbourg as the first to publish a report, in 1785, but the source was not given. In 1819, Langenbeck (see Vail, 1931) published a report on mucocele of the frontal sinus. At that time, these tumors were called *hydatids*. In the same year, a particularly detailed report was published by Keate (1819) who was surgeon to their Royal Highnesses the Duchess of Gloucester and Prince Leopold. Keate's patient was an 18-year-old girl who was first observed in March 1815. A bony protruberance three-quarters the size of an orange was present in the frontal bone over the left orbit. When a small portion of bone on the anterior surface of the mass was removed, the cystic tumor ruptured, releasing thin, colorless fluid. During the next several years, the cyst cavity was frequently reexplored, probed, and treated with both thermal and caustic cautery in unsuccessful efforts to eradicate the mass. The patient also was subjected to leeches, blistering, bloodletting, purging, and diaphoresis. On several occasions, these manipulations were discontinued because the patient became exhausted. Finally, in December 1817, all bone corresponding to the base of the tumor was sawed away; the hole that remained was 11.25 cm (4.5 in.) in diameter between inner and outer tables of the frontal bone. Through this wider exposure, all the foul contents were removed and the tumor finally was eradicated. By summer 1818 (about 3 years after the initial treatment) the patient had recovered. These harrowing events attest not only to the stamina of some patients in this era but also to the necessity for completely removing the tumor before cure is effected.

Rollet (1896) frequently is cited as the man who coined the term *mucocele*. In earlier times, long before the era of antibiotics, mucocele was a subject of common interest and frequent discussion in the combined specialties of rhinology and ophthalmology. As rhinology and ophthalmology evolved into separate fields of practice, management of this tumor seemed to fall into the domain of the rhinologist. The ophthalmologist became less concerned with the tumor's clinical aspects, and reports by either group gradually decreased. The advent of antibiotics also seemed to reduce the frequency of the tumor. In the past several decades, roentgenologists seem to have discussed the subject as often as any other specialty group.

INCIDENCE

In the previous edition of this text (1973), we commented on the wide discrepancy in the incidence of mucoceles among various surveys of unilateral proptosis, expanding lesions of the orbit, and so forth, recorded in the literature. At one extreme were the 30 mucoceles (15%) among 200 cases of unilateral exophthalmos observed by Zizmor and associates (1966) in a department of diagnostic roentgenology. Such a study would be heavily weighed with tumors that produce defects in the bony orbit but would exclude many soft tissue tumors that never erode bone. At the other extreme was the absence of mucoceles among 877 consecutive cases of orbital tumors (Reese, 1963), a finding derived from the histopathologic specimens submitted to one institution. Reese was aware of this omission, and attributing it to the common practice of not sending tissue for histologic study at the time of surgical evacuation of the mucocele. In addition, we stated that our own incidence data (based on the survey of 465 consecutive orbital tumors) seemed too low (1.5%); our explanation was that most mucoceles were explored by rhinologists and for statistical purposes were catalogued only according to sinus of origin rather than possible orbital extent. We concluded at that time that a true incidence of mucocele among a representative series of orbital tumors (excluding cases of endocrine orbitopathy) could not be stated, but we estimated the frequency to be 3 to 4%.

Since then, a detailed study of the surgical reports on all mucoceles explored within the period of our present study has revealed cases with orbital involvement that had not been included in the initial survey. Incidence data based on this more inclusive survey is summarized in Table 4.

Clinically, an incidence of 8.5% mucoceles among all orbital tumors will seem rather high to many ophthalmologists, but this figure emphasizes the point made in Chapter 3 that many cases of proptosis secondary to sinus disease receive primary care from rhinologists and are never seen by an opthalmologist. Reese included mucoceles in a later (1971) clinical series of 504 expanding lesions of the orbit treated and followed up by one group. Here, the incidence approximated 4%. He thought this incidence was low and attributed it to the successful treatment of sinusitis by antibiotics. Among the secondary orbital tumors in our survey, mucocele was next in frequency to the collective group of carcinomas but was the most frequent benign tumor secondarily producing proptosis.

The equal sex distribution and the primary location of the mucocele in the frontal, frontal-ethmoid, and ethmoid sinuses (Table 4), in descending order of frequency, agree closely with other published data in the rhinologic literature. Orbital involvement by the less frequent mucocele of the sphenoid sinus and the rare mucocele of the maxillary sinus was not observed in the period of our survey. We do not have an explanation for the nearly 2:1 predilection of mucoceles for the left side; laterality is seldom mentioned in the literature.

The age distribution of our patients (Table 4) shows a scattering among all decades, with a predominance (69%) between 41 and 70 years of age. The ages are those at the time of surgical diagnosis and do not adequately reflect the fact that some patients have symptoms of recurrent mucocele for many years before

TABLE 4.   MUCOCELES ASSOCIATED WITH PROPTOSIS (1948-1974):
SUMMARY OF INCIDENCE DATA

Number of Patients	
Total	65
Male	32
Female	33

Frequency
8.5% of all (764) orbital tumors
19% of all (343) secondary orbital tumors
40% of all (164) mucoceles surgically explored

Location	
	No. of Patients
Frontal	37
Frontal-ethmoid	18
Ethmoid	10
Right side	22
Left side	43

Age Distribution (years)	
	No. of Patients
0–20	5
21–30	7
31–40	3
41–50	19
51–60	13
61–70	13
Over 70	5

submitting to definitive surgery. Our data do not entirely support the statement frequently made in the literature that ethmoid mucoceles occur at an earlier age (young adults) than do those of the frontal sinus (older adults). Of interest are the five cases of proptosis in the first 2 decades of life, including a 16-month-old infant with the recently recognized syndrome of *mucocele associated with cystic fibrosis.*

CLINICAL FEATURES

Mucoceles frequently are discussed from the standpoint of the sinus of origin, which is important to the surgeon planning an approach. Orbital symptomatology, however, is influenced more by the specific area of bone erosion, which may be some distance from the cyst's epicenter. No matter where the mucocele is located, the slow and silent expansion may be unsuspected until bone is eroded and the cyst impinges on some other structure. The ophthalmologist becomes interested when the cyst enters the orbit, usually where the bony partition is thinnest.

Proptosis or displacement of the eye, puffiness of the upper eyelid, a mild ophthalmoplegia, some degree of visual disturbance, headache, and a palpable mass are clinical features encountered with orbital mucocele. Some degree of proptosis is common to almost all orbital mucoceles. The presence or absence of other clinical features depends on the location of the bony breakthrough. The duration of proptosis or ocular displacement may be months or years, because expansion of the tumor is insidious and pain may be absent. With cysts having a significant inflammatory component, such as pyoceles, headache is a complaint; it is usually described as being "deep" or "around" the orbit, but it may be so vague as to defy localization. In these cases, proptosis is of shorter duration. Some patients give a history of recurrent sinusitis, frequent nasal polyps, or previous sinus surgery. Fluctuations in proptosis and swelling of adnexal tissues may occur during influenza or upper respiratory infections. Variation, intermittency, or recurrence of features relating to the orbit should suggest mucocele in differential diagnosis from other tumors.

If the mucocele (usually from the frontal sinus) enters the more anterior portion of the orbital cavity, it usually does so in the upper nasal quadrant. Then the eye becomes displaced downward as well as forward, with limited excursion when looking up and nasally, the puffy soft tissues of the upper eyelid create a peculiar droopy appearance (particularly in the medial half), and a mass is palpable beneath and slightly behind the superior orbital rim. Rollet described a curious deformation wherein, from above, the bridge of the nose was flat instead of being concave downward and convex transversely; the width was increased and the palpebral fissure narrowed (Fig. 65B). Some observers have commented on slight crepitus — like the crackling of parchment or breaking of an eggshell — upon palpation; this supposedly results from shifting of thin, eroded plaques of bone that still border the protruding mass. In our experience, this sign has been infrequent. More often these tumors feel boggy, the sensation being comparable to prodding or poking a medicine ball. The mass is not tender.

Because of the forward location of the tumor, pressure causes nearly equal forward and downward displacement of the eye. The more long-standing the

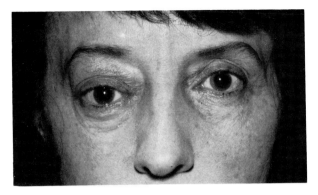

Figure 65B. Mucocele of right frontal sinus (6 years' duration) with erosion into right orbit causing signs common to frontal mucoceles: downward displacement with minimal forward proptosis of eye; puffiness and droopiness of upper eyelid producing narrowing of palpebral fissure; palpable mass in upper nasal quadrant of orbit; and flattening of sulcus between bridge of nose and bony orbital rim.

symptoms, the greater the downward deviation in proportion to forward protrusion. This downward deviation of the eye, which is partially concealed by a droopy, puffy eyelid, makes the face on the side of the tumor look heavy. In adults, some cases of advanced neurofibromatosis, neglected osteomas, and progressive meningiomas also may produce this appearance, but other clues help differentiate these tumors. Rarely, a typical-appearing mucocele may conceal an unsuspected squamous cell carcinoma of the frontal sinus. In the older literature (when surgical exploration often was deferred), photographs illustrate bizarre and advanced cases in which the eye might be pushed almost to a horizontal level with the tip of the nose by a protuberance (mucocele) along the superior rim of the orbit. Such mucoceles, which had become pyoceles by this time, often eroded the soft tissues of the upper eyelid and evacuated their contents through a tract just beneath the superior orbital rim. This drainage continued intermittently thereafter, and the fistulous tract could be reopened at will simply by pressure on the surrounding soft tissues (Fig. 66). Because of improvement in surgical techniques and the use of antibiotics, these draining pyoceles are seldom seen now, but the problem is still common in many underprivileged countries.

If the mucocele pushes into the orbit in the vicinity of the ethmoid sinus, palpation of the mass is less definite and more nondescript. Also, the eyelid is less edematous and proptosis has a different pattern from the preceding situation. The eye may be pushed so far laterally as to exceed in millimeters the amount of forward proptosis (see Fig. 8, page 18).

The symptoms of mucocele in the posterior reaches of the orbit are even more vague. Such mucoceles may arise in the sphenoid sinus and enter the orbit through posterior ethmoid cells (the area of least resistance). Headache or orbital discomfort is usually more intense and persistent than with mucoceles in other paranasal areas. Because of the proximity of the bony erosion to the apex of the orbit, variable degrees of diplopia or ptosis may occur owing to pressure on the branches of the oculomotor nerve supplying the affected muscles. A syndrome mimicking retrobulbar neuritis or pain radiating along the infraorbital portion of the trigeminal nerve may even occur. Forward proptosis rather than lateral or downward displacement of the eye is the rule, and the orbital mass is not palpable. The diagnosis may remain obscure until the mass is visualized by routine roentgenography or orbital tomography.

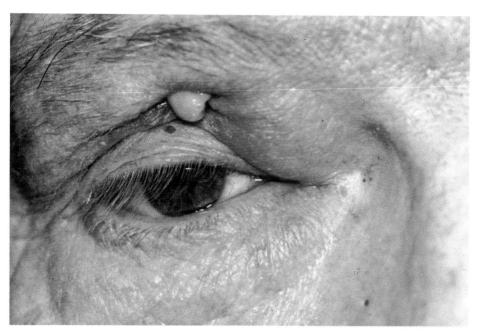

Figure 66. Intermittent drainage of pus from fistulous tract in right upper eyelid of 61-year-old man. Present for 6 months, tract was due to pyocele of frontal sinus. Note bulging mass in upper nasal portion of orbit. (Courtesy of R.W. Neault, M.D.)

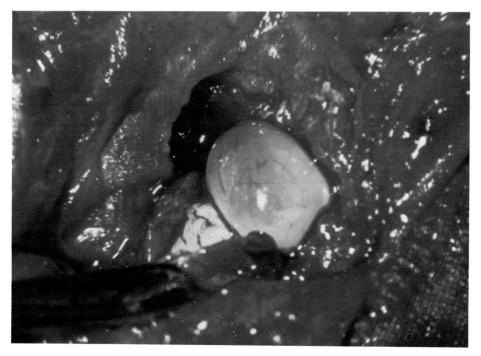

Figure 70. Echinococcus cyst. Pearly white tumor is nestled in orbital tissue of male adult. (Courtesy of H. Friesen, M.D., Kabul, Afghanistan.)

ROENTGENOGRAPHIC CHANGES

Radiographic characteristics of mucoceles have been well described. Almost every article on orbital mucoceles contains a photograph lucidly illustrating an enlarged, distorted sinus with a large bony defect that represents a breakthrough into the orbit. Radiographic changes in some of these photographs are so bizarre and obvious that any ophthalmologist with only a skimpy knowledge of roentgenology could make the diagnosis. It is the cases with minimal bony defects that pose the greatest difficulty in diagnosis; and, unfortunately, films of them cannot be photographed well enough for illustrative or teaching purposes. We have encountered, as have other clinicians, unsuspected orbital mucoceles with small bony dehiscences for which routine skull films were interpreted as negative. These examples show the difficulty of visualizing small bony defects around the orbit with routine views. Therefore, we recommend that lateral tomography be done routinely in all instances of suspected mucocele when findings on plain film roentgenography are positive or when routine views are negative but a palpable mass lies along the medial wall of the orbit.

As the cyst expands and exerts greater pressure, the walls of the frontal sinus usually lose their septate or scalloped configuration and become smoother (Fig. 67). Sometimes these defects are minimal or equivocal, but a "dished out" osteolysis along the supraorbital ridge indicates the slow expansion of the frontal sinus. Mucoceles of the ethmoid and sphenoid sinuses are more difficult to detect on standard views. Loss of translucence is the most common finding. Expansion or erosion of the affected sinus is best seen with axial tomography. Whichever sinus is affected, surrounding bone gradually becomes thinner and decalcified. Finally, especially in those mucoceles that involve more anterior

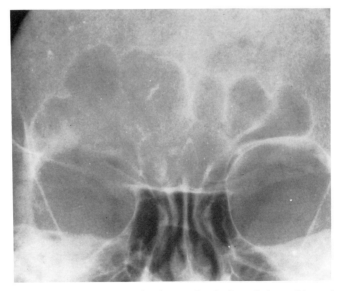

Figure 67.   Mucocele of right orbit. Enlargement of right frontal sinus with erosion of superior-nasal wall of orbit. Note configuration of right frontal sinus is less scalloped than that of left.

portions of the roof or medial walls of the orbit, a hiatus or deficiency in bone becomes apparent (Fig. 68). In a few cases, an attenuated, opercular shell of bone seems to lie loose along the advancing surface of the cyst. When any of these changes is present, the roentgenologist usually can make the diagnosis without further ado.

PATHOLOGY

Whatever the pathogenesis and cause of obstruction, the pathologic features are similar. Pseudostratified ciliated columnar epithelium gradually becomes flattened by pressure of retained secretion (Fig. 69), and the epithelium becomes more cuboidal, losing cilia. The degree of irritation that either initiates or accompanies the mucocele determines the amount of chronic inflammatory reaction in the covering wall of mucous membrane.

TREATMENT

We believe that most mucoceles should be treated by the rhinologist. Occasionally, cases with extensive involvement of the orbit (as revealed by the size of the hiatus in bone) make the inclusion of an ophthalmologist on the surgical team wise. Furthermore, there are cases in which the overall diameter of the cyst in the orbit is larger than its sinus of origin and other cases in which the mucocele, unsuspected because x-ray findings are negative, is discovered only by the ophthalmic surgeon during exploratory orbitotomy. But whichever the method or whoever the personnel, the object of surgery is the same: complete removal of the lining of the cyst and restoration of drainage from the occluded sinus into the nose.

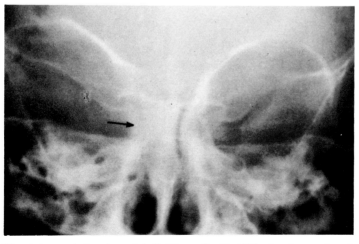

Figure 68. Anteroposterior view of skull (16-month-old child), showing erosion of medial wall of right orbit and ethmoid air cells (*arrow*). (From Robertson DM, Henderson JW: Unilateral proptosis secondary to orbital mucocele in infancy. Am J Ophthalmol 68:845–847, 1969. By permission of the Ophthalmic Publishing Company.)

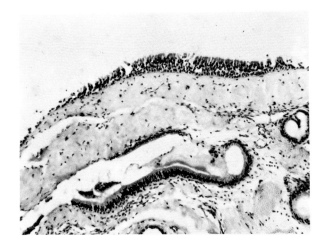

Figure 69. Mucocele. Cystic lesion is lined by ciliated respiratory epithelium with mucous glands in walls. (Hematoxylin and eosin; × 100.)

For mucoceles with obvious orbital extension from frontal sinuses, rhinologists frequently choose the external frontal approach. This is a modification of the superior orbitotomy familiar to most ophthalmologists. The skin incision parallels the superior nasal rim of the bony orbit. Rhinologists usually make the incision higher than the approach preferred by ophthalmologists. The goal is the same, that is, to reflect periosteum and periorbita and traverse the plane between the periorbita and bone. Preferably, the patient's head should be elevated to facilitate removal of the contents of the cyst and to prevent mucopus from seeping into the posterior orbit, where it is seen only with difficulty. Any loose pieces of bone are removed before the cyst is opened. If the bony defect between orbit and paranasal sinus is small, additional bone is removed, with rongeurs, to improve exposure of the sinus. Then the cyst cavity is opened and its contents are removed by suction. The next step is the important one: the thickened mucous membrane is meticulously stripped, teased, or scraped away from bone. Small ramifications and side pouches should be thoroughly explored for remnants of mucous membrane. When the diseased membrane has been removed, the bone will look white and shiny. A curved suction tip or metal probe is used to determine the approximate position of the sinus ostium. Bone is generously removed by rongeurs inferiorly into the ethmoid labyrinth and thence into the nasal cavity. Many rhinologists strive to make this bony stoma as large as possible, even converting the anterior ethmoid cells and diseased frontal sinus into one large, common cavity. A cylindrical roll of Silastic sheeting is then placed along the reconstructed passageway to maintain patency until epithelialization occurs. With drainage assured, the orbital incision may be closed tightly to minimize scar formation. If there is no involvement of the frontal sinus, an ethmoidal mucocele may be evacuated through the intranasal route.

Rhinologic texts rightly emphasize caution throughout the external frontal operation lest the eyeball be accidentally bruised or injured, but equally important is the thin belly of the levator palpebrae superioris muscle that may be close to the dependent portion of a mucocele that has protruded into the orbit from a frontal sinus. Careless handling of this muscle easily results in traumatic blepharoptosis, which is too big a price to pay for removal of a benign cyst from the orbital cavity, and sometimes a cosmetic repair is quite difficult to accomplish. Care also should be exercised not to injure the trochlea or to destroy the anchorage to the periorbita.

Most ophthalmic literature and some rhinologic literature may leave a reader with the impression that surgical treatment of frontal and ethmoidal mucoceles is final and complete. That recurrences are a real and frequent problem is not mentioned either because the writer did not follow up his surgical cases long enough or because the patient went elsewhere for the management of recurrent disease. Follow-up data of 1 year or longer were available in 42 of the 65 patients in our survey. Recurrence rate among those 42 — our own patients as well as those who had their initial operation elsewhere — was 50%. This incidence includes some multiple recurrences. A recurrence usually is manifest within 10 years after the first operation, but we know of two patients who underwent a second surgical procedure 21 and 25 years, respectively, after initial surgery.

In the management of recurrences involving the frontal sinus, some surgeons prefer to obliterate the sinus. In this procedure, the bony wall is decorticated and an autograft — usually subcutaneous fat from the abdomen — is inserted after all the diseased mucosa is removed. Theoretically, this concept is sound, but the mucocele may recur because bits of diseased mucosa remain along the wall or in the satellite ramifications of the treated sinus. For this reason, the large and eccentrically contoured cavities of many recurrent mucoceles are never completely obliterated. This brings us back to the maxim first proposed, that is, *complete removal of the cyst wall and restoration of drainage from the occluded sinus into the nose* through a wide passage probably offers the best chance of permanent relief.

PARASITIC CYSTS

Parasitic infestations of the orbit are, with one exception — hydatid disease — very infrequent. Infestations by roundworms (filaria, trichinae), trematodes (the fluke causing schistosomiasis and other river flukes), a few cestodes (sparganum, cysticercus) and larvae of several varieties of flies are uncommon. When such infestations do occur, the parasite usually is said to be encysted in the host tissue. However, such an encystment is more an inflammatory granuloma than a cyst, as the term "cyst" is used in this chapter.

Most appropriate for discussion are the orbital tumors (cysts) caused by the migrating larvae — *Echinococcus granulosus*, *Cysticercus cellulosae*, and *Coenurus* — of three tapeworms, *Taenia echinococcus*, *Taenia solium*, and *Multiceps multiceps*, respectively. The primary host for *T. solium* is man, but the reservoir for the other two tapeworms is the dog (also foxes and jackals).

The life cycles of all three tapeworms are similar. A caudal proglottid containing eggs passes out of the host's intestine among feces. Grazing animals, such as sheep, goats, pigs, cows, rabbits, and even reindeer, consume vegetation contaminated by the feces. These animals, principally the pig, become intermediate hosts. Human infestation begins when the tissues of animals containing cysts with scoleces are eaten. Or, humans may be directly infested by ingesting contaminated excreta or by fondling the principal animal host, usually the dog; this means of transmission explains the frequency of the disease in children. Once inside the human intestine, the larvae worm their way into lymphatics and blood vessels, which provide pathways for dispersion to the favored site of final deposition.

INCIDENCE

Infestation with *Echinococcus (hydatid disease)* is fairly common, cases having been noted in all continents except Antarctica. Even so, the frequency of orbital involvement cannot be accurately assessed. First, very few of the larvae migrate beyond the liver or lung or find their way to such a remote area as the orbit. Even the eye is more frequently parasitized than the orbit. Second, even in countries where echinococcus disease is endemic, the percentage of orbital hydatid disease in any consecutive survey of orbital tumors may vary from 1 to 20%. In nonendemic areas, a large series of consecutive orbital tumors may have no examples of hydatid cyst. If all these orbital surveys were combined, the incidence of hydatid disease probably would be less than 1% of total cases. The frequency of orbital involvement with cysticercus and coenurus cysts is even more rare. No case of parasitic cyst was observed in the period of our survey of orbital tumors, and our personal experience with these tapeworm infestations has been very limited. The sexes seem to be affected equally.

CLINICAL FEATURES

After the parasite has lodged in the orbit, its initial period of growth is slow. Painless progressive proptosis with some associated edema of the eyelid develops. Papilledema, visual impairment, and even optic atrophy may appear as the cystic mass enlarges. At this stage, some patients seek surgical relief because of the marked proptosis. In others, the clinical picture may suddenly change. Pain, chemosis, and congestion of the eyeball herald the stage of inflammatory response. Now, the patient seeks surgical relief because of pain. In a child, this acute picture may resemble sarcoma.

To aid differential diagnosis in endemic areas, several laboratory tests have been devised: namely, the complement fixation test, the Casoni reaction, and the indirect hemagglutination reaction. None of these three biologic tests is reliable in orbital disease.

PATHOLOGY

When the embryo reaches its destination in human tissue, a two-layered cyst is formed. The host tissue responds to this insult by forming a wall of fibrous tissue and inflammatory cells around the cyst. This barrier often is called a capsule, but it is an integral part of the host tissue and cannot easily be dissected. Instead, a cleavage plane exists between this fibrous wall and the peripheral layer (the *ectocyst*) of the offending cyst. The ectocyst (Fig. 70, page

101) is a white, chitinous, laminated layer of tissue that stains strongly with periodic acid-Schiff stain. From the inner germinal layer (the *endocyst*), broad capsules containing numerous scoleces develop. The vesicles containing these scoleces may detach from the parent endocyst and then lie free in the cystic fluid.

TREATMENT

All surgeons agree that the preferable form of treatment is surgical removal, but how this is accomplished seems to vary somewhat from one country to another. Since most cysts are large, may be attached to important orbital structures, and often are situated deep in the orbit, a lateral orbital approach usually provides the best exposure. Aspiration as the first step seems wise and has become almost routine in endemic areas. It is performed with a small-caliber needle and should be done with caution to minimize contact between the strongly antigenic cyst fluid and host tissues. Hydatid fluid is clear and has a yellowish tinge unless hemorrhage has occurred within the cyst. Microscopic examination of this fluid reveals the free-floating scoleces of the parasite. Through the aspiration needle, the interior of the cyst may be repeatedly lavaged with saline, Ringer's solution, hypertonic saline, absolute alcohol, or formalin of various concentrations, each surgeon having an individual preference.

Next, the cyst is opened and the endocyst (larvae) removed by forceps or broad-bore suction cannula. At this point, there is disagreement about whether the covering pericyst (ectocyst) needs to be removed to complete the operation. Those who do not remove this layer usually swab out the remaining cavity with one of the chemical solutions noted above.

In nonendemic areas where aspiration is not routinely practiced, attempts to excise these cysts usually result in rupture. The lining endocyst is then removed by one of the methods noted above, but the brief contact between cyst contents and host tissue causes a severe postoperative inflammatory reaction. In former years, this reaction could be so severe that an already damaged visual apparatus could be permanently compromised. In the present era, systemic administration of steroids can soften the impact of this antigenic fluid on local tissue and also lessen anaphylaxis.

These cysts are serious surgical challenges.

HEMATIC CYST

TERMINOLOGY AND ORIGIN

These cysts are infrequent but occasionally pose a challenge in the differential diagnosis of unilateral proptosis. Synonyms are *hematoma, blood cyst,* and *hematocele.* Literally, "hematoma" means a tumor containing effused blood, but practically, the term broadly indicates a visible and localized collection of blood, usually following trauma, that disappears within days. Seldom do we think of hematoma, in reference to the orbit, as a deeply placed cystic structure that may remain unchanged and unidentified for long periods. For this type of hemorrhagic condition, *hematic cyst* seems the preferable term. *Blood cyst*, as a term, also has several drawbacks. Often, it is used to explain any localized or cystic collection of blood in the orbit for which there is no ready and obvious explanation. In addition, the same term sometimes is applied to hemorrhagic extravasations within a lymphangioma or dermoid cyst. Unless the term is made more specific, it is preferably abandoned. The third synonym, *hematocele*, has never been popular.

Hematic cysts may develop as complications of a hemorrhagic diathesis, from trauma about the head, or from prolonged retention of an orbital foreign body, or they may develop so insidiously as to defy explanation. Orbital hemorrhage in cases of leukemia, thrombocytopenia, hemophilia, familial hemorrhagic disease, advanced arterial disease, scurvy, and rickets has been documented. Confusion with other orbital tumors occurs when blood cannot escape from the orbital vault, is not absorbed, and silently remains as a cystic accumulation of hematogenous debris surrounded by a wall of fibrous tissue. A history of trauma may be remote or even absent in such cases. Also, hemorrhagic systemic disease, which might otherwise furnish a clue in differential diagnosis, may be absent. In such situations, discovery of a hematic cyst at operation may be a surprise.

In the older literature, the term orbital *cholesteatoma* frequently appears. Most such cases now would be called epidermoid or dermoid cysts. However, on the basis of the histologic description and the illustrations, some of these instances of cholesteatoma would now be considered examples of hematic cysts by our standards. Rarely, the term *cholesterol granuloma* is used to designate the histopathologic features of such cases; it more nearly describes the entity of our present concern. The word "cholesteatoma" in reference to an orbital mass should be abandoned.

INCIDENCE

These cysts occur among patients of all age groups, but attempts to estimate the incidence are unreliable. One consideration is that some cases in the literature included as hematic cysts are probably examples of lymphangioma. This is particularly true of some cases appearing in youngsters in whom orbital hemorrhage suddenly occurs without obvious explanation or associated with minimal trauma. This same feature also may apply to adults, and sudden enlargement of a mass present since childhood may then require orbitotomy. In either instance, the hemorrhagic cyst is uncovered, no tissue is sent for microscopic study, and the true lymphangioma remains unsuspected. These factors would favor a lower incidence than has been noted.

Contrary to this, the absence of hematic cysts in some tumor surveys reflects interest in neoplastic growths rather than in non-neoplastic cysts and other tumors of either inflammatory or infectious origin. We also tend to disregard the reportable significance of many hemorrhagic masses obviously related to trauma. Furthermore, we tend to report the unusual case but not the commonplace. These factors would favor a higher incidence than that recorded.

In our review of 764 patients, we have included 6 cases that seem to fit the criteria of hematic cyst. All six patients were male; the youngest was 30 and the oldest was 52. All cysts were considered to be secondary to trauma. In some, the association with trauma was quite definite, and in others the incident was more remote (more than a year before onset of progressive proptosis). The trauma always involved some severe force or impact to the area of the supraorbital ridge of the affected side. Descriptions of the injury included striking the forehead on some object during an automobile accident, falling in the bathtub, the thrust of a moving rocker on a rocking chair, and injury from a baseball bat. The source of bleeding probably was the periorbita along the roof of the orbit.

CLINICAL FEATURES

Unilateral proptosis seems to be the only common sign among the various entities that produce hematic cyst. In cases of hemophilia, leukemia, and bleeding into a cavernous space of lymphangioma, the onset of proptosis is sudden and painful. Progression of proptosis may be quite rapid and be associated with chemosis, restriction of ocular rotation, and decrease of vision. The patients are frightened and aware that something serious has happened. The physician also is apprehensive and usually tries to temporize, hoping the situation will improve without need for orbital exploration or decompression.

The clinical course of hematic cyst associated with trauma is different. After the contusion and ecchymosis of the initial injury has disappeared, there is an asymptomatic period that may be longer than the interval required to litigate the consequences of the injury. Slowly progressive, forward and downward displacement of the eye then begins. At this time the defects in bone, illustrated in Figures 71 and 72, are discovered, much to everyone's surprise. This discovery probably corresponds to the time when the organizing hematoma becomes an irritant foreign to the tissues and the host begins the laborious process of exteriorizing the lesion. A palpable, vaguely defined mass may or may not be present along the superior wall of the orbit, and some restriction of upward gaze of the affected eye is present. The clinical picture is not unlike the features noted (Chapter 2) with other benign tumors of the orbit.

ROENTGENOGRAPHIC CHANGES

Hematic cysts are not visible with standard orbital roentgenography except in the peripheral zone between the periorbita and bone. The pressure of organizing hemorrhage on adjacent bone and the surrounding inflammatory reaction produce a defect in bone that varies in size and character according to the

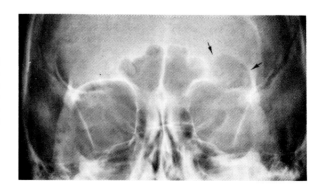

Figure 71. Hematic cyst (cholesterol granuloma). Oval lesion almost 3 cm in diameter is above left orbit (*arrows*) in 50-year-old man. Lesion is well defined, but there is very little marginal sclerosis.

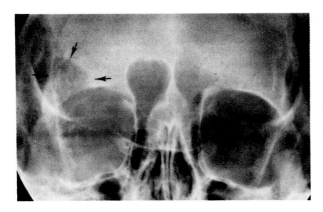

Figure 72. Hematic cyst (cholesterol granuloma). Pyramidal-shaped defect is above right eye (*arrows*) in a 39-year-old man. Cyst eroded inner table of frontal bone and was in contact with dura.

amount and duration of the hemorrhage. Smaller defects of short duration may have a slightly eroded or fuzzy contour suggesting an eosinophilic granuloma or lodgment of a malignant neoplasm. In long-standing cysts, the defects may become quite large (Fig. 71 and 72) and have distinct outlines and slightly sclerotic borders similar in appearance to those of an epidermoid cyst. The bony orbital defects of a hematic cyst have not been well publicized in either the ophthalmic or the radiologic literature, and the correct preoperative differential diagnosis often is not considered.

PATHOLOGY

Hematic cysts form because orbital hemorrhage is too great to be quickly absorbed. Incomplete or delayed clotting also may contribute to their mass. Most have a tough fibrous wall that distinguishes them grossly from the thin-walled, blood-filled, bluish cysts of lymphangioma. The contents are usually a mixture of old blood and amorphous debris. All degrees and stages of organization are encountered: cholesterol clefts, hemosiderin deposition, foreign body cells, pigment-collecting macrophages, and foam cells containing lipid (Fig. 73). The color of this material ranges through the various hues of brown and yellow. The fibrous walls are infiltrated with assorted quantities of leukocytes. An epithelial covering or lining is not present.

TREATMENT

An anterior-superior orbitotomy (see Chapter 24) was used to evacuate all but one of the hematic cysts in our series. When the incision through skin and subcutaneous tissues is completed and the superior rim of the orbit is exposed, the surgeon may easily reach the inferior extent of the cystic pouch by incising the periosteum and separating the periorbita from the roof of the orbit. Or if roentgenographic examination reveals that the bony defect is quite large, the surgeon may prefer to peel the periosteum from the frontal bone and approach the cyst directly along its anterior face, as illustrated in Figure 58. The bony partition is very thin in this area because of pressure from the expanding cyst, and it may be so soft that it can be removed by biting forceps.

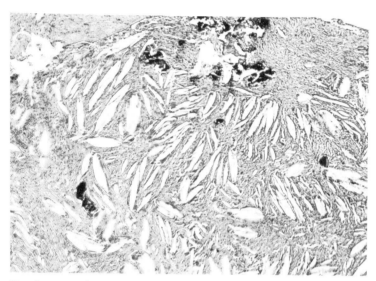

Figure 73. Organizing hematoma with degenerating blood pigment, cholesterol crystals (clefts). and scattered calcium deposits. (Hematoxylin and eosin; ×50.)

Evacuation of the cyst contents, removal of the fibrous wall lining the bony cavity, and hemostasis of bleeding points along the bared bone are sufficient. That portion of the fibrous wall attached to orbital structures, such as the levator palpebrae superioris, need not be dissected or even desiccated, as is necessary to destroy the epithelial lining of an epidermoid cyst or mucocele. Postoperative visual problems should be minimal, and the cyst will not recur if hemostasis is thorough.

SIMPLE CYSTS

Among the simple cysts we have placed several cysts that differ little from one another except in terminology. These cysts have several features in common: their extreme rarity in the orbit and their barely greater frequency in adnexal structures, such as eyelids and conjunctiva; their secondary rather than primary origin in the orbit; their lining of simple epithelium reflecting their origin; and the fact that they cause cosmetic embarrassment — but little functional impairment — of the affected eye. Three types — *serous, retention* and *implantation* cysts — are recognized.

SEROUS CYST

Serous cysts seem to arise in small and delicate bursae between tendon sheaths of ocular muscles. They develop between the superior rectus and the overlying levator palpebrae superioris and around the inferior rectus tendon as it crosses the ligament of Lockwood. For some reason they push back into the orbital cavity rather than extend forward into an adjacent cul-de-sac. The lining is cuboidal epithelium.

RETENTION CYST

These tumors originate in one of the glandular appendages of the conjunctiva, such as the glands of Krause. Obstruction of the orifices of the glands from injury, surgery, or cicatrix secondary to trachoma may be responsible for the enlarging mass. The epithelial lining of the cyst may have two layers (Fig. 74), but it also shows the simple features of conjunctival epithelium. The two examples in our survey occurred in men with downward displacement of the eye. When the upper eylid was everted, a bluish, thin-walled mass was visible in the superior conjunctival cul-de-sac. Superior orbitotomy revealed that the mass was attached to the superior fornix along its anteroinferior surface and that it extended posteriorly into the orbital cavity along the superior surface of the levator palpebrae superioris. The tumors were about the size of the distal segment of the little finger. They were cystic, filled with sticky serous fluid, and lined by cuboidal epithelium. There was no history of injury or inflammation of the eyelid. Cysts in this location are managed best by wide incision, removal of contents, and electrodesiccation of epithelial lining. Attempts to excise them needlessly traumatize the tendon of the levator palpebrae superioris.

IMPLANTATION CYST

This term implies misplacement of the surface epithelium into the orbit. These cysts are caused by external injury to adnexal structures, such as the eyelid, wherein epithelium is pushed along the tract of some penetrating wound. The lining of the cysts is modified stratified epithelium. The cysts may extend various distances into the orbit and are more difficult to eradicate than serous and retention types. All epithelium must be removed or destroyed or the cyst will recur. In superior portions of the orbit, implantation cysts usually are superior to the levator palpebrae superioris, whereas serous and retention cysts are inferior to this muscle.

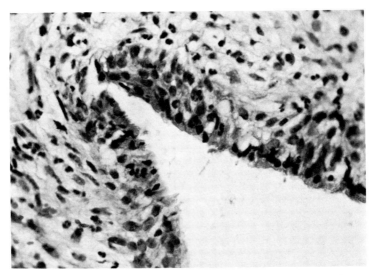

Figure 74.   Retention cyst. Lining is double-layered epithelium of dilated duct. (Hematoxylin and eosin; × 400.)

DENTIGEROUS CYST

No cysts of this type were recorded during the period of our survey. The literature on orbital aspects of these tumors also is sparse. In its strict sense, the term *dentigerous* refers to a cyst, lined with epithelium (stratified squamous) within a connective tissue wall and filled with fluid, that contains some anomalous portion of a tooth. It develops from some degenerative change in enamel epithelium after tooth formation has begun. In the broader sense of the term, referring to any cyst of odontic origin, *primordial* and *periodontal* cysts also should be mentioned. These, too, may become large enough to push on the orbit. The primordial cyst is related to the dentigerous cyst proper, but it represents degeneration of enamel anlage before the tooth is formed. The periodontal cyst is the result of inflammation, usually around the root of the tooth, after the tooth has developed. This type of cyst is found in both maxilla and mandible, but it is in the former bone, of course, that its growth may encroach on the orbit. By the time cysts have reached such a size, differentiation of one cyst from another is academic.

In cases that come to the attention of ophthalmologists, asymmetry and bulging of the face with upward deviation of the eye on the side of the lesion, suggest a malignant tumor arising in the antrum or fibrous dysplasia of maxillary bone secondarily involving the orbit. Differentiation can be made by the roentgenologist; the cyst is radiolucent, whereas the malignant tumor shows bone destruction and fibrous dysplasia is radiopaque.

These cysts should be eradicated through an inferior approach to permit dependent drainage. But if the orbit is involved, the oral surgeon is more qualified to handle the problem than is an ophthalmologist. The lining of these cysts must be completely removed. If size or multiple cavities preclude complete removal, the cysts must be marsupialized.

Bibliography

Dermoid and Epidermoid Cysts

Dayal, J, Hameed, S: Periorbital dermoid. Am J Ophthalmol 53:1013, 1962

Jakobiec, FA, Bonanno, PA, Sigelman, J: Conjunctival adnexal cysts and dermoids. Arch Ophthalmol 96:1404–1409, 1978

Jones, AC: Oil cyst of the orbit with carcinomatosis. Am J Ophthalmol 18:532–535, 1935

Pollard, ZF, Calhoun, J: Deep orbital dermoid with draining sinus. Am J Ophthalmol 79:310–313, 1975

Wright, J, Morgan, G: Squamous cell carcinoma developing in an orbital cyst. Arch Ophthalmol 95: 635–637, 1977

Teratoma

Barber, JC, Barber, LF, Guerry, D, et al: Congenital orbital teratoma. Arch Ophthalmol 91:45–48, 1974

Casanovas, R: Congenital teratomas of the orbit. Arch Ophthalmol 77:795–799, 1967

Duke-Elder, S: *System of Ophthalmology.* Vol 3. Normal and Abnormal Development. Part 2. Congenital Deformities. St. Louis, C.V. Mosby Co., 1963, p 972

Ferry, AP: Teratoma of the orbit: a report of two cases. Survey Ophthalmol 10:434–442, 1965

Hoyt, WF, Joe, S: Congenital teratoid cyst of the orbit: a case report and review of the literature. Arch Ophthalmol 68:196–201, 1962

Cephalocele

Duke-Elder, S: *System of Ophthalmology.* Vol 3. Normal and Abnormal Development. Part 2. Congenital Deformities. St. Louis, C.V. Mosby Co., 1963

Leone, CR, Marlowe, JF: Orbital presentation of an ethmoidal encephalocele: report of a case of a 62-year-old woman. Arch Ophthalmol 83:445–447, 1970

Pollock, JA, Newton, TH, Hoyt, WF: Transsphenoidal and transethmoidal encephaloceles: a review of clinical and roentgen features in 8 cases. Radiology 90:442–453, 1968

Congenital Cystic Eye

Baghdassarian, SA, Tabbara, KF, Matta, CS: Congenital cystic eye. Am J Ophthalmol 76:269–275, 1973

Dollfus, MA: Congenital cystic eyeball. Am J Ophthalmol 66:504–509, 1968

Helveston, EM, Malone, E Jr, Lashmet, MH: Congenital cystic eye. Arch Ophthalmol 84:622–624, 1970

Microphthalmos With Cyst

Bonner, J, Ide, CH: Astrocytoma of the optic nerve and chiasm associated with microphthalmos and orbital cyst. Br J Ophthalmol 58:828–831, 1974

Waring, GO, Roth, AM, Rodrigues, MM: Clinicopathologic correlation of microphthalmos with cyst. Am J Ophthalmol 82:714–721, 1976

Perioptic Hygroma

Harris, GJ, Sacks, JG, Weinberg, PE, et al: Cyst of the intraorbital optic nerve sheaths. Am J Ophthalmol 81:656–660, 1976

Holt, H: Cysts of the intracranial portion of the optic nerve. Am J Ophthalmol 61:1166–1170, 1966

Miller, NR, Green, WR: Arachnoid cysts involving a portion of the intraorbital nerve. Arch Ophthalmol 93:1117–1121, 1975

Smith, JL, Hoyt, WF, Newton, TH: Optic nerve sheath decompression for relief of chronic monocular choked disc. Am J Ophthalmol 68:633–639, 1969

Spencer, WH: Primary neoplasm of the optic nerve and its sheaths. Clinical features and current concepts of pathogenetic mechanisms. Trans Am Ophthalmol Soc 70:490–528, 1972

Mucocele

Alberti PWRM, Marshall HF, Black JIM: Fronto-ethmoidal mucocoele as a cause of unilateral proptosis. Br J Opthalmol 52:833–838, 1968

Keate R: History of a case of bony tumor successfully removed from the head of a female. R Med Chir Soc Lond 10:278–295, 1819

Reese AB: *Tumors of the Eye.* Second edition. New York, Hoeber Medical Division, Harper & Row, Publishers, 1963

Reese AB: Expanding lesions of the orbit (Bowman Lecture). Trans Ophthalmol Soc UK 91:85–104, 1971

Robertson DM, Henderson JW: Unilateral proptosis secondary to orbital mucocele in infancy. Am J Ophthalmol 68:845–847, 1969

Rollet M: Mucocèle double des orbites. Ann Ocul (Paris) 116:136, 1896

Stool S, Kertesz E, Sibinga M, et al: Exophthalmos due to pyocele of the sinus in children with cystic fibrosis. Trans Am Acad Ophthalmol Otolaryngol 70:811–816, 1966

Vail DT Jr: Orbital complications in sinus disease. Am J Ophthalmol 14:202–208, 1931

Von Leden H: Orbital mucoceles. Can J Ophthalmol 1:36–43, 1966

Zizmor J, Fasano CV, Smith B, et al: Roentgenographic diagnosis of unilateral exophthalmos. JAMA 197:343–346, 1966

Parasitic Cysts

Malek SRK, Gupta AK, Choudhry S: Ocular cysticercosis. Am J Ophthalmol 66:1168–1171, 1968

Manschot WA: *Coenurus* infestation of eye and orbit. Arch Ophthalmol 94:961–964, 1976

Sevel D. Sapeikka RJ: Hydatid cyst of the orbit. Survey Ophthalmol 22:101–105, 1977

Talib H: Orbital hydatid disease in Iraq. Br J Surg 59:391–394, 1972

Van Selm J: Some orbital swellings in children. S Afr Med J 38:590–592, 1964

Hematic Cysts

Duke-Elder SS: *System of Ophthalmology.* Volume 13. The Ocular Adnexa. St. Louis, C.V. Mosby Co., 1976, pp 819–825

5

Neoplasms of Blood and Lymph Vessels

The literature on vascular tumors (including malformations, hamartomas, and neoplasms) of the eye and adnexa is voluminous. To annotate, abstract, and record this material would be a Herculean task and on this subject alone a monograph easily could be compiled. With such an abundance of literature the orbit has not been neglected; more has been written on the orbital aspects of vascular tumors than on any other tumor in this text. Most observers, in fact, believe these are the most common tumors primary in the orbit; this would be one reason for their interest. The color of the tumors, which ranges from a striking red to a deep blue with overtones of purple, and their frequent association with other lumps and spots of similar hue scattered about the body are other factors which have attracted the interest of the color-conscious human eye from earliest time. The tumors' variable characteristics — which include soft, compressible, nonencapsulated masses, well-circumscribed firm tumors, and coils of boundless tangled vessels — have piqued the curiosity of many a clinician. Clinician and surgeon cannot help but ponder the ease with which one type of tumor is treated in contrast to the almost unsurmountable challenge of another.

HISTORICAL ASPECTS

In the earliest literature *varix* was the commonest descriptive term for this group of tumors. This broad term was clinically applicable to some growths that, because surgical techniques were limited, progressed to huge proportions. For interested historians and bibliophiles, all pertinent references to these tumors prior to 1900 can be found in the *Encyclopépedie Française d'Ophtalmologie* of Lagrange and Valude (1909). By 1860 the *cavernoma*, or *cavernous hemangioma*, was recognized as a circumscribed form of this class of tumors and von Graefe (1860) wrote an extensive review of the subject. Hodges, an American, also shared in this early history. In a report (1864) that is often overlooked, Hodges, a Boston surgeon, described removal of a cavernoma from the orbit without loss of the eye. This was a notable surgical feat because prior procedures either had included enucleation of the eye or required such extensive manipulations to staunch blood flow as to make the eye useless. Hodges removed his tumor through an incision between the lateral canthus and the lateral rim of the orbit. This encapsulated tumor was smooth and ovoid, "as large as an egg," and filled with blood.

NOMENCLATURE AND CLASSIFICATION

It is understandable that such a large clan of related tumors should encounter problems of mixed identity, selection of suitable individual designation, and subgrouping according to genesis and clinical behavior. All the tumors have in common some association with a predominantly vascular enlargement, whether it is established blood vessels, new formation of vessels, proliferation of tissue components of the vessel wall, or uncontrolled hyperplasia of cellular elements ordinarily concerned with genesis of vascular tissue. Nomenclature and classification of the tumors soon showed a mixture of clinical appearance, histopathologic patterns, anatomic location, and a generous sprinkling of eponyms. Observers frequently designate the entire group as *hemangiomas*. We prefer to call the entire group *vascular tumors*, which has a connotation reflecting broader implications of genesis and makeup. The term hemangioma, preferably, is reserved for more familiar tumors which are cellular, usually proliferative, and capillary and cavernous in type.

The classification given in Table 5 is oriented toward the main types encountered in the orbit; it includes, where applicable, a choice of synonymous appellations. It includes a closely related group, the *lymphangiomas*, which are but one step removed from an identical genesis with vascular tumors. The table excludes some types not found in the eye, eyelids, or orbit, many fibrous tissue tumors with sometimes a marked vascular component, compound tumors containing blood vessels, such as mesenchymomas, and glomus tumors, which contain elements of nervous tissue origin.

Alternate Classifications. One classification, based on histopathologic features, uses dominance of either the cellular components or vascular channels in the tumor. Those with dominant cellular patterns are termed monomorphic, and include hemangioendotheliomas and hemangiopericytomas. This group, characterized by proliferation of one cellular component of the blood vessel, comprises truer examples of neoplasia than the remainder, which are designated polymorphic; the latter include tumors showing various stages of differentiation, from simple vascular spaces to mature blood channels. Polymorphic types also are considered examples of developmental anomalies rather than neoplasia.

There is less agreement concerning classifications based on pathogenesis. Some authorities divide the family into three groups, namely, *vascular malfor-*

TABLE 5.   **CLASSIFICATION OF ORBITAL VASCULAR TUMORS**

Capillary Hemangioma (infantile hemangioma, angioblastic hemangioma, hypertrophic hemangioma, hyperplastic hemangioma, cellular hemangioma, juvenile hemangioma, benign hemangioendothelioma)
Cavernous Hemangioma
Hemangioendothelioma
Hemangiopericytoma
Vascular Leiomyoma (venous hemangioma)
Vascular Malformations
    Orbital aneurysm (arterial)
    Orbital varix (venous)
    Arteriovenous fistula
    Arteriovenous aneurysm
Lymphangioma (hygroma)

mations, hamartomas, and *neoplasms*. Malformations imply preformed, established collections of blood vessels which undergo dilation to form the tumor mass. Hamartomas refer to tumors arising from cords or islands of embryonic vascular tissue; these fail to connect in an orderly manner with the general circulation and remain, instead, as isolated, useless, enlarging vascular masses. These tumors are present at birth or appear in early infancy, but after a period of rapid growth concomitant with that of the child, most (but certainly not all) regress later in childhood. Capillary hemangiomas in the classification (Table 5) are included in this group.

The third group, neoplasms, includes hemangioendotheliomas, hemangiopericytomas, and vascular leiomyomas. Some observers would place cavernous hemangiomas among the hamartomas and others would regard them as neoplasms. A modification of this tripartite grouping is to combine hamartomas and other malformations and term them developmental anomalies. Still another modification suggests all tumors be designated as neoplasms, except those types listed as vascular malformation.

HEMANGIOMA

We prefer to apply the term *hemangioma* to the two most frequent vascular tumors, the *capillary* and *cavernous hemangiomas*, and to consider their incidence collectively. This has been the custom of our own (1973) as well as other published surveys of orbital tumors and will assist in comparing the data of one study with those of another. Other reasons for considering these benign tumors collectively have been the long-standing belief that mixtures of both histologic types occur in the same tumor and that, with increasing maturity of the host patient, a capillary hemangioma may undergo transition to a cavernous hemangioma. However, the more recent trend considers these tumors as separate entities, and, therefore, we will discuss their clinical features, histopathology, course, and treatment under separate subtitles.

INCIDENCE

The age distribution and sex of the fifty-five hemangiomas in our survey are listed in Table 6. As a group they are the third most common tumor (exceeded only by squamous cell carcinoma and mucocele) in our survey, comprising about 7% of the total 764 cases. They are the most common primary orbital tumor; 16% of tumors in this class. These data are not too different from the incidence of hemangioma (61 of 508 tumors, or 12%) in a somewhat comparable consecutive series of orbital tumors by Reese (1971). However, the Reese series

TABLE 6.   AGE AND SEX DISTRIBUTION OF 55 HEMANGIOMAS

Male	Female		Age in Years at Time of Orbital Diagnosis							
			0–10	*11–20*	*21–30*	*31–40*	*41–50*	*51–60*	*61–70*	*Over 70*
8	11	Capillary	19							
18	18	Cavernous	5	5	4	4	9	6	2	1

contained more infantile than adult hemangiomas, a finding opposite to our own survey.

From Table 6 the age differential between the infantile and adult type of hemangioma is evident. This is one factor that tends to support the concept that capillary and cavernous hemangiomas are different clinical entities. Among our patients with capillary hemangiomas the youngest was 2½ months and the oldest was 2½ years at the time of initial observation. The infantile hemangioma is not necessarily present at birth but appears soon after. The cavernous hemangioma, on the other hand, is principally a tumor of adults with peak incidence in the fifth decade. However, the time lag between onset and first observation of the adult may be quite long in some cases (Fig. 75; also see Fig. 10). Therefore, an incidence based on onset of the disease would be considerably younger than the fifth decade.

The sex incidence of both capillary and cavernous hemangioma (Table 6) was essentially equal, a finding not in total agreement with some other surveys. Harris and Jakobiec in a recent survey of 66 cases of histologically proved cavernous hemangioma noted a female predominance of 7:3.

CAPILLARY HEMANGIOMA

NOMENCLATURE

This is the striking, frequent, *strawberry mark* of the superficial tissues so familiar to pediatricians. Its principal histologic component is endothelial-lined, capillary-size vessels. In the deeper tissues of the orbit it is often a part of a less mature, more cellular endothelial cell tumor. The latter is burdened with a battery of names, including *simple hemangioma, juvenile hemangioma, hypertrophic hemangioma, cellular hemangioma, angioblastic hemangioma,* and *benign hemangioendothelioma.* The last term is preferably omitted to minimize confusion with a different tumor, malignant hemangioendothelioma. Each

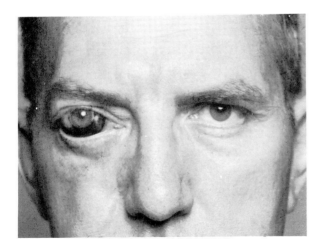

Figure 75. Cavernous hemangioma filling lower nasal quadrant of right orbit. Tumor present for 22 years with marked proptosis during last 10 years (proptosis at time of photograph, 10 mm); subconjunctival hemorrhage adjacent to inferior limbus extended across lower surface of right eye; recurrent subconjunctival hemorrhages secondary to exposure of eye and triggered by minor trauma were compelling reasons for seeking treatment; and 3 by 2 by 1 cm cavernous hemangioma excised at inferior orbitotomy.

pathologist has a favorite among this array of names but understands the nuances of the terms used by others. A further name that combines the clinical features of all these tumors in the orbit (including capillary hemangioma) but is less precise histologically is *infantile hemangioma*. We will use the latter name frequently to designate this tumor of early life that combines the transitional cellular features of an immature, benign vascular tumor.

CLINICAL FEATURES

Whereas, in *adults*, the *presenting sign of hemangioma is proptosis associated with a slowly enlarging, invisible mass*, in *infants* the *presenting sign is a visible, enlarging mass without proptosis* or displacement of the eye. Almost invariably the parents of the child will say that a swelling first appeared in the nasal portion of either the upper or lower eyelid (Fig. 76), more often in the former position. At this stage the mass is palpable, compressible, and seems to lie behind the orbital septum — but pushes the soft tissues of the eyelid anteriorly. It is not painful but its bluish overtones become more vivid and alarming when the child cries (Fig. 77). In this, the clinical picture resembles orbital varix. As the problem progresses the tumor pushes forward, the droopy lid begins to cover the visual axis, and there is displacement of the eye away from the normal horizontal or vertical plane. This is an exceptional situation among orbital tumors wherein there is an obvious large mass, the eye is displaced, but forward proptosis may almost be absent. Finally, the tumor becomes so large and the soft tissue swelling so great that the eye is hidden (Figs. 78 and 79).

Additional symptoms were the following: strabismus, minor ophthalmoplegia affecting the direction of gaze toward the tumor (suggesting a mechanical interference to ocular rotation), and enlargement and reddish discoloration of the caruncle. Also, marked astigmatism and even amblyopia of the affected eye is seen in advanced cases. Among this age group, extraorbital hemangiomas often can be found, particularly on the trunk, extremities, face or scalp.

In early cases, when only a bluish mass is evident in the upper nasal quadrant of the orbit, the question of a primary orbital rhabdomyosarcoma or a

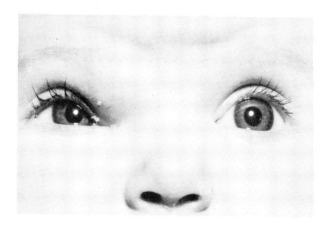

Figure 76. Features common to early orbital hemangiomas in infancy. Soft, compressible, bluish mass occupies upper nasal quadrant of right orbit but is not yet large enough to obscure vision or displace eye.

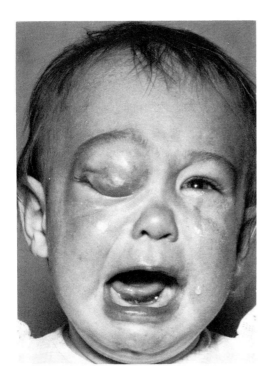

Figure 77. Infantile type of hemangioma in upper nasal quadrant of right orbit also extending into eyelid. Crying causes tumor to increase in size and cover eye as eyelid swells; adjacent tissues also may swell (in this case, the right cheek), although no gross tumor may be visible.

metastatic neuroblastoma may arise. Enlargement of these malignant neoplasms is quite rapid (measured in terms of days) as compared with the progression of infantile hemangioma (measured in terms of weeks). As the hemangioma progresses the tumor retains its bluish hue, but the skin overlying an enlarging rhabdomyosarcoma becomes a more alarming red color (Fig. 309, Chapter 19), and the skin overlying an expanding neuroblastoma may even by ecchymotic (Fig. 198, Chapter 11). The tumor of rhabdomyosarcoma and neuroblastoma does not enlarge with crying or straining. If routine orbital roentgen-

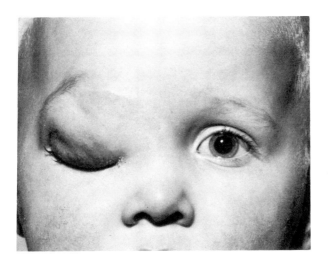

Figure 78. Large hemangioma of right orbit and eyelid. Right upper eyelid could not even be forcefully lifted; surgical scar (across medial half of eyebrow) the result of prior removal of adjacent hemangioma in forehead; treatment clearly imperative.

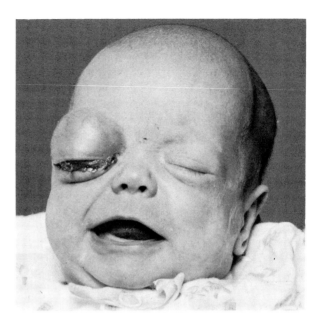

Figure 79. Huge orbital hemangioma completely hiding right eye; treatment rather than conservative observation advisable.

ography shows enlargement of the bony orbit, this would indicate an infantile hemangioma.

PATHOLOGY

Vascular tumors originate in collections of mesenchymal cells which have the potential of forming blood vessels. These primitive mesenchymal cells differentiate into endothelial cells, the latter lining the clefts and spaces which become blood vessels. Endothelial cells are common to all vascular tumors, no matter what their type or nomenclature. Endothelial cells are relatively large and flat and contain a moderate amount of cytoplasm. The nuclei are oval and resemble the nuclei of primitive fibroblasts, except for a lack of nucleoli. For some reason this embryonic vascular syncytium either remains isolated or fails to connect with other vascular anlage so that a tumor rather than an orderly, normal system of tubes and channels develops. At this stage, the isolated tumor seems to possess the potential for growth of more vascular spaces or for proliferation of the cellular components of primitive blood vessels. Sometimes both cellular and tubular structures are present in the same mass, and such mixed tumors are classified according to the predominant type of tissue.

The most immature form of infantile hemangioma consists of a nest of endothelial cells with few or no spaces and a sparse framework of connective tissue. Many of the proliferating endothelial cells are plump and arranged in solid sheets (Fig. 80). Grossly, these hemangiomas may appear solid and fleshy owing to the minimal differentiation of vascular channels, yet the tumor does not possess a true capsule, making total surgical excision unsatisfactory (Fig. 81).

In the next stage of differentiation small capillary-size channels characterize the histopathologic picture (Fig. 82). Microscopy shows that the channels

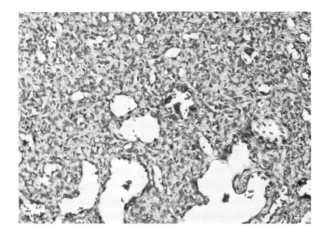

Figure 80. Hypertrophic or juvenile hemangioma: plump endothelial cells arranged in solid sheets with only occasional capillary-size channels. (Hematoxylin and eosin; × 160.)

may be segregated in clumps and clusters by connective tissue septa; sometimes diffuse, crowded, and proliferating tubes lined with endothelium may occupy an entire microscopic field. The lining of these incomplete capillaries is a single row of basic endothelial cells. Some mitotic activity usually is visible, but the usual features of malignant alteration are absent.

In many infantile hemangiomas of longer duration the vascular channels may become quite ectatic and dilated. This configuration suggests a mixed picture of cavernous-capillary hemangioma. However, these dilated channels retain the orderly lining of plump endothelial cells in contrast to the flatter, "ironed out" appearance of the endothelial lining of the true cavernous hemangioma. Also, the interstitium of the infantile hemangioma retains a delicate, more cellular character than the more fibrotic, dense interstitium seen in the adult cavernous hemangioma.

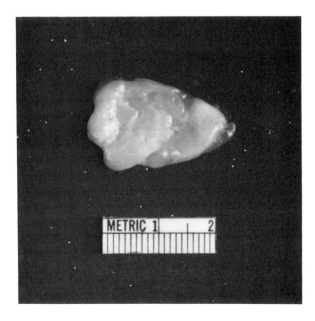

Figure 81. Hypertrophic hemangioma: surgical specimen shows solid appearance of tumor, well circumscribed but infiltrative about margins.

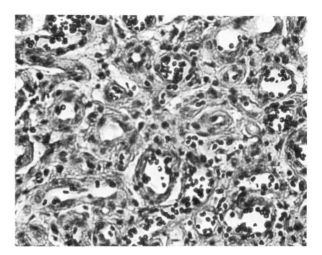

Figure 82. Capillary hemangioma: capillary-size channels are formed by endothelial cells and filled with blood. (Hematoxylin and eosin; × 300.)

TREATMENT AND COURSE

In infants and children the management of hemangioma is controversial. Many physicians believe that no treatment is required because hemangiomas may spontaneously disappear as the child becomes older. A minority advocate some form of treatment, but there is no consensus about the best treatment. The need for treatment might well hinge on the question of the natural history of all hemangiomas in this age group: Does the tumor disappear or does it persist?

In an attempt to answer this question, these aspects have been fully discussed in dermatologic and pediatric literature. Some articles report observations on thousands of cases for long periods, others include well-controlled and large studies of untreated and treated cases, and still others compare rates of resolution in various types of hemangioma. Location of the tumor also may influence the ratio of spontaneous resolution, and a survey weighted by a preponderance of hemangiomas located in the head and neck will report a smaller incidence of spontaneous resolution than would one containing a majority of similar tumors located in the trunk and extremities. Finally, the rate of regression may differ widely among publications dealing with identical types of hemangioma. Whichever figure the reader wishes to accept, a significant number of hemangiomas do not involute. Furthermore, some of them are more aggressive in growth than assumed by the family physicians and pediatricians who first see these infants. In our experience, the parents of youngsters with orbital and adnexal hemangiomas almost invariably have been told that the tumor will disappear.

How do the voluminous literature and expertise apply to orbital hemangiomas? Unfortunately, though tumors of the face often are discussed, surveys seldom mention the orbit and a controlled study of orbital hemangiomas alone does not seem to exist. The clinical course of the tumors is certainly unpredictable. Some tumors reach a certain size — 10 to 15 mm in diameter — and then remain fairly stationary; others grow at an alarmng and frightening rate, but few completely disappear. In our experience, most infants continue to have problems despite predictions of spontaneous involution. Figure 83 illustrates one such example.

However, the fact that some orbital hemangiomas do not regress is not, alone, a reason why all should be treated. After all, these are benign growths. The crux of the problem is the disfigurement and ocular disability that these tumors create as they attain a certain size. The disfigurement worries anxious parents; ocular disability alarms the ophthalmologist. The cosmetic impact of the tumors, either in the orbit or on the face, is far greater than that made by hemangiomas of similar size located elsewhere on the body. This feature was aptly illustrated by our visit with a physician who always advocated the therapeutic approach to hemangiomas of "masterful inaction" and "intelligent neglect" — until one of his own female children developed a tumor of this type in the orbit. He wanted treatment to be started promptly.

Of great concern to us is the degree of strabismus and amblyopia these tumors can cause. Once strabismus has developed, the eye seldom regains perfect parallelism, even though the hemangioma is arrested in its growth or is removed. We have observed improvement, of course, in the eye's position as the tumor recedes, but frequently normal fusion and parallelism are not recovered. Neither does an induced astigmatism entirely disappear. Not all orbital hemangiomas in infancy grow big enough to cause strabismus and amblyopia, but there is no diagnostic portent telling us which tumors will grow and harm the eye and which will stop growing before altering ocular function. In our view, orbital hemangiomas of infancy are more aggressive and conform less to the expected pattern of resolution than similar hemangiomas in any other area of the body. The ever-present possibility of permanent ocular disability strongly influences our positive approach to treatment.

Forms of Treatment.   The following six principal forms of treatment have been proposed for orbital hemangiomas in this age group: *cryotherapy, surgical diathermy, injection of sclerosing agents, radiotherapy, systemic administration of corticosteriods,* and *surgical excision.* We have abandoned the first three modalities in this list based either on our experience or observation of patients treated by others.

SURGICAL EXCISION.   Often used by ophthalmic surgeons in the past, excision sometimes is recommended today as the best method of management. Although occasionally this form of treatment may be successful, more often — at

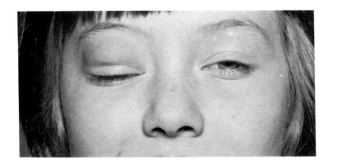

Figure 83. Hemangioma of right upper eyelid and orbit (present since birth). Right eye was displaced downward with limitation of upward rotation; at time of photograph this 6-year-old girl was still waiting for spontaneous resolution.

least in our hands — well-intentioned surgery has seemed but a triggering mechanism for embarrassing recurrence and unrestrained expansion, particularly in infants. It is as though surgical manipulation stimulates these primitive cells to even greater hyperplasia. Surgery is more appropriate in youngsters over 5 years of age in whom a hemangioma is still occupying the orbit as the result of "watchful waiting." By this time, capsule formation around the tumor is sufficient to make complete excision practicable. Surgery also may be useful when the tumor has been delimited and fibrosed by other forms of treatment, and as the last resort in cases with recurrent or progressive tumors.

RADIOTHERAPY. In some form, radiotherapy has many proponents. Its use is predicated on the basis that primitive or immature cells of this tumor are sensitive to irradiation. Clinically, we believe this is true. Placement of radium plaques over the surface of deep hemangiomas and irradiation (orthovoltage) directed to the affected orbital quadrant both have been frequently used. But both methods must be used cautiously. The infants eye must be protected by a lead shield or cataract will occur; the proliferating epithelium at the periphery of the infantile lens is nearly as radiosensitive as the tumor. For adequate protection of the eye and accurate positioning of the child, treatment should be given while the child is anesthetized, but even these precautions are not entirely protective because scatter emanations pass behind the lead shield. However, in infants irradiation does cause fibrosis or involution of the tumor. After the age of 4 years irradiation becomes less effective, and by adulthood it has almost no therapeutic effect. The critical question is whether such powerful ionizing rays should be used as the treatment of a benign tumor in an infant, considering the possible deleterious effect on both lens and bone growth. For a malignant tumor the answer is "Yes." But for capillary-cavernous hemangiomas the answer is more equivocal.

Use of Radon *

As a compromise we favor radon seeds. These have more advantages and fewer drawbacks for this particular tumor. Before the reader recalls all the hazards attributed to radon in the literature, we hasten to emphasize that we use radon of relatively weak intensity and meticulously place it in the tumor to minimize pathologic irradiation of the lens. The *objects of treatment are to arrest the growth of tumor rather than to destroy it and to initiate involution* or fibrosis.

Radon, a heavy gas, is formed in the first stage of the natural disintegration of radium. It can be collected by dissolving a soluble radium salt in water, but radon is now available from commercial laboratories and is delivered, ready for use, in small gold capsules (diameter, 1 mm approximately). Radon seeds emit only gamma rays because the alpha and beta rays are absorbed by the gold wall of the seed. The half-life of radon is only 3.8 days, so the therapeutic effectiveness is minimal 3 weeks after tumor implantation.

---

*In the therapeutic application of radon to our cases, we rely heavily on the gracious guidance and conservative counsel of a colleague in the Mayo Clinic Department of Therapuetic Radiology, Dr. Martin Van Herik.

The strength of the radon in seeds is expressed in millicuries. A single millicurie (mc) of radon effectively disintegrated will have delivered the equivalent of 132 millicurie-hours (mc-hr) of radiation; that is, this single millicurie dose would be equivalent to 1 mc of radium left in place for 132 hours. The roentgen (R) is the common unit of measurement of dose delivered; the radon seed can be considered a point source, and it will deliver 8.4 R/mc-hr at a distance of 1 cm. Thus, a single radon seed implanted in tissue would deliver, upon full decay, a dose of 1,108.8 R at a distance of 1 cm (132 mc-hr multiplied by 8.4 R per mc-hr).

As with any light source, the intensity of dose delivered will vary inversely as the square of the distance. Thus, the dose from the radon seed at a distance of 0.5 cm will be four times as much as the dose at 1 c. This brief discussion of radon physics give us the necessary knowledge to calculate in actual hemangioma implantations the dosage delivered to the lens, which is the critical tissue.

Mayo Clinic Technique

Plans for treatment of an infant usually are made 48 hours in advance. This allows time for delivery of the radon. We like to use a radon seed which, when inserted, will have a strength of from 0.22 to 0.30 mc. The gold seed is placed in the hollow tip of a spinal needle and secured by a touch of petroleum jelly (Vaseline) or lubricating jelly. Under general anesthesia we first recommend a small incisional biopsy along the extreme periphery of the lesion assisted by frozen tissue study. This area will not interfere with placement of the radon and bleeding will be more easily controlled. Before the radon is inserted, the size of the hemangioma is roughly estimated. The object is to place the seed at or near the center of the tumor. With these calculations in mind, the needle is thrust through the skin into the mass of tumor (Fig. 84). Next, the lateral or vertical distance of the needle shaft from the nearest periphery of the lens is estimated and the actual distance of the needle tip from this tissue is calculated by triangulation. We always try to have the needle tip and its contained seed at least 10 mm, and preferably a little more, from the nearest lens surface. When the

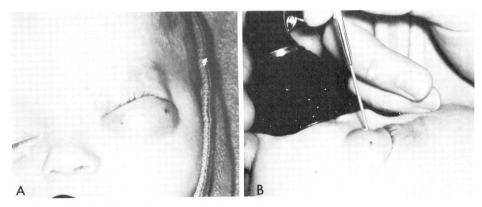

Figure 84. Technique of insertion of radon seed for treatment of hemangioma of lower quadrants of orbit. *A,* Skin is marked with suitable dye at points selected for insertion of radon; dye markers are 20 mm apart. *B,* Face mask in place for delivery of anesthetic, and spinal needle containing radon seed inserted to desired depth at nasal marker.

position seems suitable, the stylet is inserted into the needle shaft, so pushing radon seed into the tissues. Needle and stylet then are removed. Although dosage delivered to the tumor now may be calculated, the critical factor is the total roentgen dosage reaching the lens. This is the reason for such careful measurements of depth and position of the spinal needle.

Let us consider a hypothetical but rather typical case and calculate maximum amount of radiation that may reach a lens. A 4-month-old infant is observed with a hemangioma in the upper nasal quadrant of the orbit. The tumor is about 20 mm in size and has pushed the eye laterally. A seed inserted into the center of this tumor would effectively radiate all tissues in a radius of 10 millimeters. Beyond 10 millimeters roentgen dosage falls off so rapidly — because the dosage is inversely proportional to the square of the distance — that it then has virtually no effect. Let us assume that the seed is 10 mm from the edge of the lens. The maximum dosage to the nearest surface or edge of the lens would then be:

$$8.4 \text{ R. (dosage, mc-hr exposure at 10 mm)} \times 0.25$$
$$\text{(strength of seed, mc)} = 2.1 \text{ R/mc-hr} \tag{1}$$
$$132 \text{ (life of seed of 1 mc in mc-hr)} \times 2.1 \text{ R (unit per mc-hr)} = 277.2 \text{ } \gamma\text{-R.} \tag{2}$$

In this instance, the dosage delivered to the periphery of the tumor would equal the maximum dosage to the lens. If the tumor were of the same size but its center were now 15 mm from the lens periphery, the dosage to the limits of the tumor would remain the same but irradiation to the lens would decrease to:

Reciprocal of
$$\left(\frac{15}{10} \text{ mm}\right)^2 \times 277.2 \text{ R} = 123.2 \text{ } \gamma\text{-r} \tag{3}$$

the value 277.2 R being taken from equation (2) above.

For larger tumors, more seeds (of the same strength) are inserted, but they are carefully positioned in relation to the lens. The dosage from each seed is calculated separately and the sums combined to give the total irradiation to the periphery of the lens. We seldom use more than two seeds. The fact that the eye moves after recovery from anesthesia is not considered a significant influence on dosimetry.

In our experience, radiation cataract will not develop unless the lens is exposed to a radiation dosage of greater than 500 R by the techniques described previously. If the dosage is between 500 and 600 R, there is perhaps a 10% chance of a cataract developing. We prefer to use a dosage of less than 500 R when inserting one seed and we try not to exceed a total dosage of 600 R to the lens when more than one seed is inserted (Fig. 85).

CORTICOSTEROIDS. These drugs, principally prednisone, have been used for approximately 10 years. Some ophthalmologists have hailed their effect as dramatic, others have not observed long-term benefit. The object of this therapy, as with implantation of radon, is to arrest the continued growth of the hemangioma and to commence the process of involution. We encourage "wondering" parents to give corticosteroids a trial before proceeding with radon implantation

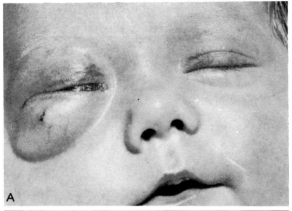

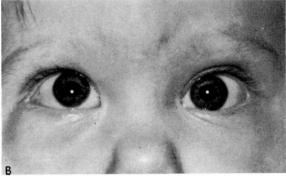

Figure 85. Results of treatment of orbital hemangioma with radon. *A*, Hemangioma filling inferior portion of right orbit and concealing eye; three radon seeds (each 0.25 mc) were inserted in triangular pattern (apex of triangle posteriorly). *B*, Appearance 4 months after insertion of radon; eye still displaced superiorly.

so as to be sure all conservative measures have been given a fair therapeutic trial.

We usually suggest a 3- to 4-week program of prednisone (dosage depending on age of child but approximately 2 mg/kg per day) followed by a 7- to 10-day tapering period. In some patients this regimen has had no effect but in others a definite decrease in the size of the tumor has been noted. However, in none of those who improved was improvement sustained; the hemangioma returned to the same size as or even larger than it was before (Fig. 86). Another course of steroids can be suggested at this pont, but there comes a time when the side effects of repeated or long-term steroid therapy outweigh their potential advantage.

CAVERNOUS HEMANGIOMA

CLINICAL FEATURES

This is the most frequent primary benign neoplasm of the orbit (age and sex incidence are noted in Table 6). As such, its clinical course is a model for the diagnostic pattern so often observed with other slow-growing neoplasms and cysts, such as epidermoid cyst, neurilemmoma, solitary neurofibroma, and

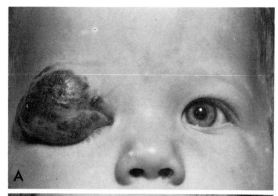

Figure 86. Results of treatment of eyelid hemangioma with steroids.

A, Hemangioma of right upper eyelid, present since birth; prednisone (25 mg daily for 19 days) was administered orally.

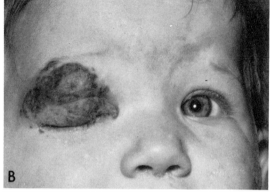

B, Appearance after prednisone therapy and before insertion of radon.

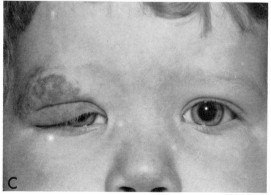

C, Ten months after insertion of two radon seeds (each, 0.32 mc).

hemangiopericytoma. The principal feature of this pattern is the remarkable ability of the eye and eyelids to maintain reasonably normal protection, visual function, and motility of the eye for long periods in the presence of a slowly progressive proptosis due to an enlarging, unyielding mass.

Initially, the problem commences as a forward protrusion of the eye which may go unnoticed for many months. One or two years later the average patient will notice some blurring or fleeting obscuration of vision due to pressure of the expanding mass on the eyeball. By this time the proptosis of the affected eye will measure about 4 to 5 mm, an induced hyperopia will be evident on refraction, and ophthalmoscopy may reveal choroidal folds along some portion of the ocular wall. At this time some restriction of ocular motility or diplopia in extreme directions of gaze may also become evident, but diplopia in the primary position is absent or fleeting in nature. As time goes on, displacement of the eye will appear in a direction opposite to the site of the tumor. A physician observing such a situation for the first time is further perplexed that no mass is palpable (about 40% of cases).

Of course, there are exceptions. Loss of central visual acuity may occur very early in conjunction with proptosis should the hemangioma be located at the orbital apex. Here, the clinical picture would resemble meningioma. Or, a mass may be palpable within the first year of onset because the tumor is more forward in the orbit. Actually, cavernous hemangioma may locate anywhere in the orbit but it tends to favor the temporal quadrants (infantile hemangioma favors the nasal quadrants), posteriorly or anteriorly, superiorly or inferiorly. On palpation the tumor is firm and smoothly contoured. Occasionally, a reddish mass will suddenly appear near the caruncle or push into the conjunctival cul de sac. These bright red tumors are a clue to the type of mischief concealed posteriorly.

Up to this point the patient may put off surgical therapy, but as the months pass, the eye and adnexa no longer compensate for the enlarging tumor. Dull headaches are noted on the side of the tumor, recurrent subconjunctival hemorrhages appear, and the induced anisometropia is no longer easily corrected. Finally, the patient realizes there is no alternative to surgical exploration.

Special Studies.   The patient's willingness to proceed with surgery has been greatly enhanced in recent years by the almost routine use of ultrasonography or computer tomography. These modalities furnish positive information to the patient that a tumor is present, information that usually was not present in former years when only roentgenology was available. It is true that standard roentgenography would occasionally show some slight orbital enlargement or fossa formation on the side of the proptosis, but this was not necessarily specific for cavernous hemangioma and did not impress the patient.

Combined A and B ultrasound will confirm the rounded, regular contour of the suspected hemangioma. Sound transmission across the tumor is good with some internal reflectivity (Fig. 46A). However, when the patient sees the round or ovoid, well-delineated mass — large in size relative to the confines of the bony orbit — on computer tomography (Fig. 36), his doubts about the need for surgery are dispelled. Enhancement of the tumor shadow with contrast techniques is not always present.

PATHOLOGY

The cavernous hemangioma is the classic, encapsulated tumor of the orbit. The capsule, which is made up of fibrous tissue, provides an excellent cleavage plane for dissection and is thick enough to give the excised tumor a firm contour, even though its interior is semi-cystic (Fig. 87). The surface of the tumor is smooth and, at times, slightly bosselated. The shape of the tumor will depend somewhat on its size and where it is located in the orbit. Small tumors are

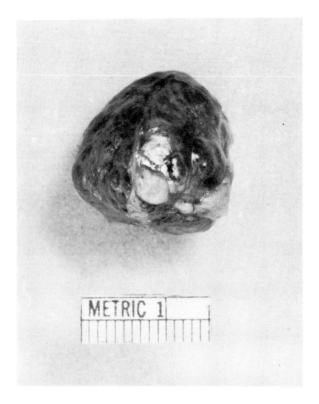

Figure 87. Cavernous hemangioma: slow expansile growth may result in capsule-like mantle, enhancing complete excision.

round or ovoid, but larger ones may be flattened along one side if they have pressed against some orbital structure that has resisted their expansion. Occasionally, a large hemangioma of long duration in the rear of the orbit will have a somewhat pyramidal shape because its surfaces have been in contact with both the optic nerve and the eyeball near their juncture. The tumors are a reddish-blue or reddish-purple color and the shortest diameter of the excised tumor seldom is less than 15 mm.

When bisected, the tumor may have an almost sponge-like consistency, the numerous dilated, cavernous-like, blood-filled spaces will be easily seen (Fig. 88). Under higher magnification the flattened endothelium lining the dilated vascular spaces is evident (Fig. 89). This endothelium may look quite attenuated and stretched in some of the larger spaces of older hemangiomas where the supporting stroma has become fibrosed secondary to pressure factors and age. In some zones of the tumor the cavernous spaces may be so numerous and so closely packed that only a thin layer of connective tissue separates one ectatic area from another. In other areas the connective tissue stroma is more loose and may contain a few fat cells, proliferating capillaries, or a small foci of inflammatory cells.

TREATMENT

If an orbital surgeon performing a lateral orbitotomy for the first time away from teacher and home training base could choose one tumor for a

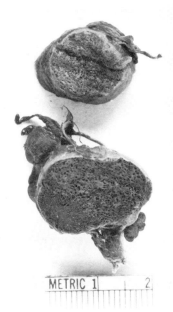

Figure 88. Cavernous hemangioma: dilated, blood-filled channels impart a sponge-like appearance to the tumor.

debut — select one tumor that would quiet the secret fear of not being able to find the tumor on the initial sally beyond the bone orbital barrier — cavernous hemangioma would be the logical choice. Its large size, its striking color, its common position in the temporal orbit make it one of the easiest tumors to locate once the soft tissues have been opened above or below the lateral rectus muscle. Its apparent attachment to other structures in the orbital cavity is deceptive because its discrete border assures intact detachment with gentle blunt

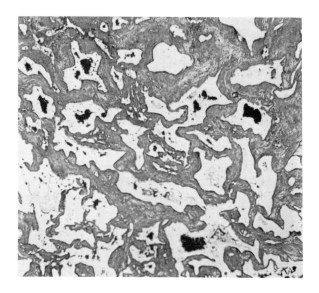

Figure 89. Cavernous hemangioma: dilated, blood-filled channels lined by flattened endothelial cells. (Hematoxylin and eosin; ×28.)

dissection. We have found the cryoprobe a particularly useful instrument for applying fixation and traction on the smooth surface of the tumor. We now use this instrument routinely for this purpose as a replacement for the tenaculums and grasping forceps of former years that so often tore the surface of the tumor in the course of its surgical mobilization. Also, we have found that cotton tip applicators are most useful devices for stripping away the tissue attachments along the visible surface of the tumor. We use them in preference to other dissectors and find that bleeding is reduced. On the masked side of the tumor, particularly when it abuts against the optic nerve or eyeball, the surgeon's forefinger is an ideal means for separating the tumor from surrounding important structures while maintaining an accurate sense of position. When the tumor is delivered there follows a gush of venous bleeding that originates from the detached feeder vessels deep in the orbit. We stop this bleeding by inserting a small gauze packing and allowing it to remain in place for the 5- to 10-minute interval required for frozen tissue study of the specimen.

Our object is always intact removal of the tumor without incisional biopsy. The effect on the preoperative proptosis is most striking and the patient's acceptance of the postoperative result is gratifying. Even so, the induced preoperative hyperopia and the acquired choroidal folds may require many months to disappear.

Some ophthalmologists will incompletely excise the tumor if they are reluctant to disturb the attachment of the tumor to structures in the apex of the orbit. We know of instances of this type where the hemangiomas did not recur and we suspect that small tags of residual tumor can be obliterated by fibrosis. However, on the basis of patients who have had regrowth of the neoplasm after incomplete excision elsewhere, we believe that recurrence is the rule. Furthermore, the growth of the tumor may be more rapid and aggressive compared with its course prior to the first surgical procedure. Removal of a recurrent hemangioma can be most difficult and one of the last things a neophyte orbital surgeon would wish to tackle on a first orbitotomy.

In the surgical approach to the hemangiomas, bleeding and capillary oozing from soft tissue structures some distance from the tumor may be surprisingly large in amount or persistent in degree. The experienced surgeon recognizes this as a tell-tale clue to a probable underlying cavernous hemangioma.

HEMANGIOENDOTHELIOMA

TERMINOLOGY AND ORIGIN

A concise and factual dissertation on this neoplasm is not easy, for several reasons. First, a revision of the nomenclature of malignant vascular tumors about 35 years ago resulted in a more restricted definition of hemangioendothelioma. Second, owing to this more restrictive terminology, the incidence of the tumor in the orbit consequently becomes meager. No one person has observed enough of these tumors in the orbit to enable him to publish an authoritative review.

In any discussion of hemangioendothelioma and its related tumor, hemangiopericytoma, the name of Stout (1943) invariably is mentioned. Stout wrote several articles on the subject of vascular tumors and, concerning orbital vascular tumors, the two most widely quoted are those of 1942 (with Murray) and 1943. Before these reports, and even for some time thereafter, most cellular vascular tumors were included under the term hemangoendotheliomas. As a result of Stout's studies, hemangiopericytoma became recognized as a separate entity. Cases of vascular tumors of the orbit in the files of the Mayo Clinic were then reviewed with attention to these revisions in classification and nomenclature. All prior cases diagnosed as hemangioendothelioma were found more nearly to conform to a classification of hemangiopericytoma. Thereafter, and up to the present time, no examples of malignant hemangioendothelioma of the orbit were observed, accounting for absence of this tumor in our study series. The infantile type of hemangioendothelioma is the tumor we already have discussed as an immature variant of capillary hemangioma. Our own preference is to eliminate the term hemangioendothelioma in reference to infantile, juvenile, or hypertrophic hemangiomas but to retain it only in conjunction with the designation malignant hemangioendothelioma. We do not consider angiosarcoma a suitable term because it implies the tumor has a nonendothelial malignant component.

Since Stout's publications, there have been few additional examples of orbital malignant hemangioendothelioma in the literature. Stout reported one case (case 12) wherein this tumor seemed primary in the orbit. Another case of malignant hemangioendothelioma of the orbit was noted in Forrest's series. Photographs of the histologic details of this case also were included, but Forrest was unable to provide information concerning clinical details. Jakobiec and Jones were aware of approximately six orbital cases that were on file at the Armed Forces Institute of Pathology and two reports, one child and one adult, have been recorded in the Japanese literature of Tsuda and Takaku 1970, Sekimoto and associates 1971. Other cases of hemangioendothelioma reported in adults, seem to be examples of arrested juvenile and hypertrophic hemangiomas or benign hemangiomas showing regressive changes (sclerosing and calcifying hemangiomas).

CLINICAL FEATURES

Stout's case (1943) seems to have been the sole source of information for this facet of malignant hemangioendothelioma. His patient was a 40-year-old woman in whom a mass in the upper nasal quadrant of the orbit caused proptosis of one eye and diplopia of 3 months' duration. The tumor extended posteriorly beneath the roof of the orbit and was 2 cm long. Partial resection was performed, and 3 years later another orbitotomy was required because of recurrence. Three years later, the patient was apparently still living, but here the trail ended.

PATHOLOGY

A review of the normal histology of the basic unit of the vascular system, the capillary, is helpful in understanding the features upon which Stout revised the classification. All endothelial-lined tubes and spaces have a basement membrane of reticulin (Fig. 90). Peripheral to this layer of reticulin are other cells and tissues which contribute to the function of vascular channels. In veins and arteries a variable layer of smooth muscle fulfills this function. In capillaries, the corresponding layer is represented by the pericyte. This cell is thought to have some contractile properties and, histologically, is similar in appearance to the endothelial cell. When either cell proliferates, as in neoplasms, differentiation may be difficult unless a reticulin binding stain is used. If proliferating cells are outside the reticulin sheath of the capillary wall, the tumor is termed a hemangiopericytoma. If many-layered, endothelial-like cells are seen within the reticulin sheath, the term hemangioendothelioma is appropriate.

The relationship of proliferating cells to either a supporting or surrounding mantle of reticulin is widely quoted in opthalmic literature as the chief differential point. It is based on Stout's suggestion that in cases of doubt with ordinary stains "the relationships can be clarified by the use of a silver reticulin stain." Stout perhaps intended this as a supplementary aid rather than the main criterion for diagnosis. Actually, in cases of hemangioendothelioma, Stout put more emphasis on the appearance of individual endothelial cells proliferating within the lumen of the capillary. Furthermore, Stout believed that the prolifer-

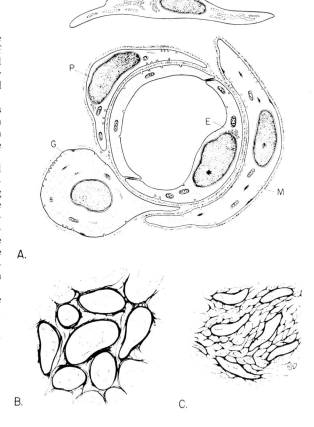

Figure 90. A, Schematic drawing of the component cells of vascular channels. Endothelial cells (E) create the capillary tubes. Pericytes (P) are arranged alongside the endothelial cells. Smooth muscle cells (M). Glomus cells (G) are specialized smooth muscle cells. Fibroblasts (F) can be found in the connective tissue adjacent to the vascular spaces. *B,* When neoplastic endothelial cells proliferate (hemangioendothelioma) they create a nesting arrangement outlined by the reticulin stain. *C,* When neoplastic pericytes proliferate (hemangiopericytoma) they occupy the interstitial spaces between the benign-appearing capillary channels. Reticulin fibers are shown surrounding the tumor pericytes. (Slightly modified from: Jakobiec FA, Howard GM, Jones IS, et al: Hemangiopericytoma of the orbit. Am J Ophthalmol 78:816–834, 1974. By permission.)

ating endothelial layer could become so exuberant in growth as to occasionally extend outside the vascular tube. In this neoplasm, the lining cell takes on the following atypical features: an increase in the number of cells that ordinarily would be required to line a vascular channel of such small caliber, alterations in size and shape of cells, and an accentuation of the usual staining properties. In addition, the vascular channels have free anastomoses and possess only a delicate framework of reticulin fibers. Based on their behavior in areas other than the orbit, these tumors are locally aggressive and have the potential for metastasis.

HEMANGIOPERICYTOMA

TERMINOLOGY AND ORIGIN

Zimmermann (1923), a Swiss histologist, described a contractile cell related to smooth muscle that wound and wrapped itself about capillaries. This cell he termed a *pericyte*. The tumor that features the abnormal proliferation of this cell is called hemangiopericytoma, the name having been coined by Stout and Murray (1942). Prior to its separate designation, cases of hemangiopericytoma were probably classified as hemangioendothelioma or hemangiosarcoma. The concept that hemangiopericytoma is a separate and distinct entity among the group of vascular tumors is now widely accepted.

INCIDENCE

A considerable volume of literature has accumulated about this tumor since it was newly named almost 40 years ago. Most of these articles have been concerned with various clinical and pathologic features of hemangiopericytoma in their more common locations — the pelvic retroperitoneal spaces and the somatic soft tissues of the neck, limbs, trunk, and paraspinal areas. Its vascular origin contributes to this ubiquitous distribution. The tumor is not common in the orbit, but a number of reports in the ophthalmic literature dealing with single cases, supplemented by a review of seven cases (Jakobiec et al 1974) and our own eleven primary hemangiopericytomas (Henderson and Farrow 1978), have added substantial information concerning the course of the tumor in the orbit. Our clinical series of 11 primary orbital hemangiopericytomas is unique in respect to total number (at time of this writing) and the long-term contact with most of the patients (eight of the patients were followed eleven years or longer).

Hemangiopericytomas may be primary in the orbit, secondarily invade the orbit from an adjacent sinus, or metastasize to the orbit from a distant focus. Our survey of orbital tumors over a 27-year period contains examples of each of these modes of orbital involvement. Incidence data relating to sex and age are summarized in Table 7.

These 13 hemangiopericytomas comprise 1.7% of the total 764 orbital tumors of our survey, and the incidence of primary hemangiopericytoma among all 340 primary tumors is 3.2%. The sex incidence is nearly equal, with a slight preponderance of females — a finding in agreement with larger surveys of

TABLE 7.   AGE AND SEX DISTRIBUTION OF 13 ORBITAL HEMANGIOPERICYTOMAS

Male	Female		Age in Years at Time of Orbital Diagnosis						
			11–20	*21 – 30*	*31–40*	*41–50*	*51–60*	*61–70*	*Over 70*
5	6	Primary		2	2	5	1		1
	1	Secondary				1			
	1	Metastatic	1						

patients with hemangiopericytomas of somatic soft tissue. In determining the age range of patients with hemangiopericytoma it is more valid to ascertain the age at onset of orbital symptoms or signs because of the long interval that may pass between onset and definitive diagnosis. Duration of symptoms was known in all but one of the eleven patients with primary orbital hemangiopericytoma. The age range recalculated on this basis was then 19 to 48 years, with an approximate median of 41 years. We have not observed an orbital hemangiopericytoma in a child or infant, but these tumors are known to occur in the somatic soft tissues of the young.

CLINICAL FEATURES

Primary Hemangiopericytoma.   This is a slow-growing, painless, circumscribed neoplasm. Progressive proptosis is the chief clinical sign but occasionally may be preceded by some puffiness of the eyelid. The course is so insidious and so uneventful from the patient's viewpoint that symptoms may extend from several years to several decades before the patient seeks medical consultation. It is not unexpected, then, that the tumor may reach considerable size. Three of our eleven patients had neoplasms that were 4 by 3 cm or larger in diameter at the time of excision. In these clinical features hemangiopericytoma resembles cavernous hemangioma.

In all but one of our eleven patients, the tumor was located in the superior quadrants of the orbit. The more anterior, palpable tumors usually were located superior-nasally but those nonpalpable, posterior masses were found in the superior temporal quadrant. In a few cases, vascularization of the caruncle or dilated vessels in adjacent adnexa served as tell-tale clues to the vascular nature of the tumor (Fig. 91), but these clues were not sufficiently specific to differentiate this tumor from a possible cavernous hemangioma or lymphangioma.

In all but one patient standard roentgenographic orbital views were negative. Enlargement of the affected orbit was noted in the one exception, but this bony alteration was nonspecific in differentiating hemangiopericytoma from other slow-growing tumors. Neither is there any feature on computer tomography which will differentiate hemangiopericytoma from a cavernous hemangioma. On ultrasonography the A-scan may show a more solid tumor than is seen with cavernous hemangioma.

Secondary Hemangiopericytoma.   The one case of secondary orbital invasion noted in our study was a 42-year-old woman who had had 2 operations in the 5 years before admission, and 2 more radical operations in the 5 years after admission because of extension of tumor into the orbit from the antrum. Metastasis to the pleura finally occurred and the patient expired 13 years after onset.

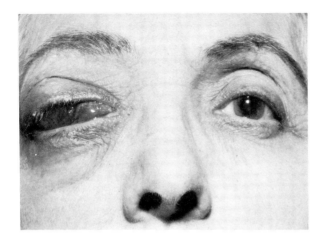

Figure 91. Hemangiopericytoma: lateral and upward displacement of right eye due to forward bulging of tumor (5 cm in diameter) in lower nasal quadrant. Reddish discoloration of overlying soft tissues suggested vascular origin of this tumor, which was excised.

Metastatic Hemangiopericytoma. The one case in our series with orbital metastasis may be unique in the literature on hemangiopericytoma. The patient was a 19-year-old girl with a mass in the upper nasal quadrant of the left orbit. A hemangiopericytoma had been removed from the primary site in the left costal area 9 months previously. Two months prior to admission, metastasis had appeared in the lung. The patient expired 3 months after admission with multiple metastasis including the other orbit.

PATHOLOGY

Hemangiopericytoma is a vascular tumor with a varying number of capillary-like spaces or channels scattered throughout (Fig. 92). The number of the channels is in roughly inverse proportion to the density of surrounding, prolif-

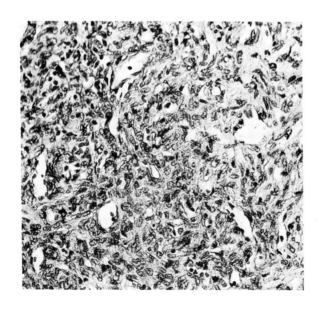

Figure 92. Benign hemangiopericytoma: capillary channels are lined by flattened endothelium, and cells proliferating around and between these channels are pericytes. (Hematoxylin and eosin; × 250.)

erating pericytes; that is, the greater the matrix of neoplastic cells, the more sparse and crowded are the acellular channels (erythrocytes excluded). A feature of the capillary spaces is the normal, unicellullar lining of endothelial cells which have narrow slender nuclei. Around the capillary and outside its reticulin sheath are closely packed, crowded aggregates of pericytes. The nuclei of these cells may show transitional forms from ovoid to elongated, spindle-shaped structures; the latter are probably but a step or two away, along the ladder of differentiation, from smooth muscle cells. In most orbital specimens we have observed, these nuclei appeared to be shaped as rounded spindles. Some authors have dubbed them plump. If silver stains are applied to this tissue, a network of reticulin fibers surrounding groups and clusters of pericytes may be observed (Fig. 93).

In the histopathologic assessment, our eleven cases were classified as *benign, borderline malignancy*, and *malignant* on the basis of composite degree of cellular anaplasia, prominence of vascular pattern, shape of the pericytes, number of mitotic figures per high power field, and the amount of reticulin. With these criteria, four of the tumors were benign, four were borderline malignant at their initial study and before recurrence, and two were malignant. In one borderline malignant case the morphologic features of the tumor remained essentially the same during the 15-year interval between successive microscopic examinations, except that the vascular pattern was less prominent in the later sample (Fig. 94). In another borderline malignant case the study of successive tissue specimens indicated a definite malignant progression during the 9-year interval between surgical procedures (Fig. 95). A malignant hemangiopericytoma at the time of initial surgical exploration is illustrated in Fig. 96.

Grossly, hemangiopericytomas are red, reddish-blue, or even pink in color. Usually the tumor is described as encapsulated (Fig. 97). Histologic study confirmed the presence of a pseudocapsule in the majority of our cases, but two of

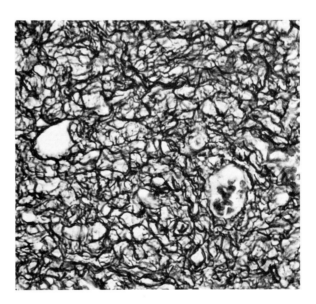

Figure 93. Hemangiopericytoma: network of black-staining reticulin fibers demonstrates that proliferation of cells is peripheral to the two vascular channels in section. (Reticulin stain; ×405.)

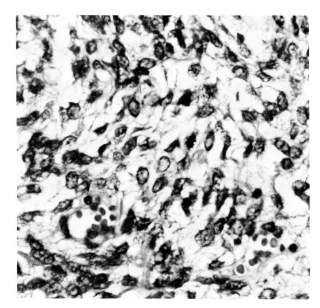

Figure 94. Borderline malignant hemangiopericytoma. Compressed, occult vascular channels containing erythrocytes are surrounded by compact mass of plump spindle cells. An occasional mitotic figure may be seen. (Hematoxylin and eosin; ×640.)

our series were infiltrative. The pseudocapsule, when present, was not as thick as the capsular tissue usually observed with cavernous hemangiomas of equal duration. The formation of a delimiting interface between the tumor and host probably depends on the resistance of orbital tissues to the growth of the neoplasm. Thus hemangiopericytomas growing in the more narrow and restrictive confines of the posterior orbit will likely possess a thicker delimiting interface than similar tumors in many other anatomic sites.

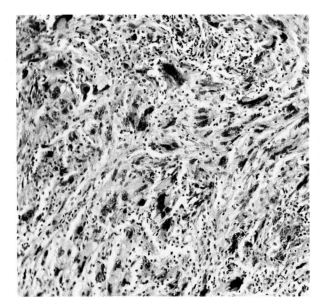

Figure 95. Highly anaplastic, malignant hemangiopericytoma recurring 9 years after incomplete excision. (Hematoxylin and eosin; ×160.)

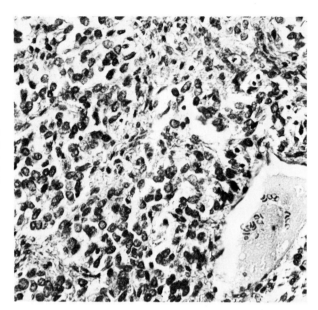

Figure 96. Malignant hemangiopericytoma. Vascular spaces are generally occult, and neoplasm is composed of bizarre hyperchromatic cells. (Hematoxylin and eosin; × 400.)

TREATMENT AND COURSE

In Table 8 we have listed data pertaining to the course and treatment of our eleven cases of primary orbital hemangiopericytoma. It is evident that the longest tumor-free survivals are in those patients who have had either a complete removal or a piecemeal excision of the neoplasm. On the other hand, in all four patients *in whom only an incomplete excision of the tumor was performed, recurrences were the rule.* Three of the deaths were among this group

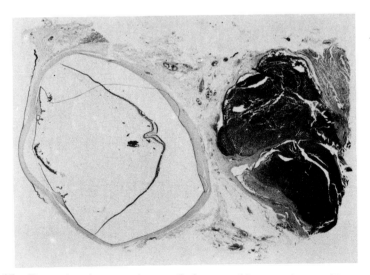

Figure 97. Hemangiopericytoma: circumscribed nature of lesion is obvious. (Hematoxylin and eosin; × 2½.)

TABLE 8. COURSE, TREATMENT, AND HISTOPATHOLOGIC CLASSIFICATION OF 11 CONSECUTIVE PRIMARY ORBITAL HEMANGIOPERICYTOMAS

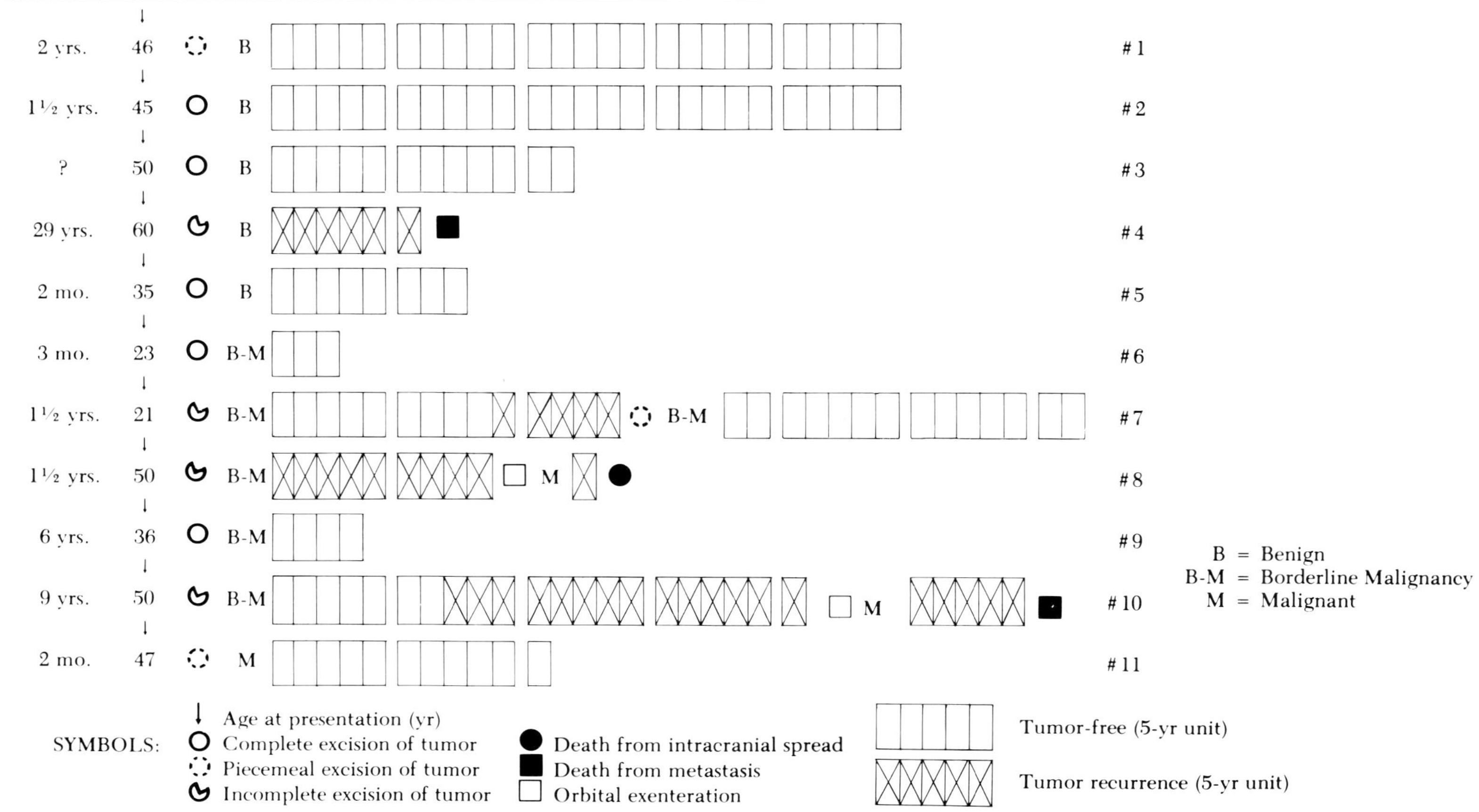

Duration of Symptoms	Age at presentation (yr)		Case
2 yrs.	46	B	#1
1½ yrs.	45	B	#2
?	50	B	#3
29 yrs.	60	B	#4
2 mo.	35	B	#5
3 mo.	23	B-M	#6
1½ yrs.	21	B-M	#7
1½ yrs.	50	B-M	#8
6 yrs.	36	B-M	#9
9 yrs.	50	B-M	#10
2 mo.	47	M	#11

B = Benign
B-M = Borderline Malignancy
M = Malignant

☐ Tumor-free (5-yr unit)
☒ Tumor recurrence (5-yr unit)

SYMBOLS:

→ Age at presentation (yr)
○ Complete excision of tumor
◌ Piecemeal excision of tumor
◗ Incomplete excision of tumor

● Death from intracranial spread
■ Death from metastasis
☐ Orbital exenteration

of four. The fourth patient (case 7), however, was tumor-free 14 years after a piecemeal excision of the first recurrence.

The circumscribed nature of most hemangiopericytomas should encourage their intact removal, but, because of their size or their location near the optic nerve, surgeons are prone either to remove them piecemeal or be satisfied with only an incomplete excision lest the surgical manipulation of an intact delivery injure the optic nerve. Although intact removal of tumor should be the ideal goal, it is satisfying to learn that the survival interval of patients who underwent piecemeal removal (cases 1, 7, and 11), so long as it is thorough, seems to approach the tumor-free period of patients who had intact excision of their tumor.

In two (cases 7 and 10) of the four patients who had only an incomplete removal of neoplasm, recurrences did not appear until a lapse of 8 or 9 years after the initial orbitotomy. This attests to the long indolent growth of many hemangiopericytomas. Therefore, we suggest that no patient who has had an incomplete or a piecemeal excision of tumor should be considered free of possible recurrence until 10 years have elapsed from the time of the initial surgery. The prognosis of patients with recurrent tumor is grave. Once a recurrrence has appeared radical surgery may be the only means of preventing fatal termination, providing occult metastasis has not already occurred.

The mortality rate of patients with orbital hemangiopericytoma of long duration or those whose tumor was incompletely removed is not generally known because most cases reported in the literature have not been followed for a sufficient number of postoperative years. This fact became known to us because it was possible to follow two of our fatal cases for a period longer than 30 years (cases 4 and 10). There are only a very few other neoplasms with malignant potential (malignant melanoma, carcinoma of the breast and ovary) where a life span of more than 30 years is possible from the time of initial surgical intervention.

Although most tumors behaved in a predictable pattern on the basis of their histologic appearance, there were several exceptions. In case 4 the tumor appeared benign but the patient was dead 6 years later. This attests to the aggressive behavior of some hemangiopericytomas even though they appear histologically benign, a fact also recognized in the behavior of hemangiopericytomas of somatic soft tissues. On the other hand was the malignant appearance of the tumor in case 11, the patient still survives 11 years after diagnosis. In case 7 the borderline malignant appearance of the tumor did not significantly change in the 14-year interval between successive histopathologic examinations. Therefore, *a definite relationship between clinical course and histopathologic classification could not be made in our limited series.*

We do not believe radiotherapy has anymore than a palliative effect on this tumor.

VASCULAR LEIOMYOMA

TERMINOLOGY AND ORIGIN

The cell type of this tumor is smooth muscle, but the smooth muscle of blood vessel walls rather than the muscular fibers of organs such as bowel or heart (Fig. 98). Although the contractile properties of the smooth muscle are similar in all structures (blood vessels as well as organs), we prefer to place this particular tumor within our vascular group rather than classify it with other smooth muscle neoplasms. We believe the blood vessel wall is the principal aberrant structure, taking precedence over the smooth muscle component as the basis for classification. In some cases, however, smooth muscle proliferation may dominate histopathologic sections. It is important to establish this difference between vascular leiomyomas and true leiomyomas of nonvascular origin, because these orbital tumors usually have been indexed under the nonvascular designation. We doubt that a true leiomyoma really exists in the orbit. Instead, we suspect that most of the very few reported examples of orbital leiomyomas are vascular leiomyomas. *Venous hemangioma* also is an acceptable term, for the majority of these neoplasms probably are associated with walls of small veins; *hemangio-leiomyoma* is another suitable synonym.

INCIDENCE

In a survey of "leiomyomas" of the orbit, Nath and Shukla (1963) reported gradual protrusion of one eye during a period of 2 years in an 18-year-old girl. An encapsulated tumor was removed from the apex of the orbit. They believed their case was the seventh to be recorded in the literature. A more recent report was that of Wolter (1965), who noted a definite example of this tumor in a 41-year-old man. This tumor also was encapsulated, which permitted complete removal from its position within retrobulbar space. It was smooth-walled, lobulated and dark red. To this group we can add the one case from our own series, already reported by Henderson and Harrison (1970). The most recent reports are those of Jakobiec and associates (1973), Jakobiec et al (1975), and Sanborn and associates (1979). Three orbital cases were recorded, a 25-year-old male, a 34-year-old female, and a 5-year-old boy, respectively. In all instances the tumor was encapsulated but incompletely excised. In the 1975 publication

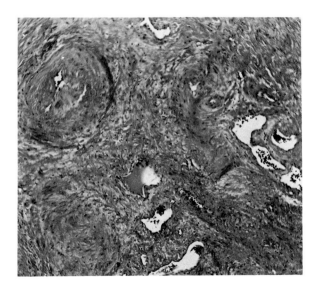

Figure 98. Vascular leiomyoma: principal tissue is smooth muscle, apparently arising from outer muscular coats of prominent, thick-walled vascular channels. (Hematoxylin and eosin; × 60.)

of Jakobiec et al another case was noted in a 17-year-old male, but the tumor seemed anterior to the orbital septum, was attached to the orbital rim, but was not associated with proptosis. We could not classify this case as originating in the orbit. In summary, there are probably no more than a dozen examples of primary orbital vascular leiomyoma in the literature. Most of these tumors have been observed in young to middle age adults.

CLINICAL FEATURES

The growth of these tumors in the orbit is characterized by slowly progressive proptosis or displacement of the eye, negligible interference with ocular functions, and definite delimitation from surrounding tissues. These features are associated with most benign encapsulated tumors in this area. Some patients also may note intermittent episodes of pain, a feature not common to other benign growth. Such pain, if present, is attributed to the vascular makeup of the tumor. Because clinical descriptions of these neoplasms are so infrequent, we summarize the features of the case encountered in our survey.

The patient was a 9-year-old girl, one of the youngest patients so far recorded. Her parents had noticed a slight upward displacement of the right eye for 3 months. A mass was palpable in the lower temporal quadrant, but it was located too posteriorly for accurate assessment of size and consistency. A history of intermittent enlargement associated with exercise suggested a possible vascular component in the mass. Roentgenograms indicated calcification of part of the tumor. An oval, encapsulated, tan tumor was then removed by inferior orbitotomy. Brisk bleeding from a profuse blood supply was observed at the time of excision. Convalescence was uneventful.

PATHOLOGY

An important criterion of correct diagnosis of these neoplasms is the demonstration of myofibrils. Identification of these fine, discrete longitudinal striations confirms that the preponderant tissue is smooth muscle, but special stains are required (Fig. 99). As such stains were not available when some earlier cases were reported, it is doubtful whether all surveyed cases are true vascular leiomyomas. Without myofibrils, the spindle-shaped cells might be confused with pericytes and the tumor might then be called hemangiopericytoma rather than a vascular leiomyoma, for both surround endothelial-lined spaces.

Electron microscopy also may be used to differentiate borderline cases. The cells of a vascular leiomyoma will show cytoplasmic filaments with fusiform densities characteristic of smooth muscle.

Smooth muscle fibers of these tumors interlace and flow in different directions, so the muscle is cut in cross section, obliquely, as well as in parallel rows (Fig. 100). Some muscle bundles are arranged around vascular spaces, but most bundles flow independently through the tissue specimen. Vascular spaces are prominent in this tumor, a pattern very similar to hemangiopericytoma.

The nuclei are long, are somewhat flattened, and have rounded ends with small nucleoli. Sometimes there is a palisade arrangement of nuclei. Reticulin fibers surrounding smooth muscle bundles and elastic fibers within the walls of small vessels also are identified by special stains. There is no anaplasia or mitotic activity to suggest malignancy.

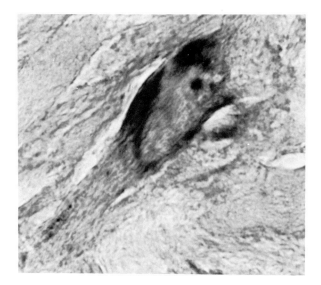

Figure 99. Vascular leiomyoma: fine, discrete, longitudinal striations (myofibrils) in section of myoma. (Phosphotungstic acid and hematoxylin; ×1,200.) (From Henderson JW, Harrison EG Jr: Vascular leiomyoma of the orbit: report of a case. Trans Am Acad Ophthalmol Otolaryngol 74:970–974, 1970. By permission of the American Academy of Ophthalmology and Otolaryngology.)

TREATMENT

The preferred management is complete excision of the tumor. This should not be difficult unless the mass is situated deep in the orbit or is attached to a vital structure. Encapsulation permits complete delivery, unless the capsule is broken during incisional biopsy. In our one case, bleeding was profuse at the time of orbitotomy, but this annoying feature was not observed in Wolter's case (1965). In one of these cases recorded by Jakobiec et al (1975) a recurrence of tumor developed seven years after incomplete excision.

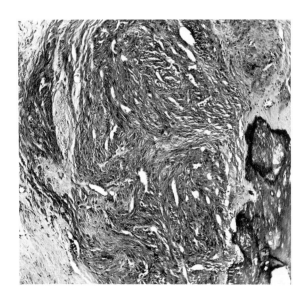

Figure 100. Vascular leiomyoma (same case as in Figure 99). Interlacing bundles of smooth muscle cells stream from wall of irregular vascular spaces lined by endothelium; the lighter staining areas are connective tissue; the darker, calcification. (Hematoxylin and eosin; ×55.)

LYMPHANGIOMA

This tumor and the infantile hemangiomas described in the first part of this chapter are siblings in the sense that they share a common parent cell; this cell has the potential for differentiation into either capillaries or lymph channels. The lymphangioma represents an aberration on the latter side of the family tree, but occasionally the two tumors are so combined as to mix the pretty color of one (hemangioma) with the ugly disposition of the other (lymphangioma). Technically, lymphangiomas also are benign but sometimes so aggressive and persistent that a less bland designation would be more appropriate. Their presence in the orbit is very annoying to the parents of a child who has such a tumor, most frustrating to the ophthalmologist who must manage such an affair, and quite cosmetically disabling to an adult who daily looks in the mirror at the blood tinged lobules that sometimes extend onto the face or eyelids.

HISTORICAL ASPECTS

Lymphangioma of the orbit, as a definite entity, has been known for over 100 years (Wecker, 1868) — a shorter period of recognition than for hemangioma. A report by Ayres, in 1895, seems to have been the first publication on this subject in the American literature. This report is one of the first in the literature and, considering the inaccessibility of foreign journals in those earlier years, the discussion is remarkably complete. Ayres noted problems of nomenclature as well as arguments about pathogenesis. To remove the tumor completely, Ayres had to enucleate the eye of his patient.

Since then, hemangioma has become known as one of the most frequent tumors primary in the orbit, but lymphangioma still remains one of the less frequent neoplasms — at least if judged solely by the literature. Up to 1959 only 34 cases of lymphangioma were recorded in the literature. Then, in 1959, Ira S. Jones, in a thesis submitted to the American Ophthalmological Society, added 29 cases of orbital lymphangioma he had studied and gave a complete dissertation on lymphangioma as it affects other ocular adnexal tissues as well. No new material of significance has appeared in the literature since this publication.

INCIDENCE

Lymphangiomas are much less frequent than hemangiomas and, considering the perverseness of the former, it is fortunate we do not have to contend with this stubborn tumor more often. Incidence statistics relating to orbital lymphangiomas are variable and subject to some scrutiny because of probable inclusion of some lymphangiomas of the eyelids and conjunctiva, cases of lymphangiectasia, and hemangiomas that have an admixture of lymphangioma. Five cases were observed in the period of our survey. This is an incidence of 1.4% of all primary tumors (342 cases) but an incidence of less than 1% of all tumors in our series. A much higher incidence — 39 cases or approximately 8% of the total 508 orbital tumors — is noted in the series of Reese (1971). The sex distribution often is not stated. Two of our patients were males; three patients were females. Lymphangiomas may be seen from early infancy on up to middle adulthood but are most prevalent in the first decade.

CLINICAL FEATURES

The symptomatology of lymphangioma closely parallels that of infantile hemangioma in the pediatric age group. Features common to both are: similarities in color and consistency; a tendency of the tumor to fluctuate in size with changes in posture, exertion, and straining; and displacement of the eye in a vertical or horizontal direction as the tumor seeks egress from the orbit. Indeed, while the tumors are still confined to the orbital cavity and covered by the orbital septum, a specific diagnosis of either neoplasm is not possible without histologic study. Actually, parts of the same mass may look like lymphangioma and others may look like infantile hemangioma. However, as the situation progresses or as the case is analyzed in more detail, several clinical features may suggest a diagnosis of lymphangioma rather than hemangioma.

Both neoplasms may be multicentric. With hemangiomas, other hemangiomas may be found on the neck, trunk, or extremities. With lymphangiomas, additional tumors more often are confined to the head and face. Soft vascular tumors in the mouth, cheek, forehead, caruncle, and eyelids, in addition to the orbital lesion, suggest lymphangioma (Fig. 101). Sometimes the entire size of an orbital lymphangioma is uncertain because of extensive involve-

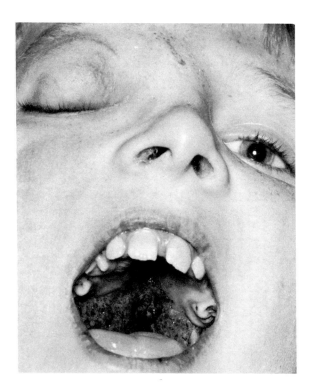

Figure 101. Lymphangioma: tumors in roof of mouth and right eye. Eye was completely covered by lymphangioma involving eyelid, forehead, and orbit.

ment of ocular adnexa and surface of the eye. Involvement of epibulbar structures is not common in infants.

The color of both tumors is so similar that it is not possible to differentiate one from the other except that, when incised or biopsied, lymphangiomas are not as vascular as their color suggests. However, lymphangiomas are more likely to bleed suddenly within the confines of the mass than are hemangiomas. Bleeding may thus cause a sudden and alarming increase in size of the orbital mass; this is more common after unsuccessful attempts to eradicate the tumor by surgery. The blood often remains unclotted and unorganized, accounting for the so-called blood cyst, when the tumor is opened or explored. Many cases of blood cysts attributed to hematomas really are lymphangiomas.

Strabismus is common to both tumors. It appears early as a tumor pushes forward in the orbit and shoves the eye in a direction opposite to the enlarging mass. With hemangioma this problem may improve or even resolve as the tumor reaches its climax and then recedes to some degree. If strabismus does persist, it often is possible to correct it surgically by the time the child enters school. The situation is less promising with lymphangioma because the tumor tends to persist or even slowly enlarge up to the stage of adolescence or older. By this time the cosmetic blemish is permanent or difficult to repair and the eye is partially amblyopic. The tumor itself may be responsible for permanent disfigurement.

Another clue to lymphangioma is recurrence of presumed orbital cellulitis, for which a child may have been treated with antibiotics. Such attacks often are associated with episodes of upper respiratory infection.

A final tragic feature of lymphangioma is the uncommon continued expansion of tumor eventually causing loss of visual function and requiring enucleation of the eye. Rarely, an expanding lymphangioma may trigger a vascular intercommunication between major vessels of the face and orbit. Such progressive, aneurysmal dilatations and varicosities may pose danger to the well-being of the patient. One such case of this type occurred among our five patients (Fig. 102). The growth of most lymphangiomas tends to halt after the patients become adults.

Lymphangioma, like hemangioma, may cause enlargement of the orbit — visible on roentgenograms — but this is not an important differential feature.

PATHOLOGY

Some histopathologists prefer to compare these tumors to hemangiomas by giving them qualifying designations such as *capillary, cavernous,* and *cystic* types. Clinically, these lymphangiomas behave similarly, and such classifications are of little practical importance. The histopathologic picture may vary according to the age of the patient and the duration of the tumor at the time it is removed. In tumors of recent origin, the stromal framework with its cellular components is relatively sparse in proportion to endothelial-lined channels. In older tumors and those subjected to therapy or surgical trauma, the stroma is thicker and contains larger collections of lymphocytes. Some nests of lymphocytes may be quite large and occasionally they will invaginate the thin

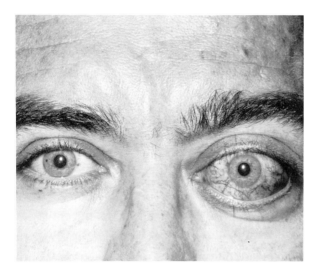

Figure 102. Lymphangioma: bluish red discoloration of left eye associated with pulsating proptosis; lymphangioma since birth with gradual development of superimposed vascular anomaly of left face, trunk, and extremities.

wall of the lymph channels (Fig. 103). We have been reluctant to designate these collections of lymphocytes as follicles. In cases of doubt, the presence of such lymphocytes favors the differentiation of lymphangioma from hemangiomas having a similar appearance.

In all specimens, lymph channels vary in size and shape. The appearance of some tissue specimens is entirely altered by collapse of the large cystic spaces that may or may not contain blood. Absence of erythrocytes and presence of a faintly pink staining matrix within endothelial channels are diagnostic, but the finding of a variable number of erythrocytes in some channels does not rule out

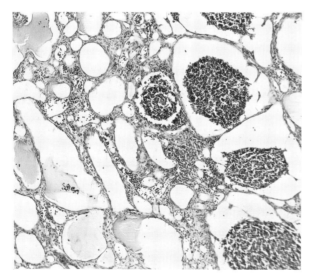

Figure 103. Lymphangioma: tumor is principally cavernous, with flattened endothelial cells lining vascular spaces, some of which contain lymph. Occasional clumps of lymphocytes seen in stromal tissue. (Hematoxylin and eosin; × 100.)

lymphangioma. In specimens designated as blood cysts, the endothelial lining will have disappeared; instead, the tissue surrounding the cavernous space contains degenerated blood and blood pigment. Sometimes the lining endothelial cells seem to hypertrophy, becoming cuboid in shape and resembling glandular epithelium. None of the tumors has a well-defined capsule.

Wright (1974) believes that the majority of cases diagnosed as lymphangioma have an underlying orbital varix, a theory based on positive venographic contrast studies. We have not had an opportunity to perform venography on our own cases of lymphangioma.

TREATMENT

Our overall experience with this aspect of the problem is limited. Treatment of lymphangiomas has not been nearly as satisfactory as treatment of hemangiomas in patients of similar age. In general, effectiveness of treatment might be expressed as being discouraging and frustrating. In several of our patients lymphangioma was more widespread than average, a factor which may contribute to our pessimism.

Radiotherapy. RADON SEEDS. In youngsters less than 18 months of age, we favor insertion of weak radon seeds, as outlined in management of infantile hemangiomas. Response to such therapy is not as dramatic as with hemangiomas but, clinically, this approach seems to have been partially beneficial. At least radon appears to have arrested or retarded expansion of lymphangioma in this age group, but we have no clinical controls to prove this point. Review of the literature suggests that there is some question whether lymphangiomas are radiosensitive or radioresistant. In infants we suspect the lesion is partially radiosensitive. Although radon treatment may not significantly shrink these masses, the delicate vascular septa between endothelial spaces probably undergo fibrosis, thus initiating the process of eventual contracture and resolution.

In patients older than 18 months, the tissues of lymphangiomas become tougher and more resistant to effects of weak irradiation. Therefore, we seldom recommend radon seed insertion for these patients except when, less frequently, expansion and growth of tumor are more rapid and alarming than average. We prefer not to advise orthovoltage or supervoltage therapy for this age group. If expansion of the tumor is slow and radon is not required, we prefer not to recommend any therapy unless pressed by the parents. Poor encapsulation of these tumors at this age does not permit clean surgical dissection; other orbital structures are still delicate and easily injured by partial surgical excision, even though well intentioned; and surgery in patients of this age may only trigger further growth.

Surgery. By school age, the cosmetic consequences of these tumors are such that most parents insist something be done. This is the time, we believe, to consider surgery. The effectiveness of excision as opposed to loss of function of adjacent structures, such as the levator muscle, from subsequent scarring needs particular consideration. An acceptable cosmetic result is especially difficult to achieve if the orbital lymphangioma also involves the upper eyelid. As a result the surgeon must be satisfied with only a partial excision, and parents must be counseled to accept a less than perfect result. The rate of recurrence is entirely unpredictable even though surgery is delayed until later childhood.

Cryotherapy.　It is for these patients that *cryotherapy* may be promising. If bleeding can be staunched or minimized after the interior of the tumor is exposed by orbitotomy, cryotherapy might well be more destructive to the vascular stromal components and less damaging to adjacent structures than either knife dissection or surgical diathermy. Intense cold has more selective effect on capillaries than on any other tissue. We have not had an opportunity to assess effects of cryotherapy on these orbital lymphangiomas adequately. Moreover, the cryopencils and probes utilized for intraocular surgery and retinal detachment procedures are small for orbital application, and present instruments need modification for use with these tumors.

Sudden bleeding within the interstices of a lymphangioma may occur at any time. It is often associated with a recurrence of tumor and is prone to follow surgical manipulation. In the latter situation, extravasated blood may show little or no tendency to absorb; therefore, we favor surgical evacuation of the resulting blood cysts. When spontaneous hemorrhage is not associated with trauma or treatment, evacuation of the blood cyst may not be required because of the tendency toward spontaneous absorption.

We disapprove of injections of sclerosing solutions.

Bibliography

Neoplasms of Blood and Lymph Vessels

Hodges RM: Cases of tumors. Boston Med Surg J 71:417–419, 1864
Hood CI: Cavernous Hemangioma of the orbit: a consideration of pathogenesis with an illustrative
　　case. Arch Ophthalmol 83:49–53, 1970
Lagrange F, Valude E: Encyclopedie Française d'Ophthalmologie. Vol 8. Paris, Octave Dion et Fils,
　　Editeurs, 1909
Von Graefe A: Zur casuistik der Geschwülste. Arch Ophthalmol (Berlin) 7 pt 2:11–24, 1960

Hemangioma

(The following references include not only articles and authors mentioned in this text but such other references as might interest a curious reader collecting information about this common tumor. No attempt is made to list the many references in the literature to this subject.)

Fost NC, Esterly NB: Successful treatment of juvenile hemangiomas with prednisone. J Pediatr 72:
　　351–357, 1968
Harris GJ, Jakobiec FA: Cavernous hemangioma of the orbit: a clinicopathologic analysis of sixty-six
　　cases. *In* Jakobiec FA: *Ocular and Adnexal Tumors.* Birmingham, Aesculapius Publishing Co.,
　　1978, pp 741–781
Henderson JW, Neault RW: The use of the cryoprobe in the removal of posterior orbital tumors.
　　Ophthal Surg 7:45–47, 1976
Hiles DA, Pilchard WA: Corticosteroid control of neonatal hemangiomas of the orbit and ocular
　　adnexa. Am J Ophthalmol 71:1003–1008, 1971
Hoehn JG, Farrow GM, Devine KD, et al: Invasive hemangioma of the head and neck. Am J Surg
　　120:495–500, 1970
Reese AB: Expanding lesions of the orbit (Bowman Lecture). Trans Ophthalmol Soc UK 91:85–104,
　　1971

Hemangioendothelioma

Forrest AW: Intraorbital tumors. Arch Ophthalmol ns 41:198–230, 1949
Jakobiec FA, Jones IS: Vascular tumors, malformations, and degenerations. *In Clinical Ophthal-
　　mology.* Vol 2. Chapter 37. Ed: T.D. Duane, Hagerstown, Harper & Row, 1976

Sekimoto T, Nakeseko H, Kondo K, et al: A case of malignant hemangioendothelioma in the orbit. Folia Ophthalmol Jap 22:535, 1971

Stout AP: Hemangio-endothelioma: a tumor of blood vessels featuring vascular endothelial cells. Ann Surg 118:445–464, 1943

Stout AP, Murray MR: Hemangiopericytoma: a vascular tumor featuring Zimmermann's pericytes. Ann Surg 116:26–33, 1942

Tsuda N, Takaku I: A case report of malignant vascular tumor of the orbit in a newborn. Folia Ophthalmol Jap 21:728, 1970

Hemangiopericytoma

Enzinger FM, Smith BH: Hemangiopericytoma: an analysis of 106 cases. Hum Pathol 7:61–82, 1976

Heckmann K: Beitrag zur Pathologic seltener Angiosarkome der Orbita: Hämangioperizytom und Hämangioendotheliom. Ophthalmologica 166:36–47, 1973

Henderson JW, Farrow GM: Primary orbital hemangiopericytoma: an aggressive and potentially malignant neoplasm. Arch Ophthalmol 96:666–673, 1978

Jakobiec FA, Howard GM, Jones IS, et al: Hemangiopericytoma of the orbit. Am J Ophthalmol 78: 816–834, 1974

McMaster MJ, Soule EH, Ivins JC: Hemangiopericytoma: a clinicopathologic study and long-term followup of 60 patients. Cancer 36:2232–2244, 1975

Zimmermann KW: Der feinere Bau der Blutcapillaren. Z Anat Entwicklungsgesch 68:29–109, 1923

Vascular Leiomyoma

Henderson JW, Harrison EG Jr: Vascular leiomyoma of the orbit: report of a case. Trans Am Acad Ophthalmol Otolaryngol 74:970–974, 1970

Jakobiec FA, Jones IS, Tannenbaum M: Leiomyoma: an unusual tumor of the orbit. Br J Ophthalmol 57:825–831, 1973

Jakobiec FA, Howard GM, Rosen M, et al: Leiomyomas and leiomyosarcoma of the orbit. Am J Ophthalmol 80:1028–1042, 1975

Nath K, Shukla BR: Orbital leiomyoma and its origin. Br J Ophthalmol 47:369–371, 1963

Sanborn GE, Valenzuela RE, Green RW: Leiomyoma of the orbit. Am J Ophthalmol 87:371–375, 1979

Wolter JR: Hemangio-leiomyoma of the orbit. Eye Ear Nose Throat Mon 44:42–46 (Jan) 1965

Lymphangioma

Ayres SC: Lymphangioma cavernosum of the orbit, with an original case. Am J Ophthalmol 12:321–331, 1895

Jones IS: Lymphangioma of the ocular adnexa: an analysis of 62 cases. Trans Am Ophthalmol Soc 57: 602, 1959

Reese AB: Expanding lesions of the orbit (Bowman Lecture). Trans Ophthalmol Soc UK 91:85–104, 1971

Wecker L: Die cavernösen Tumoren der Orbita. Klin Monatsbl Augenheilkd 6:47–49, 1868

Wright JE: Orbital vascular anomalies. Trans Am Acad Ophthalmol Otolaryngol 78:OP 606–616, 1974

6

Vascular Malformations

HISTORICAL ASPECTS

Healers, medieval barber-surgeons, and physicians from the earliest times have been fascinated by red and reddish purple enlargement, tortuosities, and sometimes intercommunications of vascular channels in various parts of the body, of either spontaneous or post-traumatic origin. According to Osler (1915), such vascular oddities on or near the surface of the body were annotated in some of the earliest medical writings. William Hunter in 1757 established the meanings of the thrill (palpable vibration) and bruit (audible vibration) of arteriovenous vascular intercommunications, and these diagnostic developments made possible an easier recognition, or at least suspicion, of vascular malformations in the deeper anatomic areas that were not associated with any external alteration of blood flow. Concomitantly, anatomists became curious as to the various locations and anomalous connections of these vascular dilations, and this led naturally to the interest of physiologists in the altered dynamics of blood flow through such vascular beds. Surgical pathologists came to study such tumors much later because the exact size, extent and components of most vascular malformations, particularly those more deeply situated, usually were not known during life. The danger of uncontrolled hemorrhage during removal of these vascular dilations discouraged surgeons from operating on patients and this nullified the role of the surgical pathologist until comparatively recent times. By the time a case came to autopsy, the significant changes that had developed in the vessels during life no longer were recognizable nor could they be accurately differentiated; the problem consequently remained in the realm only of anatomic pathology. The factor of hemorrhage and the difficult surgical approach to more inaccessible areas of the body are the reasons why the intracranial space with vascular malformations and intercommunications was one of the last anatomic sites to be studied.

In the United States, it was chiefly through the interest and publications of Dandy (1935; Dandy and Follis, 1941) that intracranial vascular dysplasia became a subject of diagnostic reality rather than clinical speculation. Anatomically and physiologically, the vascular circulation of the orbit is considered an extension of the internal carotid system. Similarly, most of the vascular malformations of the orbit have some association or interconnection with similar vascular disorders in the intracranial space. The two, therefore, usually are discussed together.

NOMENCLATURE

Before any attempt is made to describe these orbital vascular malformations, it is essential that the descriptive phrases and terms applied to them be clarified and defined. Terms such as *varix, aneurysm, arteriovenous fistula, arteriovenous aneurysm, saccular aneurysm, racemose* and *cirsoid anomalies,* and *venous angiomas* have been bandied about and used so interchangeably that to know exactly which malformation is which and what is the entity being discussed is nearly impossible. Again, the inability to uncover, dissect, or remove these vascular abnormalities during life (particularly around the head, face, and orbit) has contributed to a broad, indefinite terminology. What some have called varix would by others be designated an arteriovenous aneurysm, and vice versa. Or, a tumor designated by either name a century ago might now be described by another term. Furthermore, clinically what seemed to be, for example, either varix or arteriovenous aneurysm in life might prove at autopsy to be the opposite disorder.

All tumors discussed in this chapter are composed, either entirely or in part, of arteries, veins, or capillaries of variable size and in various combinations. From a clinical standpoint, the capillary component, if present, is of little significance, at least as it concerns the orbit. The malformation is therefore designated arterial, venous, or arteriovenous, depending on the predominant type of vascular channel in the tumor. Such tumors also are designated according to their anatomic site, for example, facial, orbital, or intracranial. The name of any given vascular malformation also may be modified according to whether its development was spontaneous (presumed to be congenital or developmental in genesis) or acquired (usually traumatic or due to vascular degenerative disease in later life).

In the past, all these vascular tumors have been called *aneurysms,* with suitable modifying adjectives designating their vascular composition and location. However, most medical dictionaries define an aneurysm as a vascular dilation or enlargement of an artery, not of a vein. A few recent editions of some dictionaries recognize a broader denotation of the word aneurysm and include malformations of veins as well as lymphatics in the definition. Thus it would be permissible to describe a vascular dilatation as an aneurysmal varix or a venous aneurysm. Similarly, *varix* — meaning an enlarged and tortuous vein — probably is as old a term as aneurysm, but in the course of centuries of use the meanings of the two nouns have been carelessly and often conveniently intermingled. Varix, strictly defined, refers to the enlargement of only one vein; practically, the word usually refers to a group or collection of dilated veins in one area. The term *angioma* we have reserved for vascular new growths (see Chapter 5); we shall not use the terms angioma and aneurysm synonymously as so frequently is done in the literature. We realize the borderline oftentimes is indistinct between angiomas (new growths) and aneurysms (malformations), particularly in the very young. Both may be considered as hamartomas, and during periods of subsequent human growth it is not unknown for external angioma-like tumors to be associated with more deeply situated aneurysmal intercommunications.

We believe, therefore, that loose usage of these terms is unfortunate. We include here the terminology that we favor:

Aneurysm: any vascular tumor of developmental or congenital origin, whose makeup — entirely or in part — is that of an artery. A tumor of the orbit whose makeup is entirely arterial will thus be termed an orbital aneurysm.

Arteriovenous aneurysm: any tumor of developmental or congenital origin in which the feeding and draining vessels are both arteries and veins.

Arteriovenous fistula: an abnormal communication between adjoining arteries and veins that is acquired through vascular disease of as a result of trauma.

Varix: any tumor that seems, on either clinical or surgical grounds, to be comprised only of venous channels. A tumor of the orbit comprising a complex of enlarged veins will thus be termed an orbital varix.

Angioma: any tumor of vascular tissue that is neoplastic.

One last clarification in terminology is necessary before proceeding with a discussion of individual vascular types. This concerns the words *cirsoid* and *racemose.* Technically, the terms are synonymous, implying dilation and tortuosity of vascular channels. In usage, the term cirsoid usually is applied only to tumors with an arterial component, whereas racemose has been used often in reference to both aneurysm and varix. The term racemose also may have some histologic implications, being used to designate malformations with significant parenchyma between vascular channels as contrasted with the more closely approximated vascular elements of the cavernous type. In an area as small as the orbital cavity it seems unnecessary to use either term as a significant descriptive adjective.

The classification of vascular malformations already has been noted in Chapter 5. In the present chapter we will note only those of the group that must be considered in the differential diagnosis of orbital tumors. Not all of these entities that produce orbital symptoms are necessarily located in the intra-orbital space. Most of the carotid-cavernous fistulas, for example, are located in the intracranial space, but they alter the dynamics of the orbital venous circulation to simulate an orbital mass. In contrast, most of the aneurysms of the proximal and intracranial portions of the ophthalmic artery can be excluded from discussion because they do not produce proptosis or orbital symptoms, although altered visual function may occur owing to pressure on the optic nerve.

ORBITAL ANEURYSM

INCIDENCE AND CLINICAL FEATURES

All the vascular entities in this chapter except carotid-cavernous fistula occur so infrequently in or around the orbital cavity that they usually are not included in statistical and clinical surveys of orbital tumors. This, and the confusion about terminology, negates accurate data on their incidence, sex ratio, and age groups. Heimburger and associates (1949) grappled with this problem in their survey of orbital aneurysms. They annotated 68 reports in the literature up to the time of their own publication, but in only 6 of the 68 cases was the diagnosis of aneurysm based on either pathologic study or surgical exploration.

Further scrutiny of the protocols of the six cases caused them to doubt whether any of the cases were true examples of orbital aneurysm. In the past several decades erroneous reports or unconfirmed examples of orbital aneurysms have become fewer, for now pulsating exophthalmos usually is recognized as being a symptom of arteriovenous fistula rather than a sign of aneurysm, as was so universally accepted earlier. More frequent use of angiography also has ruled out many tumors that once were misdiagnosed as orbital aneurysms from clinical symptoms only. Angiography also has made possible a more accurate localization of the aneurysm to either the proximal (intracranial and intracanalicular) portion of the intraorbital portion of the ophthalmic artery and its branches. It is the intraorbital aneurysm that is our chief concern because it more often produces proptosis. A brief abstract of some of the clinical cases of intraorbital aneurysm confirmed by angiography or surgical exploration in the literature follows.

Heimburger et al (1949): A 58-year-old female with congestion of left eye of 3 weeks' duration. Secondary glaucoma, proptosis, and impairment of ocular rotations also noted. No pulsation of globe. Aneurysm of lacrimal artery removed through transcranial approach.

Mortada (1961): A 51-year-old female with buzzing noises, pain, and pulsating proptosis of left eye of 7 months' duration. No congestion of eyeball. Cystic mass palpable in superior nasal quadrant of left orbit. Bruit also present. Aneurysm of intraorbital portion of ophthalmic artery noted on angiography. Treated by ligature of left common carotid artery.

Rubinstein et al (1968): A 36-year-old male with abrupt onset of burning and lacrimation of right eye soon followed by loss of vision. No bruit. No masses palpable but a central scotoma and mild pallor of right optic disc noted on ophthalmic examination. Angiography revealed a saccular aneurysm of ophthalmic artery 7 mm in diameter in retrobulbar space. Surgical management refused. Clinical picture unchanged 18 months after onset.

Meyerson and Lazar (1971): A 55-year-old male with very sudden proptosis, subconjunctival and orbital hemorrhage on right side after coughing. No light perception in affected eye. Angiography revealed a 1.3-cm saccular aneurysm of ophthalmic artery in retrobulbar space. Aneurysm removed via lateral orbitotomy.

Two of three aneurysms in our series (Table 2) also seemed to be of this type. A brief resume of the clinical features were these:

A 31-year-old female had noted prominence and bloodshot appearance of right eye for 6 weeks. No impairment of vision but some limitation of lateral ocular rotation was present. Angiography revealed an intraorbital aneurysm that filled from the orbital branch of the facial artery. Division and ligation of right external carotid and superior thyroid arteries brought about some improvement. Further surgical treatment recommended but refused.

A 63-year-old female had noted a right supraorbital headache associated with visual loss of right eye for a period of 6 months. Two months after onset a tingling of right cheek appeared associated with a pulsatile swishing noise on right side of head. Vision was reduced to hand movements, right eye, with generalized constriction of visual field and mild pallor of optic disc. Angiography showed an aneurysm of the intraorbital portion of the ophthalmic artery (Fig. 104). Surgical management was deferred because of the development of left-sided seizures.

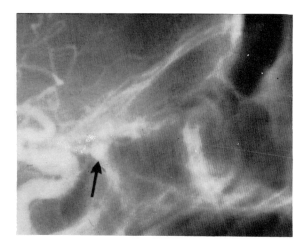

Figure 104. Aneurysm of intra-orbital portion of ophthalmic artery (*arrow*): diagnosis was made by angiography.

A uniform aneurysmal dilatation of the entire ophthalmic artery also may develop in contrast to the localized saccular aneurysm just described. Examples of these fusiform aneurysms in the literature are, briefly:

Sanford et al (1935): A 54-year-old female had noted loss of vision in the left eye over a period of 3 months. Vision was reduced to counting fingers and the visual field was severely restricted. Visual acuity in the better eye was 20/40. Craniotomy revealed bilateral enlargement and tortuosity of the ophthalmic artery extending anteriorly from its origin into the orbit. The bony optic canals were unroofed with some improvement of vision.

Pfingst (1936): A case very similar to the preceding one was noted in a 9-year-old female with a 5-month history of proptosis, diplopia, and visual loss in the left eye. The left optic canal was unroofed and the ophthalmic artery was found distended along its entire course.

The third patient of our group of three aneurysms seems to also fit in this category.

A 26-year-old female had had numerous surgical procedures since childhood to obliterate an arteriovenous aneurysm of the right eye. She sought ophthalmic consultation because of headaches. There was no proptosis. Vision was 20/20. A bruit could be heard through the closed eyelids on the right side. Angiography revealed the right ophthalmic artery was 3 mm in diameter throughout its length. Orbital venogram was negative. Also, there was enlargement of the right optic canal.

It is evident from these several cases that the *symptomatology of orbital aneurysm is extremely diverse.* There was no pattern of symptoms or signs common to any two cases. In one case (Meyerson and Lazar) the onset was sudden and the ocular consequences severe in terms of permanent visual loss. In another (Rubinstein et al) the course was relatively benign. Proptosis was present in several cases but totally absent in others. The same extremes apply to the symptomatology we so often associate with orbital vascular tumors, such as congestion of epibulbar vessels, pulsation of the eye, and bruit. In contrast to these intraorbital malformations those aneurysms of the intracranial and intra-canalicular portion of the ophthalmic artery have a more standard pattern of clinical features. Because of the proximity of the ophthalmic artery to the optic nerve in the latter area, aneurysms will produce a predictable pattern of pallor of the optic disc, central scotomas, and constriction of the visual field with supplementary features of diplopia and third nerve palsy.

The ages of the patients with intraorbital aneurysms listed above ranged from 9 to 63 years. The sex incidence was 7:2, female to male. All these cases were observed in the years prior to the widespread use of ultrasonography and computer tomography in the diagnostic work-up of unilateral proptosis; years when angiography was the only positive means for demonstrating an occult aneurysm in the retrobulbar space. Nowadays, either ultrasonography or computer tomography will provide an easier assessment of whether a patient should or should not be subjected to angiography. Where indicated, the angiogram is still the principal technical aid in mapping the extent and size of the vascular malformation.

The sum of the cases reviewed above plus proven cases of intraorbital aneurysm in the foreign literature which we have not annotated probably does not exceed sixteen.

TREATMENT

The management of these aneurysms is surgical; the object is either to excise the malformation completely or to decrease the flow of blood through the abnormal channel and thereby reduce the pressure of the aneurysm on surrounding orbital structures. If the malformation is relatively large and involves a structure such as the lacrimal artery, as did the one reported by Heimburger and associates, the vessel may be clipped both proximal and distal to the aneurysm and the tumor then excised. Interruption of blood flow along major adnexal branches of the ophthalmic artery seems to cause neither loss of vision nor major impairment of adnexal function, for the collateral circulation through remaining terminal and anastomosing branches of the internal and external carotid arterial systems is adequate. However, some impairment of visual function might well occur if similar management were recommended for the saccular aneurysms involving the main trunk of the ophthalmic artery. This is particularly germane to those aneurysms close to the ophthalmic artery and its first branch, the central retinal artery. Here, it is preferable to clip the aneurysm at its junction with the main vessel wall, but this cannot always be done because of technical and anatomic factors. It is then easier to clip the main vessel, either proximal or distal (preferably the former) to the saccular dilation in order to reduce blood flow to the abnormality, yet maintain some collateral circulation through the unclipped segment of the ophthalmic artery.

Less direct surgical methods also may be used to reduce the blood flow through the abnormal vascular channel. These techniques alone may suffice to reduce the volume of the aneurysm or they may be effective in reducing hemorrhage as a preliminary to a direct attack on the aneurysm. The oldest and most used techniques have been ligature or ligature and division of the main branches of the carotid artery that supply the aneurysm, as demonstrated by angiography.

Recently, more sophisticated refinements have evolved in this field. First, selective angiography of very small vessels, such as the ophthalmic artery, is now possible through the use of tiny caliber catheters. Utilizing the same principle, the feeder vessels close to the aneurysm or vascular malformation can be embolized with silastic pellets, silastic spheres, muscle fragments, or pieces of gel foam. Or, if the size or anatomic position of the malformation permits, liquid silicone polymers can be introduced directly to obliterate the abnormal channel. All of these newer refinements are not without danger. Even so, in the hands of a sophisticated team of neurosurgeons and neuroradiologists, some vascular intercommuncations and aneurysms of the head, face, and orbit, which were once considered hopeless, can now be treated.

ORBITAL VARIX

TERMINOLOGY

We regard the varix as a venous counterpart of the orbital aneurysm. It is the pathologic enlargement of one channel, or usually several venous channels, chiefly in the orbit. This does not preclude connection with, or often some enlargement of, the plexus of veins in areas adjacent to the orbit, such as the face, temple, forehead, and bridge of the nose. It does, however exclude malformations that have a minor arterial component, whch we believe should be classified with the arteriovenous aneurysms. In the varix, the makeup of the feeding and draining components is strictly venous in type. We realize that such terminology is open to several qualifications, but strict definition is nearly impossible to formulate solely from clinical study.

The orbital venous plexus might be considered an intermediate shunt between the intracranial and extracranial venous systems; therefore, a varix affecting orbital veins might in some cases only reflect a more posterior, distant, and hidden dilation of intracranial vessels. The primary intracranial malformation is, in such cases, most often an arteriovenous fistula or arteriovenous aneurysm, and the clinically evident orbital varix is a secondary rather than a primary orbital tumor. Also, when a varix only is suspected, it is often impossible to verify anatomically the extent of the anomaly or to remove the lesion to prove its venous makeup histologically. The different contexts of the word as used in the past also should be remembered. Some texts have used varix in its broadest sense to denote any vascular abnormality in which the venous component is more prominent than the arterial component. We realize that our preference for a more strict definition of varix cannot always be achieved, and in instances where the terminology of varix may be in question, perhaps it would be better to call the lesion a vascular abnormality with a major venous component. In infants, the borderline between a large hypertrophic hemangioma and a small, early varix might be indistinguishable. Moreover, what may commence as a hypertrophic hemangioma or a vascular capillary hemangioma may gradually become a true varix with further development of the child.

INCIDENCE

Transient and evanescent unilateral proptosis has long piqued the attention of clinicians. This "now you see it — now you don't" phenomenon is the principal sign of orbital varix. The term *intermittent exophthalmos* usually is applied to this clinical picture and has been associated with orbital varix for so long that orbital varix and intermittent exophthalmos have almost become synonymous in ophthalmic literature. Walsh and Dandy (1944) thoroughly reviewed the literature on intermittent exophthalmos and at that time found 111 cases. Brauston and Norton (1963) extended this review, commented on additional symptoms associated with the syndrome of intermittent exophthalmos, and added 20 more cases, including 2 of their own. But an estimate of incidence cannot be based on such a collection of cases because disorders other than orbital varix that may cause intermittent exophthalmos were included in the survey, and, in the majority of cases, the diagnosis was a clinical one, unsupported by angiography, surgical verification, or pathologic study. When probable cases of hemangioma in infancy, cavernous lymphangioma, and intra-orbital arteriovenous aneurysm are excluded from such surveys, the incidence of orbital varix becomes much less frequent. This factor is somewhat offset by the fact that all instances of orbital varix are not recorded as case reports; only the more startling types of orbital varix or those resulting in visual disability are the subjects of ophthalmic case studies. Many milder and nonprogressive examples of orbital varix go relatively unheeded by the patient and are of no therapeutic concern to the ophthalmologist. Therefore, the true incidence of orbital varix as related to other orbital conditions is not known and we have no constructive statistics based on our own experience. It is, however, our impression that orbital varices are more common than orbital aneurysms but less frequent than carotid-cavernous fistulas in an average ophthalmic practice.

CLINICAL FEATURES

Males and females seem affected in nearly equal numbers. Cases have been reported among all age groups, although there is a greater preponderance of orbital varix in the second and third decades of life. Orbital varix seems to affect the left orbit more often than the right orbit; proven bilateral orbital involvement does not seem to exist.

Mention has already been made of *unilateral proptosis*, and the fact that it may be intermittent. *Position also is significant.* When the patient is upright, no ocular or orbital abnormality may be manifest. In the early stages, the orbital varix may be induced by movements of the head to a dependent position or triggered by some maneuver that increases the orbital vascular pressure. Thus, in an adult, unilateral proptosis may become evident when the patient bends forward. In an infant, the eye may bulge forward precipitiously when the child cries. Aside from exertion or a change to a dependent position, proptosis can be induced by pressure over the jugular vein or forced expiration with the nose closed (Valsalva maneuver). In a case of a large varix or a varix that has been present for some years, the sudden episode of exophthalmos may evoke the oculocardiac syndrome of bradycardia, fainting, and nausea. In some of these severer cases and in cases manifesting many attacks of intermittent exophthalmos, atrophy of the orbital reticular tissue is such that in the interval between episodes of proptosis, the involved eye actually becomes enophthalmic.

The *size* of the varix, the *duration* of the attack of proptosis, and the degree of *progression* are variable and unpredictable. In some milder cases among adults the phenomenon of intermittent unilateral proptosis has been known since childhood. The patient has learned to induce attacks of proptosis almost at will and the transient bulging of the eye with its surrounding turgid appendages may be used as a parlor trick. Many of these nonprogressive and reversible cases of orbital varix are never seen by ophthalmologists and are seldom of such scientific interest as to be the subject of a case report. More often, what may commence as an apparently innocent and transient proptosis gradually progresses to frequent and unwanted episodes of ocular protrusion during a period of years. Eventually, impairment of vision owing to disturbance of optic nerve function results. Or, the onset in a young adult may be sudden and unexpected and only a few weeks or months elapse before the patient seeks consultation.

The duration of proptosis in the earlier sequences of progressive cases usually is quite short (measured in minutes); the eye recedes almost as easily and quickly as it protrudes. In time, the periods of proptosis gradually become more prolonged and the eye recedes even more slowly. Even so, the duration of these more severe attacks still is seldom longer than a few hours. Other vascular abnormalities or tumors should be considered in the differential diagnosis where the proptosis persists or is slow to regress.

Bruit, thrill, and pulsation of the globe are not signs of orbital varix as is so commonly the case with arteriovenous aneurysms and carotid cavernous fistulas. Rarely, one or several of this triad of symptoms may be noticed if the varix is a large one, situated posteriorly and associated with a dysplasia or defect in the bony partition between orbit and intracranial space. A bruit may indicate a wide communication with another similar vascular anomaly within the intracranial vault, the pulsation thus representing a transmission of the normal meningeal pulsation. It is not known which develops first — the bony dehiscence or the varix. Possibly both the abnormal bone enlargement and the varix develop concomitantly as a *forme fruste* of neurofibromatosis.

Information about other ocular and orbital signs of orbital varix is sparse. *Diplopia* may be recognized during episodes of proptosis in the milder varieties of varix. *Ophthalmoplegia* is conspicuous in more severe cases during the attack, the result of mechanical limitation of movement of the affected eye in its swollen, congested bed. As time passes and attacks of intermittent proptosis increase, permanent paresis of some of the extraocular muscles supplied by the third cranial nerve may develop; this is the consequence of irreversible damage in branches of the third cranial nerve, compressed by the orbital varix in the vicinity of the superior orbital fissure.

Dilation of the retinal venous tree is another sign, but its incidence will vary with the size and anatomic location of the varix. Similarly, dilation of the epibulbar vascular channels is an inconstant finding. As a rule, the surface of the eye does not show the corkscrew, reddish purple vessels approaching the limbus of the eye that characterize arteriovenous-type anomalies (see Figs. 18, 105, and 106). An interesting association of an orbitofrontal varix with varicosities of the legs, cutaneous hemangiectasis, and hypertrophy of all tissues in the affected limbs (Klippen-Trenaunay-Weber syndrome) has been reported by Rathbun and associates (1970).

In milder cases the patient notices no serious disturbance other than a sense of fullness during episodes of engorgement of the varix. If the degree of proptosis becomes severe, distress is proportionally increased; it may approach the

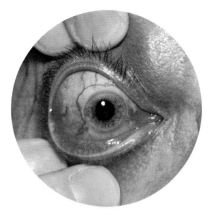 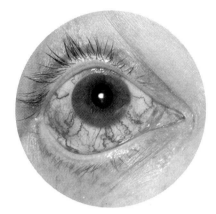

Figure 105.   Intracranial arteriovenous communication: signs were dilated, tortuous vessels on surface of eye extending to limbal area, proptosis (3 mm), and pulsating tumor of orbit.
   Figure 106.   Carotid-cavernous fistula: signs were tortuous blood vessels extending to limbal area of eye, proptosis (5 mm), bruit, and secondary glaucoma. Corneoscleral trephine had been performed at 12 o'clock limbus 3 months after onset of symptoms because of impression of primary glaucoma. Compare to Figure 18.

agonizing pain of subluxation of the eye secondary to trauma or malignant endocrine exophthalmos.

The occasional similarity, in infants, between a small orbital varix and a large hypertrophic hemangioma has been noted. The former is more diffuse and has a wider communication with the general circulation. When such a varix (usually situated in the posterior orbit) becomes engorged with blood, all tissues of the orbit participate in the ensuing swelling. The appearance is striking: the eyes of these tiny people may be pushed straightforward to such a degree that the eyes are no longer covered by the protecting eyelids. In contrast, the hemangioma is more circumscribed and less diffuse. As the tumor becomes passively congested by straining or crying, the tumor itself tends to push forward, the eye being displaced or concealed beneath the protecting eyelids in a direction opposite to that of the hemangioma.

The etiology is a matter of conjecture. Probably most cases represent an anomalous quirk in genesis of the orbital venous circulation. Trauma probably is not a factor in the development of a true orbital varix.

ROENTGENOGRAPHIC CHANGES

Improved techniques of arteriography and venography, particularly the latter, have helped to outline the size and confirm the diagnosis of orbital varix. Angiography will help determine whether the varix connects with any intracranial arteriovenous malformation. Neither technique is invariably successful and some clinical cases of varix do not show well on angiography, for reasons that are not clearly understood. Venography may be enhanced by the Valsalva maneuver just after the injection of dye. Another aid to filling of the varix with dye is movement of the patient's head to a dependent position. When the varix is filled with blood and the orbital tissues are tense and turgid, venography must be done cautiously. In such cases there is less tendency for the dye to pass into the pathologic channels.

Phleboliths may form in association with orbital varix. They probably form when there is sludging of blood in either a large or long-standing varix. Enlargement of the orbit is another possible sign, particularly in infants, and defects in the bony roof or posterior wall of the orbit already have been mentioned (see Chapter 2). In most cases of varix the standard roentgenographic views are negative.

PATHOLOGY

Well-documented reports of this feature of orbital varix are uncommon. Histopathologic studies are scarce, and most observations are based on gross appearances. In general, a plexus of thick-walled veins will be seen. Varying degrees of intraluminal thrombosis are frequent and the stroma will show areas of fibrosis mixed with foci of lymphocytes. Special stains can demonstrate some smooth muscle along the walls of these channels, but neither the amount nor the arrangement of such muscle is consistent with what would be expected in arteries. On the other hand, the walls of these vascular channels are much thicker than those in cavernous hemangioma.

TREATMENT

There is no standardization of treatment. The management must depend on various circumstances, including the size of the varix, its duration, and the presence or absence of major subjective or objective complications. Most ophthalmologists tend to follow a conservative course in the earlier stages of varix; they are hesitant to operate unless there are definite signs of progression or unless relief from some visual deterioration is necessary. When eventually it is obvious that something must be done, the surgical approach will depend on the location and extent of the varix, as outlined by venography. For those tumors chiefly confined to the posterior orbit, we recommend the transcranial approach. For those tumors that principally involve the inferior orbital venous tree, an anterior or an anterotemporal approach seems most practical. Whatever the approach, seldom is a varix so well visualized in its entirety to permit complete excision. More often, attempts are made to ligate or clip the main feeding and draining vessels in the anterior and posterior extremes of the orbital venous circulation. Or, in cases marked by a cluster of veins, thrombosis can be induced by anodal current (5 ma), as suggested by Handa and Mori (1968). In their method, the electrocurrent is applied directly to the interior of the dilated vessel by a needle of small diameter. Thrombosis causes shrinkage of the mass, making it easier to see and to ligate the limits of the varix. We have not used this method; instead, we have applied a low voltage desiccating current to the exterior of the partially dissected mass, and this has helped to shrink the varix and facilitate its surgical manipulation.

Clipping, ligation, and surgical diathermy often do not affect a complete cure because the varix usually is large by the time surgical treatment is advised, and some small feeding channel remains unseen and undetected. However, such surgery does decrease the size of the varix, with concomitant subjective improvement.

Recently, Kennedy (1978) reported the interesting management of a complicated orbital vascular malformation in a female child who was 4 years old at the time of his report. A vascular mass had been present in the right upper nasal quadrant since birth. The mass encroached on the visual axis and the affected eye was exotropic. Angiography at 15 months of age revealed 3 orbital vascular malformations supplied by the ophthalmic artery and branches of the external carotid artery. A selective transcatheter arterial embolization of the lesion with silicone pellets was performed through the right internal maxillary and external carotid artery, followed by ligation of the external carotid at its origin from the common carotid artery. Twenty-seven months later an extensive resection was performed on the residual tumor at the inner canthus and in the anterior orbit. Subsequent photographs indicated a very satisfactory cosmetic result. It is encouraging to learn of the satisfactory management of a complicated orbital vascular lesion by these newer technical procedures. It offers the ophthalmologist an additional option in the treatment of these difficult situations.

ARTERIOVENOUS FISTULA

Well-documented and proven cases of orbital arteriovenous fistula are virtually nonexistent. Most cases designated as orbital arteriovenous fistulas in the literature have no direct, acquired communication between adjoining orbital arteries and veins, and for these we prefer the term arteriovenous aneurysm. A discussion of arteriovenous fistula could well be omitted from a text on orbital tumors were it not for one arteriovenous shunt that lies outside the orbit: this is the carotid-cavernous fistula. This produces such secondary changes in orbital anatomy and physiology as to warrant its mention in this text. Anatomically, this shunt lies just posterior to the orbit proper, but the communication of the pathologic fistula with the orbital vascular plexus (particularly the veins) is so wide that a clinical picture having some features of primary orbital tumor may be seen in many cases.

HISTORICAL ASPECTS

The orbital and ocular changes associated with carotid-cavernous fistula have been widely annotated in the ophthalmic, neurologic, neurosurgical, and anatomic literature of the past. This literature is now extensive. For the physician who might be interested in the historical aspects and evolution of thought concerning these fistulas, the references in the English language, of De Schweinitz and Holloway (1908), Bedell (1915), Locke (1924), Sugar and Meyer (1940), Martin and Mabon (1943), and Henderson and Schneider (1958) will serve as a good introduction.

Travers (1811) and Dalrymple (1815) were early observers of two similar cases of pulsating exophthalmos that probably were examples of either arteriovenous aneurysm or arteriovenous fistula. A portrait of Travers' case (a 34-year-old woman with a spontaneous onset during pregnancy) is illustrated in Figure 107. Travers successfully managed the situation by ligating the common carotid artery, and he seems to have been the first surgeon to use this approach, a bold one considering the era in which he worked.

Initially, these vascular intercommunications were considered to be cirsoid aneurysms, but they were not explored surgically. It was also believed that the lesion was confined entirely to the orbit. The first autopsy study was made by Guthrie (1823), who found an aneurysm of the ophthalmic artery rather than a cirsoid malformation. This was the basis for the long-held belief in England that all cases of pulsating exophthalmos resulted from orbital aneurysm. However, it is likely that Guthrie observed an aneurysmal dilation of an ophthalmic vein rather than an aneurysm of the ophthalmic artery. In France, a contrasting point of view was held; on the basis of autopsy findings reported by Baron (1835) and other subsequent examiners, the basic disorder was considered to be a carotid-cavernous fistula. In time, it became clear that this lesion was the commonest cause of the pulsating exophthalmos syndrome. By the 20th century it was recognized that pulsating exophthalmos might result from several orbital-intracranial disorders, not all of which were vascular in type. Now, it is also known that carotid-cavernous fistula does not always produce pulsating exophthalmos.

INCIDENCE

Ordinarily, incidence factors associated with carotid-cavernous fistulas are considered in relation to other intracranial events. The total number of carotid-cavernous fistulas reported in the literature may be cited, or the frequency of

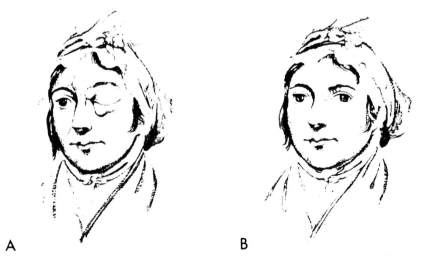

A   B

Figure 107.   A, Probably the first engraving of a patient (a 34-year-old woman) with spontaneous onset of pulsating exophthalmos during pregnancy. B, Appearance of patient 2 years after ligation of left common carotid artery. (From Travers B: A case of aneurism by anastomosis in the orbit, cured by ligature of the common carotid artery. R Med Chir Soc Lond [Med-Chir Trans] 2:1–16, 1811.)

these vascular shunts among head injuries noted. Their incidence also may be compared to the occurrence of other disorders in areas such as the chiasm. Such figures would be more pertinent if this text were concerned with intracranial tumors or diseases rather than orbital disorders, and there is reason to argue that comparisons between intracranial disorders, such as these fistulas, and orbital tumors are, from an incidence standpoint, not valid. Even so, it might be held that orbital manifestations are so commonly associated with carotid-cavernous fistulas and may so suggest other orbital vascular diseases that the incidence of the former should be included in any survey of the latter. There seems to be no well-documented and statistically significant study relating the incidence of carotid-cavernous fistulas to orbital tumors. Therefore, the data from 35 consecutive arteriovenous fistulas producing definite orbital manifestations during the 27-year interval of our tumor survey should be of interest. Sex and age factors are summarized in Table 9.

All of these fistulas were secondary in type, that is, the orbital tumor was produced by a retrograde pressure along the orbital veins from an extraorbital source. All but eight of the fistulas involved a direct communication between the internal carotid artery and the surrounding cavernous sinus (carotid-cavernous fistula), as demonstrated by angiography. In the eight exceptions the arterial source of the fistula was the tiny meningohypophyseal artery (three cases), branches from the middle meningeal artery (two cases), and terminal dural twigs of the internal maxillary artery (three cases). The 35 cases comprise 4.5% of our 764 total orbital tumors and 10% of all secondary tumors (Table 2). We have followed the convenient and common practice of dividing these fistulas into *spontaneous* and *traumatic* types. Prior to the detailed study of our cases it was our clinical impression, based on statistics in the older literature as well as the more memorable clinical features of the traumatic type, that the fistula of spontaneous origin was the least frequent of the two types. However, in our series, the spontaneous fistula was more frequent in a ratio of 4:3. Recent reports in the neurosurgical and neurologic literature support this belief that spontaneous fistulas are more common than previously stated and attribute this to more sophisticated angiography and more attentive diagnosis of suspicious cases. The age distribution of the two types is quite different (Table 9) and the sex ratios are almost reversed. The majority of the traumatic cases involved a skull fracure sustained in some accident involving moving vehicles (car, boat, tractor, or motorcycle). Other cases were head injury from gunshot wounds or severe trauma from large moving objects. None of the spontaneous fistulas occurred in pregnant females. The laterality of the fistulas was not statistically significant in either group.

TABLE 9.   AGE AND SEX DISTRIBUTION OF 35 ARTERIOVENOUS FISTULAS

Male	Female		Age in Years at Time of Orbital Diagnosis						
			11–20	21–30	31–40	41–50	51–60	61–70	Over 70
3	17	Spontaneous			2	3	8	4	3
11	4	Traumatic	6	3		4	2		

PATHOPHYSIOLOGY

Although the causative mechanism for the traumatic fistula is rather straightforward, the factors responsible for the onset of spontaneous fistulas are less clear. No doubt, some of the latter are secondary to a dehiscence or rupture in the wall of a small saccular aneurysm in the wall of the internal carotid artery or at one of its intracavernous branchings. This has been verified at autopsy. Recent refinements in angiography have also demonstrated the etiologic role of small dural malformations in the cavernous sinus (Newton and Hoyt 1970). In addition, Graf (1965) has noted spontaneous carotid-cavernous fistulas in patients with Ehlers-Danlos syndrome, a disorder of elastic tissue. Other reasons advanced as etiologic factors are more speculative and seldom proved. Moreover, none of the etiologic factors explain why the spontaneous fistula is more prevalent in women than men nor why it so often affects women in the fifth through seventh decade.

Whatever the cause, the mechanism of the orbital tumefaction is the same — a rise in the pressure of the orbital veins secondary to escape of arterial blood into the cavernous sinus. However, the severity or degree of the orbital changes will vary widely depending on the position of the shunt in the cavernous sinus, the size of the fistula, the anatomic patency of the various venous channels that communicate with the cavernous sinus, and the duration of the abnormal arteriovenous gradient. Thus, in traumatic fistulae (high flow, high pressure shunts) the orbital manifestation may be sudden and severe, but in spontaneous types secondary to dural fistulae (low pressure, low flow shunts) the symptoms and signs are relatively mild and slower in evolution. The anatomic patency of various venous exits from the cavernous sinus will determine whether contralateral or even bilateral orbital signs develop. Finally, the duration of the altered flow dynamics will determine the degree of hypoxia and ultimate visual impairment.

CLINICAL FEATURES

No other disease or tumor producing unilateral orbital tumefaction is associated with such a variety of symptoms and signs as carotid-cavernous fistula. Most of these symptoms and signs are referable to the eye and adnexa. Of all the symptoms and signs that we will now discuss, there is no one feature that will always appear in all cases of carotid-cavernous fistula. Neither will all the clinical features be present in any given case. Lastly, there is no set pattern of onset or progression that is applicable to all cases, contrary to the statements in many other publications relating to clinical diagnosis. Perhaps it is only safe to say that all patients with these fistulas will develop at least three of the features listed below, sometime between onset and angiographic diagnosis.

In Tables 10 and 11 we have listed the five most common symptoms and signs and their comparative frequency as noted in the thirty-five patients in our study. With only two exceptions the same five symptoms and signs are the most common clinical features of both types of fistulas, but their freqeuncy rate varies slightly.

Prominence of the eye and its corresponding *proptosis,* are high on the list in both Tables 10 and 11. It is one of the first symptoms observed in the trau-

TABLE 10.   FIVE MOST COMMON SYMPTOMS OF
CAROTID-CAVERNOUS FISTULA IN ORDER OF
DECREASING FREQUENCY

Spontaneous Type (20 cases)	Traumatic Type (15 cases)
Prominence of eye	Prominence of eye
Diplopia	Diplopia
Redness of eye	Head noises
Head noises	Soft tissue swelling
Headache	Redness of eye

matic fistulas, but in spontaneous fistulas its onset is often preceded by other clinical symptoms. At onset, the proptosis is straightforward, but in time the eye is displaced more inferiorly owing to persistent enlargement of the superior ophthalmic vein. The degree and amount of proptosis were greater in traumatic fistulas than spontaneous fistulas.

Diplopia and *extraocular muscle weakness* also are common symptoms and signs of orbital involvement. Diplopia frequently is the initial symptom in both the spontaneous type and the traumatic fistula of delayed onset. The close relationship of the oculomotor, trochlear, and particularly the abducens nerve to the cavernous sinus make them particularly prone to pressure early in the development of the fistula. The extraocular muscle weakness was more marked with the traumatic fistula and reflects a conduction defect along two or more of these nerves. The isolated, sixth nerve, abducens palsy was more often observed in the spontaneous fistulas.

Redness and *congestion of the eye due to dilation and tortuosity of the epibulbar venous plexus*, are in our experience the most striking and diagnostic features of carotid-cavernous fistula (Fig. 105 and 106). We have, in fact, observed a few cases wherein these changes in the epibulbar venous plexus were the principal diagnostic clue to an unsuspected carotid-cavernous fistula associated with only minimal proptosis. These corkscrew vessels, by various twists and turns or in parallel rows, extend directly to the limbus of the eye and have a brighter red hue than average venous blood. However, the intervening spaces of conjunctival and scleral tissue between the dilated vessels retain the usual flesh-white color. Some long-standing and severe cases of endocrine exophthalmos also may have dilated veins coursing up to the limbus, but the vessels are not tortuous and corkscrew-like in contour and have a purplish hue. More often, the vascular

TABLE 11.   FIVE MOST COMMON SIGNS OF
CAROTID-CAVERNOUS FISTULA IN ORDER OF
DECREASING FREQUENCY

Spontaneous Type (20 cases)	Traumatic Type (15 cases)
Epibulbar congestion	Proptosis
Proptosis*	Bruit*
Extraocular muscle paresis*	Epibulbar congestion*
Secondary glaucoma	Extraocular muscle paresis
Bruit	Secondary glaucoma

*Equal frequency

dilation of this disease is confined to the region of the lateral canthus (Figs. 19 and 20, Chapter 2).

Head noises and *bruit* are other common presentations in patients with carotid-cavernous fistula. The noises are described as buzzing, pounding, blowing, swishing, or simply strange and often are lateralized to the ipsilateral ear. They may be constant or intermittent and their intensity is usually reduced by carotid compression. Bruit is heard more often in traumatic fistulas than in the spontaneous type. A bruit may be diagnostic of carotid-cavernous fistula but does not necessarily indicate the side of the fistula.

Of the symptoms listed in Table 10, the most difficult one to assess is *headache*. There is no one descriptive feature of this head pain, other than its unilateral distribution, to distinguish it from other persistent headaches, such as migraine or those accompanying occlusive vascular disease. Another disturbing feature is that its significance frequently is unrecognized because, when present, it most often occurs as the initial symptom of the spontaneous fistula before other clues to the disorder appear. It was a much less prominent feature in our patients with traumatic fistulas.

Until we examined the details of individual cases in our series, we did not realize that *secondary glaucoma* was as common a feature of carotid-cavernous fistula as it proved to be.It was always unilateral and quite impervious to medical therapy. It was more easily controlled once the fistula was surgically treated, but the glaucoma did not entirely disappear in most of our cases. We observed one interesting example wherein unilateral glaucoma was the presenting sign of an unrecognized spontaneous fistula (Fig. 106). The person was treated with miotics as a primary glaucoma patient but the intraocular pressure remained high. Glaucoma surgery was then performed. Although the fistulizing operation remained patent, the intraocular pressure was not controlled. This ultimately lead to discovery of the true origin of the unilateral glaucoma.

The remaining symptoms and signs associated with these fistulas, such as droopy eyelid, blepharoptosis, pulsation of the eye, papilledema, dilation of retinal veins, and pupillary reflex abnormalities were infrequent and did not contribute significantly to diagnosis as compared with those features outlined in Tables 10 and 11. Pulsation of the eye occurred in only 20% of our 35 cases. Formerly, pulsating proptosis was considered to be the most obvious and frequent sign of carotid-cavernous fistula, but, as more cases of less obvious examples of fistula are recognized, the incidence of pulsation is proving to be quite low.

Another feature of arteriovenous fistula, less frequent but of extreme importance, is *visual impairment*. It seems to be proportional either to the severity of the fistula or its duration. Visual loss probably is related to the degree of hypoxia of the retina and ganglion cells. Although the progress of visual deterioration could be partially arrested by surgical treatment of the fistula, the visual status of the affected eye remained severely impaired in our patients. Fortunately, this serious complication occurred in only 14% of our cases.

SPECIAL STUDIES

Angiography is the single most important aid in the diagnosis of arteriovenous fistulas affecting the orbit. Selective angiography of the internal and external carotid system with additional selective catheterization of the external carotid system, supplemented by magnification and subtraction techniques, have become essential to the modern study of the vascular malformation. The ophthalmologist's role in this sophisticated field is entirely secondary to that of the neurosurgeon and neuroradiologist. With these techniques the site of the fistula can be localized, the direct or indirect nature of the arteriovenous communication identified, the degree of involvement of orbital veins determined, and the presence or absence of unusual fistulas (bilateral, contralateral, and alternating types) visualized.

Other special studies, such as roentgenography, axial tomography, ultrasonography, and computer tomography play a lesser role in the overall diagnostic scheme but are best used in situations where the risk of angiography is high because of the age or condition of the patient. Enlargement of the superior orbital fissure associated with erosion of the under surface of the anterior clinoid process may occur in fistulas of long duration. An A-mode scan ultrasonogram will show fast-moving echo reflections from the pulsing blood column in such rapid sequence that the display pattern appears fuzzy (Fig. 49, Chapter, 2). Computer tomography does not compare with angiography in diagnostic detail but is useful as a screening test prior to angiography in cases with borderline clinical features. The scan will usually show the dilated superior ophthalmic vein, which is the anterior extension of the extraorbital fistula. In its forward course the dilated vein may resemble the shadow of the optic nerve, except that the former passes forward and medially from the area of the superior orbital fissure in superior orbital sections, whereas the latter passes forward and laterally in midorbit sections.

COURSE AND TREATMENT

The surgical management of arteriovenous fistula is the domain of the neurosurgeon. The ophthalmologist's role is supportive and advisory. The latter, by ophthalmodynamometry, may aid in the assessment of the vascular dynamics; he should stand by to manage any postoperative glaucoma; and it may be his job to remove residual varices in the eyelids and ocular surfaces when treatment of the main malformation is completed.

The main object, of course, is to eradicate completely the offending fistula. Objectively, this is accomplished with increasing frequency. Even so, complete relief of all orbital manifestations is the exception rather then the rule. Some residual orbital or ocular problem usually remains. If the objectives of treatment are considered only on a subjective basis, it is of paramount importance to relieve the patient of those symptoms that are least tolerated. If, by surgery, the patient's headache, face pain, and distracting head noises can be eliminated, if the proptotic red eye can be reduced, the patients often will adjust to other permanent consequences of the fistula.

The management of the 35 patients in our series reflect the gamut of older and newer treatment methods over a period of 27 years. Compression of the carotid artery in the neck on the ipsilateral side may first be tried. Surprisingly, this may reduce the bruit to a tolerable level in some milder cases of the spontaneous type. Even the act of angiography alone has brought about sufficient

closure of the fistula in some patients as to make the risk of further surgery unnecessary. Ligation of the main carotid arteries in the neck supplying the
fistula, preceded or followed by intracranial trapping procedures proximal and
distal to the fistula, have long been a standard approach. More recent methods
employ selective embolization of the malformation by femoral or carotid catheterization utilizing silicone pellets, liquid silicone, and other substances. Or,
the fistula may be obliterated by an inflatable balloon. The management of
each case is judged on the angiographic pattern of the malformation and the
neurosurgeon's training background. When all these advances are considered it
is most astounding that Travers' patient — in the era of 1811 — recovered as remarkably well as Figure 101 so dramatically illustrates.

ARTERIOVENOUS ANEURYSM

TERMINOLOGY

In the past, the loose terminology associated with the diagnosis of these vascular disorders largely was based on clinical appearance or judgment. Verification of the vascular malformation by operation or autopsy usually was lacking
and angiographic mapping had not come into general use. Most of the cases
then designated as arteriovenous aneurysm we would now classify as arterial
aneurysm, orbital varix, or intracranial carotid-cavernous fistula. Indeed, as we
search explicitly for proven cases of what we define as orbital arteriovenous
aneurysm, the lesion becomes exceedingly rare. Applying our classification, we
would prefer the designation *orbital arteriovenous aneurysm* not be used unless
the arteriovenous intercommunicating mass is actually located in the orbit
rather than in adnexa such as the eyelids, or in the intracranial vault, as with
carotid-cavernous fistulas. The orbital arteriovenous aneurysm also differs from
the latter vascular shunt in that its pathogenesis is not based on a direct arterial
communication with a preexisting fixed venous sinus. Also, the diagnosis should
be reserved for those situations in which both arterial and venous components
are verified by surgical exploration, or angiography reveals strongly
presumptive evidence. Diagnosis based solely only on the clinical appearance is
insufficient and more likely the orbital condition results from one of the other
vascular malformations which have been described.

ETIOLOGY AND CLINICAL FEATURES

Arteriovenous aneurysms may be congenital or develop spontaneously; they
also have been attributed to trauma. One case that comes very close to fulfilling
our diagnostic criteria for orbital arteriovenous aneurysm resulted from trauma
and, interestingly, one that was explored and verified surgically nearly a
century ago. Lansdown (1875) described in detail the case of a man who developed proptosis, edema and discoloration of the eyelid, engorgement and tortuosity of epibulbar veins, and a pulsating tumor 6 weeks after repair of a penetrating wound of the nasal portion of the left upper eyelid caused by a glass
fragment. Although it was then customary to treat such vascular tumors by

carotid ligation, Lansdown chose a direct surgical approach to the lesion. His exploration proved there was a communication between nasal artery and vein. Ligatures placed along proximal and distal borders of the pulsating mass effected a cure. The one disturbing feature regarding precise classification of this case is that Lansdown did not state definitively whether the main tumor was located in the eyelid or orbit. As the preoperative clinical description referred to a pulsating mass immediately beneath a cicatrix in the eyelid, it is possible that this arteriovenous aneurysm was located anterior to the orbital septum and not strictly in the orbit.

Another case attributed to trauma was that reported by Sugar and Meyer (1940). A 9-year-old boy, who had been injured by orbital penetration by a pitchfork prong, showed signs and symptoms of vascular malformation that were similar to Lansdown's case; however, the diagnosis was never verified surgically. Roentgenograms of the orbit showed neither fracture nor bony dehiscence. This case was observed before angiography became a common diagnostic procedure, so the true anatomic location of the vascular shunt could not be verified. In the absence of ophthalmoplegia, a clinical diagnosis of orbital arteriovenous aneurysm rather than intracranial carotid-cavernous fistula was favored. The true diagnosis in this case, then, is uncertain. In all other orbital arteriovenous aneurysms attributed to trauma in the literature, the main shunt between artery and vein was located outside the orbit.

Cases of spontaneous onset also have been recorded. An interesting description, by Terry and Fred (1938), is that of a 23-year-old woman who developed, during 3 days, unilateral proptosis (7 mm) during the eighth month of her fourth pregnancy. She complained of a peculiar sound in the affected orbit. A murmur was heard by auscultation and a thrill was palpable over the area of the angular vein. A communication between a branch of the infratrochlear artery and a large tortuous vein in the subcutaneous tissue was verified at operation. This arteriovenous aneurysm probably was located in adnexal tissue just anterior to the orbital septum, according to the author's description, and the orbit probably was secondarily involved. In cases of spontaneous onset of this type we presume that the explanation is some form of dysgenesis due to appropriate stimuli in the normal capillary bed between nearby arteries and veins. Suddenly these intervening capillaries become arterialized, allowing more direct communication between arteries and veins, and the communication later becomes an aneursymal mass.

Jacas, Ley, and Campillo (1959) described another case of spontaneous type. A 23-year-old woman had a 2-year history of intermittent, but increasingly frequent unilateral exophthalmos associated with episodes of diplopia, transient amblyopia, and palpebral edema brought on by forward inclination of the head. Proptosis (6 mm) could be increased by pressure over the ipsilateral jugular vein. Clinically, all these features suggested a diagnosis of orbital varix, but angiography was interpreted as showing an arteriovenous anomaly with arterial supply, probably from a lacrimal artery and drainage via superior ophthalmic vein. This would point to an orbital location of this shunt, but the case never was explored surgically so the diagnosis of arteriovenous aneurysm must remain presumptive. A similar case is included in the Mayo Clinic series.

A 58-year-old woman had noticed sudden onset of vertical diplopia affecting the right eye 3 years before our observation. The original diplopia disappeared after a few days but it was followed by the gradual onset of proptosis and injection of the epibulbar vessels during the next year. During the intervening 2-year period these features did not change. Miotics were prescribed because the diagnosis of glaucoma had been made. When we examined this patient, we found pulsating proptosis (6 mm) of the right eye associated with secondary glaucoma and dilated epibulbar vessels, and we heard a soft bruit. Angiography revealed a vascular anomaly in the orbit associated with enlargement of the ophthalmic artery, a still greater enlargement of the ophthalmic vein, and an aneurysmal mass in the more anterior portion of the orbit (Fig. 108). There was no involvement of the cavernous sinus.

In the four other cases classified as arteriovenous aneurysm in our survey, the orbit was secondarily involved sometime after the diagnosis of the primary malformation. These cases are briefly annotated here to emphasize the course and problems associated with these serious lesions.

A 40-year-old male with diffuse telangiectasia from scalp to toe on left side since birth. Gradual enlargement of vascular anomaly in head and neck area. Pulsating proptosis and bluish discoloration of left eye since age 35. Angiography revealed an arterio-venous anomaly involving head and orbit with major feeder vessels from occipital artery and external carotid system. No bruit. By age 51 it was necessary to protect protruding left eye by a tarsorrhaphy of the eyelids, and the vascular anomaly now involved right orbit. Visual acuity was not impaired. Various surgical procedures to contain the anomaly were to no avail.

A 32-year-old male with a known vascular anomaly of head and neck since age 19. At age 23 he developed bilateral pulsating proptosis. Left homonymous incongruous hemanopsia developed at age 28. Angiography showed large anomaly in upper cervical

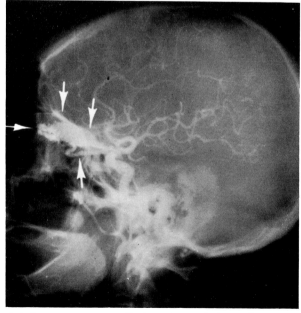

Figure 108.   Arteriovenous aneurysm (*horizontal arrow*) detected in upper, anterior orbit by angiography: also evident are enlarged ophthalmic artery (*lower vertical arrow*) and dilated superior ophthalmic vein (*upper vertical arrows*).

area with chief arterial supply from vertebral artery. A large aneurysmal-like dilation of the vein of Galen was also visible. Ligation procedures were unsuccessful in controlling the progress of the problem.

A 5-year-old male with progressive enlargement and bleeding of a vascular malformation of left forehead since birth. There was gradual displacement of left eye due to spread of varices into left orbit. Ligation of external carotid with radical excision of vascular malformation was performed. Pathologic examination confirmed arterial and venous components in the excised malformation.

A 15-year-old female with hydrocephalus since age 10. Proptosis developed in right eye at age 14. Angiography showed massive arteriovenous anomaly in right parieto-temporal area. Developed convulsive disorder and expired.

An interesting facet of these cases was that visual acuity was not significantly compromised by the obvious progression of the aneurysm. This finding is quite different from the visual disability that could result from an arteriovenous fistula of similar severity and duration.

Bibliography

Vascular Malformations

Dandy WE: The treatment of carotid cavernous arteriovenous aneurysms. Ann Surg *102*:916-920, 1935

Dandy WE, Follis RH, Jr: On the pathology of carotid-cavernous aneurysms (pulsating exophthalmos). Am J Ophthalmol *24*:365-385, 1941

Hunter W: Cited by Osler W

Osler W: Remarks on arterio-venous aneurysm. Lancet *1*:949-955, 1915

Orbital Aneurysm

Heimburger RF, Oberhill HR, McGarry HI, et al: Intraorbital aneurysm: a case of aneurysm of the lacrimal artery. Arch Ophthalmol ns *42*;1-13, 1949

Meyerson L, Lazar SJ: Intraorbital aneurysm of the ophthalmic artery. Br J Ophthalmol *55*:199-204, 1971.

Mortada A: Aneurysm of the orbital part of the ophthalmic artery. Br J Ophthalmol *45*:550–554, 1961

Pfingst AO: Anomalous ophthalmic artery with ocular symptoms. Arch Ophthalmol *16*:829-838, 1936

Rubinstein MK, Wilson G, Levin DC: Intraorbital aneurysm of the ophthalmic artery: report of a unique case and review of the literature. Arch Ophthalmol *80*:42-44, 1968

Sanford HS, Craig WM, Wagener HP: An unusual chiasmal lesion and its operative treatment. Proc Mayo Clin *10*:721-725, 1935

Orbital Varix

Brauston BB, Norton EWD: Intermittent exophthalmos. Am J Ophthalmol *55*:701-708, 1963

Handa H, Mori K: Large varix of the superior ophthalmic vein: demonstration by angular phlebography and removal by electrically induced thrombosis; case report. J Neurosurg *29*:202-205, 1968

Kennedy RE: Arterial embolization of orbital hemangiomas. Trans Am Ophth Soc *76*:266-277, 1978

Rathbun JE, Hoyt WF, Beard C: Surgical management of orbitofrontal varix in Klippel-Trenaunay-Weber syndrome. Am J Ophthalmol *70*:109-112, 1970

Walsh FB, Dandy WE: Pathogenesis of intermittent exophthalmos. Arch Ophthalmol ns *32*:1-10, 1944

Arteriovenous Fistula

Baron: Cited by Locke CE, Jr

Bedell AJ: Traumatic pulsating exophthalmos, with complete bibliography. Arch Ophthalmol *44*:139–153, 1915

Dalrymple W: A case of aneurism by anastomosis in the left orbit, cured by tying the common trunk of the left carotid artery. R Med Chir Soc Lond (Med-Chir Trans) *6*:111-123, 1815

DeSchweinitz GE, Holloway TB: *Pulsating Exophthalmos: Its Etiology, Symptomatology, Pathogenesis, and Treatment — Being an Essay Based Upon an Analysis of Sixty-nine Case Histories of this Affection.* Philadelphia, WB Saunders Company, 1908

Graf CJ: Spontaneous carotid-cavernous fistula: Ehlers-Danlos syndrome and related conditions. Arch Neurol 13:662-672, 1965

Guthrie: Cited by Locke CE, Jr

Henderson JW, Schneider RC: Ocular findings in carotid-cavernous fistula in a series of 17 cases. Trans Am Ophthalmol Soc 56:123-142, 1958

Locke CE, Jr: Intracranial arterio-venous aneurism or pulsating exophthalmos. Ann Surg 80:1-24, 1924

Martin JD, Jr, Mabon RF: Pulsating exophthalmos: review of all reported cases. JAMA‘ 121:330-334, 1943

Newton TH, Hoyt WF: Dural arteriovenous shunts in the region of the cavernous sinus. Neuroradiol 1:71-81, 1970

Sugar HS, Meyer SJ: Pulsating exophthalmos. Arch Ophthalmol ns 23:1288-1321, 1940

Travers B: A case of aneurism by anastomosis in the orbit, cured by the ligature of the common carotid. R Med Chir Soc ‘Lond (Med-Chir Trans) 2:1-16, 1811

Arteriovenous Aneurysm

Jacas R, Ley A, Campillo D: Congenital intraorbital arteriovenous aneurysm. J Neurol Neurosurg Psychiatry 22:330-332, 1959

Lansdown FP: A case of varicose aneurism of the left orbit, cured by ligature of the diseased vessels. Br Med J 1:736, 1875

Sugar HS, Meyer SJ: Pulsating exophthalmos. Arch Ophthalmol ns 23:1288-1321, 1940

Terry TL, Fred GB: Abnormal arteriovenous communication in the orbit involving the angular vein: report of a case. Arch Ophthalmol ns 19:90-94, 1938

7

Fibrous Connective Tissue Tumors

The embryonic mesenchymal cell possesses the potential to develop into any one of several tissues that support, connect, or cushion body structures of more specialized types. Thus, the cell may differentiate into angioblasts, fibroblasts, osteoblasts, and lipoblasts. From these cells, adult types of supporting tissues ultimately are derived. The most ubiquitous and adaptable cell of the entire group is the fibroblast. Neoplasms in which tissues derived from this cell are the main components may be referred to as tumors of fibrous connective tissue.

NOMENCLATURE

There are three elementary components of connective tissue: the cell itself, the supporting or connecting fiber it produces, and the matrix or ground substance of the tissue. Predominance, of any one of these components may influence the structure and hence the name of a connective tissue tumor. If the cell is abundant the tumor is likely to be soft. If the cell is particularly proliferative, almost to the exclusion of supporting fibers and matrix, a sarcomatous state prevails. If fibers are predominant, the tumor is likely to be hard and be designated fibrous. Or, matrix may be the prominent component, in which case its resemblance to primitive mesenchyme accounts for the term myxoma.

Terminology may also reflect the proportion of one component to another: the tumor is undifferentiated (cellular elements predominant) or differentiated (a greater proportion of fibers). In some tumors admixture of connective tissue components may explain a compound designation such as fibromyxoma or myxofibroma. As if this were not enough, the fibroblast tends to philander and mix with other tumors of mesenchymal origin; then more complex terms, such as fibroangioma, fibrolipoma, fibrochondroma, and osteofibroma, are the appellations. This intermingling of fibrocytic components with other tumors of mesenchymal origin, particularly malignant ones, sometimes masks the true identity of the neoplasm; a diagnosis of fibrosarcoma is made, resulting in an exaggerated incidence of this particular neoplasm. Another twist affecting both genesis and nomenclature is the recent discovery, chiefly based on tissue culture study, that not all neoplastic connective tissue necessarily is derived from fibrocytes. Other cells tracing their ancestry to primitive mesenchymal cells, such as histiocytes, lipoblasts, rhabdomyoblasts, and leiomyoblasts, sometimes possess the faculty of producing connective tissue as well as their own specialized progeny in the course of the neoplastic metaplasia. In short, these cells are facultative fibroblasts. This makes the problem of terminology even more complex and emphasizes the importance of correct diagnosis based on the true cell of origin. Finally, there is the rarer tendency to form tumors compounded of several basic tissues, each possessing pluripotential traits. To such mesodermal tumors of mixed origin the term mesenchymoma has been applied.

Another aspect of terminology concerns the manner of growth and demarcation of tumor from its host tissue. Some connective tissue tumors expand by a slow but steady cell multiplication, to which the host responds with a barrier of tough fibrous tissue. These are truly encapsulated tumors and, in the orbit, most are benign. The cells of other more aggressive tumors may insinuate among adjacent tissues so that a tough delimiting capsule never forms, yet a demarcation plane still separates the host from its invader. Such tumors are circumscribed but not encapsulated, the former arrangement frequently being associated with neoplasms of lesser malignancy. Next, some neoplasms are so infiltrative, aggressive, and malignant in character as to defeat cleavage between normal and neoplastic tissue. The surgeon may aid in tumor identification by carefully observing the gross status of the tumor when it is first uncovered. A circumscribed or nonencapsulated tumor likely will be invasive or locally malignant even though its histopathologic appearance may be benign. A myxoma represents an example of such a tumor; appearing benign under the microscope, the myxoma — through its lack of capsule — foretells invasive behavior unless it is widely excised.   Similarly, the surgeon might convert a circumscribed, less malignant tumor into a potentially invasive one by incisional biopsy of its thin exterior mantle.

The clinician should not allow all these terms to confound him. Present terminology may seem more complex but it reflects effort on the part of pathologists to correct past omissions and establish a firmer basis for common understanding.

FIBROMA

The most differentiated, benign form of the neoplasms of connective tissue is the fibroma. This is relatively common in subcutaneous tissue and is often attached to fascial and muscular structures, but in some areas of the body it is rare. The orbit is one such area.

TERMINOLOGY

Composed of fibrocytes surrounded by a dense collection of collagen fibers, the fibroma is well encapsulated. Aside from these basic characteristics, the association of fibrocytes with other tissues should be considered for clarification of terminology. Thus, vascularity is not a trait of a true fibroma; the finding of more than a few capillaries indicates that the tumor might be compound. Also, the term fibroma should not be used to designate congenital fibrous malformations, nor should it be applied to fibrous proliferations resulting from injury or prior surgery around the sinuses and intracranial vault adjacent to the orbit. If the formation of fibrous scar seems proliferative or progressive, fibromatosis would be a preferable term. Similarly, the term should not be loosely applied to fibrous collections within muscle. Fibrous admixtures with osteomas and chondromas are frequent and it may be difficult to differentiate a fibroma with cartilaginous or osseous metaplasia (fibrochondroma or fibro-osteoma) from a cartilaginous or osseous neoplasm with a fibrous component (Fig. 109).

Finally, in many cases recorded in the literature, the histopathologic descriptions or clinical course suggested neurofibroma or one of the vascular tumors with fibrous tissue components. In general it should be remarked that many case reports of fibroma are not supported by confirmatory illustrations.

INCIDENCE

In assessing frequency, one should keep all these factors in mind. Such qualifications significantly diminish the incidence based on case reports in the literature. Fowler and Terplan (1942) reviewed some thirty cases from the literature. From this group they culled sixteen cases, other than their own, that seemed to meet the histopathologic criteria of benign fibroma. This estimate may be high when assessed by modern criteria of terminology. More recent are the reports of Mortada (1971) – two male patients ages 6 and 25 years – and Case and LaPiana (1975) – a 77-year-old male. Among representative orbital tumor surveys, the incidence probably will average less than 0.5%. It seems chiefly a tumor of males.

CLINICAL FEATURES

The symptoms and signs are those of a slowly growing tumor that gradually pushes upon the eye. The direction and degree of displacement of the eye depend on the location and duration of the tumor. Since the tumor grows slowly, the patient may have had symptoms for many years.

Symptoms and signs are also related to the tumor's origin. The neoplasm usually arises from periorbita, fascial coverings of muscle or sclera, or the dural

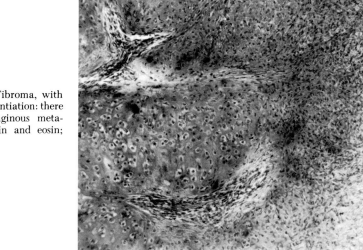

Figure 109. Fibroma, with cartilaginous differentiation: there are foci of cartilaginous metaplasia. (Hematoxylin and eosin; × 100.)

coverings of the optic nerve. In the latter situation, signs such as visual loss, papilledema, and pressure on the posterior wall of the eyeball may indicate a tumor in the retrobulbar space, but fibroma has no clinical features by which to distinguish it from other slowly growing tumors in the same location, for example, optic nerve glioma, neurofibroma, neurilemmoma, and meningioma. Since the fibroma grows slowly it may become relatively large before the patient seeks treatment (Fig. 110).

PATHOLOGY

The orbital fibroma is encapsulated and usually firm or hard in consistency. This type of tumor is definitely fibrous and shows a preponderance of collagen fibers. Its cells are uniform in size and have the spindle shape of mature fibrocytes (Fig. 111). Mitotic figures are rare because the tumor is benign. Both cells and their fibers are arranged in bundles, but these interlace and intertwine to such an extent that bundles may be cut in longitudinal, oblique, or transverse sections in any given microscopic field, hence their whorled appearance. The tumor is poorly vascularized except along fibrous tissue septa which divide the tumor into several lobes. A tumor of many years' duration or one that has long been relatively stationary in size may undergo secondary myxomatous degeneration, a change which might explain the diagnosis of fibromyxoma rather than pure fibroma. Myxomatous change might also be induced by irradiation; the literature indicates that some cases were treated by irradiation several years prior to orbitotomy.

TREATMENT

The treatment of fibroma is excision. The tumors may gradually recur if removed incompletely, and with each recurrence they become a more difficult problem of surgical eradication.

FIBROMATOSES

INCIDENCE AND ORIGIN

The fibromatoses are a newer category of fibrous connective tissue tumors. They occupy the gray zone of classification between fibrous connective tissue tu-

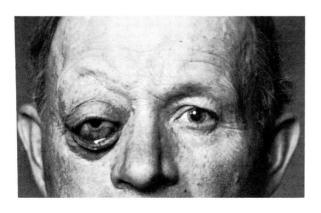

Figure 110. Fibroma: downward displacement, forward proptosis (17 mm), and difficulty in closing eye caused by palpable mass in right orbit (duration, 10 years).

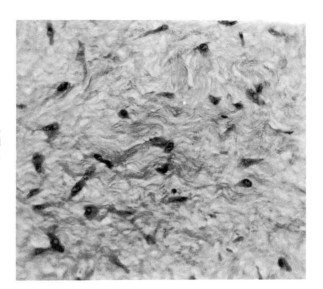

Figure 111. Fibroma: elongated fibrocytes are sparse and fibrillar collagen is abundant. (Hematoxylin and eosin; × 200.)

mors of the inflammatory, reactive type and true neoplasias. Stout believed these tumors exhibited an aggressiveness intermediate between true fibromas and fibrosarcomas. This is our reason for considering them at this point. Widely distributed in the body and variable in size and rate of growth, fibromatoses may be encountered in both young and old age groups. As a whole they have many histologic features in common but are subdivided into multiple subtypes on the basis of their clinical patterns. They tend to infiltrate and even replace tissues such as muscle and fat, and this persistent, locally invasive behavior of some tumors makes them resemble fibrosarcoma. However, they do not metastasize. Their local destructiveness and their tendency to recur if not entirely excised may be fatal if the tumor is located near a vital area. On the other hand, some of the fibromatoses may be relatively harmless.

Reports of fibromatosis affecting the orbit are exceedingly rare. One such example seems to be the case of Schnitka and associates (1958). A huge (4.5 cm in longest diameter) tumor bulging from the right orbit was noted in a newborn female. The tumor infiltrated the surrounding adnexa, displaced the nose toward the opposite orbit, and was covered by a thin layer of skin. At autopsy a normal-appearing eye was found behind the tumor. Other focal nodules of similar tumor were scattered over the child's body. The diagnosis, based on the histopathology of the tumors, was congenital generalized fibromatosis, one of the subtypes of fibromatoses according to Mackenzie (1970).

There have probably been other examples of orbital involvement by fibromatosis in the literature of the past. However, the cases were most likely designated by other terms, such as nonmetastasizing fibrosarcoma or fibrosarcoma grade 1 (desmoid type). If these cases were subject to critical review many would now be considered examples of fibromatosis, in keeping with modern terminology. Such were the circumstances resulting in the reclassification of the one case in our survey. This case seemed to be an example of the most common, musculoaponeurotic type of fibromatosis (desmoid tumor). A brief summary of the salient clinical features of this case follows.

A 5-year-old boy had had proptosis and papilledema of the left eye for approximately 5 months. Straightforward proptosis (3 mm) and papilledema (3 diopters) were observed on ophthalmoscopy. The rotations of the left eye were moderately limited in an upward and lateral direction. No palpable tumor could be elicited and roentgenograms were negative. The orbit was explored through a transfrontal approach. A hard tumor (diameter, 1.25 cm) was completely removed from the area posterior to the eye. The tumor was adherent to many soft tissue structures but seemed to originate from the lateral and superior rectus muscles.

The histopathologic features of the tumor were those of a nonencapsulated, invasive, and destructive proliferation of mature fibrous connective tissue (Fig. 112). The hallmark of the lesion was a tendency toward invasive destruction of the extraocular striated muscles, characterized by separation and isolation of individual muscle fibers. In the areas of muscle degeneration the cytoplasm assumed a glassy or refractile-like appearance. Although progressive invasive growth was prominent, histologic evidence of active fibroblastic proliferation was minimal except at the advancing periphery. Features of malignancy, such as cellular anaplasia, pleomorphism, and mitotic activity, were notably absent.

After excision of the mass the papilledema disappeared, but pallor and atrophy of the optic disk soon ensued. We were not able to follow this patient for longer than 6 months. At the end of this observation period the vision of the left eye was limited to recognition of hand movements, an enophthalmos (2 mm) was present, and considerable blepharoptosis persisted.

A second orbital example of a desmoid tumor has recently been reported (Schutz et al 1979). They observed a 69-year-old woman with 10 mm of proptosis of the right eye of six years' duration because of a palpable tumor in the superior nasal quadrant of the orbit. Owing to its invasive character and large size an exenteration was performed. The invasive character of the tumor in our case, as well as the similar behavior of many of these tumors reported in other areas of the body, suggests that it is preferable to excise the growth completely if at all possible. Irradiation does not appear to be effective.

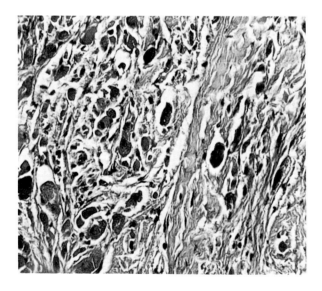

Figure 112. Desmoid: massive proliferation of fibroblasts with dense collagen production and isolation and degeneration of extraocular muscle bundles. (Hematoxylin and eosin; × 160.)

FIBROSARCOMA

TERMINOLOGY

Fibrosarcoma is the most important tumor of fibrous connective tissue. In the past, the term fibrosarcoma has been such a diagnostic refuge for sarcomas with puzzling histopathologic pictures that many malignancies mistakenly have been called by this name. This has given the neoplasm a worse reputation than it deserves. It is malignant in the broadest sense, and there seems little point in arguing the semantics of whether a definition of malignancy should include only those tumors capable of metastasis, at least as far as the orbit is concerned. Some differentiated fibrosarcomas in the orbit may be only locally aggressive when they first appear but become highly malignant when they recur. Malignancy in the orbit thus becomes a matter of degree; fibrosarcoma's effect on the eye ultimately is the same, whichever definition of malignancy is preferred.

INCIDENCE

In an earlier part of this chapter, several factors were noted that have contributed to an exaggerated incidence of fibrosarcoma. If past case descriptions in ophthalmic literature are measured by such criteria, the incidence of this neoplasm decreases sharply. Additional factors — omission or inadequate photographic documentation of the tumor in case studies, histopathologic descriptions inconsistent with a modern definition of fibrosarcoma, statistical enumeration of fibrosarcoma in tumor surveys without descriptive confirmation, inclusion of both secondary and primary neoplasms in the same statistical sample, and classification as fibrosarcoma of tumors really resulting from irradiation — lower still further the apparent incidence of this neoplasm. On the basis of past case reports, fibrosarcoma of the orbit might be considered reasonably common, but in light of modern criteria the incidence probably is relatively low. Certainly fibrosarcoma is much less common in the orbit than in many other soft tissues of the body, but comparative ratios are not known.

Our series included seven fibrosarcomas not associated with irradiation. Only three of these were primary in the orbit; four were secondary, having spread into the orbit from adjacent areas. The three primary fibrosarcomas developed in one man and two women, aged 78, 65, and 68 years, respectively. These patients were much older than those with most other orbital tumors discussed in this text, except for some of the carcinomas. The two patients (one male and one female) reported by Yanoff and Scheie (1966) also were in this older age group, being 60 and 66 years of age. These data suggest that primary fibrosarcoma of the orbit in adults is a neoplasm principally of the elderly. However, the neoplasm also occurs in children; the patient of Eifrig and Foos (1969) was a 3-year-old girl. In between these extremes of age were two of the three cases reported by Mortada (1969) — a 3-year-old boy, a 10-year-old boy, and a 10-year-old girl. A photograph supported the diagnosis in the female patient. Yanoff and Scheie critically reviewed all cases of primary orbital fibrosarcoma in the literature up to the time of their report. They rejected all cases as examples of fibrosarcoma either because no photomicrographs were included or because the histopathologic descriptions did not meet their criteria for diagnosis of this neoplasm. As for secondary fibrosarcoma, three of four patients were males, and they ranged in age from 38 to 66 years. The majority of fibrosarcomas elsewhere in the body are said to occur in males.

CLINICAL FEATURES

Primary Fibrosarcomas

In the orbit, this is a treacherous neoplasm; the clinician should not be lulled by statements in the literature that do not stress its malignant potential. Fibrosarcoma's clinical features are similar to those of other orbital malignant tumors, but the evolution and severity of symptoms may vary according to the degree of malignancy. The primary fibrosarcoma of the orbit, in its initial period of growth, shows lesser degrees (grades 1 and 2) of malignancy. Because this tumor infiltrates, significant proptosis may not become evident until the orbital spaces are extensively filled with tumor. Furthermore, the tumor tends to spread posteriorly rather than to press against fascial planes and tissues along the posterior surface of the eyelids. The palpable portion of one of these neoplasms, therefore, may represent only a small part of its entire bulk. The surgeon who rightly assumes that a palpable tumor may be removed through anterior orbitotomy often is surprised to find that this neoplasm already has spread so deeply toward the apex of the orbit that it is beyond the ken of his dissection.

The common statement that fibrosarcomas grow slowly is deceiving. In our three cases of primary fibrosarcoma, proptosis developed thus: 5 mm in 8 months, 7 mm in 3 months, and 6 mm in but 1 month. In one patient of Yanoff and Scheie (1966), proptosis of 6 mm also occurred in a period of 1 month. The degrees of malignancy in our three cases were grade 1, grade 2, and grade 3, respectively. These features certainly are not those of an indolent malignancy.

Position in the orbit influences the clinical features. In two of our cases the neoplasm was palpated in inferior quadrants of the orbit; in the third it was located in the superoposterior portion of the orbit. Other reports have noted location in the upper nasal quadrant. Ptosis and edema or swelling of the upper eyelids are the initial signs of tumors arising in upper quadrants. Often, marked ophthalmoplegia reflects the effect of the tumor's encroachment on the posterior orbit. In two of our cases the ophthalmoplegia was such, in proportion to other symptoms, as to suggest possible metastatic malignancy on initial evaluation. Roentgenograms are not helpful in diagnosis of primary fibrosarcoma. Information is too sparse to suggest any conclusions on the relationship of trauma to orbital fibrosarcomas.

Secondary Fibrosarcomas

There are several differences between secondary and primary fibrosarcomas: first, the patients with secondary fibrosarcomas seem to be younger — all four in our series (three of whom were male) were younger than the patients with primary fibrosarcoma; second, the tumors are more malignant, or become so with each attempt to eradicate them by surgery; and third, roentgenography helps to pinpoint the tumors' origins because bone destruction accompanies their growth. The orbit is only one of several areas entered by the infiltrating neoplasm. In our four patients the paranasal sinuses, the nose, and the upper jaw were areas of primary growth. In three, persistent spread into the orbit was obvious. In the remaining patient, an orbital mass was the presenting sign of a fibrosarcoma that originated in the ethmoid labyrinth.

PATHOLOGY

Although the histopathologic features of fibrosarcoma may vary from one specimen to another depending on the degree of malignancy, four components are common to all fibrosarcomas: spindle-shaped cells, elongated nuclei containing several nucleoli, a stroma of collagen fibers, and a network of reticulin. In less malignant types the spindle cells are arranged in reasonably orderly, interlacing, linear bundles and fascicles (Fig. 113); the long nuclei with rounded ends show clumping of chromatin, and the collagen stroma is abundant with the reticulin network, intertwining individual cells, becoming visible by means of special stains. As the degree of malignancy increases, the stroma of collagen becomes more sparse, the reticulin network is more irregularly distributed, the ratio of cells to stroma increases, and the nuclei become hyperchromatic (Fig. 114). The degree of malignancy often can be assessed from the number of mitoses in a given number of microscopic fields, counted under a magnification of 450 times; this is the mitotic index. The higher the index, the more malignant is the tumor and the poorer the prognosis.

Electron microscopy may be helpful in the diagnosis of doubtful cases. According to Jakobiec and Tannenbaum (1974), fibrosarcoma cells have relatively large amounts of rough-surfaced endoplasmic reticulum, and active Golgi complexes, but no basement membranes. Other characteristic features are poorly developed desmosomes and sparse intercellular interdigitations.

COURSE AND TREATMENT

The fibrosarcoma is capable of metastasis, particularly if markedly cellular and undifferentiated. The majority of fibrosarcomas originating in the orbit are less malignant types and initially remain within the orbit. After a period of

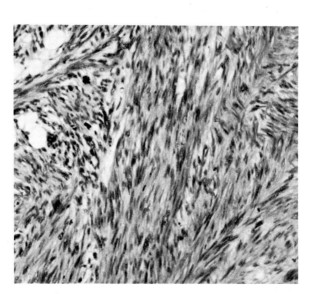

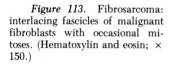

Figure 113. Fibrosarcoma: interlacing fascicles of malignant fibroblasts with occasional mitoses. (Hematoxylin and eosin; × 150.)

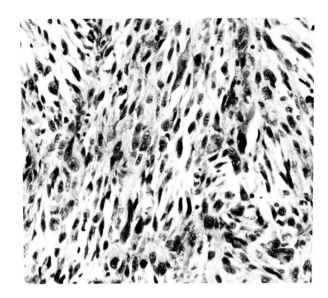

Figure 114. Fibrosarcoma: as indicators of greater malignancy (see Fig. 113) cells are larger, darker, and more varied. (Hematoxylin and eosin; × 200.)

several months, they may grow through the foramina and fissures leading to the intracranial vault. As a rule, this is interrupted by exploratory orbitotomy for the unilateral proptosis, but in most cases surgical exploration results in incomplete removal of the neoplasm. The remaining tumor then seems to become more aggressive and seeks more rapid egress by spreading to the intracranial vault or metastasizing elsewhere through the bloodstream unless interrupted or eradicated by further treatment. Definitive therapy often is deferred because the patient fears loss of the eye or the surgeon hesitates in advising and performing the radical measures necessary for possible cure. Several months or even a year may thus elapse between the initial surgical exploration and the second orbitotomy — and the length of this interval may determine whether the battle with this tumor is won or lost. The sooner the second operation, then, the greater its success. We have observed patients treated by several of these approaches; we also have observed both fatal and gratifying results. A brief résumé of the management of the seven patients in our series may help in the formulation of conclusions concerning preferred treatment. The three cases of primary fibrosarcoma are described first.

CASE 1.   A 78-year-old man had had a tumor of one orbit for 8 months. Only a biopsy was done. The histologic diagnosis was fibrosarcoma, grade 1. Despite irradiation with cobalt-60, the neoplasm spread into soft tissues, and along periosteum and periorbita on both sides of the inferior orbital rim. The patient died of a "stroke" 5 months after irradiation.

Because an autopsy was not done, the relationship of the tumor to the cerebrovascular accident could not be established. This case illustrates the radioresistance of most fibrosarcomas, a feature noted by many observers.

CASE 2.   A 65-year old woman underwent orbitotomy for proptosis of 7 mm, of 3 months' duration. A circumscribed tumor was removed, apparently in its entirety, from the superoposterior-medial portion of the orbit, and the proptosis and associated papilledema were rapidly corrected. The histologic diagnosis was fibrosarcoma, grade 2. At follow-up 14 years later this patient was living and well; vision in the affected eye was 20/20 and the optic disk was slightly pale. This case illustrates the circumscribed nature of some orbital fibrosarcomas and suggests that a cure is possible when the tumor is completely removed without preliminary biopsy.

CASE 3. A 68-year-old woman had been affected by proptosis of 6 mm for 1 month. A gray-white infiltrative mass in the posterolateral aspect of the orbital cavity was biopsied; examination proved it to be fibrosarcoma, grade 3. Next day, exenteration was performed. The neoplasm, measuring 4 by 2 by 2½ cm, had infiltrated surrounding fat, muscle, and periorbita. This treatment was supplemented with intravenous administration of actinomycin D (0.25 mg daily for 12 days) and cobalt-60 irradiation (2,400 R) in a 12-day period. Response to treatment was gratifying, and patient was tumor-free for almost 6 years. At this time a thoracotomy revealed metastatic lesions in the chest wall. The patient expired 9 years after onset with metastatic fibrosarcoma of the kidney. The vigorous approach to treatment may have been responsible for the long interval between initial surgery and metastasis, but it did not save the patient from the fatal consequences of the infiltrating tumor.

Several interesting features in the course of fibrosarcoma secondarily involving the orbit make a brief review of this group pertinent also.

CASE 4. A 38-year-old man had noted intermittent bleeding from the left side of the nose for nearly 2½ years before the diagnosis was made by biopsy. At this time a mass from the naso-ethmoid area bulged into the region of the left medial canthus and orbit. Exenteration and extensive resection of bony partitions of adjacent sinuses were performed. Histologic examination identified the neoplasm as fibrosarcoma, grade 4. Within a year the tumor had metastasized to lung and hilar nodes though the orbit and sinuses remained unaffected. The patient died from systemic manifestations of fibrosarcoma 17 months after exenteration; the orbit and sinuses were still free of tumor at that time. In this case, radical surgery seemed effective in eradicating orbital extension of the neoplasm but the long period of premonitory signs permitted the highly malignant fibrosarcoma to seed itself elsewhere beyond the scope of the surgeon.

CASE 5. A 40-year-old man had been affected by orbital invasion by a neoplasm from the left antrum for approximately 1 year before an attempt was made to destroy it. The antral mass was treated with extensive diathermy, supplemented by insertion of two radium elements (each, 50 mg). Histologic examination indicated a partially necrotic fibrosarcoma, grade 3. Exenteration of the left orbit was performed 6 months later. The patient died 2½ years after the initial antral surgery from neoplastic extension into the intracranial vault. This case was somewhat similar to the first one in regard to age, sex, tumor type, and long duration of symptoms before treatment. However, in this case surgery was not as extensive at the initial operation and when this patient died there was evidence of local recurrence.

CASE 6. A 65-year-old woman initially had complained of a pea-sized painless mass on the alveolar margin of the left upper jaw. The mass gradually enlarged but it was not until 5 years had passed that it was first resected. The tumor soon recurred and a mass was excised a second time in another 2 years. The extent of these resections was not known to us. Irradiation followed. Three years later the tumor had filled the left antrum and extended into the floor and lateral portion of the adjacent orbital cavity. At this time the tumor was identified as fibrosarcoma, grade 2. The entire maxilla was removed and the surrounding soft tissues were electrocoagulated. Local recurrence again was evident in another 2 years when the patient died of multiple metastases — 12 years after onset and 7 years following the first surgical procedure. Considering the small size of the mass and the lesser degree of malignancy in its initial stages, it seems reasonable to speculate this neoplasm might have been eradicated by either earlier or more radical resection at the time of initial surgery.

In the next case there was a happier outcome but this was in doubt at the time of local recurrence because of the proximity of the neoplasm to the intracranial space.

CASE 7.   A 54-year-old man had observed painless, progressive lateral displacement of the right eye associated with transient diplopia and blurred vision during a period of 4 months. Proptosis (7 mm) was associated wtih a firm, immovable mass which was palpably contiguous with the bony rim in the superior nasal quadrant of the right orbit. Initally we assumed the neoplasm was primary in the orbit, but roentgenograms suggested a primary locus in the adjacent ethmoid sinus, and this was confirmed at the first operation. Histologic examination identified the neoplasm as fibrosarcoma, grade 1. A "meaty" tumor filled the ethmoid labyrinth and frontal sinus, and it replaced the orbital roof and extended posteriorly to the optic foramen. A radical external fronto-ethmoid-sphenoid resection was then performed. Three years later, recurrence (diameter 2 cm) was evident along remnants of the orbital roof posteriorly, the fibrosarcoma being classified as grade 2. Two further resections were performed within 6 months. Throughout these three surgical procedures the right eye remained intact, though displaced downward. The patient was living 23 years after initial diagnosis without metastasis or local recurrence and the vision was 20/20 in the displaced eye.

From these experiences, together with the findings reported in the literature, certain statements concerning course and treatment of fibrosarcoma seem valid:

1. The longer the duration of symptoms before treatment, the greater is the chance of ultimate fatal outcome.
2. Cure sometimes follows radical removal of the tumor at the initial operation.
3. Recurrences are common after incomplete surgical removal or with other modes of therapy.
4. Prognosis becomes more guarded with each succeeding recurrence.
5. Some orbital fibrosarcomas are circumscribed.
6. The course of fibrosarcomas primary in the orbit seems to be more rapid than that of fibrosarcomas of similar malignancy elsewhere.
7. The degree of malignancy is aggravated by surgical manipulation or attempts at treatment.
8. The higher the grading of malignancy, the greater is the likelihood of metastasis.
9. The lower the grading of malignancy, the slower is the evolution and course of the neoplasm.
10. Irradiation may only be helpful for palliation of pain.

FIBROSARCOMA FOLLOWING IRRADIATION

INCIDENCE AND ORIGIN

It is appropriate here to consider sarcomas that occur in the orbital cavity and arise from orbital bones as a result of irradiation. That both carcinoma and sarcoma may follow irradiation anywhere in the body is now accepted as fact. Around the orbit, this so-called irradiation cancer usually is seen some time after extensive x-ray or gamma-ray therapy for secondary neoplasms such as squamous cell carcinomas and chondrosarcomas that invade the orbit from an adjacent sinus, and for intraocular retinoblastoma. Therapy of the latter has been the chief source for the radiation-induced neoplasms seen in the orbit or surrounding adnexa. In these situations radiotherapy usually has been administered either to prevent intracranial spread of a retinoblastoma that has extended along the optic nerve beyond the plane of section of the enucleated eye or to eradicate intraocular retinoblastoma in a child with bilateral tumors. Of the several types of sarcoma so induced, fibrosarcoma is the second most common, with osteogenic sarcoma being most frequent.

The widest experience with this problem and the most discerning reviews of the subject are the reports of Forrest (1962), Soloway (1966), Sagerman et al (1966), and Abramson et al (1976). These reports are a composite of cases reported in the literature, analyses of cases in the files of the Armed Forces Institute of Pathology, and retrospective study of the large number of patients previously treated at the Columbia-Presbyterian Medical Center Eye Tumor Clinic in New York. Emphasis was directed toward patients previously treated for retinoblastoma. As a result, some overlap of patients occurred in the successive surveys of these cases. Fibrosarcoma occurred in 16% (4 cases) of the 25 neoplasms collected by Forrest. Six fibrosarcomas (24%) were noted in the 25 radiation-induced tumors studied by Soloway. The series of Sagerman et al had 2 fibrosarcomas among their total of 21 second tumors. There was no apparent explanation in any of these surveys as to why some patients of the same age group treated with radiation in a similar manner would develop fibrosarcoma rather then osteogenic sarcoma and vice versa.

Our own experience with this problem is exceedingly limited, probably because, in an era when irradiation dosage was large, our radiophysicists and radiotherapists were quite cautious in the amount of irradiation used around the eye and orbit except in some cases of advanced carcinoma. Most of the latter never live long enough to develop a radiation-induced second neoplasm.

The one case in our series was a fibrosarcoma secondarily invading the orbit from a recurrent tumor in the maxillary sinus in a 55-year-old male. Six years previously a resection of a tumor of the cheek had been performed elsewhere, followed by cobalt irradiation of 6000 rads. The histologic makeup of this primary tumor was that of a straightforward cellullar mixed tumor of a salivary gland. Radical resection of the recurrent tumor was performed. Histologic study showed a grade 3 fibrosarcoma superimposed on residues of the mixed tumor. The cellular atypia and anaplasia were indicative of an irradiation-induced metaplasia (Fig. 115). The tumor continued to progress, proptosis became more marked, and the patient expired 1½ years after radical surgery.

CLINICAL COURSE

A firm lump appearing along the posterior wall of an anophthalmic orbit, or on the medial or lateral wall of a treated orbit, usually signifies the onset of malignant destruction. Another sign is destruction of adjacent bone, visible on roentgenograms. Those children who develop an atrophic, telangiectatic, hyperpigmented skin in or around the orbit following irradiation must be watched

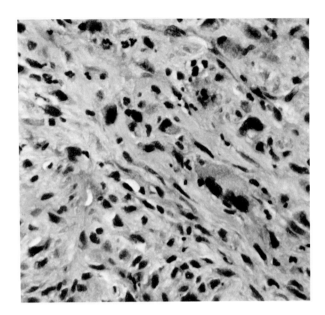

Figure 115. Post radiation fibrosarcoma in a mixed tumor. This anaplastic neoplasm contains fibrogenic spindled cells and numerous bizarre and multinucleated giant cell forms. (Hematoxylin and eosin; × 400.)

carefully for the subsequent development of any painless lump or nodule near the treated area. The patients most prone to develop this malignant change were those who had had bilateral retinoblastoma, according to Abramson et al, 78 (or 97.5%) of a total of 80 patients with second neoplasms.

A variable interval between completion of irradiation and appearance of the sarcoma was noted in all the reviews recorded above. In the four fibrosarcomas of the Forrest series the interval was as short as 5 years and as long as 27 years. In Strickland's case (1966) the latent interval was 33 years. Other conclusions common to the multiple surveys were that latent intervals were not appreciably different whether radiation was received in infancy or adulthood; that there was no direct correlation of dose with latent period; and that the prognosis was uniformly poor.

In spite of this grim picture we would like to hope that an early and wide resection of an ominous fibrosarcoma nodule, located in an accessible area, might forestall an otherwise inevitable fatality.

FIBROUS HISTIOCYTOMA

Not long ago, in 1961, Kauffman and Stout studied a group of soft tissue tumors in children in which the histiocyte was thought to be the cell of origin. These thirty-nine cases were divided into two groups, depending on the fibroblastic content of the tumor. The tumor with a large content of fibrous tissue was called *fibrous xanthoma* and the tumor with but little fibrous tissue was designated *histiocytoma*. To explain the predominant fibrous content of the majority of their cases the authors postulated that the basic histiocyte exercised its facultative character by producing fibrous tissue. This concept of a tissue cell possessing pleuripotential, tissue-forming properties was relatively new at that time.

Subsequently, Ozzello et al (1963) performed tissue culture studies of these tumor variants and found that, with time, the cells took on the features of a fibroblast. This suggested these histiocytic tumors had their origin in a more primitive precursor cell, probably related to the lineage of fibrous tissue tumors. The clinical importance of this feature was to separate these fibrohistiocytic tumors from the histiocytic tumors (histiocytosis, reticuloendotheliosis, histiocytic lymphoma) derived from the primitive reticular cell, the monocyte-histiocyte of the blood. The histiocytic tumors are multicentric disorders in contrast to the more localized character of the fibrous histiocytoma.

A latent period followed the earlier clinical observation until physicians began to place other soft tissue lesions into this new category of tumors of mesenchymal cell derivation with variable combinations of fibrous and histiocytic differentiation. Stout and Lattes (1964), in an effort to standardize the profuse and diverse nomenclature, proposed a classification wherein fibrous histiocytoma was used as the rubric for several benign and malignant tumors, such as *fibroxanthoma, atypical fibroxanthoma, nodular tenosynovitis, dermatofibroma, sclerosing hemangioma, storiform fibrous xanthoma, xanthofibroma, epithelial sarcoma,* and others. In our discussion we will use "fibrous histiocytoma" in the more limited sense as a designation for the benign and malignant forms of the fibrous xanthoma of the Stout and Lattes classification. This is in keeping with the trend in the ophthalmic literature to discuss fibrous histiocytoma as an individual tumor rather than as a multigroup designation.

INCIDENCE

In addition to many of the initial observations on this tumor, Stout also seems one of the first to describe a case of orbital involvement (O'Brien and Stout 1964). This was the case of a 51-year-old woman. A large tumor (1 by 7.5 cm) was removed from one orbit. During a period of 11 years there were three local recurrences. The orbit finally was exenterated. The exact location of this tumor was not given, except that the authors said it was "superficially placed." This term also was applied to those neoplasms with some involvement of skin or subcutaneous tissue. It is possible that in this case of Stout and O'Brien, the tumor originated in one of the adnexal tissues (eyelids) and then spread into the orbit. Its large size – 7.5 cm in one diameter – makes it unlikely that it occupied much of the true orbital space, or the eye itself would have been affected at the first operation.

No additional cases of orbital involvement were recorded until the case reported by Russman (1967). This is more likely a primary tumor in the orbit than was the case of Stout and O'Brien although the histopathologic diagnosis was much less certain. Russman's patient underwent the first orbitotomy when 28 years of age. The diagnosis then was neurinoma, but when original tissue sections again were reviewed at the time of first recurrence 27 years later, the diagnosis was changed to cellular neurofibroma. At the time of the second orbitotomy, the tumor was located in the lower temporal quadrant of the orbit and extended posteriorly to the orbital apex. The neoplasm was partially removed, the diagnosis of this specimen being low-grade fibrosarcoma. Between the first and second orbitotomies, the affected orbit was irradiated. At the third orbitotomy, 5 years after the second operation, the histopathologic diagnosis was malignant hemangiopericytoma or hemangioendothelioma. Because of such diversity in diagnosis, tissue samples were reviewed by several pathologists, and seven different diagnoses were made. Benign fibrous xanthoma was one of the seven diagnoses.

Also, in 1967, Zimmerman commented on the histopathology of orbital fibrous histiocytoma but did not include any case protocols. Zimmerman wondered if this tumor may not have been adequately recognized in the past.

Soon other reports of orbital involvement appeared. Single cases were noted by Vogel (1969), Jakobiec and Jones (1976), Rodrigues et al (1977), and Biedner and Rothkoff (1978), as well as six cases by Jakobiec et al (1974). The age of nine of these patients was stated and ranged from 1 to 59 years of age at the time of diagnosis. Sex incidence of the total 10 patients was 6:4 female to male. This would still be a meager number of cases upon which to base any incidence data were it not for a forthcoming study by Font of the Armed Forces Institute of Pathology. In something over 100 cases of fibrous histiocytoma, males and females were equally affected, and the median age was 42 years (with a range of 16 to 80 years).

Attention also should be called to a fibrous histiocytoma of the lacrimal sac (Cole and Ferry, 1978) and a fibrous histiocytoma metastatic to the orbit in a 47-year-old male (Stewart et al, 1978). So far, reports of secondary invasion of the orbit from adjacent tissues are very sparse. The one example in the Mayo Clinic survey was of this type.

A 74-year-old man was observed with a 6-month history of a mass progressively enlarging along the left superior alveolar ridge, followed by nasal obstruction, pain in the left cheek, and upward displacement of the left eye. Roentgenograms indicated a destructive lesion affecting lateral, inferior, and superior walls of the left antrum. An operation supplemented by irradiation failed to halt the progress of the malignant neoplasm and the patient died from metastasis 12 months after diagnosis.

In conclusion, what was regarded as only a new member in the clan of orbital tumors in the prior edition of this text has now become an established resident of the orbit. Its predilection for the orbit seems certain, but we are reluctant to accept the statement, based on frequency of pathologic specimens, that fibrous histiocytoma is the most common soft tissue tumor of the orbit. Its true incidence cannot be judged until a large survey of consecutive orbital tumors containing examples of the neoplasm is published.

CLINICAL FEATURES

The less than a dozen cases of fibrous histiocytoma primary in the orbit which are noted above are too few to describe a definite clinical pattern of behavior. Until follow-up data on the larger number of patients studied by Font is reported, we must be satisfied with generalities. In most cases the tumors were palpable and were described as soft, fluctuant, or somewhat cystic in contour, at least in the early stages of growth. Diplopia was uniformly present, indicating early involvement of the extraocular muscles. These two factors, if confirmed by a study of a larger series of tumors, may be of some clinical significance inasmuch as most soft tumors of the orbit, unless sarcomatous, do not affect the extraocular muscles except by the bulk of their extended growth. Pain was not a notable feature in any cases, and the character of proptosis was not different from that of other slowly growing neoplasms.

PATHOLOGY

Grossly, these tumors are soft, somewhat friable, pale in color and may be either circumscribed or infiltrative. Microscopically, the hallmark feature is a whorl-like, almost cartwheel, arrangement of proliferating spindle cells (Fig. 116). Storiform is the name most often used to describe this pattern of interwoven fascicles. In areas where this pattern is dominant the histiocytic features of the tumor may be so compressed as to be almost concealed. In other areas the polyhedral-shaped histiocytes with their foamy cytoplasm are more easily identified. The nuclei of the spindle cells will be narrow or slightly oval in shape, depending on the degree of spindling. Mitoses are uncommon. The amount of intercellular collagen and reticulin will be less in those tumors with larger zones of histiocytic proliferation. Myxomatous foci may also be noted, and a capillary component is usually a prominent feature in every tumor.

The more aggressive, atypical, or borderline malignant tumors will look more cellular, and mitoses will be more frequently seen. When the tumor becomes malignant, more bizarre, anaplastic, and pleomorphic histiocytic cells will be evident, associated with some multinucleated forms.

No matter how these tumors are described there is a wide range of histologic patterns varying from one tumor to another and sometimes within the same tumor. In the entire group, tumors are encountered which cannot be definitely classified as either malignant or benign; this has made it difficult to correlate the histologic picture with prognosis. In addition, some benign-appearing fibrous histiocytomas of somatic soft tissues have been known to metastasize, whereas some cases with malignant looking lesions have remained relatively stationary in their clinical course.

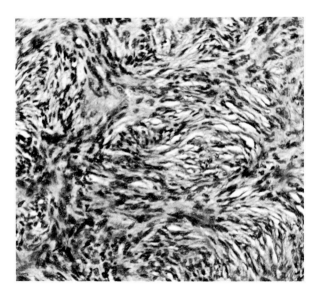

Figure 116. Fibrous histiocytoma: the fibrogenic qualities of the histiocyte predominate and cells show a cartwheel or storiform pattern. (Hematoxylin and eosin; × 170.)

In situations in which the cellular pattern is quite mixed and the diagnosis of fibrous histiocytoma is in some doubt, electron microscopy may be helpful. Although the fibrous histiocytoma cell has many ultrastructural features of the fibroblast (moderate amount of rough-surfaced endoplasmic reticulum, no basement membrane, nonspecific cytoplasmic filaments, and underdeveloped desmosomes), its prominent interdigitating cell processes differentiate it from other cells of related genre.

COURSE AND TREATMENT

There are a number of variables to consider when trying to predict the course or outline a treatment for these tumors. First, some of these tumors are circumscribed and this should encourage their complete excision. Their location also may be a determinant in the way they are managed. In most of the cases so far reported the neoplasm was located in the more anterior portion of the orbit. This factor should make an infiltrative tumor more accessible to a wide excision than would be the case if the mass were located in the posterior orbit. The soft nature of the tumor also should make it easier to manipulate and encompass than a more inelastic, hard mass, no matter where their location in the orbit. Finally, there is the problem of correlating the histopathology of the tumor with prognosis. Are the numerous recurrences of the tumor reported in the literature due to poor removal of the tumor or aggressive growth of tumor? Will widely excised but nonencapsulated tumors always recur, and, if so, what factors determine the interval of recurrence? The latter is quite variable among the recorded cases.

When faced with the dilemma of how to manage an unpredictable tumor, such as fibrous histiocytoma, the surgeon may ask what should be done if he or she were the patient. For the more accessible orbital tumors we would do a wide excision including resection of any involved extraocular muscle. If the histologic findings in the tumor were predominantly fibroblastic or if the histiocytic component were not unduly cellular or pleomorphic, we would observe the patient closely for a possible recurrence over a 5-year period. If the histologic findings were frankly malignant we would proceed with a subtotal or total exenteration, depending upon the assumed extent of the tumor beyond the plane of excision. Likewise, subtotal or total exenteration would be performed for any recurrent tumor.

The exact effect of irradiation is not known.

Perhaps only time and experience will resolve some of these questions concerning management and course.

PROLIFERATIVE NODULAR FASCIITIS

This is another tumefaction of connective tissue origin which, while resembling a neoplasm in growth and appearance, is not in fact a neoplasm. It is a benign, nodular proliferation of fibroblasts of unknown genesis which is classified among the reactive and inflammatory lesions in the "fibroblastic spectrum" of Mackenzie. It is separated from the fibromatoses, discussed earlier, on the basis of a granulomatous component. Konwaler, Keasbey, and Kaplan

(1955) were the first to report a series of such tumors. The tumor is frequently located in the subcutaneous tissue and fascia of the trunk and extremities. Some call this tumor *proliferative nodular fasciitis*; others have named it *pseudosarcomatous fasciitis*.

INCIDENCE

Two examples of orbital involvement (Levitt and associates 1969, and Perry et al 1975) have been reported and this is a reason for briefly discussing the lesion in this text. In the first case (a 14-year-old boy) the tumor was palpated beneath the superior-nasal margin of the orbit and the extent of the tumor posteriorly into the orbit was confirmed surgically. In the case of Perry et al (a 34-year-old female) the tumor was located in the posterior-superior-lateral portion of the orbit. Another thirteen cases occurring on the surface of the eye or ocular adnexa (eyelids, eyebrow, and upper face) are found in the reports of Font and Zimmerman (1966), Tolls et al (1966), Meachan (1974), and Ferry and Sherman (1974). The age range of this group was 3 to 81 years at time of diagnosis with a female to male ratio of 9:4.

CLINICAL FEATURES

The palpable tumor in the 14-year-old boy with orbital involvement was nontender, freely movable, firm, and the size of a pea. The deeper tumor in the 39-year-old female was associated with proptosis and diplopia. Symptomatology in the first case was short (3 months), but the deeper tumor had been present for at least a year. The absence of pain and discomfort in both cases was noteworthy inasmuch as this tumor, in the somatic soft tissues, often is accompanied by pain or tenderness, probably secondary to early invasion of nearby nerves. In both orbital cases the lesions were discrete and not attached to any major orbital structure. The more forward tumor in the 14-year-old was not encapsulated but the other tumor was well encapsulated and was delivered intact. In both cases the lesions were easily removed and recurrence was not anticipated.

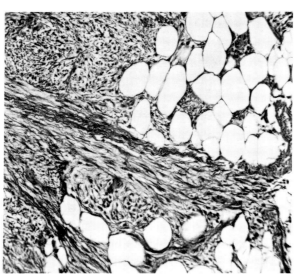

Figure 117. Proliferative fasciitis: neoplastic-like reactive proliferation of fibroblasts extending in nonencapsulated fashion into the adjacent tissues. (Hematoxylin and eosin; × 110.)

PATHOLOGY

Proliferating fibroblasts are the most prominent feature of this tumor. They may vary somewhat in shape depending on the degree of cellular density, but, in size, they are slightly larger than normal. The nuclei are oval and plump. These cells proliferate as interlacing fascicles or bundles having almost a tissue culture apearance (Fig. 117). In the more compact portions of the tumor the intercellular matrix will be collagenous, but in less compact areas the stroma will be distinctly myxoid in appearance. With silver stains a haphazard reticulin pattern can be seen. Variably sized capillaries are a frequent component of all these tumors. Mitotic activity is extremely variable but the mitotic figures look normal. A thorough search of successive microscopic sections will usually uncover zones of lymphocytes, plasma cells, and macrophages with occasional multinucleated cells. The cellularity of the tumor, the frequent myxoid stroma, and the mitotic activity are the principal features confused with sarcoma.

Bibliography

Nomenclature

Enzinger F, Lattes R, Torloni H: Histological Typing of Soft Tissue Tumors. Geneva, World Health Organization, 1969
Mackenzie DH: *The Differential Diagnosis of Fibroblastic Disorders.* Oxford, Blackwell Scientific Publications, 1970
Stout AP: Fibrous tumors of the soft tissues. Minn Med 43:455-459, 1960
Stout AP, Lattes R: Tumors of the soft tissues. In *Atlas of Tumor Pathology.* Second Series, Fascicle 1. Washington, D.C., Armed Forces Institute of Pathology, 1967

Fibroma

Case TD, LaPiana FG: Benign fibrous tumor of the orbit. Ann Ophthal 7:813-815, 1975
Fowler JG, Terplan KL: Fibroma of the orbit. Arch Ophthalmol ns 28:263-271, 1942
Mortada A: Fibroma of the orbit. Brit J Ophthalmol 55:350-352, 1971

Fibromatoses

Mackenzie DH: *The Differential Diagnosis of Fibroblastic Disorders.* Oxford, Blackwell Scientific Publications, 1970
Schnitka T, Asp D, Horner R: Congenital generalized fibromatoses. Cancer 11:627-639, 1958
Schutz JS, Rabkin MD, Schutz S: Fibromatous tumor (desmoid type) of the orbit. Arch Ophthalmol 97:703-705, 1979
Stout AP, Lattes R: Tumors of the soft tissues. In *Atlas of Tumor Pathology.* Second Series, Fascicle 1. Washington, D.C., Armed Forces Institute of Pathology, 1967

Fibrosarcoma

Eifrig DC, Foos RY: Fibrosarcoma of the orbit. Am J Opthalmol 67:244-248, 1969
Jakobiec FA, Tannenbaum M: The ultrastructure of orbital fibrosarcoma. Am J Ophthal 77:899–915, 1974
Mortada A: Rare primary orbital sarcomas. Am J Ophthalmol 68:919-925, 1969
Yanoff M, Scheic HG: Fibrosarcoma of the orbit: report of two patients. Cancer 19:1711-1716, 1966

Fibrosarcoma Following Irradiation

Abramson DH, Ellsworth RM, Zimmerman LE: Nonocular cancer in retinoblastoma survivors. Trans Am Acad Ophthalmol Otolaryng 81:OP454-457, 1976
Forrest AW: Tumors following radiation about the eye. Int Ophthalmol Clin 2:543-553, 1962
Sagerman R, Cassady J, Tretter P, et al: Radiation-induced neoplasia following external beam therapy for children with retinoblastoma. Am J Roentgenol Radium Ther Nucl Med 105:529-535, 1966

Soloway H: Radiation induced neoplasms following curative therapy for retinoblastoma. Cancer *19*:1984-1988, 1966

Strickland P: Fibromyxosarcoma of the orbit: radiation induced tumor 33 years after treatment of "bilateral ocular glioma." Brit J Ophthalmol *50*:50-53, 1966

Fibrous Histocytoma

Biedner B, Rothkoff L: Orbital fibrous histiocytoma in an infant. Am J Ophthalmol *85*:548-550, 1978

Cole SH, Ferry AP: Fibrous histiocytoma (fibrous xanthoma) of the lacrimal sac. Arch Ophthalmol *96*:1647-1649, 1978

Enzinger F, Lattes R, Torloni H: Histological typing of soft tissue tumors. *In* International Histological Classification of Tumors #3. Geneva, World Health Organization, 1969

Font; Quoted by Jakobiec FA, Jones IS

Jakobiec FA, Howard GM, Jones IS, et al: Fibrous histiocytomas of the orbit. Am J Ophthalmol *77*:333-345, 1974

Jakobiec FA, Jones IS: Mesenchymal and fibro-osseous tumors. In *Clinical Ophthalmology*. Vol 2, Chap 44. Ed: TD Duane. Hagerstown, Harper and Row Publishers, 1978

Kauffman SL, Stout AP: Histiocytic tumors (fibrous xanthoma and histiocytoma) in children. Cancer *14*:469-482, 1961

O'Brien JE, Stout AO: Malignant fibrous xanthomas. Cancer *17*:1445-1455, 1964

Ozzello L, Stout AP, Murray MR: Cultural characteristics of malignant histiocytomas and fibrous xanthomas. Cancer *16*:331-334, 1963

Rodrigues MM, Furgiuele FO, Weinreb S: Malignant fibrous histiocytoma of the orbit. Arch Ophthalmol *95*:2025-2028, 1977

Russman BA: Tumor of the orbit: a 33-year follow-up. Am J Ophthalmol *64*:273-276, 1967

Soule E, Enriquez P: Atypical fibrous histiocytoma, malignant fibrous histiocytoma, malignant histiocytoma, and epithelioid sarcoma. Cancer *30*:128-143, 1972

Stewart WB, Newman NM, Cavender JC, et al: Fibrous histiocytoma metastatic to the orbit. Arch Ophthalmol *96*:871–873, 1978

Stout AP, Lattes R: Tumors of the soft tissues. In *Atlas of Tumor Pathology*. Second Series, Fascicle 1. Washington, D.C., Armed Forces Institute of Pathology. 1967

Vogel MH: Fibröses xanthom (xanthofibrom) der Orbita. Klin Monatsbl Augenheilk *155*:552-558, 1969

Zimmerman L: Changing concepts concerning the malignancy of ocular tumors. Arch Ophthalmol *78*:166-173, 1967

Proliferative Nodular Fasciitis

Ferry AP, Sherman SE: Nodular fasciitis of the conjunctiva apparently originating in the fascia bulbi (Tenon's capsule). Am J Ophthalmol *78*:514-517, 1974

Font RL, Zimmerman LE: Nodular fasciitis of the eye and adnexa. A report of ten cases. Arch Ophthalmol *75*:475-481, 1966

Konwaler BE, Keasbey L, Kaplan L: Subcutaneous pseudosarcomatous fibromatois (fasciitis). Am J Clin Pathol *25*:241–252, 1955

Levitt JM, de Veer JA, Oguzhan MC: Orbital nodular fasciitis. Arch Ophthalmol *81*:235-237, 1969

Mackenzie DH: *The Differential Diagnosis of Fibroblastic Disorders*. Oxford, Blackwell Scientific Publications. 1970

Meacham CT: Pseudosarcomatous fasciitis. Am J Ophthalmol *77*:747-749, 1974

Perry RH, Ramoni PS, McAllister V, et al: Nodular fasciitis causing unilateral proptosis. Brit J Ophthalmol *59*:404-408, 1975

Tolls RE, Mohr S, Spencer WH: Benign nodular fasciitis originating in Tenon's capsule. Arch Ophthalmol *75*:482-483, 1966

Soule EH: Proliferative (nodular) fasciitis. Arch Path *73*:437-444, 1962

8

Osseous and Cartilaginous Tumors

These tumors are closely related to other connective tissue tumors. We have already referred to the stem cell common to connective and supporting tissues, and the ease with which one cell type of this large family may merge with another cell type — so creating a tumor that is an admixture of both. In the case of fibrous dysplasia, normal osteogenesis may suddenly change to fibrogenesis and finally, as the disease comes to a halt, the fibroblast may revert to an osteoblast. Also, it seems a matter of chance whether the malignant tumor resulting from excessive irradiation will have a predominant fibrous or bony component.

OSTEOMA

HISTORICAL ASPECTS

Osteoma is by far the most common tumor of the group of bony and cartilaginous tumors affecting the bony orbit. Owing to striking deformities of the skull (the "horned men" of ancient times) resulting from the unchecked growth of this tumor, it seems to have been the subject of published comment even before the neurofibroma. Most writers who have collected a bibliography on this tumor credit Veiga (1586) with the first description. We have not examined this reference, but it seems that Veiga first observed his case (a woman with a tumor the size of a hen's egg in the superior nasal quadrant of the orbit) in 1506, but did not publish his observation until 1586 (if this 80-year interval is true, it is quite remarkable considering the limited longevity of people, even physicians, in the 16th century). Another source attributes the first description of an orbital osteoma to Louis in 1723. By the following century reports of such tumors were not uncommon in English, German, and French publications. Many of these earlier observers referred to the tumor as an *exostosis*. Although the word *osteoma* seems to have been proposed about 1828, this term did not come into general usage until about the 20th century. Because treatment of these tumors then was limited, some malformations grew to a tremendous size. What we would consider to be a large orbital tumor by modern standards, that is, 4 by 6 cm, in those years measured 4 by 6 inches in size.

The perusal of some of these earlier reports, therefore, is interesting. A most harrowing situation was chronicled by Hilton (1836). Describing the case of a 36-year-old man, he reported a tumor originating between the nose and left eye that had been slowly enlarging for 23 years. The tumor disfigured the face by pushing the left eye aside. During the sixth year of its growth, pressure on the eyeball caused excruciating pain, which was relieved only by spontaneous rupture of the eye. In the 17th year of its growth the overlying soft tissues began to ulcerate, exposing more and more of the ivory-like tumor. Finally, all soft tissues were eroded away and to the patient's astonishment the mass spontaneously and painlessly extruded. The end-result is illustrated in Figure 118.

INCIDENCE

The Mayo Clinic series includes nine orbital cases, approximately 1% of our total orbital tumors. In other large study series (300 or more cases) the frequency of osteoma will range from 1 to 2% of orbital tumors. The frequency of the mention of orbital osteoma in the older literature is much higher because of the mistaken inclusion of exostoses. An exostosis, which looks similar to osteoma,

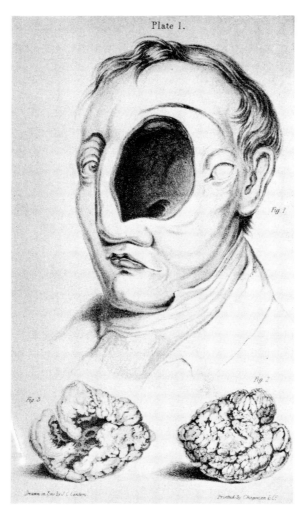

Figure 118. Osteoma: defect between nose and left orbit, the result of spontaneous extrusion of osteoma of 17 years' duration. (From Hilton: Case of a large bony tumor in the face completely removed by spontaneous separation: to which are added, observations upon some of the functions of the soft palate and pharynx. Guys Hosp Rep *1*:493–506, 1836.)

may be the natural response of bone to injury, surgery, or chronic inflammatory disease. But today, we no longer seem to see the orbital exostosis-osteoma syndrome that was prevalent 35 to 40 years ago. This was the heyday of chronic sinusitis, before the use of antibiotics, and when sinusitis was managed by repeated operations. We estimate that orbital involvement will occur in approximately 20 to 30% of osteomas arising in the walls of the paranasal sinuses and producing symptoms.

Six of the nine patients in our series were males. This is consistent with many reports in the literature, but, more recently, the reports of Wilkes and associates (1979) and Miller et al (1977) indicate a nearly equal sex distribution. Fu and Perzin (1974) found a predominance of females. The youngest patient in our series at time of diagnosis was 12 years of age; the oldest, 70 years. Four of our nine patients were in the second decade. The frontal or frontal-ethmoid area was involved in seven patients, and the left orbit was affected in all but one of the total nine cases. We do not have an explanation for the left side predominance.

CLINICAL FEATURES

The subjective symptoms are similar to those we already have encountered with other benign space-occupying masses, such as displacement of the eye, diplopia, swelling of soft tissues of the eyelids, sometimes a palpable mass if the tumor is well anterior in the orbit, and tearing if the osteoma is in a nasal location. Pain is not common in contrast to frequent headache in patients with osteomas not involving the orbit. Objective findings such as papilledema, optic atrophy, and visual loss seldom are observed unless the osteoma is unusually large, is of very long duration, or has attacked the visual pathways from its lair in the sphenoid sinus. Transient blurring of vision (Wilkes and associates) and pain (Miller et al) on movement of the eye in certain directions of gaze also should alert the clinician to a possible orbital osteoma. These are due to impingement or stretching of the extraocular muscle or optic nerve on the hard, unyielding surface of the tumor as the eye rotates in a direction opposite to the mass. We have seen similar symptoms rarely occur with nodular intraorbital meningiomas and large intraorbital tumors of many years' duration (cavernous hemangiomas and hemangiopericytomas).

Various sinus cavities seem to be affected. Although the location may vary slightly from one report to another, osteomas are most common in the frontal sinus and next most frequent in the ethmoid sinus; they less frequently originate in maxillary and sphenoid sinuses. An orbital mass is therefore most likely to be palpated or visualized by roentgenography in the nasal or upper nasal quadrant. The mass is hard and, in our experience, not tender.

When an osteoma has invaded the orbit from the sphenoid sinus, its location is too posterior for diagnostic palpation. The diagnosis will then depend on roentgenographic study. In some cases wherein osteoma has involved the orbital plate of the ethmoid bone, at operation the tumor has seemed preponderantly orbital in location with but minor involvement of the ethmoid sinus. It seems a matter of chance whether tumor cells within this thin plate of bone will cause the bone to bulge laterally into the orbit or medially into the sinus. Whether the osteoma is then primary in the orbit or truly secondary to sinus involvement is not of much practical importance, for the effect on the eye and the symptoms produced are essentially the same; an exception is that when the osteoma is largely orbital in position, symptoms tend to develop earlier. An infrequent association of an osteoma of the paranasal sinus with intestinal polyposis combined with a variety of cutaneous and subcutaneous tumors (Gardner's syndrome, 1962) has been described. Also, there is a known association between familial polyposis and intestinal adenocarcinoma. It follows that a patient with an orbital osteoma should have a colon study to uncover one of these more serious problems.

ROENTGENOGRAPHIC CHANGES

Roentgenograms are most important in the diagnostic survey. If the tumor already has been palpated, roentgenographic study will help to clinch the diagnosis. If the osteoma is situated in the posterior orbit, and is therefore not palpable, the diagnosis is made solely on the basis of the roentgenogram. Extent and size of the mass so determined also are important, for these features aid the surgeon in planning his approach and in surgical manipulation. For example, it is a comfort to the ophthalmologist who plans a surgical removal to know that the osteoma does not invade the intracranial vault (Fig. 119). Here, tomograms are very useful.

An osteoma arising in either the frontal or the ethmoid sinus is not a diagnostic problem to the practiced eye of the roentgenologist: one glance at the film suffices. To the unpracticed eye of the ophthalmologist the tumor also is

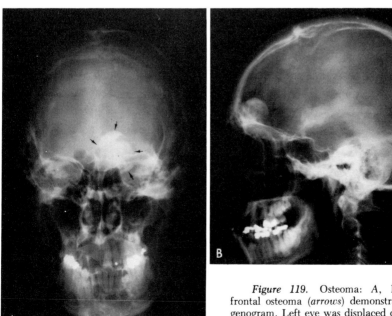

Figure 119. Osteoma: *A,* Large .orbital-frontal osteoma (*arrows*) demonstrated by roentgenogram. Left eye was displaced downward and forward, but ocular symptoms had been present only one year. *B,* Lateral projection of roentgenogram indicates major portion of mass is intracranial (*arrows*); this situation is best managed through intracranial surgical approach.

visualized easily because it is so opaque. Gradations in density of the roentgeno-graphic shadow depend on the proportion of bone and connective tissue within the tumor. The eburnated type of osteoma, which is almost solid bone, is very opaque. The spongiose type, which has more connective tissue than the former type, is less opaque: the shadow is more mottled. These gradations are visible to the roentgenologist, but they do not significantly influence the ultimate management. The opaque masses usually are round with sharply demarcated margins (Fig. 120). If osteoma has been present in a sinus cavity of irregular contour, such as an ethmoid, for some years, the surface of the mass may then become more lobulated or even knobby, rather than maintain a smooth con-tour. Whether the osteoma has a pedunculated or a sessile base is not always visible on roentgenography. The pedunculated type is more likely to arise from the ethmoid sinus, whereas the osteoma arising in the frontal sinus has a more broad-based connection to bone.

The less frequent, diffuse osteoma of the wings of the sphenoid bone, such as may supervene on a burnt-out fibrous dysplasia, is much more difficult to identify by roentgenography. The consequent hyperostosis of bone closely resembles the alteration produced by meningioma — so closely that surgical intervention probably is indicated to settle the issue. It is said that the diagnosis of osteoma probably is warranted in such situations when the individual is younger than 30 years, but if the individual is older than 30, meningioma is the likely diagnosis. However, we would not place too much reliance on this old maxim, for meningiomas have been histologically verified in individuals younger than 30 and osteomas certainly occur after the age of 30.

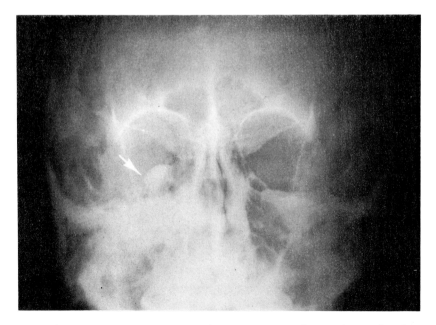

Figure 120.   Osteoma: roentgenogram indicates osteoma involving right maxillary bone with sharply demarcated mass (*arrow*) protruding into inferior nasal quadrant of orbit.

PATHOLOGY

Osteomas, grossly, could be likened to a cue ball in terms of color and consistency, except that their surface is often knobby and their contour somewhat irregular because of their tendency to conform to the confined space in which they grow (Fig. 121). Microscopically, they may be subtyped as ivory, mature, or fibrous, depending upon the proportion of bone to supporting fibrous stroma. This subdivision has no significant clinical bearing. The fibrous type is considered the more immature and actively growing variant and is said to occur in a younger age group. In our series a fibrous osteoma was seen in a 70-year-old male. This osteoma has more fibrous stroma than other subtypes and osteoblasts rim the fibrous trabeculae. As the osteoma matures the bony lamellae thicken and the fibrous stroma becomes less cellular (Fig. 122 and 123). Finally, only small islands of fibrous tissue remain as the lamellar bone hardens into an ivory-like, hypocellular bone.

TREATMENT

In the years of our grandfathers and great-grandfathers, almost every known type of surgical instrument, except obstetrical forceps, was used in the surgical destruction of osteomas of the orbit and adjacent sinuses. The literature contains a catalog of instruments: rasps, bone tongs, tenaculums, hand saws, drills, elevators, trephines, gauges, punches, rongeurs, chisels, mallets, hammers, and even a chain saw. Acids have been used to soften the tumor and caustics have been employed to destroy it. An interesting example of surgical persistence was provided by van der Meer (1829): in his case, the tumor was chipped away with a chisel, little by little, each day for 8 weeks.

At one time, removal of some of these large osteomas was quite hazardous, and bleeding, sepsis, or intracranial complications were fatal. Nowadays most

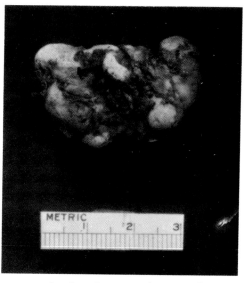

Figure 121. Osteoma: peripheral condensation of compact bone is analogous to capsule; it is often irregular and knobby.

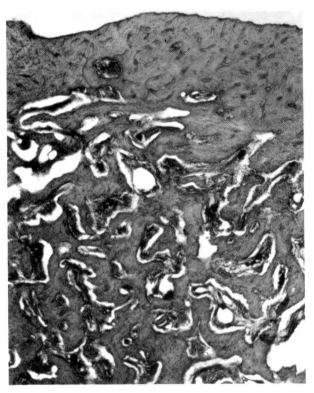

Figure 122. Osteoma: lesion consists of thickened interconnecting lamellae of bone; the bone has cortex-like surface condensation. (Hematoxylin and eosin; × 30.)

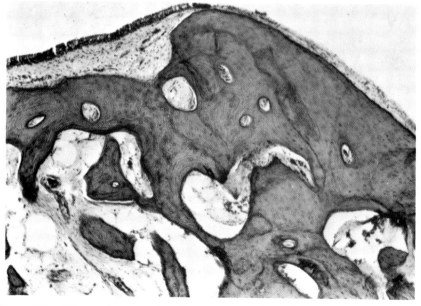

Figure 123. Osteoma: tumor projects into sinus cavity beneath intact mucosa. (Hematoxylin and eosin; × 60.)

of these hazards have been eliminated by improved surgical techniques and, after the operation, by the administration of antibiotics. Even so, an operation for osteoma is not something to be taken lightly or without good reason.

If the osteoma is small and located in the frontal, ethmoid, or maxillary sinus, the operation may be deferred until orbital symptoms appear or intracranial extension is threatened. Some tumors are discovered quite by chance during roentgenography of the skull for other reasons. They may be symptomless at this stage and show little tendency to enlarge, as shown subsequently by follow-up roentgenography. But if such an osteoma is discovered in the sphenoid sinus, immediate operation should be seriously considered in order to remove the tumor before it becomes a threat to the visual pathways as it extends beyond the sinus. Large tumors in any of the sinuses probably are best managed by the rhinologist, but if intracranial extension is evident, then a transcranial approach by a neurosurgeon is indicated.

For smaller osteomas pushing upon the eye from the frontal-ethmoid area, we use an anterior approach through the soft tissues adjacent to the superior nasal rim of the orbit. Osteomas connected to the orbital plate of the ethmoid bone are the easiest to handle. They usually are pedunculated. After incising the muco-periorbita that covers the tumor, several sharp raps with the hammer and chisel near the base of the mass usually will dislodge it. Osteomas connected to the frontal sinus may be more difficult to dislodge for they have a broader base and more chiseling is required. When bone is fractured around the base, the main mass is grasped and, by twisting and rocking, the tumor is manipulated through the incision. Or, the tumor can be debulked and removed piece meal with a Hall drill. Bleeding and infection in the postoperative period have not been problems. If the eye has not been displaced for too long, the results — from the standpoint of recurrence and relief of proptosis — have generally been satisfactory. Recurrences are most prevalent among patients in the second and third decade in whom initial surgery of the osteoma was incomplete.

OSTEOBLASTOMA

Basically, this tumor is composed of fibrous tissue and osteoid, predominantly the former; contains osteoblasts; and has a definite vascular component. Thus defined, its place in the spectrum of fibro-osseous tumors is a matter of controversy. Also, observers differ as to the diagnostic criteria that should be used to separate this tumor from others with a closely allied histology. A kinship to osteoid osteoma cannot be overlooked, and the term *giant osteoid osteoma* has been used to describe the larger size and more aggressive growth of the osteoblastoma. Microscopic sections of some osteoblastomas resemble portions of aneurysmal bone cysts, also suggesting a close relationship of these lesions. In the less recent literature a strong minority of observers contend that osteoblastoma is but a variant of fibrous dysplasia, the former differing in makeup only because of its position in cranial bones. Elsewhere, other than in bones of the skull, it has been called *osteogenic fibroma*. Finally, in the ophthalmic literature, osteoblastoma and *ossifying fibroma* may be discussed as separate tumors but the histologic descriptions and illustrations look almost identical. We have elected to follow the suggestion of Dahlin (1978) that osteoblastoma is presently the most widely accepted designation for these several variants.

INCIDENCE

Although examples of orbital involvement are diagnosed with increasing frequency, the cases are still few in number. Scott et al (1971) recorded the most detailed protocol of a patient with orbital involvement of any cases so far reported. Theirs was a 22-year-old female with a midline intracranial ossifying fibroma of bone that produced slight exophthalmos of right eye, followed two years later by moderate proptosis of the left eye due to orbital extension of tumor. In the review of seven cases of ossifying fibroma of the face and skull by Fu and Perzin (1974), two patients had exophthalmos and another patient a lateral displacement of the eye. The seven cases were discussed as a composite, so we do not know the sex or age of the patients with orbital involvement; the age range of the group was 7 to 28 years of age. One additional patient, a 12-year-old female with orbital involvement secondary to a bony tumor of the ethmoid sinus, was discussed separately by Fu and Perzin as an example of benign osteoblastoma. Another case of osteoblastoma, very nearly involving the orbit, was reported by Freedman (1975). Here the tumor produced painless epiphora secondary to expansion of the anterior ethmoid cells in a 13-year-old boy, but no proptosis was present. From this composite data we can conclude that no patient with orbital involvement was older than 28 years of age at time of diagnosis, but the data is too meager to state any sex incidence.

CLINICAL FEATURES

The cranial bones are an infrequent site for the growth of this tumor, but when the cranium is involved the bones of the midline (ethmoid and sphenoid) and the orbital portion of the frontal bone seem to be the areas of predilection. Orbital involvement could then be expected whenever the tumor expanded beyond the boundaries of these bones. The patient of Scott had a great deal of headache and pain but the growths were painless in the several patients studied by Fu and Perzin. It seems to us that pain is not necessarily a feature of orbital involvement but depends on what extraorbital structures are being pressured by the expanding tumor. Other diagnostic features associated with orbital involvement may well depend on the size of the mass and the area of the orbit first breached by the tumor. In this respect, clinical signs and symptoms will be as variable as we have already encountered with other tumors that secondarily invade the orbit from either the paranasal sinuses or intracranial vault.

ROENTGENOGRAPHIC CHANGES

In the ethmoid and frontal bones osteoblastomas are smoothly contoured, somewhat oval lesions that have radiolucent centers and a more dense but thin cortical margin. In the early stages of growth, or if the cellular component of the tumor is quite immature, the lesion may resemble an aneurysmal bone cyst.

In more mature tumors of longer duration such a degree of sclerosis may develop as to resemble the appearance of fibrous dysplasia.

PATHOLOGY

The histopathology of these tumors will vary according to the stage of development and duration of the tumor. The tumor tissue will be hemorrhagic depending on the degree of vascularity of the fibroblastic stroma, and will be granular depending on the amount of osteoid and its degree of calcification. In the younger tumors the trabeculae of bone will be sparse relative to the rapidly proliferating fibrous tissue. In these variants mitotic figures will be numerous and giant cells will be seen. In older tumors the trabeculae of bone will be thicker and more densely calcified. In all tumors the interlacing trabeculae of osteoid will be rimmed by osteoblasts with regular-contoured nuclei (Fig. 124). The periphery of the tumor will show the more dense sclerotic features of bone, but the center of the tumor will retain the more cellular features of the lesion. Scattered throughout some tumors will be small islands or spheroids of lamellar bone which have been likened to the psammoma bodies of meningioma.

COURSE AND TREATMENT

Because these tumors have a definite aggressive period of growth, treatment should be recommended if the lesion is in an accessible area of the ethmoid or frontal bone. In these situations the ophthalmologist's role is strictly secondary to either the neurosurgeon, rhinologist, or maxillofacial surgeon. In the less accessible periorbital areas curettement of the softer components of the tumor may be all that can be accomplished. Full excision of the tumor may be more of a reality for those in the more anterior portions of the orbital walls.

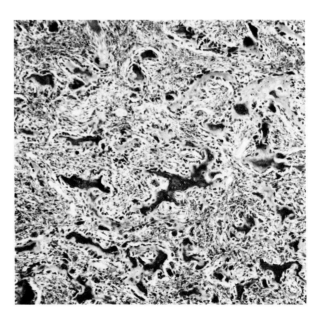

Figure 124. Osteoblastoma: irregular trabeculae of osteoid are rimmed by osteoblasts with regular nuclei. An abundant vascular, spindle cell, fibroblastic stroma is present. Scattered throughout specimen are small islands of more mature bone. (From McLeod RA, Dahlin DC, Beabout JW: The spectrum of osteoblastoma. Am J Roentgenol *126*: 321–325, 1976. By permission.)

Recurrence of tumor may depend on factors such as the stage of the tumor at the time of surgical attack and the extent of curettement or excision. A malignant transformation of an orbital osteoblastoma has not been reported, but such change has been infrequently observed in osteoblastomas in other skeletal areas.

GIANT CELL TUMOR

A discussion of this tumor is complicated by several factors. First, many fibro-osseous tumors contain giant cells. In the older literature there was a tendency to exaggerate the importance of giant cells as a criterion for diagnosis. As a result, many lesions were called giant cell tumors which would not be so designated by today's standards. Even so, the present diagnostic criteria are not so well established that total agreement is possible among all pathologists as to just what should be called giant cell tumor. Lastly, we have not found in the literature any well described and well illustrated case of orbital involvement that completely satisfies our concept of giant cell tumor. Thus, we have no cases upon which to base a meaningful discussion of clinical features or orbital course. The morphologic similarity of the giant cell of these tumors to osteoblasts is responsible for the less frequent designation *osteoclastoma*. The genesis of the tumor is not known.

Several cases in the literature have been indexed as examples of orbital giant cell tumor. The case of Babel (1973) was an 8-year-old boy with a tumor attached to the orbital rim. We believe the illustrations and protocol of this case suggest a giant cell reparative granuloma rather than a giant cell tumor of the neoplastic type. The often-quoted case of Abdalla and Hosni (1966) was a 5-year-old male with a very rapidly progressing tumor that was confined to the soft tissue structures of the orbit and in no way involved bone. This might well be a case of osteosarcoma, or a tumor now termed malignant giant cell tumor of soft parts. Cases with involvement of bones adjacent to the orbit (maxillary, ethmoid, frontal, and sphenoid bones) also have been reported. Most giant cell tumors are found in the long bones of the bony skeleton. Here they principally affect people in the third decade.

PATHOLOGY

Giant cell tumors usually are soft, rather friable, and reddish brown, hence the comparison to current jelly. The tumor usually is relatively homogeneous, but more firm, gray-yellow areas of fibrosis mixed with red or black blotches of hemorrhage may be observed in lesions of long duration.

The basic proliferating cells contain one ovoid or spindle-shaped nucleus (Fig. 125). These cells are closely approximated, with little intercellular tissue and scanty cytoplasm. Mitotic figures are almost always present. The striking feature is the generous number of multinucleated cells evenly distributed throughout the specimen, hence the name of the tumor. The multiple nuclei tend to congregate toward the center of these giant cells. The size, shape, and staining characteristics of these nuclei are similar to those of the nuclei of

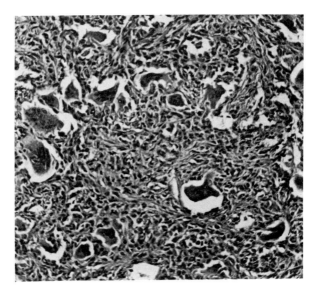

Figure 125. Giant cell tumor of bone: basic cells are small and ovoid. Numerous multinucleated giant cells are scattered throughout. (Hematoxylin and eosin; × 160.)

stromal cells; these features are responsible for the theory that giant cells are but a result of fusion of numerous stromal cells. Osteoid deposition is only rarely observed.

TREATMENT

There is little precedent upon which to base an opinion as to management of an orbital involvement. If the lesion is small and easily accessible, complete excision is strongly recommended. If the lesion is in a more inaccessible area of the orbit, a thorough curettement should be attempted. Still, the recurrence rate is high and there is an ever-lurking possibility of malignant transformation and metastasis. If recurrences develop after attempts at local removal, radical excision with sacrifice of the eye seems to be the only alternative.

OSTEOGENIC SARCOMA

TERMINOLOGY

Osteogenic sarcoma is a malignant tumor in the fullest sense of this designation. It is locally aggressive and readily metastasizes. It is the most dreaded tumor in the fibro-osseous spectrum. In the past several decades the term *osteogenic sarcoma* gradually has replaced the older, more inclusive designation *osteosarcoma* as the preferred name for this tumor. Clinically, osteogenic sarcoma is a more useful term because it emphasizes the osteoid products of this neoplasm and avoids controversy concerning the theoretical cell of origin of the tumor. The older term — osteosarcoma — was more representative of all sarcomatous tumors that evolved from connective tissue stem cells possessing osteogenic potential. In the older literature osteosarcoma would have included malignant neoplasms now classified as chondrosarcomas and fibrosarcomas of bone. Although not as inclusive a term as osteosarcoma, osteogenic sarcoma should not be considered an unduly restrictive designation because, in the pathology laboratory, it covers a wide assortment of neoplasms with varying degrees of bone formation and tissue differentiation. In anatomic areas where these malignant neoplasms are common, pathologists tend to subdivide the group into osseous, cartilaginous, and fibrous types, depending upon the predominance of tissue types and degree of osteogenesis; osteogenesis is also the basis for differentiating a fibrosarcomatous osteogenic sarcoma from a true fibrosarcoma. These nuances of terminology should be known to the ophthalmologist who wishes to make a study of bony tumors.

INCIDENCE

Orbital invasion by osteogenic sarcoma has always been considered extremely rare. At present we have more information about the orbital features of this tumor than of the preceding two tumors in this chapter, and twice as much data as was available at the time of our prior edition (1973). Case studies on four patients with osteogenic sarcoma of the orbital bones were found in the literature we have reviewed. These are the reports of Mortada (1964), Blodi (1969), Bone et al (1973), and Jakobiec and Jones (1976). Also available for review are four cases not associated with prior irradiation from our own series. The protocols of these latter four cases will be noted below. The ages of the eight patients ranged from 13 to 69 years at the time of diagnosis. The osteogenic sarcoma of the 69-year-old patient was associated with Paget's disease. The relationship of Paget's disease as a precursor of osteogenic sarcoma in the older age groups has been noted by many observers. Of the remaining seven non-Paget-associated sarcomas, three of the patients were in the sixth decade. This age distribution is considerably different from the age range of patients with osteogenic sarcomas in the more common skeletal sites (tubular long bones). In the latter, the peak incidence is in the second decade. The sex of the 13-year-old patient in this group of eight was not stated. The sex ratio was 4:3, male to female, in the remaining seven. In the group with orbital invasion the primary focus of the sarcoma was in the sphenoid bone (two cases), frontal bone (two cases), and one case each in ethmoid bone, maxilla, nasal cavity and base of skull. Additional notations of secondary orbital invasion will be found in statistical reviews of sarcomatous involvement of the bone of the face, cranium, paranasal sinuses, and so on. In these surveys the age and sex of the patient with orbital extension usually is not stated, and detailed protocols of the orbital complications are not included. Many of these composite surveys also include osteogenic sarcomas secondary to irradiation, a neoplasm that will be discussed in the following subchapter. A few osteogenic sarcomas also are tabulated in the orbital surveys of Reese (1963) and Silva (1968).

CLINICAL FEATURES

The gamut of clinical problems produced by these sarcomas in and around the orbit is well illustrated by brief details from the medical records of our four cases.

CASE 1.   A 53-year-old man was seen because of bulging of the right eye and gradual loss of vision during a 3-month period. (Forward displacement of the eye was so marked [11 mm] and so rapid in onset that a malignant tumor would be likely in this age group.) A large central scotoma had reduced vision to recognition of hand movements. No mass was palpable. Ocular rotations were limited in all directions of gaze. The retinal veins were engorged but no visible alterations were noted in configuration or color of the optic disk. Roentgenograms revealed a diffuse opacity in the area of the ethmoid sinus and along the medial wall of the orbit. Radical dissection of the frontal and ethmoid sinuses, as well as an exenteration of the orbit, was performed, supplemented by placement of five radium points along the base of the sphenoid bone for 20 hours. Histopathologic study revealed an osteogenic sarcoma, grade 2. Within 1½ years of this extensive surgery the neoplasm recurred in the upper nasal quadrant of the surgical cavity, in an area that once had corresponded to the roof of the nose. Irradiation was carried out elsewhere. After 2 years the patient died from the effects of further recurrence and spread of neoplasm into the intracranial vault.

CASE 2.   For 1 year the parents of a 15-year-old girl had noticed that the band of sclera beneath the right cornea had been wider than that beneath the left. The girl had complained of pain in the right cheek for 1 month. The initial examination showed that the right eye was displaced upward (4 mm) and proptosed (2 mm). Roentgenography indicated a destructive lesion of superior, lateral, and posterior walls of the right maxillary antrum. Exploration of this area confirmed the tentative diagnosis of malignant neoplasm, which, as histopathologic examination later proved, was an osteogenic sarcoma, grade 3. The tumor and involved bone were excised, and ramifications of the neoplasm into the pterygoid area were electrocoagulated. A recurrence, 8 months later, was treated by the insertion of two radium tubes (50 mg). The tumor soon spread into the nasal cavity, and the patient died 1 year after the initial operation (Fig. 126).

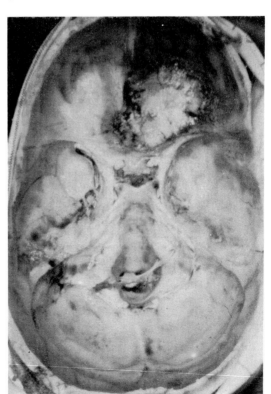

Figure 126.   Osteogenic sarcoma: extent of lesion (right orbit) emphasizes difficulties of surgical treatment.

CASE 3. A 36-year-old woman had noted relatively stationary proptosis of right eye for 18 months. Severe pain over right side of face had been present 6 months. Tomograms showed a right inferior parasellar mass causing destruction of the body of the sphenoid bone, posterior ethmoid cells, and floor of middle fossa in the region of foramen rotundum. A white meaty tumor was surgically removed from the area of sphenoid sinus and posterior ethmoid cells. Histopathologic diagnosis was fibroblastic osteogenic sarcoma, grade 3. The patient expired 11 months after surgery. At autopsy the neoplasm had spread into the right maxilla.

CASE 4. A 57-year-old male was seen because of bloody mucus discharge from left nasal passage of 5 months' duration. On roentgenography a destructive lesion was seen in the left maxilla. Exploration uncovered a 4.5 × 3.5 × 3 cm tumor arising in the left maxilla with complete filling of the sinus, infiltration of hard palate, and invasion of inferior orbit. A radical resection of the upper jaw was performed. Histopathologic diagnosis was fibroblastic osteogenic sarcoma, grade 2. At the time of death, one year later, the tumor had extended into the base of the skull around the foramen.

It is evident from the above cases that a definite sequence of clinical features is not present with orbital osteogenic sarcoma. However, the presence of any one, or a combination of any two, features of rapidly progressive proptosis, pain, or numbness should alert the clinician that a very serious orbital problem exists. Rapidly progressive proptosis, when present, reflects the ease with which a malignant neoplasm grows into the orbital cavity once it has escaped from surrounding bone or an afferent blood vessel. The more rapidly developing displacements of the eye are usually seen with the malignant sarcomas and to a lesser extent with some metastatic carcinomas (lung and kidney). Severe pain is not a common feature of primary orbital neoplasm except for some of the epithelial neoplasms of the lacrimal gland. However, such tumors are palpable by the time they produce pain. Therefore, in the absence of a palpable mass, pain should suggest a tumor infiltrating the perineural spaces of bone and periorbita. Numbness of the face or adnexa may be present alone or in conjunction with pain and is a frequent symptom of a malignant process at the base of the skull or around the orbital apex. So many clinicians place so much reliance on the diagnostic capabilities of roentgenography, computer tomography, and so on that they tend to skip over the clues provided by the patient or by the proptosed eye. The diagnostic capabilities of the roentgenogram and its modifications are not so clear-cut as may seem from the description that follows.

ROENTGENOGRAPHIC CHANGES

The density of the roentgenographic shadow immediately relates the neoplasm to bone. The shadow may vary in density from case to case, depending upon the distribution and quantity of osseous material in the tumor. If the osteoid content is high, the shadow projected is almost as dense as that of an osteoma. The central zone of such shadows may appear mottled owing to radiolucent areas of bone destruction among remaining bone trabeculae; the latter became more sclerotic in resisting the onslaught of the sarcomatous matrix. Fine linear shadows radiating from the central core, which represent filamentous fingers of neoplasm spreading toward the periphery, are further characteristics;

these impart the so-called sunray or sunburst appearance. One of the best illustrations of these roentgenographic shadows in the orbit is seen in the article by Mortada (1964) (Fig. 127). Such a clear-cut diagnostic shadow is the exception rather than the rule. The overlap of bone in this area of the skull is so great that, in the majority of cases including our own, the roentgenographic shadow of bone destruction and lysis is not specific.

PATHOLOGY

The essential tissue component of osteogenic sarcoma is a highly anaplastic sarcomatous matrix that surrounds irregular masses of osteoid and immature bone (Fig. 128). This matrix may show a predominance of osteoid, chondroid, or fibromatoid elements, but the presence of one of these subtypes does not significantly alter the course of the neoplasm. Some cells may contain several large hyperchromatic nuclei and other cells may be so large and contain such a number of nuclei as to be called giant cells. These neoplasms also are vascular, which is of relevance to the planning of surgical eradication. In many tissue specimens, tumor cells are so closely approximated to thin-walled sinusoidal spaces as to explain readily their easy blood-borne metastasis.

TREATMENT

A theme of frustration, futility, and fatality runs through most reports dealing with osteogenic sarcoma of the orbit. Frustration is typified by the diffi-

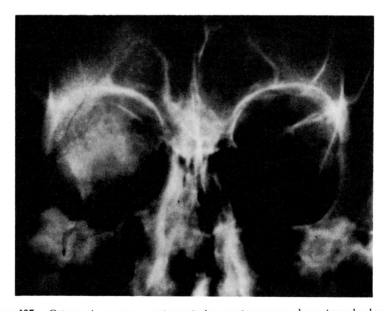

Figure 127. Osteogenic sarcoma: posteroanterior roentgenogram shows irregular bone density of greater and lesser wings of right sphenoid bone with linear, radiating "sun ray" shadows; contour of superior orbital fissure is lost. (From Mortada A: Exophthalmos and rare tumors of the orbital bones. Am J Ophthalmol 57:270–275, 1964. By permission of Ophthalmic Publishing Company.)

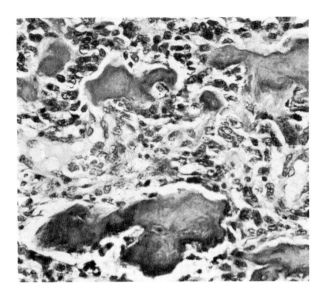

Figure 128. Osteogenic sarcoma: sarcomatous matrix of spindled cells which form irregular masses of osteoid. (Hematoxylin and eosin; × 275.)

culty of removing large portions of the sphenoid bone, should the neoplasm choose this site for growth. Futility is expressed by the seeming inadequacy of even radical eradication of these fast-growing neoplasms. By the time the diagnosis is established by orbitotomy, the neoplasms seem to have extended beyond the limits of practical removal. Recurrences usually will appear within 1 year of the initial surgery, and none of our patients lived longer than 2 years after diagnosis. Exenteration, combined with removal of as much involved bone as possible during the first surgical exploration, seems to give the only possible hope for cure. The 13-year-old patient of Jakobiec and Jones was tumor-free 1 year after an en bloc excision of the tumor at the base of the skull. This must have been a very extensive and heroic procedure. We have not been impressed with the effects of irradiation and have had no experience with chemotherapy of orbital lesions.

OSTEOGENIC SARCOMA FOLLOWING IRRADIATION

Fibrosarcomas of the orbit induced by irradiation were discussed in the previous chapter. There it was noted that osteogenic types were the most frequent of all neoplasms induced by such a modality. The majority of these cases resulted from the use of curative doses of radiation for intraocular retinoblastoma in infancy. The subject is well covered in two major reviews. Soloway (1966) summarized twenty-two cases previously reported in the literature and added three new cases of radiation-induced sarcoma. Nine of the twenty-five cases had osteogenic sarcoma. The review of Sagerman and associates (twenty-one cases) also included nine cases of radiation-induced osteogenic sarcoma. There was some overlap of patients among these two reviews. The interval between treatment and the diagnosis of osteosarcoma ranged from 5 to 22 years in the Soloway series and from 4 to 23 years in the nine patients of Sagerman and associates. The lowest tumor dose giving rise to osteogenic sarcoma in the latter series was 8000 roentgens. Once the sarcoma appeared the prognosis was grim; most of the patients were dead within a year. Death usually resulted from direct extension into the brain or metastasis to the lung. Details of the one case in the Mayo Clinic series not associated with retinoblastoma follows.

A 3-year-old boy was seen because an undifferentiated sarcoma of the right antrum, of 3 months' duration, had pushed the right eye upward. A portion of the mass also bulged into the hard palate. Two tubes of radium (60 mg and 50 mg, respectively) were inserted into the neoplasm and left there for 12 hours. Within 2 years of this treatment, nodules of recurrent sarcoma were excised from areas of the right cheek and submaxillary zone. Additional radium was applied elsewhere but the amount is not known. The sarcoma then disappeared and the patient seemed well.

At age 22 (19 years after initial treatment), the patient sought advice on cosmetic correction of atrophy of the bones on the right side of the face caused by irradiation. No neoplasm was found, and plastic surgery was not performed. He remained well for another 24 years. Then, at age 46 (43 years after the initial treatment) a mass in the right nostril began to bleed. Within 1 month of onset the right maxillary and malar bones were removed and a radical exenteration of the frontal and ethmoid sinuses was performed. Histopathologic study demonstrated a fibroblastic osteogenic sarcoma (Fig. 129), grade 2. One year later, the neoplasm recurred under the medial aspect of the right brow, and the orbit was exenterated. The neoplasm continued to recur; treatment was further surgical removal of bone, down to the dura. The patient finally died 5 years after the first radical surgery and 48 years after initial irradiation. Autopsy showed that the neoplasm had spread to the intracranial vault and had crossed the midline to invade the left orbit.

This patient showed a remarkable capacity for survival.

CHONDROMA

TERMINOLOGY AND ORIGIN

Benign cartilaginous growths composed of mature hyaline cartilage and arising in bones preformed in cartilage are termed *chondromas*. They have been subclassified as *enchondromas* if located in the central core of affected bone, and *periosteal chondromas* if they are more eccentrically positioned beneath the periosteum. Such subclassification may be pertinent in areas where chondromas are common, for example, the phalanges of fingers and toes, metacarpal and metatarsal bones, humerus, and femur. To the flat bones of the skull, such subdivisions have no practical application because the central and more peripheral zones of bone are quickly distorted by growth of the tumor. Theoretically, at least, a chondroma should not occur in membranous bones such as those constituting the major part of the bony orbit. Among the orbital bones only the body and lesser wing of the sphenoid have any significant derivation from cartilaginous precursors. Also, the trochlea attached to the superior nasal rim of the orbit is comprised of hyaline cartilage. In ophthalmic literature these neoplasms frequently are referred to as *orbital enchondromas* and their close relationship to connective tissue fibromas is reflected in the common designation *fibrochondroma*.

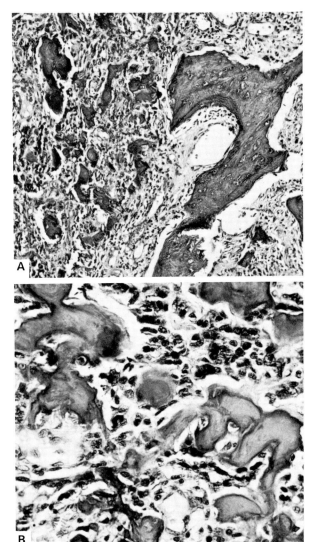

Figure 129. Post-irradiation osteogenic sarcoma.

A, Lower power magnification shows highly malignant neoplasm invading bony structure of orbit, a residual portion of which is seen to the right of the section. (Hematoxylin and eosin; × 110.)

B, A higher power shows osteoid production. (Hematoxylin and eosin; × 275.)

INCIDENCE

Orbital chondromas probably are rare, and one must have some reservations about this designation for tumors along the rim of the orbit. Such tumors are more likely to be fibromas with cartilaginous metaplasia, the so-called fibrochondromas. The infrequency of true chondromas around the orbit is reflected in the distribution of bony tumors tabulated by Dahlin (1978): of 162 cases of chondroma not one was located in the skull. Even including some fibrochondromas, there are scarcely more than a half-dozen orbital cases in the literature wherein sex and age incidence are reported. To Simões de Sá (1958) is attributed the experience of observing two cases. A well-documented case is that of Jepson and Wetzig. A small painless chondroma involved the trochlea of a 50-year-old male. There is no sex predilection.

PATHOLOGY

To the naked eye, chondromas have a pearly, bluish-white hyaline-like translucency. Under low power magnification the cartilaginous matrix appears lobulated, and blood vessels may be seen in the narrow clefts separating the lobules. In neoplasms undergoing calcification or ossification, such deposits may occur along these clefts or at the periphery of the lobules. Usually, uninuclear chondrocytes tend to collect in orderly clusters, each with its own lacunae (Fig. 130), but in chondromas arising from skull bones no such orderly arrangement is seen: the chondrocytes show more cellular atypism and binucleate forms. Cellularity generally is not a prominent feature, and, if it is present, malignant transformation must be suspected. The nuclei of the chondrocytes are round and stain darkly; the cytoplasm is pale. In some areas there is a soft mucoid-edematous matrix rather than the usual hyaline cartilage.

TREATMENT

Around the orbit, the goal of treatment should, if possible, be complete surgical removal, for chondromas may recur or undergo malignant anaplasia.

CHONDROSARCOMA

TERMINOLOGY AND ORIGIN

Chondrosarcomas are closely allied to osteogenic sarcomas and, indeed, sarcomatous features of both osseous and cartilaginous types may occur in the

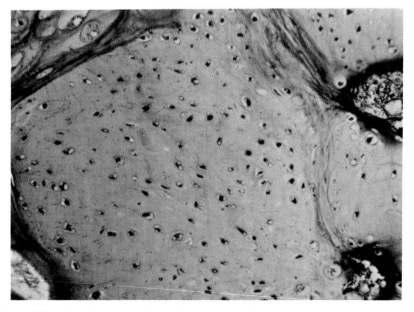

Figure 130. Chondroma: neoplasm of mature chondrocytes in matrix of hyaline cartilage. (Hematoxylin and eosin; × 170.)

same tumor. Once, compound designations were applied to such neoplasms in the belief that they were of multiple derivation. At present most such neoplasms are classified as osteogenic sarcomas, recognizing that such growths arise from an undifferentiated mesenchymal anlage that has potential for producing not only osseous tissue but cartilaginous and fibrous tissue elements as well. Chondrosarcomas, on the other hand, trace their origin to more specialized, less undifferentiated, cartilage-producing cells and contain predominantly cartilage. Osseous elements also may be seen in chondrosarcomas but, when present, are located within the lobules of chondroid rather than osseous trabeculae within the cellular matrix. Their origin from more specialized cells does not necessarily mean they are less malignant than osteogenic sarcomas, but it does explain their slower evolution and indolent progression. Chondrosarcomas favor the upper ends of long bones for their growth, but they are also found in the rib cage, shoulder girdle, and pelvis. They are quite rare in the distal portions of extremities. In the maxillary bone, chondrosarcomas appear to arise from cartilaginous structures around the nasal cavity.

INCIDENCE

This neoplasm is analogous to the osteogenic sarcoma in that both bony tumors frequently are encountered by orthopedists but are seldom observed in the domain of the opthalmologist. The report of Holland and colleagues (1961) contains the most complete bibliography on the orbital aspects of this tumor. They annotated five cases in the literature and described two cases of their own. The age and sex, where known, of these patients plus five cases from our own survey are summarized in Table 12.

In systemic distribution, chondrosarcoma is the second most frequent primary malignant tumor of bone. Although most skeletal surveys show that it is half as frequent as osteogenic sarcomas, chondrosarcomas seem at least twice as frequent as the latter in and around the bony orbit. The sex incidence is not settled. Some large skeletal surveys report a greater incidence in males; others report that the sex distribution is equal. From Table 12, the sex distribution in orbital chondrosarcomas seems to be equal, though the sample is small. More revealing is the wide age range of these patients, a finding that differs from the adult age distribution of chondrosarcomas in other skeletal areas.

TABLE 12.   AGE AND SEX DISTRIBUTION OF ORBITAL CHONDROSARCOMA

Age (yr)	
Females (N = 7)	*Males (N = 7)*
3	4
9	18
11	30
30*	35
39*	59*
"Over 40"	54
50*	55
55	62*

*From the Mayo Clinic study.

CLINICAL FEATURES

The symptoms and signs of this neoplasm when the case is first seen by an ophthalmologist seem to fall into one of three general patterns. In the first, proptosis seems to be the chief reason why the patient seeks advice. A firm mass usually can be palpated along the medial wall of the orbit, or a bulge (which is not tender) is evident at the inner canthus between the eye and the nose. Epiphora may be a feature, probably owing to pressure on the lacrimal drainage channels. In this pattern *the eye usually is displaced lateralward*, the lateral displacements measuring almost as much as the forward proptosis. Mucocele is the other tumor that may produce a very similar picture of proptosis.

The second pattern is characterized by complaints that are principally referable to the nose, such as nasal obstruction, a mass in the nose, or some nasal bleeding; the orbital symptoms are of less concern and of only moderate degree. The third pattern is the obvious one, wherein the patient has already undergone some surgery on the antrum or jaw, and upward displacement of the eye and diplopia are the reasons why the patient seeks further consultation. From these data it is evident that when tumor spreads into the orbital cavity, it usually will be palpated inferiorly, nasally, or in the lower nasal quadrant.

ROENTGENOGRAPHIC CHANGES

The roentgenographic shadow of this neoplasm may vary according to duration of the tumor, its particular location in relation to the orbit, or its histologic makeup. Thus a tumor of recent onset located in an area of thin bone, such as the floor of the orbit or the ethmoid portion of the bony orbit, may show only bone destruction. The irregular outline so caused in the normal contours of this area is similar roentgenographically to the defect of a mucocele. The roentgenographic shadow of this type of chondrosarcoma is not specifically diagnostic except to raise the possibility of a malignant neoplasm. When the tumor originates in an area of thicker bone, or when it is of such duration as to have undergone calcific degeneration, the shadow is more opaque, mottled, or fuzzy in character. Such a shadow in the sphenoid bone is illustrated in Figure 131. However, even this shadow is not so distinctive as to make diagnosis of chondrosarcoma as easy as with a similar tumor in the ribs, pelvis, or long bones.

PATHOLOGY

The cell common to all these neoplasms is the chondrocyte that has changed from a benign to a malignant phase. Certain alterations in appearance signify malignancy. Normally, the chondrocyte is a relatively large cell neatly tucked away in a lacuna of hyaline-like matrix which, in fixed sections, tends to assume a polyhedral shape. As it becomes malignant there is a significant change or malformation in the shape of one cell as compared to another. The nuclei become hyperchromatic and some cells may have two or more nuclei (Fig. 132). The matrix of the neoplasm is variable and may show features of other mesenchymal derivatives. Islands of hyalinized cartilage may merge into a stroma not unlike fibrosarcoma, or even a loose myxoid tissue (Fig. 133); if there are portions of hyaline matrix in the specimen the cellularity is greater

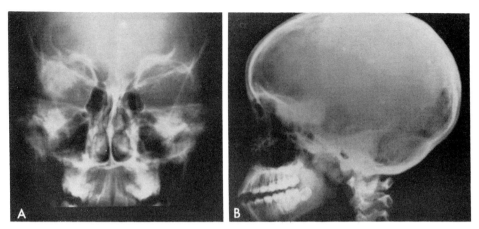

Figure 131. Chondrosarcoma: *A*, Posteroanterior roentgenogram showing densely calcified tumor arising from lateral portion of greater wing of right sphenoid bone. *B*, Lateral projection. (From Holland MG, Allen JH, Ichinose H: Chondrosarcoma of the orbit. Trans Am Acad Ophthalmol Otolaryngol 65:898–905, 1961. By permission of the American Academy of Ophthalmology and Otolaryngology.)

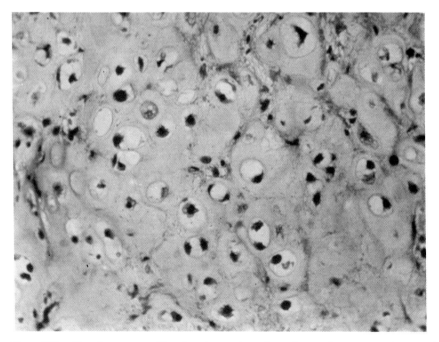

Figure 132. Chondrosarcoma: Chondrocytes are irregular and many lacunae contain more than one cell; matrix is hyaline cartilage. (Hematoxylin and eosin; × 185.)

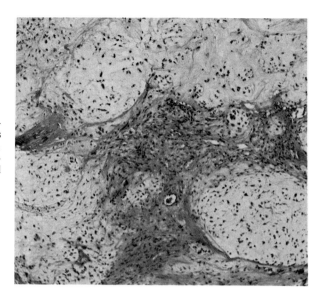

Figure 133. Chondrosarcoma: malignant chondrocytes with stroma of myxo-cartilage. Increased cellularity typifies malignancy. (Hematoxylin and eosin; × 120.)

than normal and the lacunae are closely apposed; and if the tumor is long-standing, focal necrosis and central deposits of amorphous calcium are the main features. A myxoid stroma is an ominous sign, strongly suggestive of malignancy. Grossly, the specimens usually are gray, tend to be gelatinous in consistency once the surface has been incised, are vascular, and seem to erode the bone in a locular manner. In current terminology any tumor containing these anaplastic chondrocytes is designated a chondrosarcoma, even though the tissue may contain fibrosarcomatous areas and show myxomatous change. Formerly such tumors with a mixture of these mesenchymal derivates were designated by compound terms, for example, fibrochondrosarcoma and myxochondroma.

TREATMENT AND COURSE

Surgical excision, various modalities of irradiation, and surgical diathermy have been used in an attempt to suppress this neoplasm, but complete removal of tumor should be the initial and preferable goal of treatment. In the long bones, orthopedic surgeons often accomplish this objective by amputation. A similar eradication of a neoplasm involving the bones of the orbit and adnexal areas requires an en bloc resection. In some cases of orbital involvement this is possible, but it requires an understanding patient and an experienced and resourceful maxillofacial surgeon to carry off successfully such an event. Around the orbit such operations involve much loss of bone and the patient must have the courage to accept such cosmetic consequences of radical surgery. Even the loss of an eye at the initial operation must sometimes be accepted as necessary to an adequate access to the lesion.

The surgeon's role also is a difficult one. He or she must be bold with the chisel and saw to remove the required bone, adaptable to staunch the sudden bursts of bleeding from moderate- to large-size vessels, and ever mindful of the proximity of the intracranial space. The knowledgeable surgeon knows that anything short of complete removal of tumor will inevitably result in recurrence. Even a careless biopsy may negate an otherwise successful surgeon's attack because of the ease with which malignant chondrocytes implant themselves in the surgical field.

One patient salvaged by such major surgical endeavors was the 59-year-old female (Table 12) in our Mayo Clinic survey. Her chondrosarcoma arose from the face of the sphenoid at its junction with the nasal septum. At initial surgery the entire nasal septum and left ethmoid cells were removed, and the sphenoid sinus was exenterated. Eleven years later a dome-shaped tumor bulged into the medial and inferior orbit on the left side. The tumor was removed by a rhinotomy combined with resection of the orbital floor and rim along the inferior, temporal, and posterior border of the neoplasm. Another eight years have passed without recurrence and the patient still retains a useful but downwardly displaced eye.

Some excerpts from the other case histories in the Mayo Clinic study illustrate the evil and perverse disposition of chondrosarcoma. In the 30-year-old woman, the tumor initially was removed from the left antrum. Six years later the upper jaw and all maxillary bone except along the floor of the orbit were resected because of recurrence. During the next 5-year period, irradiation was used on many occasions. Twelve years after the initial operation, recurrent neoplasm had grown along the floor of the left orbit and the left eye was immobile. A complicated cataract was present in the opposite eye.

In the male patient, age 62, the tumor first was resected in the upper jaw around the teeth. During the next 6 years, six radical resections, including exenteration of the orbit, were performed because of frequent recurrences. By the end of this interval, the maxillary bone and the lateral and medial walls of the orbit also had been excised. Recurrences of tumor extending into the pterygoid fossa and along the posterior wall of the orbit affected vital areas beyond surgical ken; they were treated with surgical diathermy and implantation of radon. The patient died 7 years after the onset from extension of neoplasm into the intracranial spaces.

The other male patient, age 39, had an incomplete removal of a chondrosarcoma involving right maxillary sinus, right ethmoid bone, nasal septum and turbinates. Fifteen months later there was obstruction of the left nasal passages and progressive proptosis of the left eye due to extension of tumor across the midline. Supervoltage radiation therapy of 2000 roentgens was administered, followed in six months by another 4680 roentgens. Two years after the initial operation, partial removal of tumor in the nasopharynx was performed to relieve the obstructed airway. In another year the left eye was blind because of extension of tumor into the orbital apex and along the sphenoid ridge. When the patient died from extension of the chondrosarcoma into the intracranial cavity 4½ years after diagnosis, the vision was decreasing in the remaining useful right eye.

The situation in another woman, age 50, was similar, the patient having undergone seven operations in 8 years. By the end of this period the neoplasm had crossed the midline to involve the sinus and orbit on the side opposite to its original site. Extension across the midline with bilateral involvement of the orbits has been noted among other cases in the literature. This patient died 10 years after onset due to intracranial spread.

These excerpts illustrate the common features of extended intervals between recurrences: the slow but obstinate spread from one bone to another, the lack of distant metastases, and the failure to eradicate the neoplasm even with radical operations. In this area of the body the tumor finally kills by reaching the brain. The patients with bilateral spread also are nearly blind.

MESENCHYMAL CHONDROSARCOMA

This neoplasm and the fibrous histiocytoma discussed in the prior chapter share the "new tumor of the orbit" designation in this edition of our text. Both neoplasms were observed — but designated as variants of a larger parent class of tumor — prior to their description as separate entities in the same time period, 1959-1961. Both were initially considered quite rare, but they have become less so as more pathologists have become aware of the criteria necessary for their diagnosis. In each tumor the first orbital case was reported after a 5- to 7-year interval from their initial description. Since then case reports of orbital involvement have been "coming out of the woodwork," relatively speaking, and each neoplasm now has an established niche in the panorama of orbital tumors.

INCIDENCE

The tumor was first described by Lichtenstein and Bernstein (1959). They reviewed a group of twenty-five unusual chondroid tumors. Two of these had such distinctive histologic patterns as to warrant a separate classification. One tumor was from a thoracic vertebra and the other from a parietal bone. Dowling (1964) reported two similar neoplasms from an extraosseous source and agreed that mesenchymal chondrosarcoma was an appropriate name. Subsequently, references to orbital involvement appeared (Trzcinska-Dabrowska et al 1969, Cardenas-Ramirez et al 1971, Guccion et al 1973, Salvador and associates 1971, Sevel 1974). Some confusion has resulted as to the total number of patients with orbital involvement because the same case has been counted in more than one reference and because a case reported by Reeh (1966), under a different name, was not recognized as an example of mesenchymal chondrosarcoma until much later. According to our count there are now a total of six cases of orbital mesenchymal chondrosarcoma. Five of these six were females, aged 19, 22, 26, 27, and 34 years at time of orbital diagnosis. The one male was 39 years of age. Three of these cases seemed to be extraskeletal examples of this neoplasm, one was a recurrent neoplasm definitely involving orbital bone, and the origin of two cases was not stated.

CLINICAL FEATURES

Proptosis of a nonspecific type seemed to be present in all cases and, except for the case of recurrent tumor of bone (Trzcinska-Dabrowska et al), the tumor was of such size as to suggest a reasonably rapid progression. Two of the tumors could be palpated in the more anterior orbit but the tumor in Reeh's case was not recognized until exploration of the posterior-temporal orbit. Some restriction of ocular rotation was also noted in several cases. Standard roentgenographic views of the orbit were negative in those tumors of soft tissue genesis. The x-rays of the bony tumor showed an irregular mass with several cloud-like calcinations characteristic of cartilaginous tissue.

PATHOLOGY

Grossly, these tumors are gray in color, firm, slightly lobulated, and poorly circumscribed. On cut surface the center of the tumor has a bluish cast because of the cut sections of cartilage. Larger tumors may contain zones of necrosis and hemorrhage. The principal cellular features are the sheets of undifferentiated mesenchymal cells in which are scattered small islands of hyaline cartilage (Figs. 134 and 135). When examined under low power magnification the mesenchymal tissue is seen to grow in a pattern very suggestive of hemangiopericytoma. The cells have small, round to oval, hyperchromatic nuclei and the cytoplasm is very scanty.

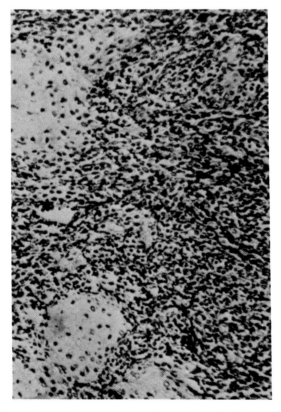

Figure 134. Mesenchymal chondrosarcoma: islands of well-differentiated cartilage are surrounded by undifferentiated mesenchymal cells arranged in hemangiopericytoma pattern (× 170). (From Reeh MJ: Hemangiopericytoma with cartilaginous differentiation involving orbit. Arch Ophthalmol 75:82–83, 1966. By permission.)

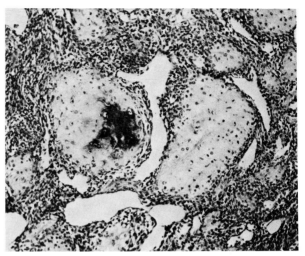

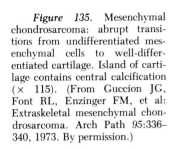

Figure 135. Mesenchymal chondrosarcoma: abrupt transitions from undifferentiated mesenchymal cells to well-differentiated cartilage. Island of cartilage contains central calcification (× 115). (From Guccion JG, Font RL, Enzinger FM, et al: Extraskeletal mesenchymal chondrosarcoma. Arch Path 95:336–340, 1973. By permission.)

TREATMENT AND COURSE

Complete surgical removal of tumor seems to be the preferable method of treatment based on the limited number of protocols available for study. Anything short of complete excision will subject the patient to recurrences, continued local spread of the tumor, and possible metastasis. The most successful examples of management were the cases of Reeh and Sevel, with survival intervals of 10 and 5 years, respectively. Exenteration of the orbit was performed in both cases. The exact effect or role of radiation and chemotherapy in the management of these tumors is not known at this time.

FIBROUS DYSPLASIA

At present, most observers agree that fibrous dysplasia of bone is non-neoplastic but disagree as to the genesis of the disease and its correct place in the spectrum of fibro-osseous tumors. We will follow what seems to be the majority's preference and discuss the lesion among the osseous and cartilaginous tumors. We will avoid the debate as to histogenesis and simply repeat the opinion of many that the lesion represents an anomaly or arrest in the development of bone.

Lichtenstein (1938) first used the term *fibrous dysplasia* for the bony lesion and this name has been widely accepted through the intervening years. Dahlin (1978) suggests that *fibro-osseous dysplasia* is a term that is gaining acceptance for many of the defects of this type that involve the base of the skull and jaw-bones. We prefer to limit our narrative to the monostotic form of the disease associated with proptosis that simulates other orbital tumors. For those with further interest in either the polyostotic form or the nonskeletal components of the disease we are appending the references of Pritchard (1951), Harris et al (1962), and Albright et al (1938).

INCIDENCE

We do not believe this orbital disorder is as infrequent as the reader might assume from a perusal of the ophthalmic literature. Some of the larger surveys of orbital tumors do not mention the disorder but this omission may be due to closer orientation to neoplasms and less attention to non-neoplastic tumors that may simulate neoplasms. The most comprehensive review of orbital involvement by fibrous dysplasia associated with exophthalmos is that of Moore (1969). He summarized data from eight cases in the literature from three different sources and added two cases of his own. Our Mayo Clinic series includes five cases. In Table 13 we have summarized the sex and age data from the composite ten cases in the report of Moore plus our own five cases. In the Moore report age data is recorded at time of diagnosis whereas the age data from our cases is recorded in terms of age of onset. Age at time of diagnosis sometimes is misleading because the symptoms and signs of the disease may have been present for several years before the child or adolescent comes to the attention of an ophthalmologist. It is evident from this data (Table 13) that the disease is one of childhood and adolescence. In cases involving the orbit as well as adjacent paranasal sinuses there seems to be a slight predominance in females.

CLINICAL FEATURES

When the dysplasia involves the orbit it usually does so through one of the major (maxillary, malar, ethmoid, frontal, or sphenoid) bones contributing to the orbital contour. Sometimes contiguous orbital bones are involved and it is our impression that, when this happens, the frontal and sphenoid bones more often share this arrangement. Four of the five cases had neither obvious bony involvement other than the orbit nor known endocrine disturbance. In the one remaining case an additional diagnosis of dyschondroplastic dwarfism was made.

The ocular and orbital symptoms produced by this disease vary according to which bone is affected and how dysplasia affects the bone. Orbital bones seem to be affected in one or a combination of two ways. In thinner portions of

TABLE 13.   AGE AND SEX DISTRIBUTION OF ORBITAL FIBROUS DYSPLASIA

Age (yr)	
Females (N = 9)	*Males* (N = 6)
3	6*
3	8
7*	8
9*	8*
12	11
12	13
19	
19*	
23	

*From the Mayo Clinic study.

orbital bones — the orbital plates of maxillary, ethmoid, and frontal bones, for example — the thin cortex tends to expand more rapidly and to a greater degree from the dysplasia than do thicker portions of the bone. It is these same thin surfaces that are adjacent to other cavities. The bone tends to bulge into either the orbital space or the sinus, and cystic spaces then develop within the expanding mass. The body and wings of the sphenoid bone, as well as thicker portions of the previously mentioned bones, seem to react differently. Bony overgrowth is more solid and sclerotic, causing a harder, more unyielding thickening of bone. When this change affects the sphenoid bone in the region of the optic nerve, the optic canal gradually and uniformly narrows. Impairment of function of the optic nerve follows as the tissue is affected by a boa-like squeeze. The malar bone along its orbital surface seems capable of either response.

When the orbital maxilla is affected, the eye is pushed upward, and when the roof of the orbit is involved, the eye will be pushed downward; the eye is always displaced in a direction opposite to the source of the expanding mass. This horizontal or vertical displacement may be disproportionately greater than forward proptosis — a feature not common to the majority of other tumors. Prominence of the face, cheek, forehead, temple, or area around the bridge of the nose on the side of proptosis results from the participation of the remainder of the involved bone in the process of dysplasia. This unilateral bony asymmetry makes the patient's face look lopsided (Fig. 136).

Although such a displacement of the eye causes some mechanical interference with rotation, the eye, as a rule, does not come to serious harm as the result of such an expanding mass. There may be some blurring of vision simply due to the effect of proptosis and pressure on refraction. After the mass has been removed there is reasonable return of ocular function and some improvement in the position of the eye in most cases. The growth of the tumor usually is painless unless the eye has been displaced for many years; patients may then describe a dull ache around the orbit. The duration of symptoms before the child is brought for consultation usually is several years; this is a much longer interval than the average for other orbital tumors among this age group. The marked

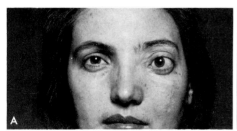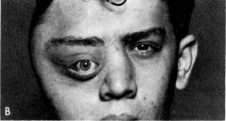

Figure 136. Fibrous dysplasia. *A,* Prominence of left malar bone (contiguous sclerosis and deformity of maxilla), progressive proptosis and lateral deviation of left eye (gradually advancing fibrous dysplasia since age 5), involvement of ethmoid and frontal bones, and eventual blindness in left eye (involvement of greater and lesser wings of sphenoid and optic canal deformity) were characteristic in this 36-year-old woman. (Courtesy of Dr. R. W. Neault.)

B, Gradual progression of proptosis and displacement of right eye (since age 8) and deformity of right face (since age 10) in a 19-year-old man; fibrous dysplasia affected temporal, malar, zygomatic, ethmoid, and sphenoid bones slowly and progressively during a 12-year-period after this photograph.

forward-horizontal or forward-vertical displacement of an eye of several years' duration associated with *bony asymmetry of the face or head* is quite diagnostic of fibrous dysplasia. The diagnosis might well be suspected upon first observation of the child as he enters the consultation room. Roentgenograms may well cinch the diagnosis.

When the sphenoid is affected, proptosis is less severe and more straight-forward. But visual function usually becomes impaired owing to interference with transmission of nerve impulses along the optic nerve; pallor of the disk or marked optic atrophy is then noticeable. We observed one child who was blind with advanced atrophy of the optic disk when first brought for consultation. In this case dysplasia had progressed so insidiously and painlessly for so long that unilateral blindness had developed without the child's realizing it. In some patients, marked visual failure develops without any proptosis. In such instances the dysplasia strangles the nerve posterior to the orbit. In the *differential diagnosis* of the optic atrophy and visual loss, glioma of the optic nerve also should be considered. In earlier years some reports of meningioma in children probably were examples of this type of fibrous dysplasia. Bony asymmetry of the face or head usually is not as marked with meningioma.

ROENTGENOGRAPHIC CHANGES

The roentgenographic changes in cranial bones range from small translucent zones to large diffuse areas of sclerosis. The latter may extend through several adjoining bones without regard to suture boundaries. The diffuse sclerosis type is the change we have most often encountered in our patients with orbital involvement although, in one, a cystic zone about 2½ cm in diameter had expanded the thin orbital plate of the frontal bone. In routine skull views the orbital deformity usually is quite evident at first glance (Fig. 137). Changes in the sphenoid bone are most easily seen in lateral views (Fig.

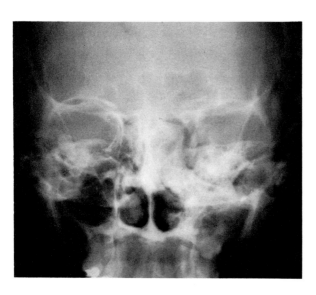

Figure 137. Fibrous dysplasia: roentgenogram showing marked deformity of left orbit and left maxilla.

138); the body and wings show dense sclerosis with some overall thickening, a change that may be quite diffuse throughout this bone. This appearance closely resembles a meningioma. Tomograms also help to reveal the more radiolucent center of a mass, a feature which is related to the content of fibrous tissue. In cases of pallor of the optic nerve, special views usually reveal narrowing or constriction of the bony optic canal due to sclerosis of the surrounding bone (Fig. 139).

PATHOLOGY

The principal feature is a proliferation of relatively uniform spindle-shaped fibroblasts producing a collagenous matrix and surrounding interconnecting or sometimes isolated spicules of osteoid. The latter is arranged haphazardly through the tumor (Fig. 140). In some lesions of more sclerotic consistency the osteoid, or even islands of chondroid, may be more predominant than the proliferating fibrous tissue. Also, the center of some tumors may be predominantly fibrous in character but the periphery may show a greater profusion of osteoid. These imperfect spindles of bone are responsible for the gritty sensation the surgeon encounters in opening into a more radiolucent area of the tumor. The osteoid content also will determine the degree of radiodensity. Mitotic figures may be few or moderate in number but there is no cellular atypia. As the lesion progresses, areas of degeneration may develop in the tumor characterized by an acellular fibrous or myxoid tissue. The islands and trabeculae of osteoid are not covered by a layer of osteoblasts (Fig. 141) such as would be seen in the closely related osteoblastoma and ossifying fibroma. It is the absence of osteoblasts in

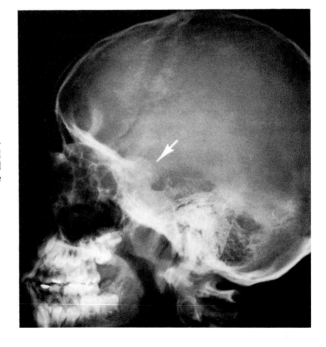

Figure 138. Fibrous dysplasia: roentgenogram (lateral projection) showing sclerosis and deformity of sphenoid bone surrounding sella turcica.

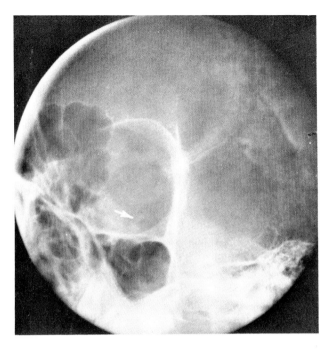

Figure 139. Fibrous dysplasia: roentgenogram showing marked narrowing (3 mm) of right optic canal (*arrow*). The right eye of this 9-year-old boy was blind.

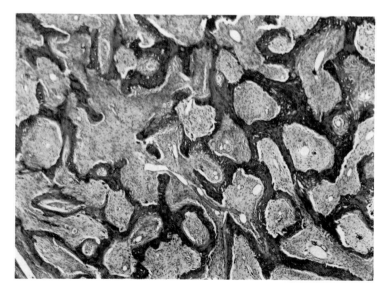

Figure 140. Fibrous dysplasia: irregular, imperfect osteoid trabeculae dispersed in fibrous tissue. (Hematoxylin and eosin; × 40.)

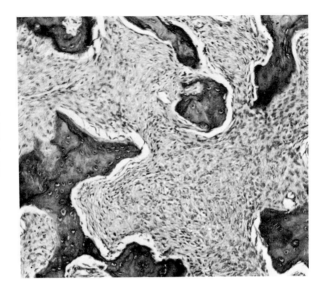

Figure 141. Fibrous dysplasia: osteoid trabeculae are formed without intervention of osteoblasts by apparent metaplastic phenomenon of fibroblasts. (Hematoxylin and eosin; × 125.)

fibrous dysplasia which supports the theory that the lesion represents an arrest in the development of immature woven bone into more mature lamellar bone.

TREATMENT AND COURSE

Whereas the treatment of several of the tumors previously discussed in this chapter was dictated by the fear of possible metastasis and the prevention of an aggressive local recurrence, these factors are minimal or nonexistent in the case of fibrous dysplasia. Surgical removal of the latter can be deferred until proptosis of the eye or the deformity of orbital bone reaches a degree where the cosmetic liability of the disease is no longer acceptable. Here, the principal goal is to remove that portion of the mass which will bring about a satisfactory reduction of proptosis or reduce the offending bulk of the fibrous overgrowth. Biting forceps are used for removal of the sclerotic or cortical bone and a scoop or curette for removal of the less dense fibrous component. Such a debulking procedure may need repeating after a lapse of several years for those cases that continue to progress contrary to the often repeated statement that the disease stops progressing after puberty. One of the patients under our observation had undergone three surgical procedures for an orbital fibrous dysplasia by the age of 21 years and the lesion still was showing roentgenographic evidence of progression at age 29.

If the dysplasia involves the sphenoid bone with subsequent narrowing of the optic canal and pressure on the optic nerve, surgical intervention becomes mandatory in an effort to restore visual function to the affected eye. Prognosis for recovery of vision in such cases must be guarded because of the consequences of long-continued pressure on the optic nerve prior to surgery or the surgical trauma to the nerve in the course of the bony decompression.

We do not recommend irradiation because of the possibility of inducing a malignant transformation in an otherwise benign but sometimes aggressive process.

INFANTILE CORTICAL HYPEROSTOSIS

TERMINOLOGY

This is generally considered to be a benign disorder of bone which, by the tumefactions and histologic alterations it produces in soft tissues adjacent to the lesion, may be mistaken for neoplasm. More than 100 reports of this disease could probably be assembled by combing the literature in the fields of pediatrics and roentgenology, but ophthalmologists probably are less familiar (considering its frequency) with this disorder than with any other discussed in this text. The disease has been attached to any one of several eponyms, such as Caffey-Silverman, Caffey-de Toni-Silverman, Caffey-Smyth, and simply Caffey. Caffey (1957) was not the first to describe the disease — it has been known since 1930 — but he did assemble a significant number of cases and he established the disease as a new entity; he seems also to be responsible for the name by which it is presently designated. The most recent and well-documented orbital examples of the disease are to be found in the publications of Iliff and Ossofsky (1962), Bywaters and colleagues (1963), and Minton and Elliott (1967), and Galyear and Robertson (1970).

CLINICAL FEATURES

Since the disease usually appears before the age of 5 months, the pediatrician is most likely to see the condition first. The mean age at onset is reportedly 9 weeks. To observe this disease the ophthalmologist must be on the lookout for some puzzling swelling of the soft tissues of the face, jaws, eyelids, or tissues adjacent to the eye in a tiny infant. But in such a situation the diagnosis already may have been established and the ophthalmologist's role will be to observe the course of proptosis. At onset the soft tissues overlying the affected bone become swollen and firm. The disease seems prone to affect some bones more often than others. The mandible is the bone most frequently involved, then the clavicle; the scapula, ribs, and tubular bones also may be affected. The bones at the base of the skull seldom are affected, hence the scarcity of case reports in the ophthalmic literature. More than one bone may be affected before remissions and exacerbations run their normal course. When the jaws are affected the soft tissue swelling may be so exquisitely tender as to interfere with the infant's feeding. If both jaws are swollen, the tumefaction, from a front view, is not unlike the appearance of mumps in older children (Fig. 142). This swelling may extend up into the lower eyelids to give the picture of orbital cellulitis. Irritability and fever and an accelerated sedimentation rate indicate systemic reaction to the illness. Proptosis is the consequence of direct involvement of one of the orbital bones. Involvement of one of the orbital bones as a first manifestation of the disease is very rare and, when it occurs, the cause of proptosis might be puzzling unless roentgenograms are made.

The swelling of soft tissue usually subsides during a period of several months; the roentgenographic changes do not finally disappear until several years have elapsed, but no significant permanent dysfunction remains. The cause of the disease is not known, although there are many theories. In a few cases death has been attributed to the disease, so the disorder may not be as

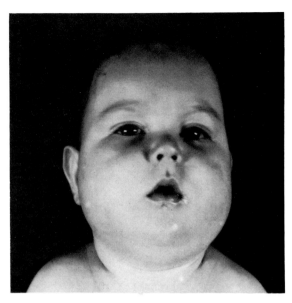

Figure 142. Infantile cortical hyperostosis: classic facial appearance. (From Minton LR, Elliott JH: Ocular manifestations of infantile cortical hyperostosis. Am J Ophthalmol 64:902–907, 1967. By permission of the Ophthalmic Publishing Company.)

benign as is generally considered. We found no cases of orbital involvement in our series, nor is the disorder mentioned among statistical surveys of other large series of orbital tumors.

ROENTGENOGRAPHIC CHANGES

If there is any guess or puzzle about the meaning of the clinical symptoms, roentgenograms quickly will provide a solution. Hyperostosis of the involved bone is so marked as to make the bone appear sclerotic. The increased density is particularly striking when compared to the shadows of other bones of the infant's skeleton. The involved bone may be irregularly thickened so that the usual smooth contour of the bony shadow is lost. The shadow in the mandible is somewhat laminated owing to attempts by the periosteum to form new bone. The swelling of the soft tissues precedes the changes in the bone and roentgenographic marks persist for many months after the inflammatory process in the adjacent soft tissues had disappeared.

PATHOLOGY

The basic inflammatory process seems to affect the periosteum. This proliferates with consequent hyperplasia of adjoining cortical bone (Fig. 143). If the periosteum is biopsied during the acute phase of the inflammatory reaction, the number of mitoses may be so great as to raise the question of osteogenic sarcoma; pathologists must be aware of this, lest radical surgery be mistakenly performed. The overlying soft tissues are edematous and are infiltrated with a variable number of inflammatory cells.

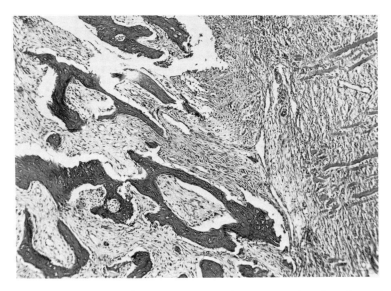

Figure 143. Infantile cortical hyperostosis: section from periosteal surface shows chronic inflammatory reaction with fibrous tissue proliferation and marked reactive new bone formation. (Hematoxylin and eosin; × 100.)

TREATMENT

Most reported cases have resolved with only nonspecific supportive treatment. It is generally agreed that surgical manipulation is not required. Steroids have been used, but opinion differs on their efficacy or need. For cases marked by remissions and exacerbations involving multiple sites, the pediatrician is likely to turn to the steroids for possible help in suppressing the disease. We do not know of any case of permanent damage to the eye as the result of proptosis secondary to swelling of the orbital soft tissues.

PROGRESSIVE DIAPHYSEAL DYSPLASIA

This is another non-neoplastic dysplasia that may affect orbital bone and thereby simulate an orbital neoplasm by producing proptosis. Several aspects of its orbital and ocular symptomatology are similar to fibrous dysplasia. It is a rather rare symmetric hyperostosis of bone chiefly affecting the diaphyses of long bones, the base of the skull, and clavicles, with a frequent familial expression. The disease is seldom noted in the ophthalmic literature.

NOMENCLATURE

Cockayne (1920) described a scrawny, malnourished 9½-year-old boy with slender extremities and prominent eyes who, on x-ray examination, proved to have marked thickening of the bones at the base of the skull and the frontal bone, and new bone density in the femurs, humeri, tibias, and fibulas. Cockayne and associates puzzled over the cause of the problem but gave the condition no name. Subsequently, the disease was noted by other observers but, in the gamesmanship of eponyms, Cockayne's name was never used in later terminology of this dysplasia. Next, in 1922, Camurati noted x-ray findings similar to those in Cockayne's patient in a father and son, both with painful lower extremities. This hereditary aspect of the disease was later confirmed in many other cases. Engelmann (1929), a radiologist in Vienna, documented the muscular wasting so often associated with the bony involvement and named the disease *osteopathia hyperostotica (sclerotisans) multiplex infantilis*. With such a complex name it is little wonder that subsequent observers simply referred to the condition as *Engelmann's disease*, the term still in most common use. Other proposed names are *hereditary multiple diaphyseal sclerosis, hyperostosis corticalis generalisata familiaris*, and the name we have used as our title.

CLINICAL FEATURES

It is the frequent involvement of the cranium with thickening of the frontal bone and marked sclerosis of the bones at the base of the skull which are responsible for the orbital changes with which we are concerned. As the frontal bone thickens, the space in the orbit is reduced, causing the proptosis. As the bone at the base of the skull becomes sclerosed (Fig. 144) the optic canals are narrowed, eventually causing loss of vision secondary to compression of the optic nerve. In these respects the symptomatology is very similar to fibrous dysplasia involving similar periorbital sites. In a 5-year-old boy reported by Krohel and Wirth (1977) the roof of one orbit was 22 mm thick. Thickening of

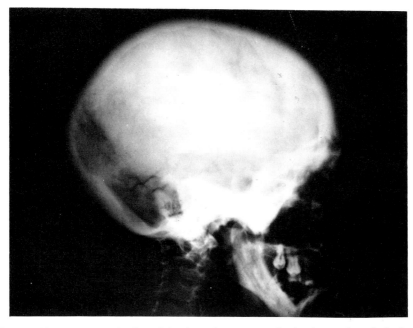

Figure 144. Progressive diaphyseal dysplasia: hyperostosis of calvarium and marked sclerosis of bones at base of skull. (From Murray RO, Jacobson HG: *The Radiology of Skeletal Disorders*. Baltimore, Williams & Wilkins Co, 1971. By permission.)

the calvarium also may occur, causing an overall enlargement of the skull (Fig. 145). The progressive hyperostosis of frontal bones may reach such a degree as to cause marked proptosis; exophthalmometer measurements in the patient of Krohel and Wirth were 28 mm on the right side, 25 mm on the left side. Additional cases with orbital or ocular involvement will be found in the reports of Mottram and Hill (1965), and Morse et al (1967).

The disease has its onset in childhood, usually between the ages of 2 and 12 years. In younger children the onset is most often associated with poor muscle development, leg pain, difficulty in walking (waddling gait), and fatigue. On roentgenography the leg bones will show symmetric sclerosis and fusiform widening of the diaphyses which usually extends proximally and distally with advancing age. The orbital and ocular symptoms develop later. Excellent retention of vision in some and blindness in others have been reported in patients who exhibited long-standing disk edema and pallor. The origin of the disease is not known.

TREATMENT

There does not seem to be an established treatment. Analgesics can be offered in an effort to reduce pain in the extremities, and an attempt should be made to improve the child's nutritional status and well-being. In the latter respects administration of corticosteroids in low maintenance doses may prove helpful. The effect of such treatment on the underlying bone disease can be followed by roentgenography.

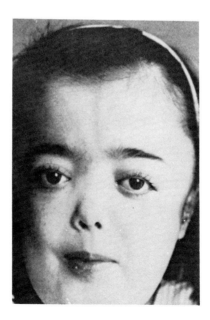

Figure 145. Progressive diaphyseal dysplasia: photograph of face, demonstrating large head, prominent forehead, and exophthalmos. (From Morse PH, Walsh FB, McCormick JR: Ocular findings in hereditary diaphyseal dysplasia (Englemann's disease). Am J Ophthalmol 68:100–104, 1969. By permission.)

Management of the orbital and ocular complications is conservative but expectant. If the proptosis becomes too extreme an effort should be made to remove some of the hyperostotic bone impinging on the orbital cavity. In patients in whom this has been attempted, surgeons have noted that the diseased bone is very hard and more difficult to remove than in cases of fibrous dysplasia. If the function of the optic nerve is compromised because of stenosis of its bony canal secondary to sclerosis of the sphenoid bone, a decompression of the bony canal will have to be considered. Surgeons disagree as to the expected help from such a procedure, some contending it may extinguish what little visual function remains in the compressed nerve. Each case of progressive visual loss will have to be judged on individual factors, and on the overall question of whether there is more to gain or lose by a transcranial unroofing of the optic canals. The patient of Krohel and Wirth underwent a two-stage unroofing of the optic canals. On one side there was no postoperative change in the degree of optic disk edema, but on the other side marked improvement occurred. Too few cases with orbital involvement have been followed for long-term intervals to provide firm data on the eventual prognosis of these patients.

ANEURYSMAL BONE CYST

TERMINOLOGY AND ORIGIN

This is a strange, benign lesion of bone which seldom affects the bony orbit. It now is considered to have such distinctive clinical and histologic features as to warrant a separate designation, but it is a comparatively new member among the family of osseous and cartilaginous tumors. The name *aneurysmal cyst* first was applied by Jaffe and Lichtenstein in 1942 to differentiate the lesion from solitary unicameral bone cyst, which was the main subject of their publication. They noted the course of these aneurysmal cysts in two patients. In the following 15-year period, Lichtenstein further clarified the concept of aneurysmal bone cyst and differentiated it from other benign lesions of bone, such as giant cell tumor, fibrous dysplasia, and giant cell reparative granuloma. The word *aneurysmal* immediately brings to mind a sac-like dilatation of a blood vessel, but Lichtenstein used this term to denote a distinctive type of "blowout" contour in roentgenograms of tubular bones affected by the tumor. The term *bone cyst* refers to cavernous-like spaces occurring within the tumor when its thin covering shell of bone is penetrated.

The pathogenesis of the tumor is not understood. It is not considered a neoplasm because it has been known to regress after incomplete removal. Although a minority contends that the tumor is a type of hemangioma affecting bone, we prefer to discuss the lesion in relation to bony lesions rather than with vascular neoplasms. It most commonly affects the long tubular bones and vertebrae. Here, we intend to enumerate the few features that are known concerning its occurrence in the bony orbit.

INCIDENCE

Examples of aneurysmal bone cyst are not mentioned in most large surveys of orbital tumors. There are approximately a dozen cases in the literature reporting involvement of one of the walls or bones rimming the orbital cavity. Not all of these cases are associated with proptosis because the expanding cyst may push into the anterior or middle fossa of the skull, or invade another sinus without significant compromise of the orbital cavity. In such instances ocular signs, such as decrease in central acuity, papilledema, ocular muscle palsies, and so on, may occur without an orbital mass. Recent reviews on the orbital and ocular manifestations of aneurysmal bone cyst are those of Powell and Glaser (1975), and Yee and colleagues (1977).

The age distribution of those patients in the literature associated with unilateral proptosis range from 8 to 31 years of age at time of diagnosis. There is a slight predominance among females. The roof of the orbit is most frequently involved. The medial wall and posterior borders of the orbit are next in frequency. One of the two cases under our observation seems to be the only example of tumor involvement along the floor of the orbit.

CLINICAL FEATURES

Painless progressive proptosis with displacement of the eye in a direction opposite to the position of the cyst protruding into the orbit is the cardinal feature of orbital aneurysmal bone cyst. Other signs, such as a palpable mass or limitation of ocular rotation in a given direction, will depend on the orbital position of the expanding mass, its rate of growth, and duration. The clinical data from the two cases in our survey follows.

Case 1. A 15-year-old girl was seen because of prominence of the right eye of indefinite duration. The right eye was proptosed 6 mm and displaced upward 3mm. Vision was not impaired. On ophthalmoscopy, choroidal folds were present along the posterior wall of the eye. A mass could be palpated in the posterior-inferior temporal quadrant. X-rays revealed bony expansion of the floor of the orbit extending upward into the orbital cavity and downward into maxillary antrum (Fig. 146). Through an inferior orbitotomy a bone-colored, dome-shaped mass was found in the peripheral orbital space inferiorly. When the eggshell-like wall was removed a cystic space filled with a marrow-like tissue

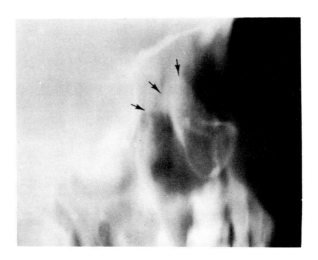

Figure 146. Aneurysmal bone cyst: tomogram (lateral projection) to show dome-shaped mass (*arrows*) along floor of orbit.

containing spicules of bone was entered. All soft tissue contents were removed and the bony wall lightly curetted. At the end of a 3-year period there was no recurrence, but slight upward displacement of the eye was still present.

Case 2. We saw this 5-year-old girl first in January 1970. Proptosis of the left eye had been present for 7 months. Approximately 6 weeks after onset (July 1969) anterior orbitotomy was performed elsewhere because of suspected orbital malignancy. Tissue removed from a reportedly soft tissue mass in the superior portion of the left orbit was shown by histopathologic examination to have a fibro-adipose structure. Proptosis progressed but more slowly than before operation. When the child came under our observation, the displacement of the left eye was as illustrated in Figure 147. Significant ocular findings were these: forward protrusion, 1 cm; vision (affected eye), 20/40; and chronic papilledema, 2 D. Roentgenograms (Fig. 148) indicated obvious enlargement and bony erosion of the left orbit due to an expanding but slow-growing, destructive tumor. A definite mass could not be palpated. Anterior orbitotomy through the brow approach was performed soon after admission. Just posterior to the overhanging lip of the superior bony rim was a firm, bone-like mass filling the upper nasal quadrant and the midportion of the orbital roof and extending posteriorly for an indefinite distance. Our initial impression was that a neoplasm had pushed the orbital roof downward against the eyeball, in a manner similar to that of an osteoma or fibrous dysplasia. However, the bony surface shattered easily when touched by dissecting instruments; it proved to be a shell-like lamina of frontal bone comprising the floor and anterior wall of a cyst-like cavity filled with soft, pulpy, vascular tissue. The latter ws easily removed by curette; it contained gritty spicules of bone similar to the contents of some tumors associated with fibrous dysplasia. A tough fibrous lining was peeled away from the inner surfaces of the bony cavity. Bleeding was sharp but not sustained as soon as all soft tissue was removed. The roof of the cavity proved to be an eroded, thinned-out lamina of frontal bone constituting the floor of the intracranial frontal fossa. The total area of the emptied cavity was approximately one-third of the normal orbital space. The thin bony partition pushing against the eye was removed with rongeurs. The dura was not exposed. There has been no recurrence in the follow-up interval of 8 years.

Roentgenographic Changes

The distinctive roentgenographic pattern of this lesion, as it affects long bones, was one of the features suggesting to Jaffe and Lichtenstein (1942) a separate classification for this tumor among other bone cysts. The radiolucent, eccentric, ballooned-out area covered by a thin layer of bone cortex also was

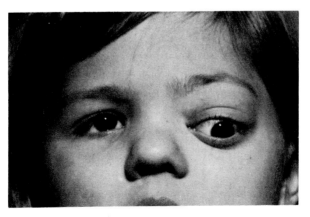

Figure 147. Aneurysmal bone cyst: obvious displacement of left eye from aneurysmal bone cyst occupying upper one-third of orbital space.

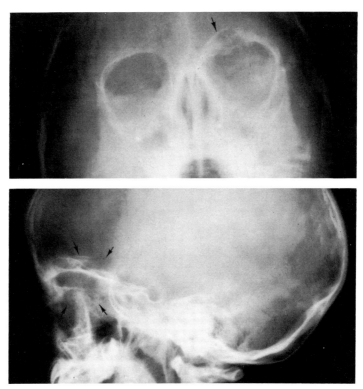

Figure 148.   Aneurysmal bone cyst: Above, Roentgenogram (Waters projection) showing asymmetry of left orbit with bony erosion (*arrow*) of orbital roof from aneurysmal bone cyst of 7 months' duration. (Same patient as in Fig. 147.) Below, Lateral projection showing aneurysmal bone cyst occupying upper portion of left orbit and upward extent expanding toward intracranial space (*upper arrows*); on stereoscopic projection, thin shell-like layer of bone is visible, representing inferior wall of cyst (*lower arrows*).

responsible for the name of the tumor. These and other characteristic roentgenographic traits are well documented in many other texts and publications. In flat bones of the calvarium, with which we are most concerned in this text, such roentgenographic changes seldom are seen. The roentgenographic features of our two cases (Figs. 146 and 148) are exceptional in this regard.

PATHOLOGY

The soft, friable, reddish-brown tissue beneath the thin shell of bone is composed of a fibrous tissue containing spicules of osteoid and honeycombed by variable sized cavernous spaces. Most of the multiple anastomosing spaces contain fresh blood or blood-tinged fluid, but some will contain only a clear fluid or even appear empty. The lining of these spaces may vary from a condensation of flattened spindle cells to a simple endothelium, but in the latter there are no other features of normal vascular channels (Fig. 149). The fibrous matrix is composed of fairly dense spindle cells that show mitoses but no anaplasia. The spicules of osteoid scattered throughout the matrix may have some covering of osteoblasts similar in appearance to osteoblastomas. Benign, multinucleated

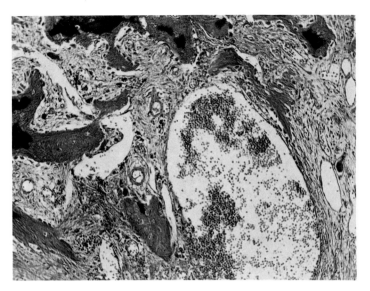

Figure 149. Aneurysmal bone cyst: blood-filled spaces, separated by fibrous septa containing bony spicules, are lined by flattened endothelium. (Hematoxylin and eosin; × 110.)

giant cells also are scattered throughout the matrix, a feature responsible for the inclusion at one time of these lesions among the giant cell tumors.

TREATMENT

Complete removal of the soft tissue contents of the bony cyst seemed adequate in our two cases, but these tumors were more accessible than some other orbital lesions reported in the literature. Complete resection may not be possible for some of the cysts along the posterior wall or the apex of the orbit because of danger of trauma to the structures passing through the superior orbital fissure. Here, a compromise is justified because, in some cases, the tumor does not seem to recur if incompletely removed. However, there is no firm data on this point in regard to orbital cases. When the bony wall of the cyst is opened bleeding may be quite sharp, but it is not alarmingly sustained as the surgeon proceeds with evacuation of the cyst contents. Irradiation is not recommended.

CHORDOMA

This tumor is better known to neurosurgeons and rhinologists than to ophthalmologists. It is an uncommon midline neoplasm arising from remnants of the notochord situated in the region of the dorsum sella and clivus. Its growth is very slow and it may remain asymptomatic for many years. Its direction of expansion is exceedingly variable, but if it grows upward, anteriorly, or sidewise it will affect some extension of the visual apparatus (optic nerve or optic chiasm) or one of the cranial nerves innervating the extraocular muscles. Therefore, clinical features such as progressive hemanopsia or quadrantanopsia, papilledema, optic atrophy, or diplopia — when associated with persistent head-ache — may occur early in the puzzling symptomatology of these tumors. In contrast, orbital involvement, as manifested by unilateral or bilateral proptosis, is very rare and, when present, usually occurs late in the course of the problem. The neoplasm must become quite large before the orbital cavity is invaded, and many patients do not live long enough to experience this complication.

Orbital involvement secondary to massive growth of the neoplasm is illus-trated by two of the very few case reports in the literature. Crikelair and McDonald (1955) recounted the trouble that a 19-year-old boy had had with a nasopharyngeal chordoma since he was 11. Initially the patient had a sixth nerve palsy, eye pain, and nasal obstruction secondary to a nasopharyngeal tumor. The mass subsided with roentgen therapy. Over the next few years there were several recurrences, each responding to radiation treatment. Even so, roentgenography showed continued destruction of the floor of the middle fossa and erosion of bone at apex of left orbit. At age 15 the left eye was enucleated. At age 16 a subtotal resection of a mass in left orbit was performed. The recur-rent tumor at age 17 is depicted in Figure 150A. Two years after excision of this mass the patient was still living (Fig. 150B).

Binkhorst et al (1957) observed a 70-year-old female with headaches, forward-lateral displacement of both eyes, and a huge midline chordoma pro-truding through one nostril. X-rays showed destruction of the medial and inferior walls and lateral nasal walls. The nasal septum was missing. When the

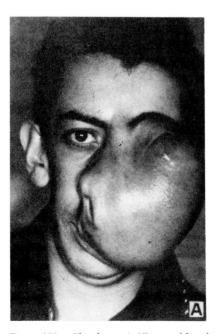 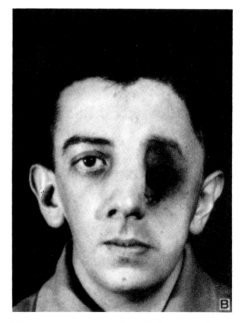

Figure 150.   Chordoma: *A*, 17-year-old male with massive distortion of face. Left eye enucleated two years previously because of orbital involvement. *B*, Appearance two years after removal of recur-rent tumor. (From Crikelair GF, McDonald JJ: Nasopharyngeal chordoma. Plast Reconstr Surg *16*: 138–144, 1955. By permission.)

protruding nasal mass was manipulated, movement was transmitted to both protruding eyes. The patient was known to have had bilateral optic atrophy and complete blindness for twenty years.

Other cases of orbital involvement with proptosis are those of Zeitlin and Levinson (18-year-old female), Argaud and colleagues (3-year-old male), and Roche and colleagues (76-year-old female). These reports give us some idea of the very wide range of these neoplasms as they affect the orbit. Almost all other reports of chordomas in the ophthalmic literature are concerned with neuro-ophthalmic manifestations.

ROENTGENOGRAPHIC CHANGES

Early in the course of the tumor, standard roentgenographic views of the skull may be normal. In such cases patients with persistent, progressive head-ache, extraocular muscle palsy, a visual field defect, and failing vision in one eye may undergo an intracranial surgical exploratory procedure before the neo-plasm is discovered. More often, bone destruction of some portion of the sella turcica is seen on roentgenography which tends to progress slowly, depending on the direction of the neoplasm's expansion. As time passes radiopaque amorphous masses also appear in the zones of bone destruction. At this stage the roentgenographic aspects of chordoma closely resemble chondroma in the same area.

PATHOLOGY

These are soft, smooth-surfaced, lobulated gray tumors varying in hue from red to blue. The cells are large, round or oval, with large central nuclei and a vacuolated cytoplasm (physaliferous cells). The intracytoplasmic vacuoles are filled with a mucin-like substance and may become so distended as to be twice the diameter of the cell's nucleus (Fig. 151). The cells may grow in cords, nests, or alveolar arrangement and are surrounded by a mucinous matrix of variable density. The periphery of the tumor is circumscribed where it pushes against soft tissue structures but is frankly infiltrative in areas of bone invasion.

TREATMENT AND COURSE

Complete excision of the neoplasm is the ideal goal but is very rarely possible in the area of the dorsum sella or clivus. Still, an effort should be made to remove the more accessible areas of the tumor in those patients with increased intracranial pressure, headache, or decreasing vision. Those firmer nodular portions of the neoplasm which balloon into the orbital cavity, intra-cranial space, or a paranasal sinus may be excised, but the more myxoid, soft portions infiltrating bone can only be removed by suction, curettes, or swabs. Such subtotal resections may provide a gratifying, albeit temporary, remission of symptoms.

We have already noted that some chordomas that expand anteriorly along the midline may be compatible with survival for a period of several decades,

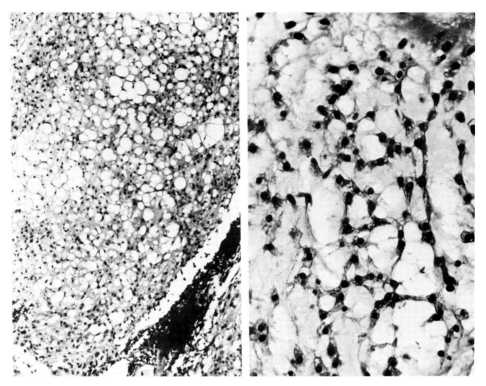

Figure 151. Chordoma: Left, Mucous vacuoles in cytoplasm of chordoma cells, so-called physaliferous cells (× 100). (From Dahlin DC, MacCarty CS: Chordoma: A study of fifty-nine cases. Cancer 5:1170–1178, 1952. By permission.) Right, Cells occur in syncytial anastomosing strands of cytoplasm (× 350). (From Dahlin DC: *Bone Tumors, General Aspects and Data on 6,221 Cases.* Springfield, Illinois, Charles C Thomas Publishers, 1978. By permission.)

although the patient may be severely disabled. However, those chordomas that expand superiorly, inferiorly, or posteriorly into the intracranial space usually are fatal within 3 to 5 years from the first onset of symptoms.

Radiotherapy may be useful for the inoperable tumors and recurrences.

EWING'S TUMOR

To complete this chapter we mention a not uncommon, nonosteogenic neoplasm occurring in bone which may come to the attention of ophthalmologists because of its tendency to metastasize to other bones, including the bony orbit. When the latter occurs, progressive proptosis will signal the event and the ophthalmologist may be called upon to measure the ocular displacement and to assess the patient's visual status. Otherwise the ophthalmologist's role is strictly as a standby because the diagnosis of the primary tumor has already been made, the lytic lesions in the skull or bony orbit have been recognized, and treatment has been instituted by the orthopedic oncologist.

Briefly, Ewing's tumor probably arises from undifferentiated mesenchyme and usually occurs in the long tubular bones of young people in the 5- to 25-year-old age group. Metastasis to the orbital bones is not common and only sporadic reports of such cases are found in the ophthalmic literature. The most informative of such reports is that of Albert and associates (1967). They recorded five patients with known Ewing's tumor who developed unilateral proptosis due to clinical orbital metastasis. The male to female ratio was 3:2 and the age of the five patients ranged from 9 to 17 years. The interval between the diagnosis of the primary lesion and the appearance of the metastasis averaged 14 months, with a range of from 4 to 38 months. Survival following orbital metastasis ranged from 1 to 14 months. The proptosis occurring in this malignant disease does not have any clinically distinctive features.

Reports of a primary Ewing's tumor in the orbit must be regarded with considerable reservation.

Bibliography

Osteoma

Fu YS, Perzin KH: Non-epithelial tumors of the nasal cavity, paranasal sinuses, and nasopharynx. A clinicopathologic study. II. Osseous and fibro-osseous lesions, including osteoma, fibrous dysplasia, ossifying fibroma, osteoblastoma, giant cell tumor, and osteosarcoma. Cancer 33:1289–1305, 1974

Gardner EJ: Follow-up study of family group exhibiting dominant inheritance for a syndrome including intestinal polyps, osteomas, fibromas, and epidermal cysts. Am J Hum Genet 14:376–390, 1962

Hilton: Case of a large bony tumor in the face completely removed by spontaneous separation: to which are added, observations upon some of the functions of the soft palate and pharynx. Guys Hosp Rep 1:493-506, 1836

Louis J: Cited by Váncea P, Lázărescu D

Miller NR, Gray J, Snip R: Giant mushroom-shaped osteoma of the orbit originating from the maxillary sinus. Am J Ophthalmol 83:587-591, 1977

Teed RW: Primary osteoma of the frontal sinus. Arch Otolaryngol 33:255-292, 1941 (This reference contains the most complete bibliography of any publication in the English language up to this time.)

Vancea P, Lázărescu D: L'ostéome de l'orbite. Ophthalmologica 136:225-238, 1958

Van der Meer G: Cited by Teed RW

Veiga T: Cited by Teed RW

Wilkes SR, Trautmann JC, De Santo LW, et al: Osteoma: an unusual cause of amaurosis fugax. Mayo Clin Proceed 54:258-260, 1979

Osteoblastoma

Dahlin DC: *Bone Tumors, General Aspects and Data on 6,221 Cases.* Springfield, Charles C Thomas Publishers, 1978

Freedman SR: Benign osteoblastoma of the ethmoid bone. Am J Clin Path 63:391-396, 1975

Fu YS, Perzin KH: Nonepithelial tumors of the nasal cavity, paranasal sinuses and nasopharynx. A clinicopathologic study: II. Osseous and fibro-osseous lesions, including osteoma, fibrous dysplasia, ossifying fibroma, osteoblastoma, giant cell tumor and osteosarcoma. Cancer 33:1289-1305, 1974

Lehrer HZ: Ossifying fibroma of the orbital roof. Its distinction from "blistering" or intra-osseous meningioma. Arch Neurol 20:536-541, 1969

Scott M, Peale AR, Croissant PD: Intracranial midline anterior fossae ossifying fibroma invading orbits, paranasal sinuses and right maxillary antrum. Case report. J Neurosurg 34:827-831, 1971

Sherman RS, Sternbergh WCA: The roentgen appearance of ossifying fibroma of bone. Radiology 50:595-609, 1948

Giant Cell Tumor

Abdalla MI, Hosni F: Osteoclastoma of the orbit: case report. Br J Ophthalmol 50:95–98, 1966

Babel J: Osteoclastome et granulome à céllules géantes du rebord orbitarie. Ann Ocul 206:725–729, 1973

Osteogenic Sarcoma

Blodi FC: Unusual orbital neoplasms. Am J Ophthalmol 68:407-412, 1969
Bone RC, Biller HF, Harris BL: Osteogenic sarcoma of the frontal sinus. Ann Otolaryngol 82:162-165, 1973
Jakobiec FA, Jones IS: Mesenchymal and fibro-osseous tumors. In *Clinical Ophthalmology.* Volume 2, Chapter 44, Ed: TD Duane, Hagerstown, Harper & Row Publishers, 1978
Mortada A: Exophthalmos and rare tumors of the orbital bones. Am J Ophthalmol 57:270-275, 1964
Reese AB: *Tumors of the Eye.* Second edition. New York, Hoeber Medical Division, Harper & Row, Publishers, 1963
Silva D: Orbital tumors. Am J Ophthalmol 65:318-339, 1968

Osteogenic Sarcoma Following Irradiation

Sagerman R, Cassady J, Trotter P, et al: Radiation-induced neoplasia following external beam therapy for children with retinoblastoma. Am J Roentgenol Radium Ther Nucl Med 105:529-535, 1966
Soloway H: Radiaton-induced neoplasms following curative therapy for retinoblastoma. Cancer 19: 1984-1988, 1966

Chondroma

Dahlin DC: *Bone Tumors. General Aspects and Data on 6,221 Cases.* Third Edition. Springfield, Charles C Thomas, Publisher, 1978
Jepson CM, Wetzig PC: Pure chondroma of the trochlea. Survey Ophthalmol 11:656–659, 1966
Reese AB: *Tumors of the Eye.* Second edition. New York, Hoeber Medical Division, Harper and Row Publishers, 1963
Simões de Sá A: Cited by Reese AB

Chondrosarcoma

Holland MG, Allen JH, Ichinose H: Chondrosarcoma of the orbit. Trans Am Acad Ophthalmol Otolaryngol 65:898-905, 1961

Mesenchymal Chondrosarcoma

Cárdenas-Ramirez L, Albores-Saavedra J, de Buen S: Mesenchymal chondrosarcoma of the orbit. Report of five cases in orbital location. Arch Ophthalmol 86:410-413, 1971
Dowling EA: Mesenchymal chondrosarcoma. J Bone Joint Surg 46A:747-754, 1964
Guccion JG, Font RL, Enzinger FM, et al: Extraskeletal mesenchymal chondrosarcoma. Arch Path 95:336-340, 1973
Lichtenstein L, Bernstein D: Unusual benign and malignant chondroid tumors of bone. Cancer 12: 1142-1157, 1959
Reeh MJ: Hemangiopericytoma with cartilaginous differentiation involving orbit. Arch Ophthalmol 75:82–83, 1966
Salvador AH, Beabout JW, Dahlin DC: Mesenchymal chondrosarcoma — observation on 30 new cases. Cancer 28:605–615, 1971
Sevel D: Mesenchymal chondrosarcoma of the orbit. Br J Opthal 58:882–887, 1974
Trzcinska-Dabrowska Z, Witwicki T, Zielinski K: Primary mesenchymal chondrosarcoma of the orbit treated by biological resection. Ophthalmologica (Basel) 157:24–35, 1969

Fibrous Dysplasia of Bone

Albright F, Scoville B, Sulkowitch HW: Syndrome characterized by osteitis fibrosa disseminata, areas of pigmentation and gonadal dysfunction — further observations including the report of two more cases. Endocrinology 22:411-421, 1938
Dahlin DC: *Bone Tumors. General Aspects and Data on 6,221 Cases.* Springfield, Charles C Thomas Publishers, 1978
Harris WH, Dudley HR, Jr, Barry RJ: The natural history of fibrous dysplasia: an orthopedic, pathological and roentgenographic study. J Bone Joint Surg 44a;207-233, 1962
Leeds N, Seaman WB: Fibrous dysplasia of skull and its differential diagnosis: a clinical and roentgenographic study of 46 cases. Radiology 78:570-582, 1962
Lichtenstein L: Polyostotic fibrous dysplasia. 36:874-898, 1938
Moore RT: Fibrous dysplasia of the orbit. Surv Ophth 13:321-334, 1969
Pritchard JE: Fibrous dysplasia of the bones. Am J Med Sci 222:313-332, 1951

Infantile Cortical Hyperostosis

Bywaters TW Jr, Bailey RW, Carroll CJ, et al: Infantile cortical hyperostosis presenting with exophthalmos: case report. Mich Med 62:285-288, 1963

Caffey J: Infantile cortical hyperostosis: a review of the clinical and radiographic features. Proc R Soc Med 50:347-354, 1957

Caffey J, Silverman WA: Infantile cortical hyperostoses: preliminary report on a new syndrome. Am J Roentgenol Radium Ther Nucl Med 54:1-16, 1945

Galyear J, Robertson W: Caffey's syndrome. Some unusual ocular manifestations. Pediatrics 45: 122-124, 1970

Iliff CE, Ossofsky HJ: Infantile cortical hyperostosis: an unusual cause of proptosis. Am J Ophthalmol 53:976-981, 1962

Minton LR, Elliott JH: Ocular manifestations of infantile cortical hyperostosis. Am J Ophthalmol 64: 902-907, 1967

Progressive Diaphyseal Dysplasia

Camurati M: Di un raro caso di osteita simmatrica ereditaria degli arti inferiori. Chir degli Organi di Movimento 6:662-665, 1922

Cockayne EA: Case for diagnosis. Proc Royal Soc Med 13:132-136, 1920

Engelmann G: Ein Fall von Osteopathia hyperostotica (sclerotisans) multiplex infantilis. Fortschritte auf dem Gebiete der Rontgenstrahlen und der Nuclearmedizin 39:1101-1106, 1929

Krohel GB, Wirth CR: Englemann's disease. Am J Ophthalmol 84:520-525, 1977

Morse PH, Walsh FB, McCormick JR: Ocular findings in hereditary diaphyseal dysplasia (Engelmann's disease). Am J Ophthalmol 68:100-104, 1969

Mottram ME, Hill HA: Diaphyseal dysplasia: report of a case. Am J Roentgen 95:162-167, 1965

Sparks RS, Graham CB: Camurati-Engelmann's disease. Genetics and clinical manifestations with a review of the literature. J Med Genet 9:73-85, 1972

Aneurysmal Bone Cyst

Jaffe HL, Lichtenstein L: Solitary unicameral bone cyst: with emphasis on the roentgen picture, the pathologic appearance and the pathogenesis. Arch Surg 44:1004-1025, 1942

Powell JO, Glaser JS: Aneurysmal bone cyst of the orbit. Arch Ophthalmol 93:340-342, 1975

Yee RD, Cogan DG, Thorp TR, et al: Optic nerve compression due to aneurysmal bone cyst. Arch Ophthalmol 95:2176-2179, 1977

Chordoma

Argaud, Gorse, Calmette: Chordome intraorbitaire chez un infant de trois ans. Ann Anat Pathol 14:419-422, 1937

Binkhorst CD, Schierbeek P, Petten GJW: Neoplasms of the notochord: report of a case of basilar chordoma with nasal and bilateral orbital involvement. Ophthalmologica 133:12-22, 1955

Crickelair GF, McDonald JJ: Nasopharyngeal chordoma. Plast Reconstr Surg 16:138-144, 1955

Roche, Thiers, Martin: L'Aspect ophthalmologique d'un cas de chordome. Bull Soc Franc Ophtal 50:70-79, 1937

Zeitlin H, Levinson SA: Intracranial chordoma. Arch Neurol Psychiat 45:984-991, 1941

Ewing's Tumor

Albert DM, Rubenstein RA, Scheie HG: Tumor metastasis to the eye. Am J Ophthalmol 63:727-732, 1967

9

Tumors of Mesenchymal
and Adipose Tissue

In chapter 8 we discussed several tumor families that share a common precursor, or parent, the undifferentiated *mesenchymal cell*. Here, we will note the *myxoma*, a direct progeny of this cell, two neoplasms, *lipoma* and *liposarcoma*, which frequently have myxomatous tissue in their makeup, and *mesenchymoma*, composed of two or more tumor families of mesodermal heritage which have merged into one neoplasm.

MYXOMA

TERMINOLOGY

Myxoma probably originates in remnants of primitive or embryonic mucinous tissue which does not undergo adult differentiation. Also, it is possible that the stem cell is an altered fibroblast that has lost its ability to produce mature collagen. Some contend there is no such tumor as a true myxoma because there are no cells such as myxoblasts and myxocytes. This argument need not detract from their designation as separate tumors because their origin may be traced directly to the mesenchymal cell, mother of all connective tissue tumors. A common synonym is *fibromyxoma*, which indicates how frequently and how closely they are associated with the connective tissue tumor of the fibromatous type. Terminology becomes even more complex when a possible malignant analog of this tumor is considered. Some believe that myxomas are incapable of metastasis and are opposed to the term myxosarcoma. They further contend that those tumors reported as myxosarcomas were, in reality, primary malignancies of another connective tissue type, the tumors containing much myxoid substance.

A recent case report by Blodi (1969) illustrates some of these problems of classification and nomenclature. His patient was a 42-year-old woman with unilateral proptosis (6 mm) caused by a soft tumor that filled the entire retrobulbar space. The tumor was too extensive to permit total excision. Blodi classified the tumor as a myxosarcoma, but the histopathologic description referred to a large lipomatous component also. This tumor recurred, and after 1 year another orbitotomy became necessary. By the time of the second operation the neoplasm had spread to the temporal fossa, extending toward the brow outside the orbit. This proved its locally invasive character. A radical operation

248

including exenteration was required to remove the recurring mass and to prevent further spread. On the basis of mitosis in tissue sections as well as the locally invasive character, Blodi seems justified in having judged the tumor malignant. However, some pathologists would deny its malignancy because of the lack of metastasis and they would, instead, call it a benign myxoma showing the usual locally invasive trends. Still other pathologists, rather than describe the tumor as a myxoma, would classify it as a lipomatous neoplasm with myxoid features, that is, a myxoid liposarcoma.

INCIDENCE

Myxomas of the orbit are rare. Blegvad (1944) collected five cases between 1913 and the time of his own case report, but these tumors were not all located in the orbit, as so often has been mistakenly quoted. The initial case — Mauricione (1913) — originated in the subcutaneous tissue at the medial commissure of the eyelids; if the orbit was involved, it was affected secondarily. Lamb (1928) referred to another reported case in which the orbit was secondarily involved by a myxoma arising in a frontal sinus. Including Blegvad's case, then, there was a total of five myxomas primary in the orbit. Interestingly, the five cases were in women of 40, 16, 29, 25, and 29 years of age, respectively. Kreuger et al (1967) added a 31-year-old male to this series. Also to be considered are cases, never more than two in each, scattered among the larger surveys of orbital tumors, but the clinical details of these cases are unknown. According to the review of Kreuger and associates, the duration of symptoms prior to the first exam will vary from 3 to 33 years in the majority of cases.

CLINICAL FEATURES AND PATHOLOGY

Our knowledge of the clinical picture must depend largely on the few descriptive reports in the literature. Most agree the neoplasm is gray or white. In one report the tumor was described as yellow, and this raises the possibility of a lipomatous tumor. It is quite common for orbital lipomatous tumors to have myxoid features and, as already noted, some of these mistakenly are classified as myxomas. The tumor is soft and mucoid in consistency; some observers have called them slimy (Fig. 152). A true capsule is lacking, though a pseudocapsule or connective tissue membrane seems to partially cover the lobulated tumor in most cases. Gifford (1931) reported a somewhat different structure in that the tumor consisted more of separate, multiple lobules rather than a conglomerate mass: "a bunch of grapes" was Gifford's description. At the first operation a cluster of 7 tumors was removed and, at the time of recurrence several years later, 10 lobules were excised.

The main component is a mucinous matrix interspersed, through a delicate framework of reticulin and collagen fibers, with stellate cells resembling parent mesenchyme (Fig. 153). The mucinous matrix — chemically, in large part mucopolysaccharide — stains red with mucicarmine and this staining reaction is essential to diagnosis of myxoma. Most of these neoplasms occur in the upper quadrants of the orbit, but in long-standing cases the mass may fill the entire retrobulbar space. Their growth is exceedingly slow and the eye can leisurely adapt to the pressure of the tumor. Therefore, the pattern of proptosis and dis-

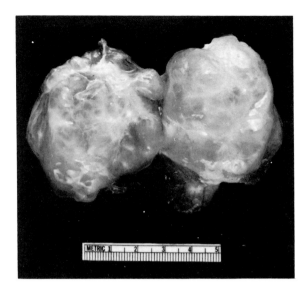

Figure 152. Myxoma: tumor is soft and mucoid, with jelly-like material exuded from the cut surface. (This specimen, from lower extremity.)

placement will be that of a benign orbital tumor (Chapter 1). Diplopia also will be noted when the malposition of the eye becomes more marked. Ultrasonography is useful in outlining the extent of the tumor prior to surgical intervention.

TREATMENT

The soft structure of this tumor and its very slow growth do not pose any serious threat to the function of those structures passing through the orbital space, but the bulk of the tumor and degree of proptosis finally make orbitotomy mandatory. The less vascular nature of the tumor makes it easier to

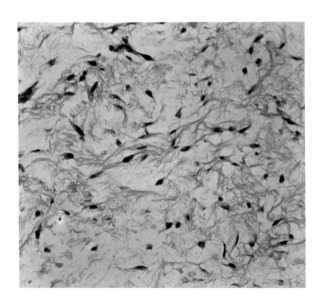

Figure 153. Myxoma: sparse stellate cells in delicate framework are dispersed in mucinous matrix. (Hematoxylin and eosin; × 200.)

remove than most orbital tumors; this advantage is offset by the frequent absence of a well-delineated cleavage between tumor and surrounding orbital fat. A further problem may be seepage of mucinous material from the periphery of the tumor during the course of dissection. These several factors militate against a complete, intact removal of tumor. Recurrence of tumor, therefore, might be expected, but data on the orbital aspect of this is very meager. The multiple lobulated, large tumor of Gifford's recurred 30 months after apparent complete removal. The case of Kreuger was followed for three years postoperatively. At this time there was 1-mm proptosis of the affected eye but ultrasonography was equivocal on the question of recurrence. In all other cases in the literature the follow-up interval was too short to permit valid conclusions. There have been no reported instances of metastasis from orbital myxomas nor any spread beyond the confines of the orbital bones.

MESENCHYMOMA

TERMINOLOGY

Klein (1932) seems to have been the first to use the term, *mesenchymoma*, in reference to a somewhat loose group of tumors composed of primitive mesenchymal cells. Klein preferred that the term not be applied to any sarcomas that might contain spindle cells destined to form fibrous tissue or bone. Theoretically, Klein's mesenchymoma would contain such uniform, undifferentiated mesenchymal cells that the pathologist would not be able to state the ultimate path of cellular differentiation. This classification was not easy to follow becuase many sarcomas, even at a very early stage, contained cells in various stages of differentiation and differing tissue specificity.

Later, Stout (1938) found it a convenient term for sarcomas that contained two or more malignant elements of mesenchymal derivation not ordinarily associated in the process of neoplasia. Most pathologists have subsequently respected Stout's wish to restrict the term to tumors of this type. Of the two or more tissue types required to fulfill the definition, one component may be composed of unclassifiable mesodermal elements.

CLINICAL FEATURES

Orbital cases of mesenchymoma are so sparse as to make impossible a meaningful assembly of data on either incidence or clinical features. Stout, in his 1967 fascicle written with Lattes, assembled, through the year 1959, such a number of cases of malignant mesenchymoma representative of all areas of the body as to make one wonder why this neoplasm has not been reported more often. He suspects that mesenchymomas have, in the past, been classified on the basis of predominant or most easily recognized tissue component.

Stout listed six cases located in the orbit. Two of these six were in children; they were probably the same two cases noted in his joint publication with Nash in 1961. No details of the remaining four adult patients seem to have been included in any of his publications. This is regrettable because these four cases might have formed the basis for some opinion about the clinical features of the neoplasms as they affect the orbit. Little more is known about the two children. Each child was 6 years of age; one was a boy and the other a girl. In one, the mesenchymoma was a mixture of rhabdomyosarcoma, leiomyosarcoma, and undifferentiated tissue, and in the other it was a mixture of chondrosarcoma and undifferentiated tumor. The tumor was fatal in both children.

Elsewhere in the literature is the report by Valvo (1968). This concerns a 28-year-old man with proptosis of 2 months' duration. The neoplasm was located in the posterior portion of the orbit and had elements of both rhabdomyosarcoma and liposarcoma. An exenteration was performed and, 1½ years after surgery, the patient was living, without signs of recurrence. Valvo believed his case was the fourth to be reported in the literature, counting the two children of Nash and Stout, and one adult noted by Reeh (1966). Reeh's case eventually was classified as a mesenchymal chondrosarcoma. Therefore, Reeh's case should no longer be considered a mesenchymoma.

LIPOMA

Owing to the wide distribution of adipose tissue throughout the body, the benign lipoma may occur anywhere. It is most common in subcutaneous tissues of the extremities and trunk or in deeper areas, such as retroperitoneum, mediastinum, and inguinal canal. As a rule, it is a solitary growth, but occasionally two or three lipomas may be found in the same person. They vary widely in size: some lipomas are but small nubbins; others expand to approach or even exceed the weight of the host. In essence, the lipoma seems to be a circumscribed collection of apparently mature fat.

INCIDENCE

The orbital space not occupied by the eye is generously endowed with adipose tissue, but the question of whether all masses containing lipomatous tissue should be called lipomas accounts for the statistical discrepancy of orbital lipomas in the literature. Nineteen lipomas were listed in Forrest's series of 222 orbital neoplasms. At the other extreme are the two series of Moss (230 orbital tumors) and Silva (300 tumors) in which no lipomas are listed. Offret noted 1 lipoma in his series of 110 tumors, and 2 cases were observed in our Mayo Clinic series of 764 tumors. A middle ground is represented by the series of Reese (1963), in which 6 lipomas were recorded among a total of 877 cases. However, in a later series of 504 cases (1971), Reese does not list any lipomas.

One reason for such extremes in incidence is that many cases in Forrest's series probably were not true lipomas. Forrest was aware of this problem and noted that, histologically, a capsule was not apparent in some of the tumors. Since these tumors were indistinguishable from normal orbital fat, the diagnosis of lipoma often was based only on a surgeon's statement. Many such cases probably represent instances in which fat was removed in the belief that such tissue represented the true tumor, or suspicious, edematous adipose tissue was excised to justify an otherwise negative exploratory orbitotomy.

Orbital lipomas seem most common in middle-aged and elderly adults. Our two cases occurred in 37- and 59-year-old men. The sex incidence is about equal.

CLINICAL FEATURES

The number of authentic cases in the literature is insufficient for one to assemble significant data on this facet of the tumor. In our two cases the lipoma was located in the posterior-superior portion of the orbit with straightforward proptosis as the presenting and principal clinical feature. Johnson and Linn (1979) describe what was called a spindle cell lipoma in a 42-year-old female which had been present 5 years. It was a well-circumscribed mass with a rich vascular supply located in the superior nasal quadrant of the orbit. The tumor was totally excised and there was no recurrence in the 16 months after surgery. Evolution of the tumor is slow.

PATHOLOGY

Lipomas frequently are described as being yellow. In the orbit, the intensity of their hue may be less than in the surrounding adipose tissue, and they appear to be yellowish white. This feature, and the fact that lipomas are circumscribed should permit proper identification and removal. The mature fat cells are arranged in lobules with variable amounts of connective tissue and capillaries in the intercellular septa. If mucoid or myxoid-like components are seen within the tumor, malignancy should be suspected.

In the ordinary paraffin section of tissue the fat globule is not visible within the hollow profile of the cell membrane, but if a section is fixed first with osmium tetroxide, the fat content of the tissue will be visible as black droplets. By special techniques, fat may also be stained red by dyes such as scharlach R or Sudan III.

TREATMENT

Unless subject to prior biopsy or irradiation, orbital lipomas should be sufficiently circumscribed and unattached to other ocular and orbital structures to permit removal by careful dissection.

LIPOSARCOMA

The malignant member of the family of adipose tissue tumors — the liposarcoma — is an ugly neoplasm: unsightly in appearance, unpleasant to contemplate, and unrelenting in its growth. It is regarded as a relatively common soft tissue tumor; it may occur anywhere in the body but tends to favor deeper areas of the thigh, leg, gluteal region, and retroperitoneum. Like its kin, the lipoma, it may reach a considerable size.

INCIDENCE

Assessment of incidence is hampered by many of the factors that have been discussed in relation to the sarcomas with mesenchymal anlages. Some compound tumors have been designated liposarcomas that more properly should be classified as malignancies of the other mesenchymal derivation, and not all tumors containing fat should necessarily be regarded as tumors of adipose tissue. A liposarcoma, properly, is a neoplasm of malignant lipoblasts, a definition emphasized by many writers. In recent literature, neoplasms that may qualify as liposarcomas of the orbit are infrequent. Quéré and associates (1963) and Cilotti (1964) have observed this neoplasm primary in the orbit in children. In adults, Mortada (1969) briefly reported a case in a 37-year-old man and Schroeder et al (1976) in a 47-year-old male. The malignant tumor in a 42-year-old female reported by Blodi (1969) also has many features of a primary orbital liposarcoma. Jakobiec and Jones (1976) have observed two cases in adult females, 19 and 51 years of age, respectively. Abdalla and associates (1966), and Enterline and his colleagues (1960) reported instances of liposarcoma metastasizing to the orbit from a primary focus in the thigh; in the former case (a 43-year-old male), metastasis developed 2 years after discovery of tumor in the thigh, and in the latter (a 53-year-old female), metastasis became evident 16 years after the initial diagnosis of liposarcoma. Some liposarcomas of the orbit believed to be metastatic may actually be examples of multicentric origin of the neoplasm. Liposarcoma is noted for its tendency to occur in unusual locations and is not always a unicentric neoplasm.

Considering the scarcity of reported orbital cases, it is unusual that we should have observed four cases during the period of our survey. Two of our four patients were aged 61 years at the time of onset of unilateral proptosis; the other two patients were aged 14 and 29 years. This age range, combined with the two cases observed in children already noted, suggests that liposarcomas of the orbit may occur at any age, and this is consistent with data on the age range of patients with liposarcoma occurring elsewhere in the body. As for the sex ratio, three of our four patients were males. The sex ratio of liposarcomas in other body areas is approximately equal, although some surveys do report a slight predominance among males. In three of our patients the liposarcoma was considered primary in the orbit, and in the fourth the neoplasm extended from the adjacent antrum into the orbit. Liposarcomas primary in the paranasal sinuses seem equally infrequent as those primary in the orbit.

CLINICAL FEATURES

Because it is such a malignant tumor, rapid onset and aggressive orbital growth might be expected. Such seems to be the case in the patient described by Quéré and associates (1963) (Fig. 154) in whom the liposarcoma reached a size of 12 by 9 by 9 cm in a 10-month period. On the other hand, growth of the liposarcoma in one of our patients (a 29-year-old man) was so slow that in a 3-year period the affected eye developed proptosis of only 3 mm. Variation in malignancy between one patient and another probably explains such a diversity of clinical behavior. In the former case a more anaplastic and pleomorphic type of liposarcoma might be anticipated, whereas in the latter case, malignancy of only grade 1 or 2 might be present. Proptosis or puffiness and edema of the upper eyelid are likely to be early signs, followed by impairment of ocular muscle function as the tumor expands. In all three of our cases of primary liposarcoma the tumor was palpable in the superior nasal quadrant of the orbit. None of these clinical features, however, is so distinctive of liposarcoma as to differentiate this tumor from many other nonspecific orbital masses before operation. It is likely that the diagnosis of liposarcoma will not be made until orbitotomy.

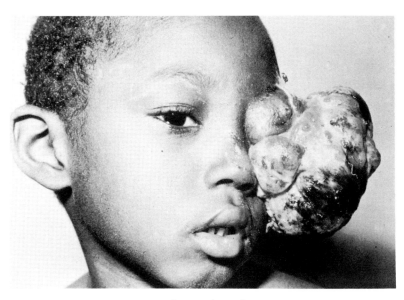

Figure 154.   Liposarcoma: tumor was large and rapidly progressive. The child was 5 years old. (From Quéré MA, Camain R, Baylet R: Liposarcome orbitaire. Ann Ocul [Paris] *196*:994–1003, 1963. By permission of Gaston Doin & Cie.)

Because information concerning the clinical features and long-term course of orbital liposarcomas is so infrequently reported in the literature, some details from our cases are instructive. The clinical course in two of these was quite different, though the tumors were histopathologically similar, and each was believed to have a myxoid liposarcoma, grade 2, primary in the orbit.

CASE 1.   A 29-year-old man had a slowly progressive proptosis for 3 years. A painless mass was palpated in the superior quadrants of the left orbit. At orbitotomy a soft circumscribed tumor (3 by 2 cm) was removed. Convalescence was uneventful, and 13 years have passed since orbitotomy without signs of recurrence.

CASE 2.   A 17-year-old boy had noticed symptoms referable to the orbit, also for about 3 years. Four months prior to our observation an anterior orbitotomy was performed because of slight proptosis of the right eye and a mass in the superior orbit. A biopsy only was done but a definite pathologic diagnosis was not established. The tissue specimen was examined by different pathologists, but no agreement was reached as to the true character of the neoplasm. Meantime, orbital symptoms became more marked owing to accelerated growth of the tumor. Our initial examination of the eye revealed forward proptosis (4 mm), downward displacement (2 mm), and a soft mass with diffuse borders that was palpable in the superior nasal quadrant. Following exenteration, gross examination of the specimen showed that it was a fatty myxoid tumor with infiltrating, indefinite margins (approximately 5 by 3 by 2.5 cm) (Fig. 155), and it later proved to be a liposarcoma. The tumor had infiltrated adjacent orbital fat and the superior rectus muscle. A distressing feature was the forward extension of neoplasm along the tract of the earlier biopsy, permitting infiltration of soft tissues of the upper eyelid. Recurrences appeared 5 years later along the forehead, just above the right orbit and in the temporal fossa. At this point the patient preferred not to pursue further attempts to eradicate the neoplasm by radical surgery. The tumors continue to enlarge slowly. Figure 156 depicts the situation 6½ years after exenteration.

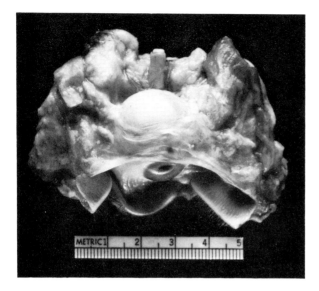

Figure 155. Liposarcoma: nonencapsulated fatty-myxoid tumor that encompassed globe, surrounding optic nerve and invading extraocular muscles.

Onset, early course, and histopathologic classification were essentially the same in the two cases but the outcome was vastly different. The first case illustrates that some of these orbital liposarcomas can be completely removed; moreover, cure seems to have been achieved. The second case indicates the more persistent and perverse nature of orbital liposarcomas. In this case an opportunity to cure the patient might well have been lost at the time of initial orbitotomy, when biopsy was performed in preference to surgical resection. Even though simple resection of the tumor might have proven too big a challenge, an earlier exenteration might have provided a better prognosis.

A third patient with liposarcoma primary in the orbit was lost to follow-up after undergoing a subtotal exenteration as the initial surgical procedure. The fourth patient among this series died 6 years after the onset of symptoms referable to liposarcoma in one antrum. Exenteration performed late in the course

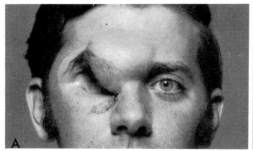
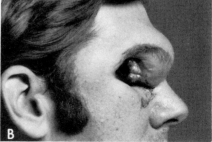

Figure 156. Liposarcoma: recurrent tumor 6½ years after exenteration of right orbit. *A*, Anterior view: large tumor (6 by 4 by 3 cm) infiltrating tissues beneath skin of forehead, and less prominent tumor filling right temporal fossa. *B*, Lateral view.

also was of no avail. Both cases of Jakobiec and Jones had recurrences 1 year after local excision of the neoplasm. In one of these patients the liposarcoma was fatal 6 years after orbital presentation.

PATHOLOGY

Liposarcomas vary greatly in makeup, ranging from circumscribed differentiated tumors to infiltrative, highly pleomorphic malignancies. The former also are more uniformly yellow and are soft in texture, but more malignant tumors show a mixture of adipose tissue and myxoid matrix interspersed with ugly areas of hemorrhage and necrosis. When cut they appear slimy. Grossly, this more embryonic, myxoid stroma is a rough indication of the degree of malignancy: the greater the myxoid component the more malignant the tumor. Microscopically, the degree of malignancy is judged on the basis of the number and types of bizarre, immature lipoblasts as well as the content of embryonic mucoid matrix (Fig. 157). The adipose tissue cell is the basic component of these tumors but their structure varies greatly. The more differentiated, less malignant neoplasms contain a greater number of mature fat cells, the nuclei being eccentrically positioned along the peripheral cell membrane (Fig. 158). The more malignant tumors contain a larger number of abortive, signet-cell lipoblasts and, in some areas, nuclei are arranged in flowing bundles, suggesting the appearance of myoblasts. The fat cells have foamy cytoplasm, readily identifiable by special fat stains. A distinctive feature of these neoplasms are the giant cells which usually are unicellular and contain pyknotic nuclei (Fig. 159). The pyknotic feature helps to differentiate them from giant cells occurring in other malignancies derived from mesenchymal anlage.

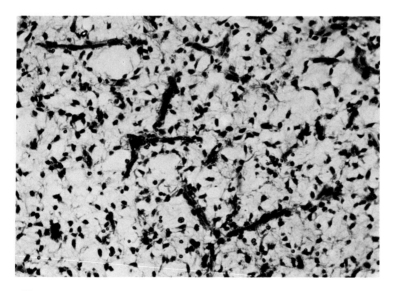

Figure 157. Liposarcoma: tumor is well differentiated and myxoid. In this common histologic variant, fat is minimal and small stellate cells produce myxoid stroma rich in mucopolysaccharides. (Hematoxylin and eosin; × 245.)

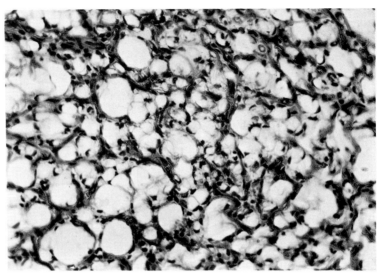

Figure 158. Liposarcoma: neoplasm consists of rounded cells which contain a large cytoplasmic fat globule resembling embryonal lipoblasts. (Hematoxylin and eosin; × 245.)

TREATMENT

The less malignant and more circumscribed liposarcomas probably can be completely removed from the more anterior portions of the orbit with a reasonable chance of cure, as illustrated by the successful course of one of the patients in our survey. If a liposarcoma is situated posteriorly, complete excision is hampered by nerves and important ocular structures; it probably is wiser to advise exenteration and proceed as soon as possible (Fig. 160). Incomplete excision of liposarcoma in this area only delays, rather than arrests, its growth and seriously compromises the patient's chance to escape this lethal neoplasm.

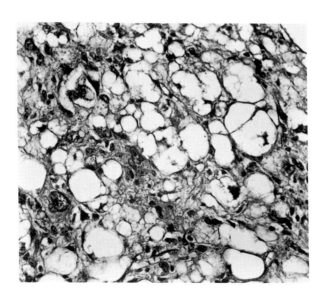

Figure 159. Liposarcoma: pleomorphic type. Highly malignant, anaplastic neoplasm with giant cells and foamy lipoblasts. (Hematoxylin and eosin; × 275.)

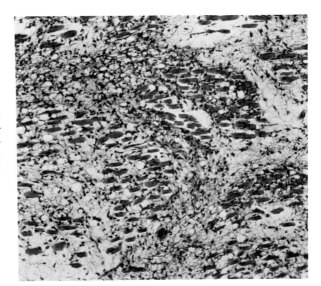

Figure 160. Liposarcoma: extensive invasion of extraocular muscles. Anything short of exenteration unlikely to effect cure. (Hematoxylin and eosin; × 110.)

Bibliography

Myxoma

Blegvad O: Myxoma of the orbit. Acta Ophthalmol (Kbh) 22:131–140, 1944.
Blodi FC: Unusual orbital neoplasms. Am J Ophthalmol 68:407–412, 1969
Gifford SR: Multiple myxoma of the orbit. Arch Ophthalmol 5:445–448, 1931
Kreuger EG, Polifrone JC, Baum G: Retrobulbar orbital myxoma and its detection by ultrasonography. J Neurosurg 26:87–91, 1967
Lamb HD: Myxoma of the orbit, with case report and anatomical findings. Arch Ophthalmol 57: 425–429, 1928
Mauricione: Cited by Blegvad O

Mesenchymoma

Klein W: Mesenchymoma. J Med Soc New Jersey 29:774–778, 1932
Nash A, Stout AP: Malignant mesenchymomas in children. Cancer 14:524–533, 1961
Reeh MJ: Hemangiopericytoma with cartilaginous differentiation involving orbit. Arch Ophthalmol 75:82–83, 1966
Stout AP: Mesenchymoma, the mixed tumor of mesenchymal derivatives. Ann Surg 127:278–290, 1948
Stout AP, Lattes R: Tumors of the soft tissues. In *Atlas of Tumor Pathology.* Second Series, Fascicle 1. Washington, D.C., Armed Forces Institute of Pathology, 1967
Valvo A: Malignant mesodermal mixed tumor (mesenchymoma) of the orbit. Am J Ophthalmol 66: 919–923, 1968

Lipoma

Forrest AW: Intraorbital tumors. Arch Ophthalmol ns 41:198–230, 1949
Johnson BL, Linn JG: Spindle cell lipoma of the orbit. Arch Ophthalmol 97:133–134, 1979
Moss HM: Expanding lesions of the orbit: a clinical study of 230 consecutive cases. Am J Ophthalmol 54:761–770, 1962
Offret G: *Les Tumeurs Primitives de l'Orbite et Leur Traitement.* Paris, Masson and Cie, 1951
Reese AB: *Tumors of the Eye.* Second edition. New York, Hoeber Medical Division, Harper & Row, Publishers, 1963
Reese AB: Expanding lesions of the orbit (Bowman lecture). Trans Ophthalmol Soc UK 91:85–104, 1971
Silva D: Orbital Tumors. Am J Ophthalmol 65:318–339, 1968

Liposarcoma

Abdalla MI, Ghaly AF, Hosni F: Liposarcoma with orbital metastases: case report. Brit J Ophthalmol 50:426–428, 1966

Blodi FC: Unusual orbital neoplasms. Am J Ophthalmol 68:407–412, 1969

Cilotti P: A particular form of liposarcoma of the orbit with striking morphological changes in the course of its evolution. Ann Ottalmol Clin Ocul 90:325–337, 1964. (Abstract Excerpta Medica 19, Section 12:207, 1965)

Enterline HT, Culberson JD, Rochlin DB, et al: Liposarcoma: a clinical and pathological study of 53 cases. Cancer 13:932–950, 1960

Jakobiec FA, Jones IS: Mesenchymal and fibro-osseous tumors. In *Clinical Ophthalmology*. Volume 2, Chapter 44. Ed: TD Duane, Hagerstown, Harper & Row, 1976

Mortada A: Rare primary orbital sarcomas. Am J Ophthalmol 68:919–925, 1969

Quéré MA, Camain R, Baylet R: Liposarcome orbitaire. Ann Ocul (Paris) 196:994–1003, 1963

Schroeder W, Kastendieck H, von Domarus D: Primäres myxoides Liposarkom der Orbita. Ophthalmologica 172:337–345, 1976

10

Tumors of Nerve Sheath Origin

This chapter will be devoted to a discussion of the orbital manifestations of tumors of nerve sheath origin. Among these tumors, neurofibroma in its various forms is by far the most common. This tumor belongs to a small family of growths that are designated hamartomas. Neurofibroma holds a tenuous kinship with another hamartoma — the hemangioma — because of its wide distribution throughout the body, its popularity as a subject for publication and photography, its frequency, its potpourri of forms, and its position among the family of tumors as one of the first to be described in detail in the era of the printed word.

HISTORICAL ASPECTS

Cheselden, in 1740, seems to have been among the first to publish a distinct descripion of one of the systemic forms of neural tumors; and one can infer that these tumors were recognized even earlier. According to the Scottish surgeon, Wood (1829), a tumor of this type was removed as early as 1773. Wood also credited Odier, of Geneva, with coining, in 1803, the term *neuroma* to designate tumors formed by enlargement of nerves. This term was applied to all tumors associated with nerves, including those arising from the sympathetic nervous system as well as those that might have resulted from trauma or amputation. It is important for the reader, who may peruse the older literature, to know that neuroma was about the only designation for this class of tumors for more than half a century. Technically, neuroma refers to a tumor of the nerve itself, but writers who used this term recognized that most of these tumors had their true origin in the connective tissue or sheaths surrounding nerves. It is not clear who first used the word *neurofibroma*, although this name appeared in the title of an article by Billroth, a Viennese surgeon, in 1869. By the time of von Recklinghausen's publication (1882), neurofibroma was replacing neuroma as a more correct designation for the common type of peripheral nerve tumor. During this interval it became evident that such tumors varied widely in their character and distribution, so that no single descriptive term was adequate.

Virchow (1867), as he did with so many human neoplasms, clarified the nosology of these "nerve tumors" by studying their histopathology. The essential feature of his study was the classification of this family of tumors on the basis of structure rather than clinical behavior. He realized that some tumors originated from the nerve itself (true tumors), whereas others were derived from the sheath of the nerve and were predominantly connective tissue in their makeup (false tumors). He thought that the former were more common but time has shown that the latter (the false tumors) predominate. Still, attempts to designate some tumors by their clinical characteristics persisted, for it was in this same era that the term *plexiforme neuroma* came into usage. Verneuil (1861), of France, seems responsible for this term that is still used today. Verneuil's *néurome cylindrique plexiforme* is essentially the same tumor as the one Bruns (1870), in Germany, designated *Rankenneurom*. Von Recklinghausen's contribution was in emphasizing the role of cutaneous nerve endings in the makeup of multiple fibromas of the skin (*molluscum fibrosum*) that were present in so many cases. By this time interest in these neurofibromas had become so widespread in Europe that the literature abounded with reports of the disorder and its bizarre manifestations; and most hallmarks of the disorder as we know it today had been recognized by this era. These were

1. neuromatous tumors of peripheral and sympathetic nerves;
2. café-au-lait spots;
3. molluscum fibrosum;
4. plexiforme tumors; and
5. diffuse hypertrophy of the skin and subcutaneous tissues.

As more physicians became aware of the widely disseminated character of the disorder in many people, there grew a greater need for some clinically descriptive, inclusive term. This seems to account for the origin of the term neurofibromatosis, which was in widespread use by 1900.

What of orbital forms of the disease? It is not certain who described the first case of orbital involvement. Descriptions of orbital nerve sheath tumors are found in the case reports and discussions of Billroth (1869), Bruns (1870), and Marchand (1877). The respective ages of these patients were 18, 20, and 12 years. All patients had shown some manifestations of neurofibromatosis since birth and the orbital tumor was of the plexiform type with involvement of the adjacent eyelid.

NOMENCLATURE AND CLASSIFICATION

The terminology of some of these tumors may depend upon the observer's viewpoint regarding their histogenesis. For the tumor that seems almost exclusively to be a proliferation of nerve sheath, the majority prefer the name *schwannoma* or *neurilemmoma*. This implies that the tumor is derived from neurilemma which traces its origin to neuroectoderm. A minority believe the same tumor to be a proliferation of supporing mesodermal elements within the nerve bundle and designate its peripheral position by the name *perineural fibroblastoma*. *Neurinoma* also has been applied to this tumor, but such a term should be reserved for a proliferation of nerve fibers rather than their sheaths.

Origin of the closely allied tumor, *neurofibroma*, is less controversial, but attempts to classify this tumor on the basis of its varied histology — its single or multiple growth pattern, its anatomic distribution, or its protean forms — and clinical manifestations may only confuse the problem. The present trend is to regard all such related tumors as a manifestation of neurofibromatosis and to designate each individual case by modifying adjectives appropriate to the particular form of the growth. Thus, *plexiforme neuroma* persists as a name for a particular form of neurofibromatosis where hamartomatous-like hypertrophy of nerve bundles is a prominent feature.

Finally, some related growths, by their anaplasia, cellular pleomorphism, and aggressive behavior, must be regarded as malignant. These have been called, among other terms, *neurofibrosarcoma, malignant schwannoma, neurogenic sarcoma,* and *malignant neurilemmoma.*

NEUROFIBROMA AND NEUROFIBROMATOSIS

It will not be long before an ophthalmologist in either training or clinical practice encounters some manifestation of neurofibromatosis affecting the eye or adnexa. In regard to the relatively small area of body surface that they occupy, the eye and adnexa may shown an unusual assortment of features of this disorder, and scarcely any structure or tissue within or around the eye, except possibly the lens, seems immune to this congenital or developmental, and often familial, overgrowth of neural supporting structures. Of more concern, in some cases, to patients, parents, and relatives are manifestations of neurofibromatosis in the eyelids and adjacent soft tissues of the face because of resulting cosmetic disfigurement. The skin in this area may show a coffee-colored pigmentation and there may be such a pendulous hypertrophy and thickening of the upper eyelid as to obscure the eye completely. Or, the disease may manifest lump-like tumors (molluscum fibrosum) in this zone. The bony structures of the face may show asymmetry; and the orbit, with which we are chiefly concerned, may share in these distortions and disturbances of eyelids and eye or may be the site of but a single manifestation of the disease.

INCIDENCE

It is difficult to obtain an accurate assessment of the incidence. Surveys that touch upon this statistical point vary widely. First, there are differences in source material upon which tumor surveys are based, a variable common to the incidence ratios of many tumors in this text. Second, in many surveys, both recent and older, neurilemmomas have been included with neurofibromas in the total count. Third, there are many instances wherein adnexal neurofibromas, particularly of the upper eyelid, are loosely included with orbital cases; and indeed, some manifestations of neurofibromatosis of the eyelids are so ponderous as to create also the false impression of orbital involvement. In our own survey we were careful to exlude such cases. Lastly, a further separation of orbital cases into solitary neurofibromas or diffuse neurofibromatosis is not often attempted. Eighteen of these tumors were observed in our survey of 764 cases, an incidence of 2.3%. In five of these patients the neurofibroma was a solitary tumor and the single manifestation of the disease. In the remaining 13 patients the neurofibroma was of the plexiform type and associated with neurofibromatosis. The sex ratio of the total group was equal.

The orbital form of neurofibromatosis is predominantly a disease with its presentation in the first two decades. Although patients may not be seen at the initial visit until adolescence, questioning will reveal the onset of symptoms much earlier in childhood. The orbital disorder may be the presenting sign of the disease but, on closer examination of the child, other manifestations, particularly café-au-lait patches, will be found. In other words, in the majority of infants and children the disorder already is generalized by the time orbital symptoms are recognized. The age distribution of our patients with solitary neurofibroma, however was quite different: three were past 50 years of age at the time of onset. This difference in age distribution of the diffuse and solitary orbital neurofibromas suggests the former is more of a hamartomatous tumor whereas the solitary neurofibroma is more of a neoplasm.

CLINICAL FEATURES

Those cases in our survey which were examples of *the diffuse or multiple form* of the disorder (the majority) differed little in their clinical manifestations from many reported cases of this type in the literature. This is the form of the disease with heredofamilial aspects and represents a congenital aberration of many different tissue systems and organs. Whereas with most orbital tumors among children and infants the presenting sign of orbital mischief is proptosis or displacement of the eye, with neurofibromatosis the initial symptom more frequently is a visible or palpable mass. Less frequently, an enlarged or displaced eye is the reason for initial consultation and the orbital mass is discovered later. Trauma seldom is a feature of the anamnesis, as so often is the case with sarcomatous tumors of the orbit. The orbital mass is painless and frequently described as "lumpy," "rubbery," or a tumor of "cords" and "nodules." The tumor commonly is palpated in one of the superior quadrants of the orbit and causes downward displacement of the eye. The most frequent accessory stigma is drooping and hypertrophy of the lateral half of the eyelid on the affected side, due to a plexiform type tumor in soft tissues of the eyelid (Fig. 161).

In such cases, the margin of the affected eyelid has been likened to an S-curve, but such an extreme degree of curvature is somewhat an exaggeration; at this age it is more sinuous. As the disease progresses and the plexiform mass increases in size, the entire lid may become so thick and redundant as to conceal the proptosed eye (Fig. 162). By adolescence or adulthood the orbital masses and eyelid tumors have become so fused that it is difficult to separate one from another. Other less frequent, stigmata associated with the orbital tumor may be seen; the eye may show one or a combination of several of the following:buphthalmos or congenital glaucoma; megalocornea without glaucoma;

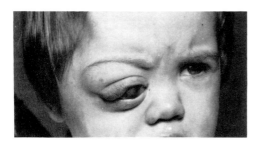

Figure 161. Neurofibroma: plexiform type in lateral portion of right upper lid; right eye displaced and buphthalmic.

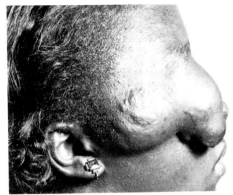

Figure 162. Neurofibromatosis: side view showing marked deformity, thickening, and ptosis of right eyelid associated with neurofibromatosis; right eye completely obscured.

neurofibromatous nodules near the optic disk, within the iris, and along the perilimbal areas; and infiltration of ciliary nerves. Tumors of the optic disk (a very rare association) were not found in any of our patients. As the child grows older, the tumor enlarges slowly, steadily, and relentlessly in most cases. Attempts to remove the offending orbital mass usually are undertaken before the eye reaches extreme displacement. However, either because of trauma associated with repeated surgery or because of continued growth of the tumor, the eye usually becomes useless as a visual organ and also a cosmetic liability. The frequent hypertrophy of the adjacent soft tissues of the face and eyelids make the resulting facial deformity particularly bizarre. Figure 163 illustrates an individual who had only a moderate deformity compared to many, but he was, for more than 18 years, futilely seeking a physician who could completely relieve him of the unsightly hypertrophied flesh.

The *solitary orbital form* of neurofibroma that seems to affect an older age group often has, by contrast, a course as bright as that of orbital neurofibromatosis is dismal. These patients usually notice a slowly progressive, painless proptosis. The duration of proptosis is from 1 to several years depending upon the patient's concern about the problem; progression is so slow that visual disturbance is only minimal. The tumor usually is found in the superior or superopos-

Figure 163. Neurofibromatosis: a 16-year-old boy who had undergone numerous operations to correct deformity of left eyelids but to little avail.

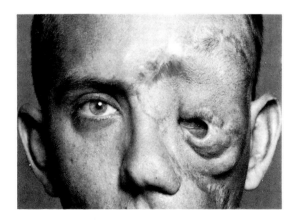

terior portion of the orbit causing forward and downward displacement of the eye. Weakness of ocular rotation may be noted in upward gaze. The overall picture is similar in these respects to other benign neoplasms and cysts (as described in Section I). When uncovered surgically the tumors among our patients were encapsulated or well circumscribed and of medium size (Fig. 164); they were firm, rubbery, tan or flesh-colored, and could be dissected from adjacent orbital tissues without the bothersome bleeding so characteristic of diffuse neurofibromatosis. Once removed, the tumors do not recur but displacement of the eye does not always recede. Multiple solitary neurofibromas may also occur in the orbit.

ROENTGENOGRAPHIC CHANGES

Several years after the discovery of x-rays it was observed that certain defects in the bony orbit might be associated with neurofibromatosis. Rockcliffe and Parsons (1903–1904) told of a child in whom an eye had been enucleated together with removal of an orbital tumor because of severe pulsating proptosis. The child did not survive. The tumor proved to be a plexiform neuroma, and at autopsy, the roof, orbital portions of the lesser and greater wings of the sphenoid, and lacrimal plate of the ethmoid were found to be missing. Many years passed before enough similar cases were collected in such a way as to establish a definite association between this bony orbital defect and the generalized disorder. Some writers attribute the first adequate roentgenologic description of the defect to LeWald (1933) of New York. But Moore (1931), of London, had earlier made a relatively complete description of the roentgenographic changes in an individual with pulsating proptosis and neurofibromatosis. These observations, oriented to the roentgenographic alterations, were important for several reasons. They established a basis for pulsating proptosis other than the commonly accepted cause, a vascular aneurysm or anomaly. In addition, they served as a warning that such a deficiency of orbital contours should not be mistaken for a generalized erosion of bone such as might occur with an orbital sarcoma in childhood; thus patients might be saved unnecessary operations. Figure 165 is a diagrammatic representation of the most common form of the bony defect.

These bony changes are most easily seen on routine posteroanterior views of the skull (Fig. 166). In patients with extensive defects, normal landmarks along

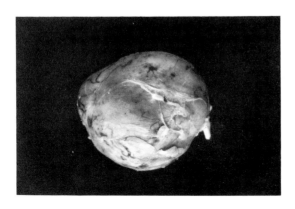

Figure 164. Neurofibroma: solitary form, well encapsulated; at right is segment of nerve trunk from which it arose.

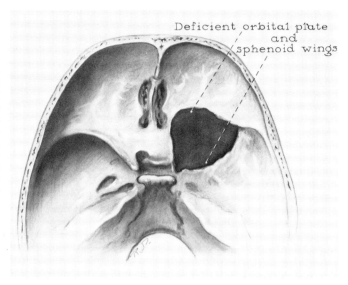

Figure 165. Neurofibromatosis: drawing of deficient development of lesser and greater wings of sphenoid and of orbital roof; this allows cerebral contents to herniate into the orbit. (From Bruwer AJ, Kierland RR: Neurofibromatosis and congenital unilateral pulsating and nonpulsating exophthalmos. Arch Ophthalmol ns 53:2–12, 1955. By permission of the American Medical Association.)

the posterior aspects of the bony orbit, such as the temporal line and sphenoid ridge, may be absent or altered in position. Bruwer and Kierland (1955) aptly designated such change as a "blank" appearance. An enlargement of the bony orbit, particularly in children (Fig. 167), also is common. On lateral views the most prominent feature is an enlargement of the middle cranial fossa and a "scooped out" configuration of the sella. The optic canal also may be enlarged, and this may be a clue to involvement of the optic nerve by neurofibromatosis.

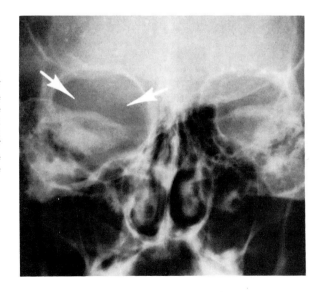

Figure 166. Neurofibromatosis: roentgenogram of orbit of 21-year-old man with progressive displacement of right eye since birth. Absence of lesser and greater wings of right sphenoid bone (*arrows*) and enlargement of bony orbit; clinically, progressive displacement of right eye since birth and some pulsation of eye.

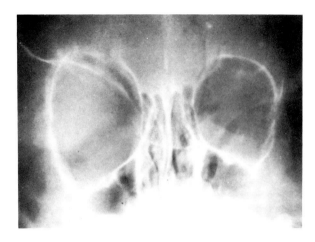

Figure 167. Neurofibromatosis: marked enlargement of right orbit in a 4-year-old child.

Not all patients with these defects necessarily show pulsation of the proptosed eye. The pulsation, of course, is transmitted from the intracranial vault through the bony defect. The pulsation is synchronous with the radial pulse, but no bruit is heard, as would be the case with a vascular anomaly such as arteriovenous fistula. It has not been established how large the bony defect must be before pulsation of the eye appears. Just how neurofibromatosis brings about this bony dysplasia is not known. Roentgenographic evidence of such dysplasia was present in 4 of our series of 13 patients.

Decalcification of the bony orbit wall, caused by pressure of the expanding tumor, is another common feature. Erosion and destruction of bone due to invasion of tumor is seen in cases of longer duration or more advanced degree. We have seen this occur in all four walls of the orbit but the change is less frequent along the inferior wall. Small areas of calcification in the orbital cavity also may occasionally be visible. Some thickening of orbital bone also may be seen in some cases of solitary neurofibroma.

PATHOLOGY

Neurofibroma is a variable mixture of axons, covering Schwann cells and supporting endoneural cells. The latter proliferate in a pattern of wavy, fibrillar, interlacing strands separated by a myxomatous or scanty collagen matrix (Fig. 168). In the more diffuse and plexiform neurofibromas the hyperplasia results in a greater thickening and tortuosity of tumor bundles with a larger proportion of axis cylinders. The result is a mass of thickened, sometimes nodular, nerves resembling masses of knotted twine (Fig. 169). Running through the convoluted cords of tumors are axons of the nerves (Fig. 170); these are best seen when sectioned and specially stained. All these proliferating components of the nerve are nestled in a tangled mass of connective tissue which, in the more diffuse forms of neurofibromatosis, is highly vascular. Vascularization is, in fact, to be reckoned with when a surgical approach to the plexiform type is planned. In the isolated, encapsulated neurofibroma of the orbit, such vascularization is not prominent. Occasionally, and by diligent search through the tissue sections of the plexiform variety, areas resembling the histologic

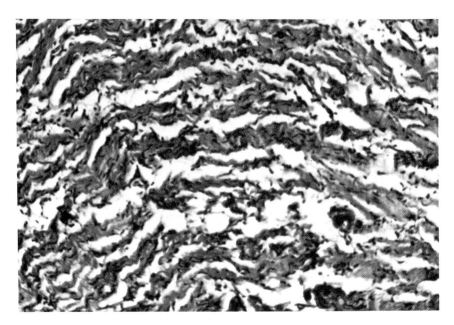

Figure 168. Neurofibroma: basic proliferating cells are fibroblasts from endoneurium and perineurium. (Hematoxylin and eosin; × 130.)

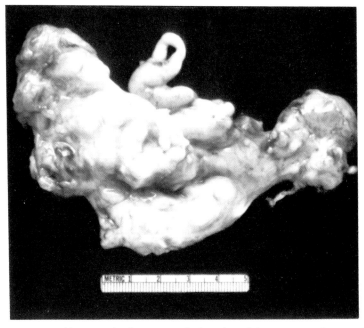

Figure 169. Neurofibroma: plexiform type; thickened, nodular nerve trunks resemble knotted twine.

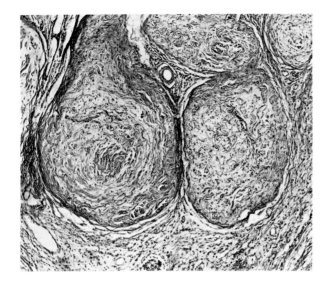

Figure 170. Neurofibroma: plexiform type; gigantic nerve-like structures are nestled in matted mass of connective tissue. (Hematoxylin and eosin; × 35.)

makeup of tactile corpuscles may be seen (Fig. 171). In some of the more advanced cases the tumor may show signs of degeneration. The enlarged nerve bundle then loses some of its cellular detail and looks more myoxomatous.

TREATMENT AND COURSE

The management of the *isolated form* of neurofibroma in the orbit does not seem to be a major problem. The tumor can be removed through any of the surgical approaches to the orbit, depending on its location. With careful dissection it can be entirely removed without leaving any permanent, functional embarrassment to the eye. Bleeding is not unusually profuse. If not removed completely it will continue to grow.

Removal of the *diffuse* and *plexiform tumor* is a different matter and a greater challenge. Aside from total exenteration, seldom is it possible to remove these tumors completely. The remaining vermiform cords of tissue slowly increase in size, to taunt the surgeon again. Several factors contribute to such a disappointing situation. The tumor is much more diffuse than its solitary counterpart. Ultimately, it may invade and destroy bone, traveling into the intracranial vault, the temporal fossa, or paranasal sinuses. Also, it may entangle muscle bundles such as the levator palpebrae superioris (Fig. 172), or grasp adjacent blood vessels and nerves in its search for living space. Thus, no single surgical approach always assures complete visibility of the tumor and the surgeon must move along cautiously with the tip of the finger of one hand guiding the scissors held in the other. Bolder dissection, beyond the average ken of visibility, entails irreparable damage to other important orbital structures that are enmeshed in the tenacles of the tumor. If this alone were not enough to promote restraint, bleeding may be a major complication, and the vascular supply of some tumors is so extensive and diffuse that bleeding is not easily quenched.

Still, there are situations wherein proptosis becomes so marked or ocular motility so strangled that something must be done for the patient. Then the orbit may be approached anteriorly through an incision just inside and parallel

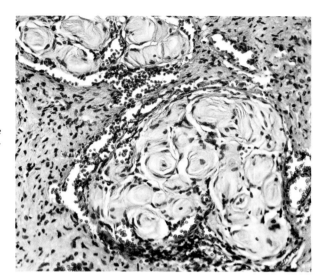

Figure 171. Neurofibroma: some areas may resemble tactile corpuscles within neoplasm. (Hematoxylin and eosin; × 200.)

to the temporo-inferior rim of the orbit. This approach bypasses the lacrimal gland and permits better visibility; less bleeding is encountered here and less harm is done to the levator palpebrae superioris. In other cases the bulk of the tumor lies in another quadrant and so must be uncovered by an incision elsewhere. Whatever the approach, dissection must be limited to the more bulky cords of tumor so as to decompress the orbital space yet avoid the hinterlands of the optic nerve and superior orbital fissure. In little children, in whom the disease is associated with a proptosed, enlarged, blind eye, enucleation alone usually is sufficient. At a later age, if a prosthesis cannot be worn owing to continued slow expansion of the plexiform mass, additional pieces of the tumor along its anterior face may be removed so as to permit reinsertion of the artificial eye. The philosophy of such an approach to treatment is to remove what-

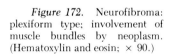

Figure 172. Neurofibroma: plexiform type; involvement of muscle bundles by neoplasm. (Hematoxylin and eosin; × 90.)

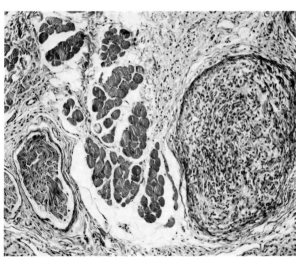

ever tumor is easily accessible but no more. In so many of our cases, the involvement of the eyelid has been so extensive and disfiguring that cosmetic correction of this fault has taken precedence over the less obvious orbital neurofibroma.

Whatever is done, the resulting cosmesis seldom approaches the level of expectancy. So far as orbital surgery is concerned, we have never observed other than an expression of disappointment when the bandages are removed and the victim views again the still distorted eye and adnexa.

Four of our thirteen patients with orbital neurofibromatosis underwent an enucleation of one eye during the long course of the disease. Another two patients have undergone an orbital exenteration. One of these, at age 16 (Fig 162) also had an excision of the tumor extension from the right temple at the time of exenteration. In subsequent years she seemed more content with her facial disfigurement than others of a similar age group who were undergoing yet another surgical procedure on their plexiform neurofibroma in the hopes of either restoring the visual function of an almost blind eye or capturing the ever elusive symmetry of the normal face and orbit. Two of our patients with neurofibromatosis since birth have had neurologic and x-ray evidence of intracranial spread since age 1 and 15 years, respectively. Both are living, the former at age 20, the latter at age 28.

We have observed a few of our patients for a period of three decades. It is our clinical impression that the orbital form of the disease seems to be less progressive after the age of 30 years.

NEURILEMMOMA

HISTORICAL ASPECTS

If Virchow had recognized this member of the family of neural tumors, he would have classified it within his group of "false tumors" for this also is a tumor of supporting structure of the peripheral nerve. It was during a study and regrouping of neural tumors by Verocay (1910) that the subject of neurilemmoma was described. Verocay, of Prague, affixed the name *neurinoma* to this new tumor and separated it from the large family of neurofibromas, and this, until recently, was the designation favored by European opthalmologists. Since Verocay's publication several other names have been proposed. Among these, names such as *perineural fibroma* and *schwannoma* stemmed from efforts to describe the cellular anlage of the tumor; usage depended on whether the tumor was regarded as mesodermal or neuroectodermal in origin. The final refinement in nomenclature was the work of Stout (1935). He pointed out that the term *neurinoma* meant nerve fiber tumor; the growth in question was, however, derived from the nerve sheaths. It was but a logical step, then, to name the tumor for the encompassing sheath of the nerve, the *neurilemma*. (The term offers scope for variations in spelling: the letter *m* sometimes appears twice, sometimes thrice, in the spelling of the tumor; also the *i* is sometimes replaced by an *o*.) Subsequently, electron microscopy of these tumors identified the Schwann cell as the principal proliferating unit of the nerve sheath, and schwannoma has regained support as the preferable designation.

INCIDENCE

Many publications still regard orbital neurilemmoma as a rare or unusual tumor, but histopathologic criteria for the correct diagnosis of this tumor have been clarified and surgeons are more aware of the lesion than formerly. No longer is neurilemmoma the curiosity it once was supposed to be. The tumor has a relatively wide anatomic distribution, for it may grow along any peripheral or cranial nerve. The auditory nerve is the commonest single site among the cranial nerves; here it is well known as the acoustic neuroma. Among peripheral nerves, the neurilemmoma often is found along the flexor surfaces of extremities, brachial plexus, the neck, hands, mediastinum, and spinal cord.

Schatz (1971) reviewed nine series of orbital tumors totaling 2,196 cases. There were 25 cases of neurilemmoma in this composite number. This is an incidence of 1.1%. In our own survey of 764 consecutive orbital tumors there were 8 neurilemmomas, an incidence of 1%. Seven of the latter were primary in the orbit and the other neurilemmoma invaded the orbit from the maxillary antrum. The sex distrubution of these cases was equal. The youngest patients at time of initial orbitotomy was 20 years of age and the oldest was 67. This range corresponds to statements in the literature to the effect that orbital neurilemmoma may occur at any age. The ratio of neurofibromas to neurilemmomas is roughly 2:1.

CLINICAL FEATURES

Neurilemmomas are usually solitary tumors that grow slowly, are benign, and may be associated with neurofibromatosis. Rarely, they may be multiple in the orbit. Because the tumor is benign it may reach a considerable size before surgical identification (Fig. 173).

In one of our patients the tumor problem had been present 15 years. Tumors in the posterior quadrants of the orbit cause the patient to seek attention sooner (6 to 12 months) owing to blurring of vision, the consequence of proximity of the growth to the optic nerve. Central or paracentral scotomas in the visual field may even suggest a diagnosis of retrobulbar neuritis. In these cases striae may be seen along the posterior wall of the eye. Forward proptosis is the chief clinical sign, with some displacement of the eye in a direction opposite the site of the tumor. Neurilemmoma may occur anywhere in the orbit. Other ocular signs, such as marked ophthalmoplegia, ptosis of the upper eyelid, pain,

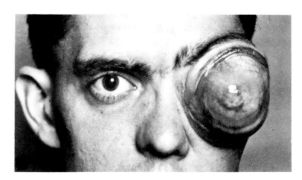

Figure 173. Neurilemmoma: Appearance of solitary neurilemmoma of orbit; eye completely engulfed by neoplasm, present for 12 years, measured 7 by 6 by 5 cm.

and loss of vision, are not common with orbital neurilemmomas unless the tumor is quite large or has been present over a period of many years. Roentgenograms usually are negative.

Orbital neurilemmoma is a solid, smooth, sometimes nodular, benign, encapsulated, white or yellowish gray tumor (Fig. 174). Older and larger growths may show areas of hemorrhagic necrosis or cystic degeneration on the cut surface. The yellow color of some neurilemmomas may lead the exploring surgeon to conclude the tumor is a lipoma or a cyst containing fatty material. They are variants of neurofibroma with dominance of the proliferating Schwann cell but scanty collagen formation. The tumor grows by simple fusiform expansion. The axons of the affected nerve may be stretched over the surface of the tumor, like thin wisps of thread, or the relatively intact axonal bundle may be located eccentrically along one surface of the expanding mass. The Schwann cells are long and fusiform, with tapering poles (Fig. 175). The nucleus also is spindle-shaped. The architecture of the entire tumor has more pattern and order than has the neurofibroma.

Two histologic types, Antoni (a German pathologist) types A and B, are recognized. In the former type (the commoner) the cells are arranged in wavy, flowing, interlacing cords or whorled bundles. The elongated nuclei, which may vary in size, tend to arrange themselves in rows with intervening spaces devoid of nuclei. This is referred to as *palisading* and has been likened to the appearance of "staves on a barrel" (Fig. 176); it is considered to be the most typical feature of these tumors. In some areas an alveolar-like pattern is seen and this has been likened to the appearance of sensory corpuscles (Verocay bodies). Throughout such specimens of tumor the supporting stroma is sparse. In the type B tumor there are fewer cells and their nuclei do not assume a palisade arrangement. The cells may run in any direction; no bodies of Verocay are

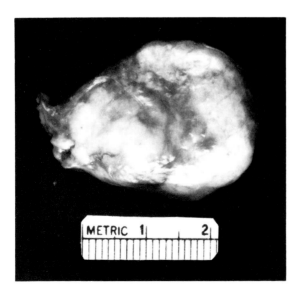

Figure 174. Neurilemmoma: nodular, well-encapsulated tumor; light areas were bright yellow in fresh state.

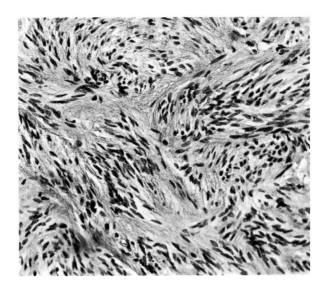

Figure 175. Neurilemmoma: neoplasm is composed of interlacing bundles of spindle-shaped cells with tapered nuclei. (Hematoxylin and eosin; × 225.)

seen. Also, the entire stroma appears more loose and reticular, giving the specimen a myxomatous appearance. Here and there foci of cystic degeneration are visible. Identifying features of Schwann cells under electron microscopy are sinuous cellular processes, basement membranes, minimal rough-surfaced endoplasmic reticulum, and banded basement membrane material.

TREATMENT

Removal of a small neurilemmoma can be one of the more satisfying experiences in orbital surgery. The tumor is benign; it is usually delimited from adjacent orbital structures; and for the patient the results also are satisfying and

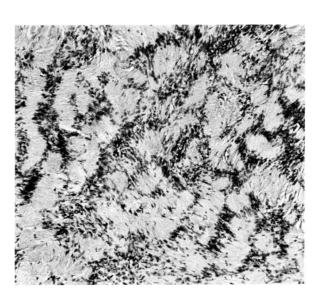

Figure 176. Neurilemmoma: nuclei may proliferate in rows, giving palisaded appearance. (Hematoxylin and eosin; × 100.)

rewarding, as proptosis is relieved and, if dissection has been meticulous and complete, there is no undue damage to ocular function. Some difficulties may be encountered if the tumor is large, is of long duration, and is situated close to the optic nerve. In such cases the tumor has compressed the optic nerve so firmly that the capsule of the tumor becomes fused with the sheath of the nerve. Dissection of the neurilemmoma from the adjoining nerve is then hazardous because of the danger of injury to the latter or rupture of the capsular barrier of the former. In such a dilemma, complete excision of the tumor probably must be abandoned in favor of preservation of the nerve. However, the tumor may grow further in several months or years, and another surgical procedure may be required; the optic nerve may then have to be resected during the second operation. Also, both surgeon and patient must realize that incomplete excision of a neurilemmoma, or piecemeal enucleation of the tumor from within its capsule, entails some risk of malignant transformation. This may have contributed to the malignant transformation and death of a 27-year-old woman in whom a benign neurilemmoma was removed piecemeal from the supraorbital nerve, as reported by Schatz (1971). He believed this case to be the only example in the literature of sarcomatous metaplasia of an orbital neurilemmoma. In our own experience, resection of small orbital nerves attached to the neurilemmoma during complete excision of the tumor has not been followed by any serious sequelae. These tumors are not unduly vascular so that bleeding is not the threatening complication commonly observed during surgical manipulation of neurifibromatosis.

NEUROFIBROSARCOMA AND MALIGNANT SCHWANNOMA

We will discuss these two neoplasms together because, clinically, they are essentially the same tumor. They differ only in the prevalence of the malignant Schwann cell in the cellular pattern of neoplasia, their antecedence in either neurofibromatosis or neurilemmoma, and the preference of terminology of the pathologist. Those who prefer the term *neurofibrosarcoma* point out that malignant transformation of a neurofibromatosis is frequent but a *malignant schwannoma* evolving from a prior neurilemmoma is unusual.

INCIDENCE

In the survey of Schatz of 2,196 cases tabulated from nine sources (noted above), there were 14 of these malignant neoplasms.

Additional case reports in the literature are those of Calvet and Coadau (1949) (a 4-year-old girl), Cerveira (1953), Ginde (1953) (a 25-year-old man), Mortada (1968) (a 50-year-old woman and a 55-year-old man), Schiff-Wertheimer and Loisillier (1954) (a 2-year-old girl), Grinberg and Levy (1974) (47-year-old male), Jakobiec and Jones (1976), and the unusual case of Schatz (a 27-year-old female) of sarcomatous transformation of a benign neurilemmoma. However, we have some reservation classifying the case of Ginde in the malignant category. Also of interest is the case of Radnot 1963) of secondary involvement of the orbit by a tumor on the surface of the eye. Lastly, there are two cases of neurofibrosarcoma from our own series. From this collection of cases it is evident the malignant tumor may occur at any age without sex predilection.

CLINICAL FEATURES

Data from the tabulated cases (above) is so meager, and so incomplete from some of the reported cases, that it is difficult to construct a uniform pattern of clinical features. In some, where there is no associated neurofibromatosis, the development of the malignant phase of the orbital neoplasm is rather rapid, an interval of several months. In this short period the degree of proptosis is relatively great and its progression alarming. Soon there is limitation of ocular rotations in all directions of gaze with consequent diplopia. In cases where the neoplasm seems to arise along the frontal or supraorbital nerve there is pain and tenderness on palpation in the superior nasal quadrant of the orbit with anesthesia or paresthesias over the area of nerve branch distribution. The interval between the initial surgical procedure and first recurrence also is relatively short, less than a year, and metastasis of the neoplasm is soon fatal.

A different clinical pattern is observed in patients with the diffuse and plexiform types of neurofibroma. Here the diagnosis of nerve sheath neoplasm is known some years prior to the time of sarcomatous transformation. Usually, in this interval, the patient has had one or more surgical procedures to excise or debulk some manifestation of the neurofibroma somewhere in the body. The course is slow, indolent, and recurrent. The longevity of these patients is considerably greater than the prior group and more dependent on the degree and grading of the malignancy. In one of our patients the neurofibrosarcoma was fatal at age 45, 8 years after the initial surgical procedure. The other patient was still living with multiple recurrences at age 83, 7 years after the first histologic verification of sarcoma in an neurofibromatosis of many decades duration.

In the case of Ginde (1953), wherein we have some question as to the diagnosis of neurofibrosarcoma, the neoplasm was well encapsulated (not usually a feature of malignancy), and showed no evidence of recurrence 1 year and 7 months after incomplete excision (a feature more compatible with a nonmalignant process).

PATHOLOGY

A tumor may appear de novo as a solitary growth along the course of a nerve or it may be discovered as a malignant transformation of a neurofibromatous nodule that has suddenly undergone a change in size or growth pattern. White or gray, the solitary tumor is poorly circumscribed and tends to grow along tissue planes of the nerve, causing a nodular or bulbous enlargement. In tumors associated with neurofibromatosis, the malignant focus may proliferate adjacent to the neurofibromatous nodule, it may infiltrate or invade the nodule, or there may be a gradual transition between benign and malignant zones. In the last arrangement the neurofibromatous nodule may show cellular, atypism or hypercellularity in an area adjacent to the malignant focus. In cellularity, pleomorphism, and hyperchromatism of the spindle-shaped cells (Fig. 177). The cells may be clustered in a loose syncytium, but more often they are arranged in whorls and interlacing fascicles. Occasional small islands of

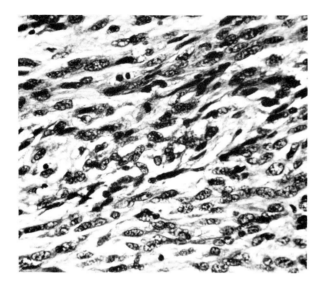

Figure 177. Neurofibrosarcoma: main features are increased cellularity, hyperchromatism, mitotic activity, and cellular pleomorphism. (Hematoxylin and eosin; × 300.)

epithelioid cells are interspersed in the tumor matrix. Scattered multinucleated giant cells also may be present. Histologically, these neoplasms resemble fibrosarcoma. Electron microscopy will help to differentiate them on the basis of the differing ultrastructural features of the Schwann cell and the fibrocyte already described.

TREATMENT

Whether the neoplasm arises de novo or as a sarcomatous change in preexisting neurofibroma, the ultimate outcome, sooner or later, is fatal. Efforts to eradicate the lesion either by total excision or exenteration of the orbit seem to be to no avail. Radiation also is ineffective. Information is lacking in regard to the effectiveness of chemotherapy.

Bibliography

A reader who may have time to browse through earlier publications on the subject of nerve sheath tumors will find the following references most helpful, not only for the information provided but also for references to even earlier source material. The English monographs of Smith and Thomson will appeal to the majority of readers. The text of Smith contains some beautiful illustrations; they have been reproduced in many subsequent publications. Smith's monograph has an additional point of interest. It is said that this monograph is the largest text ever published in Dublin; its cover measures 65 by 46½ centimeters (approximately 26 by 18 inches). The German and French references also are important but some are long.

Billroth T: Plexiformes Neurofibrom des oberon Augenlides und der Schläfengegend. Arch Klin Chir 11:232–234, 1869
Bruns P: Das Ranken-Neurom. Virchows Arch [Pathol Anat] 50:80–112, 1870
Cheselden: Cited by Smith RW
Marchand R: Das plexiforme Neurom (cylindrische Fibrom der Nervenscheiden). Virchows Arch [Pathol Anat] 70:36–55, 1877

Odier L: Cited by Wood W: Observations on neuroma. Edin Med Chir Trans Vol 3, 1829
Smith RW: A Treatise on the Pathology, Diagnosis, and Treatment of Neuroma. Dublin, Hodges and Smith, 1849
Thomson A: On Neuroma and Neuro-fibromatosis. Edinburgh, Turnbull & Spears, 1900
Verneuil A: Observation pour servir a l'histoire des altérations locales des nerfs. Arch Gen Med *108*:537–552, 1861
Virchow R: Die krankhaften Geschwülste. Vol 3. Berlin, A Hirschwald, 1867, pp. 233–305
Von Recklinghausen FD: Ueber die multiplen Fibrome der Haut und ihre Beziehung zu den mutliplen Neuromen. Berlin, A Hirschwald, 1882
Wood W: Cited by Thomson A

Neurofibroma and Neurofibromatosis

Bruwer AJ, Kierland RR: Neurofibromatosis and congenital unilateral pulsating and nonpulsating exophthalmos. Arch Ophthalmol ns *53*:2–12, 1955
LeWald LT: Congenital absence of the superior orbital wall associated with pulsating exophthalmos: report of four cases. Am J Roentgenol Radium Ther Nucl Med *30*:757–764, 1933
Moore RF: Diffuse neurofibromatosis with proptosis. Br J Opthalmol *15*:272–279, 1931
Rockliffe WC, Parsons JH: Plexiform neuroma of the orbit. Trans Pathol Soc Lond *55*:27–35, 1903–1904

Neurilemmoma

Masson P: Experimental and spontaneous schwannomas (peripheral gliomas). II. Spontaneous schwannomas. Am J Pathol *8*:389–417, 1932
Rottino A, Kelly AS: Specific nerve sheath tumor of orbit (neurilemmoma, neurinoma): report of a case with review of literature. Arch Opthalmol ns *26*:478–488, 1941 (This article contains a very complete bibliography on the subject.)
Schatz H: Benign orbital neurilemoma: sarcomatous transformation in von Recklinghausen's disease. Arch Opthalmol *86*:268–273, 1971
Stout AP: The peripheral manifestations of the specific nerve sheath tumor (neurilemoma). Am J Cancer *24*:751–796, 1935
Verocay J: Zur Kenntnis der "Neurofibrome." Beitr Pathol Anat *48*:1–69, 1910

Neurofibrosarcoma and Malignant Schwannoma

Calvet J, Couadau A: Schwannome malin de l'orbite Bull Soc Ophtalmol Fr *1*:285–287, 1949
Cerveira A: Cited by Mortada A
Ginde RG: Case of neurogenic sarcoma, successfully operated without recurrence. J All India Ophthalmol Soc *2*:29–31, 1953
Grinberg MA, Levy NS: Malignant neurilemmoma of the supraorbital nerve. Am J Ophthalmol *78*:489–492, 1974
Jakobiec FA, Jones IS: Neurogenic tumors. In *Clinical Ophthalmology*. Volume 2, Chapter 41. Ed: TD Duane. Hagerstown, Harper & Row, 1976
Mortada A: Solitary orbital malignant neurilemmomas. Br J Ophthalmol *52*:188–190, 1968
Radnót M: Malignes neurilemmom. Klin Monatsbl Augenheilkd *143*:869–875, 1963
Schatz H: Benign orbital neurilemoma: sarcomatous transformation in von Recklinghausen's disease. Arch Ophthalmol *86*:268–274, 1971
Schiff-Wertheimer S, Loisillier P: Neurilemome malin de l'orbite chez une enfant: traitement chirurgical. Bull Soc Ophthalmol Fr No *4*:314–317, 1954

11

Neurocytic and Neurogliogenic Tumors

In this chapter we will note the neoplasia of several neural, neuroglial, and neuroganglionic tissues which share an ancestry from the primitive epithelium of the neural tube. In this somewhat heterogenous group are tumors that may involve the orbit either as primary, secondary, or metastatic growths. Three of the tumors — retinoblastoma, optic nerve glioma, and neuroblastoma — are well known to ophthalmologists. The remainder of the group are curiosities in the average ophthalmic practice.

RETINOBLASTOMA

Retinoblastoma is so standard a term and has been so common during the past several decades that some ophthalmologists may not know that this designation is relatively recent. The term was proposed by the American pathologist Verhoeff in 1922 and came into general usage several years later.The neoplasm has been known for more than 200 years and it has been called by many other names. The history and story of retinoblastoma have been well described by Dunphy (1964); so interesting and complete is his report that the interested physician should read it, and no attempt will be made to summarize or abstract this information here.

The name retinoblastoma refers to the undifferentiated nature of the cells that constitute the tumor. After the careful study of Parkhill and Benedict (1941), the genesis of the tumor was associated with the glial or supporting component of the neuroepithelium. More recently, based on ultrastructural studies, histologists think that the tumor has a neuroblastic rather than a glioblastic genesis.

INCIDENCE

Since our manuscript on orbital retinoblastoma was assembled over 9 years ago in preparation for the first edition of this text, data on the cases of intraocular retinoblastoma observed and treated at the Edward S. Harkness Eye Institute in New York has been analyzed. This study encompasses over 1100 cases (the total varies slightly in several publications depending on the features selected by the author for study) in a period of 49 years and, because of its size, supersedes all prior statistical studies pertaining to incidence, treatment, complications, and survival of retinoblastoma patients. Reference to this study has appeared in several publications by physicians who have had access to the voluminous case files. Among the several reports in the ophthalmic literature of this type are those of Ellsworth (1974), Jakobiec and Jones (1976), and Rootman and colleagues (1978). Data on the incidence and course of orbital extension of retinoblastoma in these reports is particularly germane to our discussion.

Orbital involvement varied from 8 to 10% of the total sample, depending on whether the diagnosis was based on histologic proof or clinical assumptions. The average age of the patients at onset of orbital extension was 22 months, with an age range of from 1 month to 12 years. The occurrence of either intra-ocular or orbital extension of retinoblastoma after the first decade is quite unusual. There is no significant sex predilection.

In regard to the incidence of orbital retinoblastoma in a consecutive series of orbital tumors, statistical extremes are represented in our own and the Reese (1963) survey, wherein similar orbital conditions were included in the total sample. In our series the incidence was less than 1% (6 cases among 764 tumors); in the series of Reese the incidence was 5.5% (49 cases among 877 tumors). This discrepancy is easily explained on the basis of the large number of cases of intraocular retinoblastoma referred to Reese at the Edward S. Harkness Eye Institute. Our own incidence statistics would have been higher had not the management of retinoblastoma been so concentrated elsewhere.

CLINICAL FEATURES

Orbital extension begins with the escape of tumor cells from the eye, for which there are several routes other than careless rupture of the eyeball during the course of enucleation. The route that has received most attention is through the lamina cribrosa, with slow intraneural dissemination until the subarachnoid space is reached either by spread along the central retinal vessels or focal erosion of the pial covering of the optic nerve (Fig. 178). The neoplasm reaches the central nervous system via the subarachnoid space and is then rapidly fatal. Another route is spread of tumor from the choroid along the emissary nerves and vessels that pass through the scleral barrier, finally gaining access to the posterior surface of the eye (Fig. 179). In the absence of gross tumor it is this route that is so easily overlooked yet so difficult to detect. Hence, microscopic search should be made for tumor cells in the soft tissues attached to the back surface of the eye following enucleation, particularly in advanced cases of intra-ocular retinoblastoma with secondary glaucoma. If tumor cells are found in these soft tissues attached to the eye, orbital recurrence is likely. The choroid also is the means for hematogenous spread of the tumor to distant sites. Hematogenous metastasis to the viscera or other sites distant from the eye may have already occurred in many cases in which the only obvious sign of trouble is a lump in the orbit.

Whatever route the tumor chooses to leave the eye, the presenting symptom of orbital recurrence is a lump, usually in the rear of the orbit. The lump may be of any size, depending on how closely the child is observed by the parents or the physician after enucleation. If an implant is placed in the socket following enucleation (the usual procedure) the symptoms may be more subtle. In these

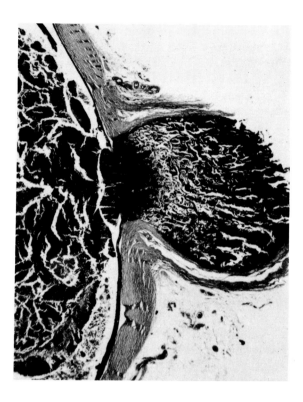

Figure 178.   Retinoblastoma: orbital involvement most commonly results from penetration through lamina cribrosa and spread in optic nerve. (Hematoxylin and eosin; × 10.)

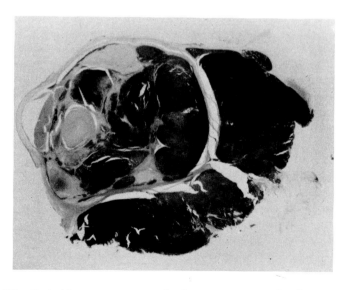

Figure 179.   Retinoblastoma: massive orbital invasion apparently along emissary vascular channels rather than via optic nerve. (Hematoxylin and eosin; × 2½.)

cases the prosthetist may see the child on several occasions for adjustment of the prosthesis before it becomes obvious that an enlarging orbital mass is responsible for the misalignment or extrusion of the artificial eye. These orbital masses, however large they may be when first discovered, are not tender. As the mass enlarges it becomes red — owing to a rich blood supply — and friable. In these features the tumor resembles other orbital neoplasms of childhood, such as rhabdomyosarcoma and neuroblastoma, but the retinoblastoma does not grow as rapidly as the latter tumors. Growth of retinoblastomas is assessed in terms of weeks or months; orbital recurrence in children almost always makes its presence known within 6 months of enucleation. In contrast, rhabdomyosarcomas and neuroblastomas enlarge so rapidly that their growth may be measured in terms of days.

Such a sequence of signs, however, is not the rule among African children. Here, the extension of the neoplasm from the eye into the surrounding orbit goes unnoticed, and the progressive proptosis of the affected eye is at first ignored. Gradually, the orbital situation becomes so extreme, the child so listless and weak, that even the tribal witch doctor can do no more. Then the affected child is brought to the nearest regional medical facility. In short, the presentation of the disease has become orbital rather than intraocular. The orbital mass has become so large — capped by the necrotic, smashed-looking eye — that it is a clinical horror difficult to imagine by a non-African resident. This presentation is almost pathognomonic of retinoblastoma, except that some neglected Burkitt's lymphoma of the orbit may also reach such a monstrous size. However, in the latter disease there is often some involvement of the jaws and face on the side of the lesion, giving the child an even more grotesque appearance.

A type of orbital presentation also should be mentioned wherein the socket on the side of the enucleated eye is normal but proptosis of the opposite eye heralds the initial sign of metastasis. Although retinoblastoma affects virtually only infants and children, retinoblastoma occasionally has been noted in adults. Also, while retinoblastoma is not truly an orbital tumor, Guinaudeau (1951) reported a retinoblastoma that he thought was primary in the orbit. An intraocular tumor was not observed. The cells of this tumor were described as stellate, with fine prolongations connecting one cell to another. This could have been a tumor originating in nervous tissue, but the histopathologic description was not typical of retinoblastoma.

PATHOLOGY

The histologic features of intraocular retinoblastoma are more important than those of orbital recurrence, for the initial and definitive diagnosis is based on the features of the intraocular lesion. Information about the orbital patterns of growth is scant. But it is important to be able to recognize retinoblastoma, either in its earliest sojourn outside the eye or when it is submitted as a biopsy specimen from an orbit in which the enucleated eye, having been removed elsewhere, is not readily available for examination. In the former situation a careful search should be made at the time of enucleation not only for small clusters of retinoblastoma cells along the septa of the optic nerve but also in the connective tissue that may be clinging to the surface of the enucleated globe. Usually, cells of the retinoblastoma within the eye appear relatively uniform. The cell stains a bluish purple, the oval or round nuclei with their abundant chromatin are prominent, and most nuclei are about the same size. Pseudorosettes, clusters of cells proliferating around a central blood vessel, are common but should not be confused with true rosettes. The latter are rings of cells showing some photoreceptor differentiation (Fig. 180).

Most of these features change as the neoplasm leaves the eye; for example, the rosette patterns tend to disappear (Fig. 181). If the tumor proliferates within the sclera the cells vary in size. Some nuclei are small and appear almost solid with the purple dye; others may be relatively large, larger than some of the nuclei of the original tumor, but retain their oval or round contours with a distinctive pattern of chromatin staining. These features may also be seen among the neoplastic cells proliferating in the reticulum of the orbital cavity. Here the small, densely staining nuclei that are surrounded by a thin rim of cytoplasm may resemble a small cluster of lymphocytes. If the growth of the neoplasm meets with resistance, such as a barrier of fibrous tissue, the cells become more irregular and smaller and tend to advance along the tissue septa in sheets and wisps. These sheets may stain so densely as to make it difficult to identify individual nuclei. If there is less resistance to cell proliferation the tumor may find a pocket where it can grow exuberantly. In these foci the nuclei remain small but their contours are round and uniform. They are so densely packed as to suggest a diagnosis of small cell undifferentiated carcinoma (Fig. 182). If such zones are found, some areas of necrosis likely will be present. As a rule, such foci are either removed or treated before calcification develops. Taktikos concluded from a histologic study of 287 nonorbital cases that no histopathologic classification could, at present, be correlated with prognosis.

TREATMENT

Potential or possible orbital extension of retinoblastoma should be considered when the diagnosis of intraocular retinoblastoma is first made. Computer tomography of the orbits may show a shadow behind the involved eye that

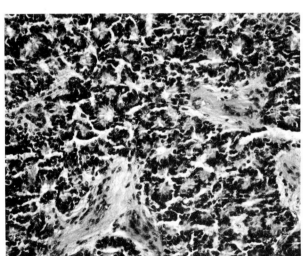

Figure 180. Retinoblastoma: well-differentiated example composed of uniform cells with prominent rosettes. (Hematoxylin and eosin; × 150.)

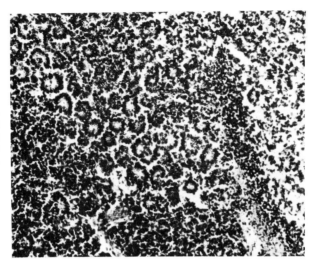

Figure 181. Retinoblastoma: less-differentiated example in which cells are not so uniform and rosettes are not as well developed; compare with Figure 180. (Hematoxylin and eosin; × 155.)

represents a small focal extension of neoplasm that otherwise would not be expected in the absence of proptosis. This should alert the surgeon to the logic of an exenteration rather than an enucleation as a means for complete surgical removal of the neoplasm at the initial operation.

Another cardinal objective in treatment is to obtain a long portion of the optic nerve at the time of enucleation—if this can be designated as treatment rather than as prevention. Since the purpose is to sever the optic nerve nearer the optic foramen than its attachment to the eyeball, the scissors or clamp should be directed straight posteriorly and parallel to the medial wall of the orbit rather than following the contour of the eyeball as in the usual enucleation procedure.

If the surgeon is unfamiliar with the feel of the optic nerve in this direct approach, excision of a long section of the optic nerve is still possible by the following modification of the usual maneuver. When all six muscles have been severed at their tendinous attachment to the eye, either 4-0 silk sutures or small hemostats are placed on the stumps of the medial and lateral recti muscles still

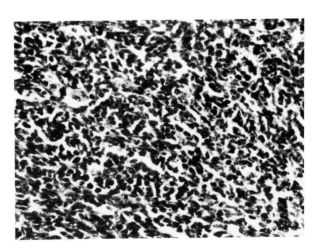

Figure 182. Retinoblastoma: highly undifferentiated and irregular, small and often spindled cells. (Hematoxylin and eosin; × 250.)

attached to the eye. With traction on the sutures or hemostats the eye is pulled forward as far as possible. At the same time the enucleation scissor is pushed posteriorly along the nerve until the surrounding soft tissues no longer yield to traction and countertraction along the anteroposterior axis of the orbit. The nerve is interrupted at this point. An effort should be made to obtain a tail of optic nerve, still attached to the eyeball, of at least 10 mm in length. Section of the optic nerve at such a point usually is well beyond the extent of retinoblastoma cells along the nerve fiber bundles, except when the intraocular neoplasm is advanced and has been present many months.

One other point related to the enucleation procedure should not be overlooked. This is the need to palpate the orbital cavity for residual tumor after the eye has been removed. In the early stages of its orbital growth, retinoblastoma is the same color as its supporting medium, in contrast to the more reddish hue of the advanced case. Therefore, a small nodule of orbital retinoblastoma might go unnoticed if the surgeon relies only on a visual inspection of the orbital tissues.

If an orbital nodule or an enlarged proximal stump of optic nerve is discovered during enucleation, we would perform a complete excision of the mass and recommend local radiotherapy and systemic chemotherapy postoperatively. A similar combined approach of surgery, radiotherapy, and chemotherapy is also followed for "delayed" orbital recurrence observed some months after enucleation. If an examination of the enucleated tissue shows some neoplastic cells along the surface of the eye, spread of tumor along the scleral emissaria, or tumor approaching the limits of the optic nerve section, we would proceed with local radiotherapy and adjuvant chemotherapy but defer further surgery. In these latter hypothetical situations, orbital seeding cannot be positively demonstrated but we consider orbital recurrence so likely that all therapeutic modalities should be employed to thwart further spread of neoplasm.

Before starting combined radiotherapy–chemotherapy treatment, the child should be surveyed for possible metastasis. Radiography of the optic canals (if not already performed prior to enucleation) may show enlargement indicating proximal spread of neoplasm along the optic nerve. Bone marrow and spinal fluid examinations should be done in search of tumor cells. If evidence of metastasis is found, therapy becomes palliative rather than curative.

In recommending local radiotherapy and adjuvant chemotherapy to these situations with both equivocal and unequivocal orbital spread we realize there is no well-controlled study of a large number of treated cases upon which to base positive conclusions. Turning again to the large series of patients from the Institute of Ophthalmology in New York, their data strongly suggests these combined modalities of therapy are a major factor in the improved survival rates of their patients in the period 1959–1974 as compared with prior years. Also, we recognize that such combined therapy is the future trend in an effort to attain cure.

Wolff (1978), who has had extensive experience in this field, anticipates that various Cancer Study Groups in this country will join in a unified, aggressive treatment protocol for these difficult situations. Such a protocol might provide for the administration of three chemotherapeutic agents (cyclophosphamide, vincristine, and adriamycin), each drug every 3 weeks for 21 months, combined with local radiotherapy in the first six-week period for patients with biopsy-proven orbital recurrence or microscopic evidence of tumor at the cut edge of the optic nerve at time of enucleation. The total dose of radiotherapy would be 5,000 rads. The suggested intravenous dosage of the several drugs are: vincristine 0.05 mg/kg, cyclophosphamide 20 mg/kg, and adriamycin 2 mg/kg. The adriamycin would be discontinued after 21 months (the eighth injection) but the vincristine and cyclophosphamide would be continued for another 14 to 24 months. Patients with only equivocal orbital spread (tumor cells in scleral emissaria or in episcleral tissues at time of enucleation) would not be given radiotherapy or adriamycin. Instead, vincristine (0.05 mg/kg) would be given with a larger amount of cyclophosphamide (30 mg/kg) every 3 weeks for a 57-week period.

PROGNOSIS

Through the many years that physicians have been grappling with the management of intraocular retinoblastoma there has been a gradual improvement in survival rates chiefly based on earlier recognition and treatment of the neoplasm. However, once the tumor appeared in the orbit it was almost 100% fatal. Well-documented records of survival of children with histologically proved orbital retinoblastoma were exceedingly rare.

Most noteworthy in this respect is the case reported by Oliver (1962). The patient, a child, was living and well 5 years after treatment. The eye had been enucleated when the child was 9 months old. At 22 months of age a pea-sized nodule of recurrent retinoblastoma was confirmed in the left orbit. Exenteration of the orbit was performed and therapy supplemented with irradiation (3,496 R) and TEM (12.5 mg) during a period of several months. After an interval, treatment was repeated (irradiation, 2,095 R; TEM, 19 mg). Reese and Ellsworth (1963) reported four patients they regarded as being cured, but no details of the treatment program of these four cases were included in their publication. Two of these four are probably the cases referred to in the Reese text (1963). One was living 7 years and the other 20 years after treatment by exenteration and x-rays alone. In neither of these cases was the orbital tumor examined histologically. Reese also referred to an "authenticated" cure observed by Moore.

But now there is an encouraging glimmer. Rootman and colleagues (1978) report, in their series of more recently treated patients, that 9.4% lived more than two years after diagnosis. Of the fatal cases the longest survival was 42 months; 80% of the fatalities were dead within 10 months of the diagnosis of recurrence. Orbital retinoblastoma still is a very grim affair.

MEDULLOEPITHELIOMA

This rather rare neoplasm has many similarities to the preceding retinoblastoma. The medulloepithelioma (the *diktyoma* of older literature) arises from the medullary neuroepithelium of the inner wall of the secondary optic vesicle just anterior (pars ciliaris retinae) to the area of retinblastomas. Also, it may arise from embryonal medullary neuroepithelium near the optic nerve head. Like the retinoblastoma, medulloepithelioma presents in childhood as an intraocular tumor, may extend into the orbit as a malignant neoplasm, has a high mortality rate, and may show cellular rosettes in its histopathology. It differs from retinoblastoma in its presentation in older children; in a much slower rate of growth; and in a tendency to form heteroplastic, teratoid-like tissue not normally observed in the eye, such as cartilage, skeletal muscle, and brain tissue.

Broughton and Zimmerman (1978) have studied fifty-six medulloepitheliomas. Thirty-seven of these were considered malignant. Among the latter were eight cases showing definite orbital involvement. A child with orbital involvement is described by Malone (1955), and the several cases with known involvement of the orbital portion of the optic nerve are detailed in the reports of Reese (1957) and Green and colleagues (1974). The mean age at the time ocular symptoms are first noted is in the range of 3½ to 5 years. However, the interval between the initial suspicion of the neoplasm and definitive diagnosis or orbital spread may be very long, attesting to the very slow growth of the neoplasm. In the case of Rubino (1941) an intraocular tumor was suspected at age 3, but the eye was removed only when an extrabulbar mass appeared at age 19. In Andersen's (1948) case the tumor was suspected at birth but the eye was not removed until the patient was 16. There is no sex predilection.

At present, there are no uniform criteria for determining whether the intraocular tumor is benign or malignant; this is of little concern to our discussion because, by the time of orbital invasion, the tumor has become malignant. In the eye the proliferating embryonal cells throw the single-layered neuroepithelium into numerous folds so that, on cut sections, the tumor has a multi-layered appearance (Fig. 183). With further growth and crowding the multi-layered cells may partially fuse and circumscribe an empty space or a cavity filled with a colorless coagulum. The empty spaces will be lined by the outer cellular border corresponding to the external limiting membrane. The spaces filled by colorless tissue will be lined by the inner cellular membrane corresponding to the internal limiting membrane of the ciliary epithelium. The colorless coagulum will stain intensely for the acid mucopolysaccharide of the primitive vitreous. When orbital extension occurs the histologic pattern is replaced by masses and sheets of poorly differentiated cells with hyperchromatic nuclei and scant cytoplasm resembling the picture of retinoblastoma (Fig. 182). If rosettes are observed they will be larger than those of retinoblastoma and may be multilayered rather than single-layered. Mitotic figures are frequent.

Cases of survival of histologically proven orbital involvement are quite rare. The patient of Green and associates, a 6-year-old female, was living without metastasis 18 months after exenteration of the orbit. The medulloepithelioma was found at the level of the optic nerve section at the time of enucleation. Broughton and Zimmerman describe two cases that were treated for presumed orbital involvement on the basis of histopathologic evidence of extraocular extension at time of enucleation. One of these patients underwent orbital exenteration within two weeks after enucleation and was well five years later without additional therapy. The other patient was treated with orbital radiation and systemic chemotherapy and was well two years after enucleation. Death from medulloepithelioma is usually attributed to intracranial spread. Therefore, the key to prognosis is the prevention or treatment of orbital extension.

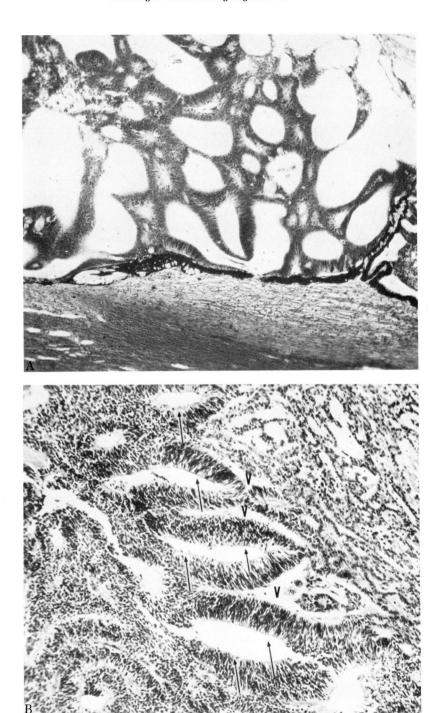

Figure 183. Medulloepithelioma (*A*). The medulloepithelioma arises from the nonpigmented ciliary epithelium and produces intricate convolutions enclosing lumina of various shapes and sizes. (Hematoxylin and eosin; × 80.) (*B*) The multicellular bands are polarized, forming a sharply defined structure analogous to the external limiting membrane of the retina along one surface (*arrows*); the less well-defined opposite surface is in contact with primitive vitreous (V). (Hematoxylin and eosin; × 115.) (From Zimmerman LE: Verhoeff's "Terato-neuroma." Am J Ophthalmol 72:1039–1057, 1971. By permission.)

OPTIC NERVE GLIOMA

The nervous tissue that extends from optic papilla to optic chiasm is familiar to all as the optic nerve. This structure is not in fact a true nerve because it possesses neither sheaths nor cells of Schwann and the neuronal components are not supported by endoneurium; instead, it is surrounded by the same coverings as the brain, and the intrinsic supporting structures are true neuroglial cells. This "nerve" is morphologically and functionally a tract of the central nervous system comparable to the white matter of the brain. The nerve tract differs somewhat from this white matter in that its fibers are separated into bundles by vascular connective tissue septa extending into the tract from the surrounding pia.

It is the abnormal proliferation of supporting neuroglial cells to which the term *glioma* has been applied. Gliomas may arise anywhere in the central nervous system. Neoplasms arising in the anterior portion of the visual pathways are differentiated from similar growths elsewhere in the brain by the designation *optic nerve gliomas*. Likewise, this term is useful to separate this glioma from those described as occurring in the orbit and retina. Still, the designation is not strictly specific in that it does not confine the glioma to that portion of the tract extending from the optic papilla to the optic chiasm. Instead, in practical usage, optic nerve glioma is an inclusive term designating a primary tumor arising in any portion of the anterior visual pathways, that is, the optic nerve, optic chiasm, and optic tracts.

This discussion is mainly concerned with the glioma in the optic nerve proper rather than its manifestations in the chiasm and optic tracts. It is the glioma of the intra-orbital portion of the optic nerve, in particular, that may mimic the clinical features of a true orbital tumor. This is the basis for discussing the optic nerve glioma among the orbital tumors.

HISTORICAL ASPECTS

One of the first physicians to remove a tumor of the optic nerve was no less than a surgeon to the King of Scotland. The surgeon, Wishart, related in 1833 the story of a 13-year-old girl with an orbital tumor; the right eye, in his words, "projects considerably" beyond the orbit. Treatment with leeches applied over the eyebrow and blisters to the temple was unsuccessful and the eye became so prominent as to warrant its removal. Because a mass could be palpated behind the protruding eye, the entire contents of the orbit were extirpated. The eye was found to be "perfectly sound" but it had been pushed forward by a large tumor distending the optic nerve (an engraving of the eye and the attached nerve with its tumor was included in his publication). The cut surface of the tumor resembled "cerebral substance." Wishart was impressed not only by discovery of the tumor but also by the fact that the patient survived the operation. Wishart was aware of another patient who might have had a tumor similar to the one removed in his patient. He referred to Panizza (1821), who described a 6-year-old girl in whom small tumors surrounded each optic nerve, with a still larger cerebral mass growing in the base of the brain. Soon after Wishart had described his case, Middlemore (1838), of England, reported another instance of surgical removal of an optic nerve tumor from a 3-year-old boy. This was followed by the description of the clinical characteristics and the pathologic examination of optic nerve tumors by von Graefe (1864, 1866) and by anatomic classification of these tumors into intradural and extradural types by Leber (1877).

During the next 50 years there was lively controversy as to the embryogenesis of these tumor types, discussion as to whether they represented neoplasms or hypertrophy of normal structures, and speculation as to whether the tumors were benign or malignant. Throughout this period a host of descriptive terms applied to the tumors reflected the diversity of microscopic patterns described by different pathologists. The discovery of special stains, which brought out the distinctive features of various neuroglial cells,helped to bring some order out of confusion. The present pathologic concept that intradural or intrinsic tumors of the optic nerve are gliomas related to those occurring in the brain was developed by Verhoeff (1922). Even so, some continued to believe that these tumors were a form of degenerative gliomatosis.

Throughout the last century of interest in this tumor, many fine reviews were written; each updated the extensive bibliography and summarized current concepts. Among these should be mentioned the reports of Hudson (1912), von Hippel (1923), Davis (1940), Dodge and associates (1958), Wagener (1959) and Chutorian and associates (1964).

INCIDENCE

The tumor always has been considered to be rare. Davis (1940), from his survey and those of others, estimated the incidence to be 1:176,000 of all patients with ocular disorders. Perhaps this infrequent incidence stimulated others to tabulate cases more closely. Whatever the reason, the sum total of cases frequently has been recalculated and updated in succeeding reviews. This concern with total cases seems greater with this tumor than with any other in this text. Hudson (1912), in his exhaustive report, was one of the first to make a detailed count: up to his time 118 optic nerve gliomas were found. Marshall (1954) reviewed 660 cases. Lloyd's review (1973) brought the total to 1,076 cases. We see no basis for continuing to designate this tumor as rare or uncommon. In most of the larger surveys the incidence of this neoplasm among all orbital tumors is approximately 1% to 2%. In our study there were 19 cases of glioma affecting the intra-orbital portion of the nerve (2.4% of the total tumors and 5.5% of primary tumors in the series) (Table 2, Chapter 3). This proportion of gliomas in the total study would be larger if those affecting the chiasmal or intracranial portion of the nerve had been included. Of this type we found 49 cases in a similar period of observation, a ratio of almost 2.6:1 chiasmal to orbital gliomas. This ratio differs from that observed by Chutorian and colleagues (1964): among their 56 patients observed during a 29-year period, 30 had chiasmal gliomas and 26 had optic nerve gliomas. In the Lloyd series of 41 optic nerve gliomas, chiasmal involvement was noted in 32 patients.

Optic nerve gliomas chiefly affect children, the majority of cases being either diagnosed or treated by the age of 15 years. Occasionally the symptoms of this tumor may not appear until the patient is much older; thus, one of our patients was 45 years of age when proptosis and loss of vision first were noted. Others also have observed optic nerve gliomas in patients of the middle age group; Hoyt and Baghdassarian (1969) found a chiasmal and optic nerve glioma in a 64-year-old woman at autopsy. An even older patient, a 79-year-old woman, was reported by Condon and Rose (1967). In the youngest patient of our series (2 months of age), proptosis was first noted at the age of 6 weeks. The age range of our 19 patients with gliomas of the intraorbital portion of the optic nerve are listed in Table 3, Chapter 3. The tumor has traits of a congenital hamartoma.

Most observers have reported that the tumor is commoner in females. Of our 19 patients, 12 were females.

CLINICAL FEATURES

A favorite locus of origin for the orbital type of this tumor is near the optic foramen. From this point it may extend in either a centrifugal or centripetal direction. However, in cases of several years' duration, it may not be possible to determine just where the tumor started. The chief clinical signs are *gradual, painless, unilateral proptosis associated with loss of vision*, due to growth of tumor within or along the optic nerve. Early in its growth, proptosis is straightforward; and pressure also is soon exerted on the neuronal components, causing early visual failure.

Usually it is proptosis that first brings the infant or child to the attention of the physician (Fig. 184) because the preceding visual loss is not noticed by either patient or parent. Duration of proptosis often is only a few months or even a few weeks in the very young. And, because the symptoms are of short duration, proptosis is not advanced. These two features — the duration of symptoms and the degree of proptosis — are less than with those of meningioma of the optic nerve sheath in a comparable age group of children, though there are exceptions. Proptosis may be extreme and visual loss advanced in cases in which the approach to diagnosis is conservative, the therapy tried is irradiation, or an optic nerve tumor simply is not suspected. In these cases the clinical picture more resembles that of meningioma.

If the neoplasm develops in the intracanalicular side of the foramen rather than on its orbital side, visual loss may precede proptosis or it may be advanced by the time proptosis appears. In an alert adolescent or adult, for example, the presenting symptom may be visual blurring with but minimal proptosis. In gen-

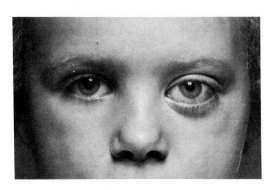

Figure 184. Optic nerve glioma: upward deviation and slight proptosis of left eye of 1 month's duration; left eye was nearly blind (light projection only) and chronic papilledema and moderate pallor of left disk were ophthalmoscopic findings.

eral, among the younger patients, no other orbital tumor brings about such early impairment of vision in relation to proptosis as does optic nerve glioma. Among a series of 36 patients with optic nerve gliomas (Hoyt and Baghdassarian, 1969), visual loss was already severe in 45% of eyes at the time the tumor was diagnosed. In 13 of our 17 children with gliomas of the intraorbital portion of the optic nerve, measurements of visual acuity were possible. In 10 (77%) of the 13, visual acuity was reduced to light perception or amaurosis in the affected eye. In only 3 of the 13 patients was the visual acuity better than 20/80. Such severe visual loss contrasts with some statements in the literature that less than 50% of the patients will have visual loss at the time they are first seen and the visual decrease is relatively static.

Definite assessment of visual dysfunction is not always possible in these young patients, but other clues may help to differentiate the proptosis from that of other types of orbital tumors. A principal sign is roentgenographic evidence of enlargement (9 of our 17 children) of the optic foramen on the affected side, as shown by optic canal views. The intrinsic disturbance within the nerve also may produce papilledema (12 of our 17 children) and the expanding tumor even may indent the posterior pole of the eyeball (induced hypermetropia). Pallor of the disk, without prior papilledema, also may occur, but usually this is not seen until the growth is advanced. Strabismus frequently is noted as an additional sign, but this often is a sign of other orbital tumors in childhood. It is more common among the younger than among the older childhood age groups. Accurrate perimetry, if possible, demonstrates irregular or altitudinal contractions of the visual fields, unless the tumor already has involved the chiasm; then, visual fields show bitemporal defects. Seldom will the tumor be palpable.

Several authors have commented on the relationship of optic nerve gliomas to von Recklinghausen's disease and there seems to be a clinical basis for assuming a more than coincidental association. The incidence of von Recklinghausen's disease among patients with optic nerve glioma varies widely among reports in the literature and may depend on the diligence of the search for manifestations of neurofibromatosis. Therefore, any youngster with the skin manifestations of neurofibromatosis who also has unexplained loss of vision should be observed not only for orbital neurofibroma but also for possible optic nerve glioma. The presence of neurofibromatosis does not seem to alter the course or prognosis of the optic nerve tumor.

A quite different clinical sequence may be seen in some adults. Here, the *onset of visual loss is sudden* (suggesting the diagnosis of optic neuritis); progression of visual loss, proptosis, papilledema, and headache is quite rapid (a few weeks or several months); and death occurs 6 to 12 months from the onset of ocular symptoms. A malignant form of astrocytoma is found in these cases, either on surgical exploration or autopsy. Hoyt and associates (1973) have summarized most of the well-documented cases of this aggressive form of the disease in the literature, including five cases of their own. The age range of these malignant cases extends from 22 to 70 years of age with a sex ratio of approximately 2:1, male to female. However, not all malignant cases occur in adults.

The striking nature of these adult cases, and the number reported, may suggest a higher incidence of this form of optic nerve glioma than would be present if they were viewed only within the context of a large number of gliomas in all age groups. The benign optic nerve glioma also may occur in adults, but their course is not so different from the childhood type of gliomas as to warrant separate descriptions. Two of our nineteen intraorbital optic nerve gliomas were in adult females, aged 21 and 46 years, at time of surgical diagnosis. In both cases, successive decrease of vision and proptosis over a period of 19 to 30 months brought the patient to the ophthalmologist. Intermittent orbital pain in one and increasing hypermetropia in the other patient were additional symptoms. Enlargement of the optic canal was noted only in the 21-year-old patient. An intraorbital, well-encapsulated, grade 1 astrocytoma was removed from each patient. The patients have been followed for 19 and 9 years, respectively, without recurrence of tumor.

Some estimate of the incidence of benign versus malignant optic nerve gliomas in both adults and children is possible from a study of sixty-six histologically proved tumors involving the chiasmal, intracranial, intracanalicular, and intraorbital portions of the optic nerve in the 27-year time period of our orbital tumor survey. The statistical sample does not include 6 cases in which a presumed glioma was identified in the chiasm at time of surgical exploration but not biopsied. Fourteen (21%) of the 66 patients were 20 years or older (adults). There were 9 (13%) malignant (grade 3 or 4 in the histologic grading scale) gliomas in the total sample. Five of the 9 malignant gliomas were in adults, and the remaining 4 cases were in patients 4 months, 8 years, 10 years, and 15 years of age, respectively.

ROENTGENOGRAPHIC CHANGES

Concentric enlargement of the optic foramen with preservation of a well-corticated margin is the principal roentgenographic sign of glioma involving the orbital portion of the optic nerve. Such enlargement is not exclusive to gliomas in this location and it also may result from forward extension of glioma originating around the optic chiasm or intracranial portion of the optic nerve. Also, enlargement of the optic foramen may be associated with orbital neurofibromas and craniopharyngiomas affecting patients of the same age group. However, when clinicians note an enlarged optic foramen in infants or young children, their first consideration usually is optic nerve glioma of the orbital type.

For purposes of comparison, similar views of both optic foramina are necessary (Fig. 185). Since optic foramina may not be exactly symmetric in diameter and configuration, the question arises as to what difference is significant. Some observers consider a difference in diameter of 1 mm as diagnostic, but such asymmetry may have only presumptive value. More often, a diameter of one optic foramen exceeding 6.5 mm is considered significant. Another helpful feature is the polished sclerotic appearance of the bony foramen surrounding a glioma, an appearance produced by slow, steady pressure of the neoplasm. The optic foramina of children tend to show relatively greater enlargement than those of adults with a tumor of similar size and duration. And in infants, in particular, the optic foramina may become relatively large. The optic canal of one patient in the series of Chutorian and associates (1964) was enlarged to a circular lumen of 11 mm, with intact cortical margins. Ten (58%) of the 17 children of our survey with intraorbital tumors showed enlargement of the optic foramen or canal. Although enlargement is diagnostic in cases in which it occurs, many ob-

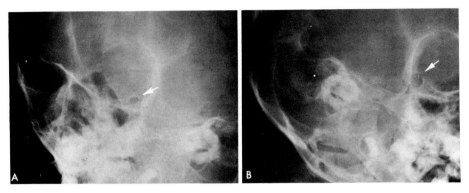

Figure 185. Optic nerve glioma: roentgenograms of optic canals of 2½-year-old boy with slowly progressive lateral deviation and proptosis of left eye of 8 months' duration. *A,* Right optic canal (*arrow*) is normal. *B,* Left optic canal is approximately twice normal size, due to growth of glioma.

servers have emphasized that absence of enlargement is not conclusive evidence that a tumor does not exist in suspected cases. Neither is the presence or absence of enlargement necessarily of prognostic significance. Negative optic canal roentgenograms are particular pitfalls in adults who harbor a glioma but show minimal or equivocal proptosis. The visual blurring and pallor of the optic disk mistakenly may be diagnosed as optic neuritis in such cases.

Tomography of the optic canals either at right angles or parallel to the long axis (Fig. 29, Chapter 2) may reveal abnormalities not evident on routine optic canal views Such techniques permit visualization of the length of the canal, comparison of the contours of the right and left optic canals, and may show enlargement of the posterior meatus of the optic canal. Such information is important in determining the extent of an orbital glioma. A positive tomogram might well be considered a positive indication for surgical exploration, whereas, with both negative tomography and routine optic canal views, surgery might be deferred in a case of suspected orbital glioma.

In recent years either computer tomography or ultrasonography have become routine diagnostic supplements in confirming the size and configuration of suspected orbital gliomas.

Rarely, in the very young, standard orbital views may show only orbital enlargement without alteration of the optic foramen. Other roentgenographic changes seen on routine skull views, such as gourd-shaped and J-shaped sellae, are more diagnostic of the chiasmal gliomas.

PATHOLOGY

Optic nerve glioma has been a popular and widely used term in the medical profession to designate a tumor associated with a well-known clinical entity. The noun, *glioma,* also has served well as a designation for the morphologic structure of the tumor since a glial genesis was accepted approximately 70 years ago. In the intervening years most pathologists have accepted the astrocyte as the major cellular component of the tumor, and the more specific term, *astrocytoma*, has been used in many publications as a replacement for the older, glioma. However, these same observers agree that another glial cell, the oligodendrocyte, is a frequent part of the tumor, and some pathologists continue to prefer the less specific term, glioma, to include the tumor with a mixed glial structure. Whether the oligodendrocytes are a true part of the neoplasm or residual cells of the involved optic nerve "along for the ride" is not settled. Also, in respect to whether the tumor is benign or malignant, astrocytoma is no more specific a term than glioma. There is currently a trend to classify optic nerve tumors more precisely; the more common benign astrocytoma is now designated a *juvenile pilocytic astrocytoma.* Such a term is useful in differentiating the histologically benign tumor from the less frequent but more anaplastic fibrillary astrocytoma.

Pilocytic (hair-like) refers to the elongated, fusiform or spindle-shaped cells that interlace and intersect in various directions (Fig. 186). Some nuclear pleomorphism is common. In some areas the cells have oval, vesicular nuclei and in other areas the nuclei are round and dark (Fig. 187). Cell outlines are indistinct. Mitotic figures are not usually found but, if present, must be regarded as a sign of increasing anaplasia with an ominous prognosis. In large tumors of long duration, where the fibrillary astrocytes are densely packed, degenerative changes in the form of eosinophilic, irregular shaped, amorphous densities (Rosenthal fibers, Verhoeff's bodies) may be present (Fig. 190). These amorphous structures, which may be intracellular or extracellular, represent the degenerative residues of astroglial cytoplasmic filaments. They are not seen in nerve sheath tumors. Less compact tumors have a more lacy appearance because of dilated intercellular spaces of edema fluid or a mucocoid substance (see Fig. 189). A circular arrangement of cells around a blood vessel in a pseudo-rosette fashion is a feature that may suggest a more aggressive type of neoplasm.

The tumors may be classified into four groups based on histopathologic appearance with a gradual transition from the most benign, grade 1, to the most malignant, grade 4. In grades 1 and 2, simple proliferation of astrocytes results in an increase in the number of glial cells as compared to a normal section of optic nerve (Fig. 188). Cell outlines are more prominent and distinct with more numerous and thicker fibrillar processes and the nuclei also are larger and more

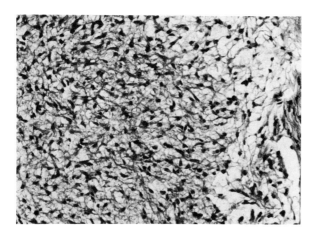

Figure 186. Optic nerve astrocytoma: neoplasm composed of fine fibrillary astrocytes. (Hematoxylin and eosin; × 155.)

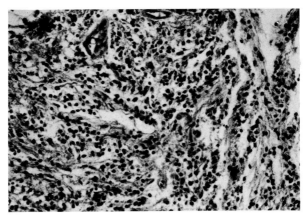

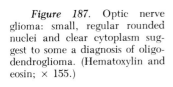
Figure 187. Optic nerve glioma: small, regular rounded nuclei and clear cytoplasm suggest to some a diagnosis of oligodendroglioma. (Hematoxylin and eosin; × 155.)

hyperchromatic than normal. Pleomorphism is minimal, mitotic figures and giant cells are absent. The difference between grade 1 and grade 2 is only a matter of degree (Fig. 189). Tumors with these cytologic features are considered benign but this designation should not mislead clinicians into the belief that these tumors are all innocuous.

Grades 3 and 4 astrocytomas are considered malignant. Criteria of malignancy are based on further increase in cell size, thicker fibrous proliferation, and more intense hyperchromatic appearance of cell nuclei: in short, there is increased anaplasia and pleomorphism (Fig. 190). Mitotic activity and giant cells first appear in these more malignant grades. A compensatory increase in vascular tissue is evident and perivascular rosettes and zones of necrosis may be found within the tumor. Metastasis from neoplasms of any of the grades is exceptional.

Several components are involved in the growth and expansion of these tumors. Initially there is simple hyperplasia of astrocytes and an increase in size and thickness of the associated fibrillary processes. Because mitosis is scarce in most specimens this cellular proliferation within the nerve must be very slow. Gradually the pial covering of the nerve is penetrated and beyond this barrier the texture of the neoplasm is looser. Arachnoid and connective tissue adjacent to the expanding tumor undergo reactive proliferation, often called collateral hyperplasia (Fig. 191). This collateral hyperplasia may alter the diameter, length, and microscopic appearance of the tumor. When the tumor originates in the intracranial portion of the optic nerve, arachnoidal proliferation along the nearby sphenoid ridge may be so great as to suggest meningioma. As growth continues the dural covering of the nerve finally is stretched, but dura is not invaded as with meningioma.

Grossly, such growth usually causes a smooth-surfaced, bulbous, fusiform, or spindle-shaped enlargement of the optic nerve between eyeball and optic foramen (Figs. 192 and 193). Cross section of such a mass shows that the central, more solid, intraneural portion of the tumor tends to be gray as contrasted to the white, more loosely textured, extraneural portion of the growth (Fig. 194). Occasionally, growth of the tumor is asymmetric in relation to the nerve. In such cases the nerve, almost normal in appearance, passes tangentially along one surface of the mass.

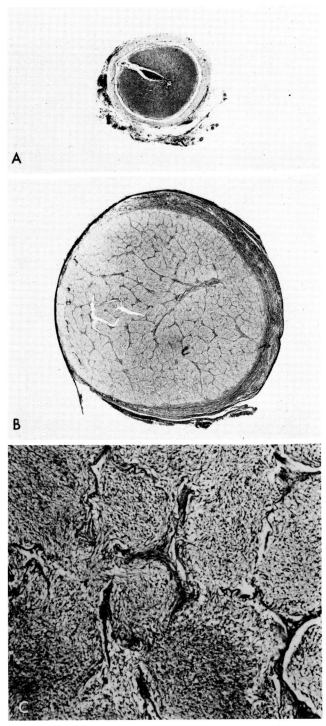

Figure 188. Comparison of normal optic nerve astrocytoma. *A*, Normal optic nerve: note diameter and arrangement of nerve fascicles. (Hematoxylin and eosin; × 6.) *B*, Optic nerve astrocytoma, grade 1: compared with *A* (at same magnification), enlargement of nerve is marked; this is symmetric and reflected in increased thickness of individual nerve fascicles. (Hematoxylin and eosin; × 6.) *C*, Optic nerve astrocytoma, grade 1: diagnosis is based also upon demonstration of increased numbers of astrocytes within nerve; appreciable anaplasia and pleomorphism are absent. (Hematoxylin and eosin; × 65.)

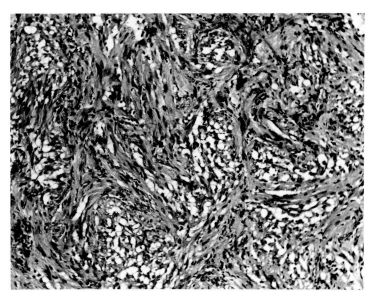

Figure 189. Optic nerve astrocytoma, grade 2: neoplasm is more cellular and cytoplasmic processes are coarser, imparting more fibrous appearance. Less dense microcystic areas are evident. (Hematoxylin and eosin; × 100.)

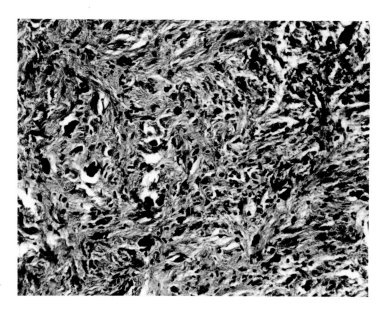

Figure 190. Optic nerve astrocytoma, grade 3: increased cellularity and, more significantly, cellular anaplasia and pleomorphism; mitosis can be found in this section. Irregular-shaped, amorphous, dense-staining structures are Rosenthal fibers. (Hematoxylin and eosin; × 55.)

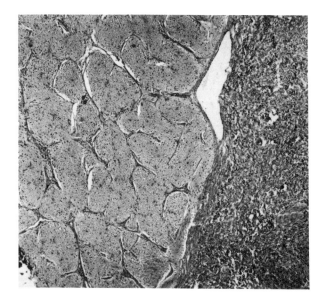

Figure 191. Collateral hyperplasia: secondary proliferation, about optic nerve, of arachnoid cells and connective tissue that is not part of optic nerve glioma. (Hematoxylin and eosin; × 40.)

TREATMENT AND PROGNOSIS

In this text, discussion of treatment and prognosis will be chiefly centered on the tumor as it affects the intra-orbital portion of the optic nerve. Perusal of the literature suggests three possible choices of management. The first is conservative. This entails *observation* of the patient with a diagnosis either based on clinical judgement, positive neurologic evidence or surgical biopsy of a small piece of tumor. The second possibility is *radiotherapy*, the diagnosis again being based on either of the above methods. The third approach would be *surgery*, in an effort to remove the tumor. All three methods have their staunch advocates and, in each, case records can be cited to support the favored approach.

This variance in methods of treatment should alert the reader immediately to a possible difficulty in predicting the behavior and course of an optic nerve glioma. The one factor common to the majority of gliomas is their exceedingly slow, and sometime unpredictable, rate of growth. An observer therefore should

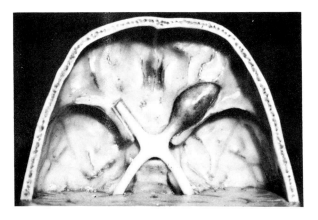

Figure 192. Model of typical glioma of orbital portion of optic nerve.

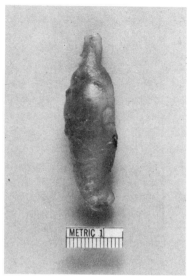

Figure 193. Optic nerve astrocytoma, grade 1: fusiform enlargement of right optic nerve in 2-year-old girl who had had lateral deviation of right eye for 6 months; papilledema and proptosis had been observed for 2 months before operation.

scrutinize closely the stated interval of follow-up study in any report. Any retrospective study not based on a period of follow-up observation of 15 years or more is subject to some reservation as to the true efficacy of the recommended management; many published reports suffer this deficiency. Had some patients been followed for a few more years the outcome might have been different from that based on a shorter interval of observation. A case reported by Donahue (1955) illustrates some of these points. A 3-year-old girl underwent enucleation of one eye with its attached tumor because of glioma of the optic nerve. A little more than 1 year later, recurrence was evident from extrusion of the implant placed in the orbit at the time of the first operation. Exenteration was performed. About 21 years then elapsed before the patient returned with a second recurrence. By this time the tumor had reached the size of a tennis ball and filled the orbital cavity. However, this mass was neither biopsied nor surgically

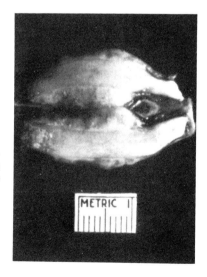

Figure 194. Optic nerve astrocytoma: on cut section, central portion of nerve is still somewhat preserved; neoplasm has extended extraneurally along sheath structures.

removed, so histologic diagnosis is lacking. Also, it is possible the mass was a collateral hyperplasia of the arachnoid at the stump of the sectioned nerve. Such hyperplasia would not be considered a true tumor recurrence. The long interval between exenteration and presumed recurrence also illustrates the indolent but persistent nature of some of these tumors. This patient did not seem in the least incapacitated by local growth of the tumor, a point that might support a more conservative attitude toward treatment. Finally, the case illustrates lack of metastasis of this tumor. Spencer (1972) noted a case of A.R. Irvine in which an optic nerve glioma was excised from the chiasm to the point of entry of the central retinal artery. The tumor recurred after 7 years, 2 years thereafter, a third time in another 3 years, and a fourth time the following year.

Other, more secondary, factors also should be considered in selecting a plan of management. Features such as *proptosis*, degree of *visual loss*, *age* of patient, and *histopathologic grading* of the tumor should be examined against the background of probable slow course of the tumor. We believe a child with progressive proptosis is of more concern to anxious parents than a child otherwise afflicted with a similar tumor but without proptosis. Persistent proptosis is not only a cosmetic liability to a female child but a source of guilt for the parents if some treatment is not attempted. Since proptosis is a positive sign of the intraorbital position of the tumor, surgical removal may be recommended, particularly if loss of vision has been established or pallor of the optic disk is present. On the other hand, some parents might rather procrastinate if radiologic proof of intracanalicular spread is lacking and there is no assurance that vision will be improved by surgical management. The attitude and role of the parents toward the child's glioma is seldom discussed in the literature as a factor in management.

What of visual failure? Many recommend a conservative approach so long as useful vision remains in the affected eye and strongly disapprove of removal of the optic nerve unless the eye is blind. Here, age of the patient is another determinant, for adults are more likely to favor such a nonsurgical approach until vision is more seriously compromised. Children have less say about the problem and, furthermore, loss of vision usually is much more advanced than in adults when the tumor is discovered. Sometimes the debate is settled by an increased proptosis which tips the scales in favor of surgery.

The meaning of the histopathologic designation *benign astrocytoma* or *juvenile pilocytic astrocytoma* should be considered. We already have remarked that this term is reserved for astrocytomas, grades 1 and 2. Most reports that recommend a conservative approach stress the benign appearance of the intraorbital glioma. But the histologic appearance of this tumor does not necessarily assure the clinician the tumor will behave in this manner. The appearance of the tumor and the actual realities of its growth are two different facts. Surveys that stress the benign behavior of gliomas tend to gloss over the fact that children succumb to this tumor, even when the tumor is considered benign. Parents who have watched their children die, while a program of watchful observation is being followed, find it exceedingly difficult to believe that the tumor was as benign as they were originally informed.

Three of our 17 children died because of intracranial extension of a grade 1 or 2 astrocytoma. One, a boy 2 months of age at the time of attempted surgical removal, died less than 1 year after exploration. Another boy had been treated with radium at the age of 2 years because of optic nerve glioma. By the age of 12 years progressive proptosis was so disfiguring that partial excision of the tumor was performed for cosmetic reasons. The tumor was a grade 1 astrocytoma. Within 4 years the patient died from intracranial spread. The third patient, a lad of almost 3 years at the time of subtotal removal of tumor, died a little more than 3 years later from extension.

Such events do not necessarily mean that surgery is positively better than conservative waiting. However, parents seem more willing to accept the finality of death if removal of tumor is attempted as contrasted to nonsurgical observation. They frequently rationalize the tragedy by remarking that everything possible was done, and we agree.

The next question is whether complete removal always is mandatory or whether incomplete resection, sometimes easier to perform is equally satisfactory. Well-documented instances of long-term survival after incomplete removal of tumor have been recorded., How may this be explained? One possibility is that the tumor is larger than its neoplastic core because of a surrounding meningeal gliomatosis (collateral hyperplasia). Section may pass through this peripheral zone of reactive hyperplasia and thus removal appears to be incomplete, but the plane of section still is beyond the active nucleus of growth. This also possibly explains roentgenographic evidence of enlargement of the optic foramen in cases of intraorbital glioma in which tumor was removed through a lateral orbital approach without subsequent recurrence. Here, the enlarged foramen was secondary to collateral hyperplasia and not due to actual extension of tumor into the intracanalicular portion of the optic canal. Still, this explanation does not satisfy all situations. We must assume that spontaneous arrest occurs in some cases following surgery or that the tumor had reached a stage of self-limited growth prior to surgery. Since it is not possible to predict such a fortuitous event, the surgeon should strive for total removal if at all possible.

What of the survivors? Their course and management is summarized in Table 14. Those patients whose tumor was of such size and extent as to permit total removal have done well and are free of recurrence in the stated follow-up interval. Those patients whose tumor was too extensive to permit total removal have done less well. Two of these patients are having problems related to intracranial spread of the tumor. The one remaining patient whose tumor was partially excised has lived 6 postoperative years without recurrence. Although tumor was identified at the proximal end of the nerve section no gross tumor was visible beyond the line of surgical dissection. Although this was classified as a partial excision it is possible that surgical removal was total.

Among the survivors, there were all degrees and ranges of proptosis and loss of vision before operation. In some, the proptosis was minimal but the visual loss severe. In others, proptosis was marked but signs such as visual impairment, papilledema, and pallor of disk were disproportionately less marked. The duration of the tumor could not be assessed in some of the very young. The factor, then, that seemed to influence the prognosis to the greatest degree was the position, extent, and resectability of the tumor. In all surviving patients the intraorbital glioma was approached through the transcranial route.

TABLE 14.   SURVIVING CASES OF ORBITAL OPTIC NERVE GLIOMA

Sex and age (yr.) at time of surgical diagnosis	Treatment	Follow-up observation (yr.)	Remarks
M, 11	Biopsy and irradiation	6	Spread to chiasm. Light perception affected eye
F, 4	Partial excision, irradiation	22	Intracranial recurrences. Under treatment for convulsive disorder
F, 2	Complete excision	3	No recurrence
F, 8	Complete excision	15	No recurrence
M, 4	Complete excision	17	No recurrence
F, 2	Complete excision	21	No recurrence
F, 21	Complete excision	18	No recurrence
M, 7	Partial excision, irradiation	6	Eye blind. No recurrence
M, 12	Complete excision	11	No recurrence
F, 12	Complete excision	8	No recurrence
F, 12	Complete excision	2	No recurrence
F, 46	Complete excision	8	No recurrence
F, 5	Complete excision	7	No recurrence
F, 5	Complete excision	10	No recurrence
F, 2	Complete excision	5	No recurrence
F, 13	Complete excision	17	No recurrence

Although sacrifice of the intraorbital portion of the optic nerve is the expected consequence of complete removal of an optic nerve glioma, many surgeons attempt to preserve the eye as a cosmetic appendage. Such an orphaned eye may be a more suitable appendage than an artificial eye for some time. An attempt to preserve the eye was made in twelve of the patients in Table 14 who had a complete removal of their tumor. Nine of the twelve still retained the blind eye at the time of the last follow-up observation. In the remaining three patients the eye was enucleated for cosmetic reasons.

Debate about the proper surgical approach to intraorbital gliomas would fill many a page of print. These tumors may be removed through either transfrontal craniotomy or lateral orbitotomy. Some cases without enlargement of the optic canal are approached routinely, as are other orbital tumors, through a lateral route. For those cases showing roentgenographic evidence of an enlarged optic foramen on presurgical assessment, we recommend transfrontal exploration. Our only preference for route is influenced by cosmetic considerations. If the tumor can be delivered without removal of the orbital roof, downward displacement of the remaining blind eye after the operation is likely to be less. We have observed both gratifying success and disappointing failure with each method.

We do not believe that radiotherapy is indicated for the orbital type of optic nerve glioma.

NEUROEPITHELIOMA

It is embarrassing not to know with certainty the meaning of the tumor about to be discussed. We refer to the term *neuroepithelioma*. We are not alone in this respect because neuropathologists, who might be expected to have some agreement on the subject, seem equally confused. In one text on neuropathology, neuroepithelioma is used only as a synonym for retinoblastoma, a usage not common in ophthalmology for many years. Another text states the majority of cases given the name of neuroepithelioma are probably ependymomas. Other neuropathologists disagree with this concept and prefer to reserve neuroepithelioma as a designation for the most undifferentiated tumor of neuronal elements, rather than the primitive tumor of glialepithelial (ependymoma) lineage. Those who agree the name is most appropriate for a type of neuronal tumor disagree as to whether it is a separate entity. Some believe the neuroepithelioma is the most undifferentiated form of the family of tumors whose other members are *neuroblastoma* and the more differentiated *ganglioneuroma*. Others reduce the family to two tumors, ganglioneuroma and neuroblastoma, but use neuroepithelioma synonymously with the latter term. Our only reasons for mentioning this problem are as preparation for the discussion of neuroblastoma and ganglioneuroma and to note an orbital case of neuroepithelioma reported by Howard (1965).

The only basic agreement in the disagreement above is that neuroepithelioma is probably the most undifferentiated of the tumors derived from the primitive neuroepithelium of the neural tube. It is in this context that Howard reports his case, a curiosity in the ophthalmic literature. The patient was an eight-month-old boy with a mass in the right inferior orbit that proved to be multilobular on excision. The tumor recurred, finally metastasized, and the patient died 14 months after the first surgical procedure. Exenteration and radiation therapy were of no avail.

Microscopically, the tumor was composed of small, oval almost cuboid cells with basophilic cytoplasm and indistinct cell borders. In areas where tumor infiltrated orbital tissue the cells grew in cords and islands suggestive of carcinoma (Fig. 195). In other areas of less constricted growth the cells may grow in a monocellular membrane around clear spaces without formation of neurites (Fig. 196). The latter is a principal differential feature from the rosettes seen in neuro-

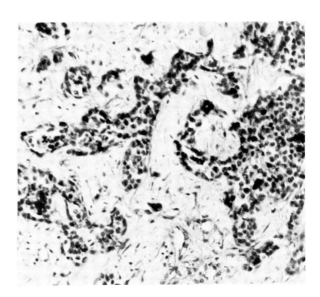

Figure 195. Neuroepithelioma: tumor infiltrated the surrounding fibrous tissues in cords, mimicking the type of growth noted in some carcinomas.

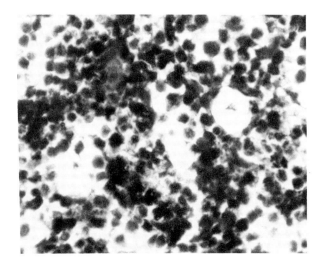

Figure 196. Neuroepithelioma: a cellular area of tumor which showed no formation of neurites by the cells around the central clear lumina. (Both Figures 195 and 196 reproduced from Howard GM: Neuroepithelioma of the orbit. Am J Ophthalmol 59:934–937, 1965. By permission.)

blastoma. Zones of necrosis were present in the tumor and atypical mitoses were commensurate with the malignant character of the tumor.

NEUROBLASTOMA

This is a malignant neoplasm of primitive neuroblasts normally destined to form the sympathetic nervous system and ganglia. It is considered a very undifferentiated neoplasm, but on the ladder of cell differentiation it is one rung above the preceding neuroepithelioma. In several respects it is the peripheral nervous system counterpart of retinoblastoma. These tumors, with few exceptions, involve the orbit as metastatic neoplasms.

Neuroblastoma was the name proposed by Wright, a Boston pathologist, in 1910. The problem of how to classify this fatal neoplasm in an earlier era is illustrated by the remarks of Dalton, who reported one of the first cases in 1885. He speculated that the disease might be a type of sarcoma, an exaggeration or diffuse form of "leucocythaemia," or some unusual manifestation of syphilis. Wright proposed that the sympathogonia, the primitive sympathetic cells, gave origin to these tumors. This viewpoint subsequently was supported by other pathologists, though as more cases were observed, some variations from the histopathologic picture described by Wright were noted.

In 1927 came the startling report of Cushing and Wolbach, who described the case of an adolescent boy in whom a tumor removed during laminectomy proved to be ganglioneuroma, a benign tumor composed of more mature sympathetic ganglia. This boy had been operated on elsewhere 10 years previously for the same paravertebral tumor, but at this time the mass had been considered to be a sarcoma. Review of the histologic specimens taken during the first operation indicated that the tumor was an example of Wright's neuroblastoma. This confirmed the differentiation of an immature malignant neuroblastoma into a benign mature ganglioneuroma, an observation since corroborated by others. This suggested also a correlation between the histologic appearance of the tumor and the clinical course.

INCIDENCE

Neuroblastoma is second to rhabdomyosarcoma as the most frequent malignant tumor affecting the orbit of infants and children. The occurrence of neuroblastoma in the orbit is sufficiently frequent (though not common) that most ophthalmologists are aware of the possibilities of the neoplasm in an infant or child with either unilateral or bilateral proptosis. Also, this aspect of the neoplasm is given full coverage in most ophthalmic texts.

In the period of our survey, 11 neuroblastomas were observed among a total of 764 orbital tumors, an incidence of 1.4%. This agrees closely with the incidences of 1.6% (14 neuroblastomas among a total of 877 orbital tumors) and 1.1% (6 neuroblastomas among 504 consecutive orbital lesions in the 1963 and 1971 surveys of Reese, respectively. Other surveys in the pediatric and ophthalmic literature relate the ratio of orbital metastasis to the total number of cases of neuroblastoma in a given period. In one of the larger studies of this type, Albert, Rubenstein, and Scheie (1967) found orbital metastasis in 41 of 108 patients with neuroblastoma, an incidence of 38%. This exceeds the incidence given by Stowens (1957) among 105 cases (incidence, 17%), and that from our own 11 cases occurring among 75 patients with neuroblastoma (incidence 11%). Pocheldy (1976) points out that frequency of orbital metastasis varies according to primary site of the neoplasm. In his study of 64 patients with abdominal neuroblastoma, incidence of orbital involvement was 45% (29 patients), whereas, if the primary site was in the thoracic sympathetic chain, orbital metastasis dropped to 14% (2 of 14 patients).

Neuroblastoma is mainly a disease of infants and children, and the neoplasm may be present even at birth. Nelson, Vaughan, and McKay (1969) estimated that 25% of patients with neuroblastoma will have initial manifestations during the first year of life and 75% before the age of 5. Bodian (1959) estimated the incidence of initial symptoms to be as high as 40% in the first year of life, and Dargeon (1962) gave 60% as the incidence of initial symptoms during the first 4 years of life. Exelby's (1978) estimates were 50% of cases under age 2 and 75% under age 4 at time of diagnosis. It is less well known that neuroblastoma also may occur in adolescents and in adults, but orbital symptoms in these older patients are much less frequent. In view of the frequency of orbital involvement in the very young, it is curious that intraocular invasion is so rare.

In most surveys, sex distribution of the neoplasm is approximately equal, and there seem to be no familial trends. Neither does the metastasis seem to favor one orbit over the other. At one time it was believed that orbital metastasis would occur on the side ipsilateral to the primary growth, but further scrutiny of a large number of cases has not confirmed this selectivity. The frequency of bilateral orbital involvement is noteworthy. Albert and associates found the ratio of bilateral to unilateral orbital metastasis to approximate 4:3.

Several authors also have contended that neuroblastoma is primary in the orbit, but most of the authors' claims have not been supported by autopsy reports in the exclusion of more common primary growths in the cervical, thoracic, or abdominal portions of the sympathetic chain. Levy (1957) believes that his case (a 3-year-old boy) was an example of neuroblastoma primary in the orbit and cited autopsy findings to confirm his reasoning. Presumably these neuroblastomas primary in the orbit arise in the ciliary ganglion.

CLINICAL FEATURES

Neuroblastoma most often reaches the orbit as a colony of cells that have metastasized from a primary locus either in the retroperitoneal area of the abdomen or from a zone adjacent to the adrenal gland. As a rule, there are some simultaneous metastases to bones of the skull; should such a route of spread involve the orbital portions of the malar and maxillary bones, there might be some argument whether the neoplasm is located principally in the soft tissues of the orbit or whether the tumor has invaded the orbital space secondarily from adjacent bone. In practice, it makes little difference because the orbital signs of this rapidly growing neoplasm in each case are closely similar, except for some variation in direction of displacement of the eye. Some ocular signs also may accompany a neuroblastoma whose growth is primary in the neck. A syndrome similar to Horner's on the ipsilateral side particularly should, in the absence of other orbital pathology, alert the examiner to possible new growths in the cervical region among this group of patients.

In patients with metastases to the soft tissues of the orbit or to adjacent bone (Fig. 197), the initial manifestations usually will be observed either as abnormalities in the eyelids or as alterations in the position of the eye. The orbital neoplasm may grow so rapidly that proptosis and changes in the adnexa, such as the eyelids, may occur almost simultaneously or within a few days of one another. Edema, swelling, or puffiness of one of more eyelids often is the first indication of disorder. Redness and swelling may suggest an inflammatory lesion, but an increase in local heat or induration, typical of orbital cellulitis, is lacking. The clinical picture at this stage may resemble rhabdomyosarcoma primary in the orbit (see also Figs. 308 and 309, Chapter 19), but a rhabdomyosarcoma usually feels firmer than a neuroblastoma. Instead of appearing inflamed, the eyelids may appear ecchymotic (Fig. 198; compare with Fig. 309, Chapter 19). The latter feature is more common in cases of neuroblastoma than rhabdomyosarcoma but it also may be seen in the leukemias. Ecchymosis is secondary to necrosis and hemorrhage within the tumor. In general, these early changes in the eyelids are quite similar for the several types of malignant neoplasms of the orbit in infants and children. The problem is not so much to differentiate these several neoplasms on the basis of the appearance of the orbital adnexa as to make the diagnosis of a serious malignancy rather than an inflammatory disorder.

The proptosed eye may be displaced in any direction; it will be straightforward if the neoplasm has lodged in the soft tissues of the posterior orbit, or to one side or another in a direction opposite to a metastatic colony contiguous to the orbital bony wall. As the eye becomes displaced, the epibulbar tissues become chemotic and congested, further delineating the picture suggestive of inflammation. The eye also becomes increasingly immobile.

Such a clinical picture is observed more often among those patients in whom the orbital metastasis either is the presenting symptom of a hidden primary tumor elsewhere or has occurred very early during the growth of an abdominal mass. When orbital metastases develop late in the course of neoplastic dissemination the child usually has become so ill and anemic that the adnexal tissues do not respond to the challenge of an invasive malignancy by an

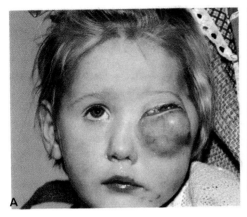
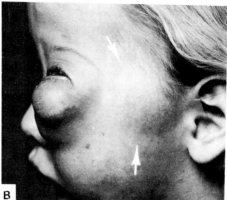

Figure 197. Orbital neuroblastoma: *A*, Frontal view showing progressive swelling of left lower eyelid and palpable mass in inferior orbit (duration, only 2 months). *B*, Side view showing additional mass of neuroblastoma (*arrows*) along lateral aspect of left orbit (duration, 1 month). The orbital portion of the zygomatic bone is a frequent locus for metastatic neuroblastoma.

inflammatory type of response. Instead, the ecchymosis is superimposed on pale, edematous eyelids and there is an associated boggy chemosis.

Other ocular changes, such as impairment of vision, corneal desiccation, papilledema, dilatation of retinal veins, and the formation of retinal striae, have received scattered mention in the numerous case reports in the literature, but such alterations are not specific for the tumor. They are so overshadowed in practice by orbital and adnexal changes that they are much less important in either diagnosis or management. All these ocular and orbital changes become manifest over a period of several weeks; the rate of progression is so rapid and alarming that 4 or 6 weeks seldom elapse before the child sees a physician. In their study of 108 cases of neuroblastoma, Albert, Rubenstein and Scheie (1967) noted that orbital metastasis occurred at an average interval of 3 months after diagnosis of the primary locus of malignancy. Only in a minority of these cases (2.8%) did orbital metastasis precede discovery of the primary neuroblastoma.

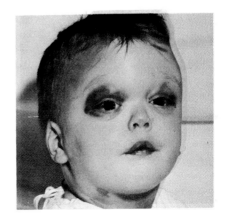

Figure 198. Metastatic neuroblastoma: bilateral ecchymosis of eyelids with asymmetric proptosis (R > L). (Courtesy, Dr. E. O. Burgert, Jr.)

In those few patients in whom orbital metastasis is the initial manifestation of a still undiscovered or unrecognized neuroblastoma, it behooves the ophthalmologist to know some of the common systemic manifestations of the disease. First, these children are sick. They may have varying degrees of pallor, irritability, weakness, fever and malaise. Limping, or pain on walking, or general body aching is a very frequent clinical feature. Because metastases to the skull often occur at about the same time as orbital metastasis, the child may have some enlargement of the skull with dilated veins coursing over soft lumps scattered around the cranium. If palpation of the abdomen is equivocal the consulting pediatrician may suggest orbitotomy rather than abdominal exploration as the easier method of establishing a histopathologic diagnosis. A useful test is the chemical analysis of the urine to determine the excretion of catecholamines, which is increased in cases of neuroblastoma. Of the catecholamines, the metabolites 4-hydroxy-3-methoxyphenylacetic acid (homovanillic acid, HVA), 3-methoxy-4-hydroxyphenylethyleneglycol (HMPG), and 4-hydroxy-3-methoxymandelic acid (vanilmandelic acid, VMA) are the most conspicuous.

ROENTGENOGRAPHIC CHANGES

Several radiographic features are suggestive of neuroblastoma, and these may be most helpful if an obvious tumor is not palpable or visible. Among these, changes in the roentgenographic appearance of the skull are quite common and of interest to ophthalmologists. Phillips (1953) has estimated that metastasis to the cranium occurs in 74% of cases. Alfano (1968), in his study of 29 neuroblastomas with ophthalmologic signs, found that approximately 65% showed radiographic changes in the skull or orbit. In these areas evidence of both destructive and reactive lesions in bone may be seen and, when accompanied by sutural separation (Fig. 199), the picture is almost pathognomonic. The zygoma is the bone most frequently involved in orbital metastasis. Abdominal films may reveal the primary tumor as a soft tissue mass which displaces the kidney downward and laterally. About 50% of such cases show focal areas of calcification in the areas of the adrenal gland. Skeletal surveys also may show areas of destruction alternating with zones of proliferation of new bone in the vertebrae, ribs, and long bones.

PATHOLOGY

Descriptions of these tumors as encountered in the orbit have varied. There seems to be no constant gross appearance. Levy (1957) described the tumor in his case, which was believed to be primary in the orbit, as a bluish, smooth-walled, cystic mass with a tough outer coat. Others have described the tumor as a firm, gray, vascular mass. We have found the metastatic lesion to be a rather soft, poorly circumscribed, friable neoplasm with a red-gray or bluish red color; the appearance is not unlike that of malignant lymphoma, in both children and adults, and of leukemic infiltrates in children. Some of these orbital neuroblastomas contain specks of calcium in the stroma, causing them to feel gritty when dissected. Others are somewhat cystic, with clumps of necrotic tissue mixed with clotted and semi-clotted hemorrhagic tissue.

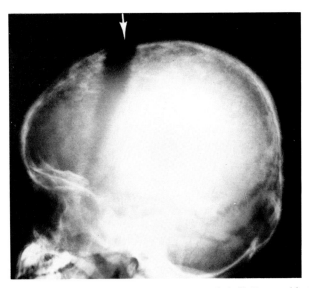

Figure 199. Metastatic neuroblastoma: roentgenogram of skull (2-year-old girl) showing wide separation of cranial suture line (*arrow*), secondary to increased intracranial pressure from growth of metastasis, and destructive and reactive lesions in skull.

In the more immature, malignant, metastatic tumor, the basic cell is an embryonal neuroblast—sometimes referred to as a *sympathoblast*. These cells are small (about the size of a lymphocyte) and round or slightly elongated, with poorly delineated cell boundaries that usually are arranged in sheets or clumps (Fig. 200). A connective tissue framework may support a group or clump of

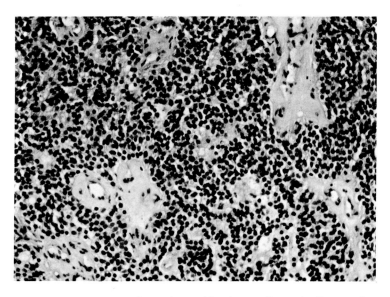

Figure 200. Neuroblastoma: embryonal neuroblast is a small round cell, generally arranged in clumps with indistinct cell boundaries. (Hematoxylin and eosin; × 165.)

cells, but connective tissue septa and stroma are not present between individual cells (Fig. 201). The nuclei are prominent, hyperchromatic, and oval and contain dense stippled chromatin. Sometimes, the cells array themselves in a ring around a central tangle of fibrillary cell processes (rosettes). These cytoplasmic fibrillary processes are analogous to the neurofibrils of more mature nerve cells. Mitotic figures are common. There is a striking tendency for these tumors to undergo necrosis.

Many tumors show features indicating some attempts toward more mature differentiation. More acellular zones in the tumor may indicate attempts to form glial tissue and, in some areas where such fibrillary matrix is present, larger and more differentiated, ganglion-like cells will be observed (Fig. 202). Such a tumor may be designated a *ganglioneuroblastoma*, or partly differentiated neuroblastoma, but this type of neoplasm still possesses nearly the same degree of malignancy in children as a less differentiated type.

COURSE AND TREATMENT

The unpredictable course (often poor but occasionally surprisingly good) and response to therapy of neuroblastoma long have intrigued physicians. Ophthalmologists chiefly are involved only with those cases that show orbital metastasis sometime during the course of neoplastic growth. Initially, some of the many variables that affect prognosis and influence treatment should be enumerated.

First, there seems to be a definite indication that the disease is less lethal in cildren under 1 year of age. Second, the anatomic site itself also may influence survival, probably because, surgically, some tumors are more approachable and, pathologically, more circumscribed. The tumors originating in areas of the

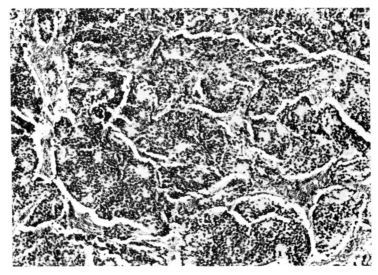

Figure 201.   Neuroblastoma: fine connective tissue septa may group cells and create an organoid appearance; within cell clumps are poorly developed rosettes. (Hematoxylin and eosin; × 100.)

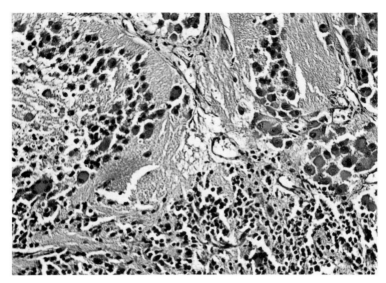

Figure 202. Ganglioneuroblastoma: immature neuroblastic cells (bottom of field) merge with variably differentiated sympathetic ganglion cells, suggesting a degree of maturation in primitive cell. (Hematoxylin and eosin; × 130.)

mediastinum and adrenal gland would be of this type. Third, the extent and location of metastasis when the patient first is seen also may alter the success of therapy. Bony metastasis, in particular, is considered to be a sign of relatively poor prognosis. Fourth, the degree of cytologic differentiation of the tumor may definitely influence rate of dissemination and ultimate course. Finally, there is the unpredictable but amazing fact that spontaneous resolution has been reported, even in cases of known metastasis.

Next, the ways in which the orbit is involved should be considered. These determine treatment. A case may fall into one of two categories.

1. *Rarely, an orbital mass is the initial and only manifestation of neuroblastoma.* Careful systemic search fails to reveal tumor elsewhere. In this case, the orbital tumor should be removed completely if possible. If its location, configuration, or size does not permit its intact removal, exenteration should be considered. In either situation supplementary chemotherapy should be attempted in the hope of eradicating any undetected dissemination. The child should be observed thereafter, but radiotherapy should be withheld until there is definite evidence of extraorbital spread.

2. *The orbit is but one of several metastatic loci,* after the primary neoplasm has been removed or treated. Then the treatment consists of irradiation to the orbit and the systemic administration of steroids, if the critical total dose of radiation has not already been reached during irradiation to other areas.

Radiotherapy

Radiation usually is given in increments that are proportional to the age of the child. Larger doses of radiation are given to older children, not only because their tissues are more mature and more tolerant to such dosages but also because the prognosis of neuroblastoma in these patients is poorer. In general, the dosage is as follows: For youngsters under 1 year of age, a total of 1,000 to 1,500 R, in daily amounts of 100 to 200 R; for patients age 1, a similar program, but with a total dose of 2,000 R; for patients in the 2- to 3-year age group, a total dose of 2,400 R, over a period of 2 to 3 weeks; and as the child matures, further increases in dosage to a maximum dose of about 4,000 R in patients aged 9 to 16 years.

Chemotherapy

Of the several chemical agents that have been tried, vincristine sulfate, dactinomycin, chlorambucil, methotrexate, triethylenemelamine, adriamycin, and cyclosphosphamide are currently the most widely used. These potent drugs are given intravenously. They may have serious side effects, and their administration is not in the field of the ophthalmologist. The dosage schedule and the most effective combination of these agents have not been standardized.

Whether radiotherapy or chemotherapy is used alone or in combination, the child's progress may be judged not only by the clinical response but also by the measurement of urinary catecholamines. In patients who respond satisfactorily to treatment, the urinary excretion of catecholamines is likely to decrease; but later, if the concentration of catecholamines in the urine either suddenly increases or does not decrease progressively over a period of weeks, further therapy is likely to be needed.

Before 1940, the prognosis of neuroblastoma was considered hopeless — except for those almost miraculous instances of spontaneous resolution. The latter probably came about either because of necrosis (the neoplasm having outgrown its blood supply) or because of cellular differentiation to a less malignant or a benign type of sympathetic nerve tumor, such as Cushing and Wolbach (1927) described. As time has passed, survival rates have improved. Most prognostic surveys in the literature are based on 2-year intervals following diagnosis and treatment. If the child survived that long a cure seemed likely. In Bodian's series (1959) of 129 cases in the period 1925 to 1958, the survival rate was 33%. Among the fatal cases, death occurred within 6 months in more than 60% of the total, and within 1 year in 99%. In Alfano's (1968) smaller series (53 cases), the survival rate was 45.2%. This survival rate seems rather high on the basis of our own clinical observations. Nelson, Vaughan, and McKay (1969) estimated an overall survival rate of 35%. All these survival rates must be analyzed further according to patient age, because survival rates seem higher in younger infants.

Another means of judging prognosis is the hypothesis of Collins, Loeffler, and Tivey (1956). They accounted for the age of the child at discovery of the tumor and offered a less arbitrary basis for estimating prognosis than the 2-year cure interval. These authors assumed that each tumor has a constant rate of growth which is equated in terms of its "doubling time"; they also assumed that childhood tumors like neuroblastoma begin their growth at or near the time of conception. Thus, the tumor already is 9 months old at or near the time of birth. In a theoretical case, if the patient is 6 months old at the time the neoplasm is discovered, the age of the tumor would be 15 months (6 + 9). If treatment is effective in eradicating all but one tumor cell, then the remaining cell possesses the potential to grow at a constant rate and, consequently, the tumor should again appear by the time the patient is twice as old plus 9 months. In this theoretical case, cure would be achieved if the child reached the age of 21 months (doubling the postnatal age of 6 months, at which time the tumor was discovered, plus 9 months) and was free of disease. However, if this concept of doubling time is applied to an older child who is 2 years old when the tumor is first discovered, then before cure is pronounced, it is necessary to wait until another 2 years and also 9 months have elapsed — in other words, until the child is 4 years and 9 months of age.

From our limited clinical experience with neuroblastoma having orbital involvement, we have formed the impression that orbital metastasis indicates a poor prognosis. Albert, Rubenstein, and Scheie (1967) found that the survival period after orbital metastasis averaged 3½ months (range, 2 weeks to 24 months). Present-day chemotherapy probably has lengthened the average survival interval but cure remains an elusive goal.

GANGLIONEUROMA

The ganglioneuroma is the most mature member of the group of tumors originating from sympathetic cells that normally are destined to form sympathetic ganglia. The well-differentiated form of the tumor is benign and encapsulated. The principal histopathologic features are a mixture of mature ganglion cells and glial tissue (Fig. 203). As was noted in the earlier part of this chapter, tumors whose origins are traced to sympathicoblasts may vary greatly in their

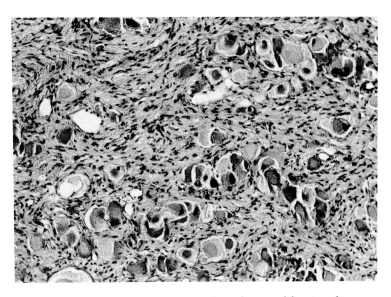

Figure 203.   Ganglioneuroma: this benign neoplasm shows proliferation of mature sympathetic ganglion cells. (Hematoxylin and eosin; × 110.)

cellular composition and degree of differentiation. For this reason some ganglio-neuromas show a mixture of less mature cells and such tumors are capable of metastasis. Such neoplasms really are less malignant neuroblastomas; perhaps it is better to designate such pleomorphic sympathetic cell tumors as well-differ-entiated neuroblastomas, so as not to confuse them with the nonmetastatic ganglioneuromas. Theoretically, ganglioneuromas might arise in the orbit in the area of the ciliary ganglion but no proven cases have been reported. Walsh and Hoyt (1969) recorded a case of possible ganglioneuroma of the orbit in an infant boy who, at 2 months of age, was first noted to have progressive painless en-largement of the right anterior cervical nodes. At 1½ years of age, a mass in the left thigh was biopsied, and a diagnosis of metastatic tumor of neurogenic origin was made. At age two, 17 mm of proptosis of the right eye was recorded, but no histologic examination of the orbital mass was made. Subsequently, the cervical masses were biopsied with a diagnosis of ganglioneuroma. It is likely this case is an example of a neuroblastoma that underwent maturation (a not infrequent occurrence) to a ganglioneuroma, with metastases occurring to the orbit and thigh sometime during its less differentiated stage. Toppozada (1958) reported a 4-year-old girl with a proven ganglioneuroma of a maxillary sinus that caused pressure destruction of the upper maxilla with secondary involvement of the orbit. The origin of the tumor was along the infraorbital nerve.

CHEMODECTOMA

This is a neoplasia of neuronal cells and supporting tissues of the para-sympathetic nervous system. Theoretically, these tumors may arise in the orbit from the ciliary ganglion; clinically, they are usually found attached to one of the extraocular muscles. Morphologically similar tumors are found in the carotid body (their most common site), the ganglion nodosum of the vagus nerve, the glomus jugulare, and the parasympathetic cells in the adventitia of the aortic arch (aortic bodies).

These tumors are a subclass of *paragangliomas* in the sense that tumors of parasympathetic structures usually are divided into two groups on the basis of their histochemical differences. Paraganglionic cells of one type contain chromaffin granules. This chromaffin material is involved in the production of norepinephrine and epinephrine, and such tumors are hormonally active. These parasympathetic tumors usually occur in association with the visceral sympa-thetic chain and are of no concern to the orbit. They are named *pheochromo-cytomas* or *chromaffinomas* to differentiate them from hormonally inert tumors the *nonchromaffin paragangliomas*. Terminology becomes more complex if the latter neoplasms are further subdivided into benign and malignant subclasses based on the belief that both types are variants of the same tumor. However, malignant transformation of a benign nonchromaffin paraganglioma seldom is observed, and other pathologists are reluctant to call the malignant variant a paraganglioma. Our choice of the name, *chemodectoma*, was made to avoid this confusion and to make clear that our discussion will be limited to the benign, encapsulated, nonchromaffin form of paraganglioma. Discussion of the malignant paradigm will be deferred to Chapter 23.

INCIDENCE

Those reports of nonchromaffin paraganglioma in the literature which seem to reflect the picture of a well-differentiated, well-circumscribed chemodectoma are those of Tye (1961), Fisher and Hazard (1952), Hughes and Ambrose (1944), Deutsch and Duckworth (1969), Thacker and Duckworth (1969), Goder (1970), and Zawirska and Drozdowska (1970). Two of these reports seem to refer to the same patient, so the final total is six patients. All but one were females, and the age range was 4 to 55 years. We have not seen an orbital chemodectoma in the 27-year period of our study, and these tumors are rarely mentioned in most orbital tumor surveys.

The case of Lattes and associates (1954) may or may not belong to this group. A 35-year-old man had had a tumor in the area of the right neck for 15 years. A few months before surgical exploration, proptosis of the right eye and a definite bulging of the right temporal area were observed. A diagnosis of carotid body tumors was made after biopsy of the neck and orbital masses. The patient died within 2 years of surgical intervention because of continued growth of the mass in the neck. The authors believed the neck and orbital masses represented multicentric foci of paraganglioma rather than metastasis of the neck tumor to the orbit. In their histologic description of the tumor they noted occasional "round empty spaces" amidst the organoid clusters of cells, a feature similar to descriptions of the alveolar-like component of soft part sarcomas. Because of its long duration in the neck the tumor might be considered benign, but the orbital mass was of shorter duration and seemed more aggressive in growth. Perhaps this case represents a tumor that underwent malignant change during its growth. All remaining reports of nonchromaffin paraganglioma in the literature describe malignant, destructive, and often fatal tumors. These will be noted again in Chapter 23.

CLINICAL FEATURES

Several features in the above case reports might alert the clinician to a possible chemodectoma during the preoperative assessment. In three of the six cases the tumor was attached to one of the extraocular muscles. Such a tumor will move in the same direction as the proptosed eye moves, or become invisible in the conjunctival fornix as the eye rotates in extreme gaze into the orbital quadrant opposite the tumor. The vascular nature of the tumor is suggested by the throbbing orbital pain of one patient and an arcade of dilated conjunctival vessels overlying the orbital position of the mass in another patient. In the latter, the clinical picture closely resembled cavernous hemangioma. The case of Zawirska and Drozdowska had a noteworthy feature. A 33-year-old woman had a recurrent chemodectoma removed 20 years after an initial incomplete excision. Neither tumor infiltration nor metastasis was found at time of the second surgical procedure. Chemodectomas also may arise in the nasal passage and invade the orbit secondarily.

PATHOLOGY

The tumor varies from red-brown to light tan in color and is slightly lobulated. The polygonal cells are arranged in "clusters," "islands," or "nests." The

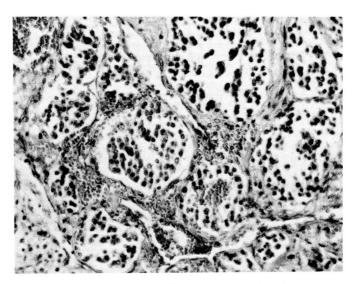

Figure 204. Chemodectoma (nonchromaffin paraganglioma): cells are arranged in clusters bounded by vascular reticulin framework. (Hematoxylin and eosin; × 245.)

terms *organoid* and *alveolar* have been used to describe this arrangement (Fig. 204). The nuclei are round or oval and somewhat vesicular. These nuclei are prominent against a background of pale, lightly eosinophilic-staining, finely granular, abundant cytoplasm. Each group or lobule of cells is surrounded by a connective tissue-reticulin framework or by sinusoidal endothelial network. Mitotic figures are quite rare.

TREATMENT

Complete removal is recommended if at all possible. There have been too few orbital cases to permit any prediction about the rate of growth or interval of recurrence after complete excision.

OLFACTORY NEUROBLASTOMA

This is a malignant tumor arising from the neurosensory receptor cells of the olfactory mucosa. It is histologically similar to several tumors already discussed in this chapter, and also arises from cells of neuroectodermal origin. This tumor is seldom discussed in the ophthalmic literature, and it is even more infrequently that an ophthalmologist participates in the management of a given case. Large or aggressive olfactory neuroblastomas may invade the orbit and it seems appropriate to discuss the tumor at this place.

In its present costume it has been known for only a little over 50 years. It was first named *esthésioneuroépithéliome olfactif* by Berger and associates (1924). A few years later a slightly different tumor was called *esthésioneurocytome olfactif*, and, still later, another histologic variant was named *esthésio-*

neuroblastome. This immediately alerts us to a tumor capable of wearing several masks and this fact, combined with its concealed location and its infrequent occurrence, has made diagnosis difficult and equivocal. We have followed the recent trend to use the noun, *neuroblastoma*, as an inclusive term for the tumor and the adjective, olfactory, to pinpoint its site of origin.

INCIDENCE

Approximately 150 cases have now been reported in the world literature but there are only a few publications that review more than 10 cases. Some of the latter are the reports of Kadish and associates (1976), Momose and associates (1978), Oberman and Rice (1976), and Djalilian and associates (1977). Even here, the frequency of olfactory neuroblastoma may not average more than one case per year over a 10- to 20-year period. However, the incidence of this tumor will increase in the future because of earlier recognition by sophisticated neuroradiologic diagnostic techniques. In the not too distant past, cases of olfactory neuroblastoma were not diagnosed in the lifetime of some individuals. A review of the world literature by Skolnik and colleagues (1966) also should be noted.

Olfactory neuroblastomas are not listed in larger surveys of orbital tumors. In the 27-year period of our study, four cases with orbital involvement were seen. This number represents an incidence of approximately 2% of all olfactory neuroblastomas seen in a similar time period at the Mayo Clinic. In the study of Momose the incidence of orbital involvement was 1.2% (3 of 25 verified olfactory neuroblastomas). The age of our patients with orbital invasion ranged from 22 to 57 years at time of histologic diagnosis. Three of these patients were female. The overall age range of patients with olfactory neuroblastoma in the world literature extends from 3 to 77 years. Some reviews say the tumor is more common in males, other reviews show a preponderance of females. When all case reports are lumped together there is probably no significant sex predominance.

CLINICAL ASPECTS

Nasal obstruction and nose bleed are the two most common symptoms of olfactory neuroblastoma. At this time the tumor may be seen high up in the nasal vault as a pinkish-grey or red, friable, polypoid mass. If the neoplasm extends posteriorly into the intracranial space, anosmia, rhinorrhea, headache, and pain will occur. A tumor that grows anteriorly may eventually cause epiphora. Orbital involvement comes late in the course of the disease and is characterized by progressive proptosis, ocular motor nerve paresis, and loss of vision. The type of orbital symptomatology will depend on whether the neoplasm invades the orbital space through the ethmoid plate or destroys bone around the apex of the orbit. The tumor will not be palpated in the orbit unless the case is very advanced.

The duration of the disease prior to orbital invasion is extremely variable. Some tumors are most aggressive, extending into the orbit within a few months after onset. Other cases are most indolent, with nasal obstruction and slight epistaxis extending over a period of many, many years before diagnosis is made.

ROENTGENOGRAPHIC CHANGES

In the early stages of the neoplasm, standard roentgenograms of the skull are usually negative. In such views erosion or destruction of bone will not be evident until the tumor invades the lateral wall of the nasal fossa or contiguous structures medial, superior, or posterior to its origin. As the situation progresses standard views also show an opacification of one of the paranasal sinuses, usually the ethmoid, owing to occlusion of the ostium of the sinus. When tomography came into routine use, bony changes could be detected at an earlier stage than was possible with routine views, but computer tomography has been the single most important refinement in noninvasive diagnosis. Computer tomography not only has permitted earlier diagnosis and treatment but outlines the extent of the tumor (Fig. 44, Chapter 2) to such a degree as to facilitate greatly the surgical approach.

PATHOLOGY

Microscopically, these tumors have quite a varied morphology, ranging from the immature neuroblast to the more differentiated, benign-appearing neurocyte. These variable features plus the presence or absence of cellular rosettes and pseudorosettes were responsible for the various names given to the tumor. Such a classification also was encouraged because of possible correlation with prognosis, but most pathologists now believe such microscopic subdivisions have no clinical value. The one feature most helpful in differentiating this neoplasm from other malignancies in a similar anatomic area is the organization of tumor cells into nests and clusters separated by vascular fibrous tissue (Fig. 205). The individual cells within these compartments are small and have hyperchromatic nuclei and scant cytoplasm such as already noted in nonolfactory neuroblastomas (Figs. 200 and 201). In more differentiated zones the cells are

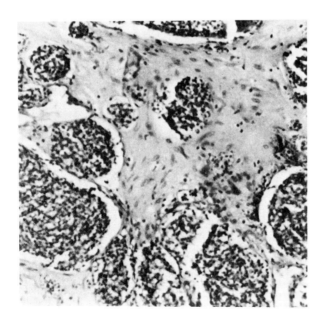

Figure 205. Olfactory neuroblastoma: tumor shows organoid pattern; islands of tumor cells separated by fibrous septae. (Hematoxylin and eosin; × 100.)

larger, with a more abundant eosinophilic cytoplasm that seems to merge into the surrounding fibrillar matrix (Fig. 206). Areas of necrosis are frequent; mitoses are infrequent.

TREATMENT AND COURSE

Although olfactory neuroblastoma is a radiosensitive neoplasm it is not radiocurable. Radiotherapy alone may prolong survival but will not prevent local destruction of bone, spread of tumor into the intracranial or retrobulbar space, or metastasis. The logical alternative is surgical excision of the tumor, with radiotherapy reserved for inoperable recurrences, primary tumors too advanced for surgical excision, and metastasis.

When surgery is undertaken the surgeon should be strongly motivated toward complete removal of all gross tumor. The more extensive the resection the less residues of tumor there will be for recurrence, and the longer the survival of the patient. Our surgical associates in this field use the rhinotomy as the preferred approach. In this procedure the nasal and lacrimal bones, orbital plate of the ethmoid, floor and anterior wall of the frontal sinus, and medial half of orbital floor are rongeured away to gain access to the tumor. For those who have not participated in the surgical attack on these tumors the description of Devine in the report of Djalilian and associates provides some inkling of the hurdles that must be overcome. Devine usually removes the cribriform plate and will pursue the tumor into the intracranial vault if necessary. Because of almost continual oozing of blood from the many areas of resected bone, the frequent lacerations of the dura, the flow of spinal fluid, and the occasional need for overlays of mucosal grafts or placement of free skin grafts, this is not an area for timid souls.

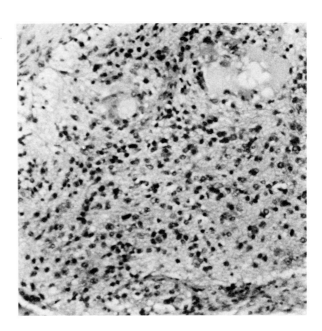

Figure 206. Olfactory neuroblastoma: tumor cells are large with abundant cytoplasm that blends imperceptibly into surrounding fibrillar matrix. (Hematoxylin and eosin; × 100.) (Both Figures 205 and 206 reproduced from Djalilian M, Zujko RD, Weiland LH, et al: Olfactory neuroblastoma. Surg Clin North Am 57:751–762, 1977. By permission.)

Just as there is a wide difference in the rate of progression prior to diagnosis, so there is considerable variation in the course of the disease after definitive excision. There are no uniform standards upon which to base a firm prognosis. Also, most case samples in the literature are too small to support meaningful statistical data. Several observers agree, however, that a follow-up interval of five years is inadequate for judging patient survival or cure. Many patients do quite well and have many useful years of life, although they are not cured of neoplasm. Even if the neoplasm recurs near its primary site another rhinotomy can be performed and the recurrence removed. A common area of metastasis is the cervical area and, in the absence of other metastases or intracranial spread, the metastasis can be debulked and the area irradiated.

No cases of spontaneous regression of this neoplasm have been reported as they have with the nonolfactory neuroblastoma.

Bibliography

Retinoblastoma

Dunphy EB: The story of retinoblastoma: the XX Edward Jackson memorial lecture. Am J Ophthalmol 58:539–552, 1964

Ellsworth RM: Orbital retinoblastoma. Trans Amer Ophthalmol Soc 72:79–88, 1974

Guinaudeau MP: Rétinoblastome de l'orbite. Bull Mem Soc Fr Ophtalmol 64:4–6, 1951

Jakobiec FA, Jones IS: Secondary and metastatic tumors of the orbit. In Clinical Ophthalmology Volume 2, Chapter 46. Ed: TD Duane. Hagerstown, Md, Harper & Row, 1976

Oliver DS: Recurrent retinoblastoma: a case with five-year survival. Am J Ophthalmol 53:376–377, 1962

Parkhill EM, Benedict WL: Gliomas of the retina: a histopathologic study. Am J Ophthalmol 24:1354–1373, 1941

Reese AB: Tumors of the Eye, Second edition. New York, Hoeber Medical Division, Harper & Row, 1963

Reese AB, Ellsworth RM: The evaluation and current concept of retinoblastoma therapy. Trans Am Acad Ophthalmol Otolaryngol 67:164–170, 1963

Rootman J, Ellsworth RM, Hofbauer J et al: Orbital extension of retinablastoma: a clinicopathological study. Can J Ophthamol 13:72–80, 1978

Taktikos A: Investigation of retinoblastoma with special references to histology and prognosis. Brit J Ophthalmol 50:225–234, 1966

Verhoeff FH: Cited in Minutes of the Proceedings. Trans Am Ophthalmol Soc 24:38–39, 1926

Wolff JA: Chemotherapy of retinoblastoma. In Jakobiec FA: Ocular and Adnexal Tumors. Chapter 16. Birmingham, Ala, Aesculapius Publishing Co, 1978

Medulloepithelioma

Andersen SR: Medulloepithelioma, diktyoma, and malignant epithelioma of the ciliary body. Acta Ophthalmol 26:313–330, 1948

Broughton WL, Zimmerman LE: A clinicopathologic study of 56 cases of intraocular medulloepithelioma. Am J Ophthalmol 85:407–418, 1978

Green WR, Iliff WJ, Trotter RR: Malignant teratoid medulloepithelioma of the optic nerve. Arch Ophthalmol 91:451–454, 1974

Malone RGS: Dictyoma. Brit J Ophthalmol 39:429–436, 1955

Reese AB: Medulloepithelioma (dictyoma) of the optic nerve. Am J Ophthalmol 44:4–6, 1957

Rubino A: I tumori della pars ciliaris retinae (dictiomi di Fuchs). Ann Ottalmol Clin Ocul 69:385–437, 1941

Zimmerman L: Verhoeff's "terato-neuroma." Am J Ophthalmol 72:1039–1057, 1971

Optic Nerve Glioma

Chutorian AM, Schwartz JF, Evans RA, et al: Optic gliomas in children. Neurology (Minneap) 14:83–95, 1964

Condon JR, Rose FG: Optic nerve glioma. Brit J Ophthalmol 51:703–706, 1967

Davis FA: Primary tumors of the optic nerve (a phenomenon of Recklinghausen's disease): a clinical and pathologic study with a report of five cases and a review of the literature. Arch Ophthalmol ns 23:735–821; 957–1018, 1940

Dodge HW Jr, Love JG, Craig WM, et al: Gliomas of the optic nerves. Arch Neurol Psychiatry 79: 607–621, 1958

Donahue HC: An exceptional lesion of the orbit. Arch Ophthalmol ns 54:259–261, 1955

Hoyt WF, Baghdassarian SA: Optic glioma of childhood: natural history and rationale for conservative management. Br J Ophthalmol 53:793–798, 1969

Hoyt WF, Meshel LG, Lessel S, et al: Malignant optic glioma of adulthood. Brain 96:121–133, 1973

Hudson AC: Primary tumours of the optic nerve. R Lond Ophthalmic Hosp Rep 18:317–439, 1912

Leber: Cited by Hudson AC

Lloyd LA: Glioma of the optic nerve and chiasm in childhood. Trans Am Ophthal Soc 71:488–535, 1973

Marshall D: Glioma of the optic nerve: as a manifestation of von Recklinghausen's disease. Am J Ophthalmol 37:15–33, 1954

Middlemore R: Extirpation of the eye: on account of a tumor developed within the optic sheath. Lond Med Gaz 22:897–899, 1838

Panizza B: Annotazioni Anatomico-chirurgiche sul Fungo Midollare Dell'occhio, e Sulla Depressione Della Cateratta. Pavia, Italy, P Bizzoni, 1821

Spencer WH: Primary neoplasms of the optic nerve and its sheaths: clinical features and current concepts of pathogenetic mechanisms. Trans Am Ophthal Soc 70:490–528, 1972

Verhoeff FH: Primary intraneural tumors (gliomas) of the optic nerve. Arch Ophthalmol 51:120–140; 239–254, 1922

Von Graefe: Cited by Hudson AC

Von Hippel E: Die Krankheiten des Sehnerven. In *Handbuch der gesamten Augenheilkunde*. Volume 7. Pt 2. Ed: A von Graefe, ET Saemisch. Berlin, Julius Springer, 1923, pp 535–574

Wagener HP: Gliomas of the optic nerve. Am J Med Sci 237:238–261, 1959

Wishart JH: Case of extirpation of the eye-ball. Edinb Med Surg J 40:274–276, 1833

Yanoff M, Davis RL, Zimmerman LE: Juvenile pilocytic astrocytoma ("glioma") of optic nerve: clinicopathologic study of sixty-three cases. In Jakobiec FA: *Ocular and Adnexal Tumors*. Chapter 48. Birmingham, Ala, Aesculapius Publishing Co, 1978

Neuroepithelioma

Howard GM: Neuroepithelioma of the orbit. Am J Ophthalmol 59:934–937, 1965

Neuroblastoma

Albert DM, Rubenstein RA, Scheie HG: Tumor metastasis to the eye. Part II. Clinical study in infants and children. Am J Ophthalmol 63:727–732, 1967

Alfano JE: Ophthalmological aspects of neuroblastomatosis: a study of 53 verified cases. Trans Am Acad Ophthalmol Otolaryngol 72:830–848, 1968

Bodian M: Neuroblastoma. Pediatr Clin North Am 6:449, 1959

Collins VP, Loeffler RK, Tivey H: Observations on growth rates of human tumors. Am J Roentgenol Radium Ther Nucl Med 76:988–1000, 1956

Cushing H, Wolbach SB: The transformation of a malignant paravertebral sympathicoblastoma into a benign ganglioneuroma. Am J Pathol 3:203–216, 1927

Dalton N: Infiltrating growth in liver and suprarenal capsule. Trans Pathol Soc Lond 36:247–251, 1885

Dargeon HW: Neuroblastoma. J Pediatr 61:456–471, 1962

Exelby PR: Solid tumors in children: Wilms' tumor, neuroblastoma, and soft tissue sarcomas. Ca Cancer J Clinicians 28:146–163, 1978

Levy WJ: Neuroblastoma. Br J Ophthalmol 41:48–53, 1957

Nelson WE, Vaughan VC III, McKay RJ: Textbook of Pediatrics. Ninth edition. Philadelphia, WB Saunders Company, 1969

Phillips R: Neuroblastoma. Ann R Coll Surg Engl 12:29–48, 1953

Pochedly C: *Neuroblastoma*. Acton, Mass, Publishing Sciences Group, 1976

Reese AB: *Tumors of the Eye*. Second edition. New york, Hoeber Medical Division, Harper & Row, Publishers, 1963

Reese AB: Expanding lesions of the orbit (Bowman lecture). Trans Ophthalmol Soc UK 91:85–104, 1971

Stowens D: Neuroblastoma and related tumors. Arch Pathol 63:451–459, 1957

Wright JH: Neurocytoma or neuroblastoma, a kind of tumor not generally recognized. J Exp Med 12: 556–561, 1910

Ganglioneuroma

Toppozada HH: Ganglioneuroma of the left maxilla and orbit. J Laryngol 72:733–742, 1958
Walsh FB, Hoyt WF: *Clinical Neuro-ophthalmology.* Third edition. Baltimore, Williams & Wilkins Co, 1969, p 2293

Chemodectoma

Deutsch AR, Duckworth JK: Nonchromaffin paraganglioma of the orbit. Am J Ophthalmol 68:659–663, 1969
Fisher ER, Hazard JB: Nonchromaffin paraganglioma of the orbit. Cancer 5:521–524, 1952
Goder G: Das nichtchromaffine paragliom der orbita. Zentrabl Allg Pathol 113:167–172, 1970
Hughes LW, Ambrose A: Retro-orbital adrenal rest tumor. JAMA 126:231–232, 1944
Lattes R, McDonald JJ, Sproul E: Non-chromaffin paraganglioma of carotid body and orbit. Report of a case. Ann Surg 139:382–384, 1954
Thacker WC, Duckworth JK: Chemodectoma of the orbit. Cancer 23:1233–1238, 1969
Tye AA: Non-chromaffin paraganglioma of the orbit. Ophth Soc Australia 21:113–114, 1961
Zawirska B, Drozdowska S: Le chemodectome recidivant de l'orbite. Ann Ocul 203:361–370, 1970

Olfactory Neuroblastoma

Berger L, Luc R: L'esthésioneuroépithéliome olfactif. Bull Assoc Fr Etude Cancer 13:410–421, 1924
Djalilian M, Zujko RD, Weiland LH, et al: Olfactory neuroblastoma. Surg Clin North Am 57:751–761, 1977
Kadish S, Goodman M, Wang CC: Olfactory neuroblastoma. A clinical analysis of 17 cases. Cancer 37:1571–1576, 1976
Momose KJ, Weber AL, Goodman ML: Radiological and pathological findings of esthesioneuroblastoma. Adv Otorhinolaryngol 24:166–169, 1978
Oberman HA, Rice DH: Olfactory neuroblastoma: a clinicopathologic study. Cancer 38:2494–2502, 1976
Skolnik EM, Massari FS, Tenta LT: Olfactory neuroepithelioma: review of the world literature and presentation of two cases. Arch Otolaryngol 84:644–653, 1966

12

Malignant Melanoma

Dark brown, sometimes coal-black, capricious in behavior, and evil in portent, malignant melanoma probably is familiar to more ophthalmologists than any other tumor discussed in this text. Several factors contribute to this. The first is its color. Most patients and practically all physicians recognize the evil portents of this type of enlarging mass. When it occurs on the epibulbar area or the eyelid, or the surface tissues of a socket that has lost its eye, its presence is quickly noticed and the patient will seek advice more quickly than with any other tumor of similar size. Only the stationary brown nevus may mimic the color of malignant melanoma in these areas. But since the nevus may become transformed into the melanoma, many consider it wise to remove all tumors of such color even though they prove benign on histopathologic study.

The second factor is one of its probable consequences — enucleation. For this reason, more attention is given to this tumor when it grows inside the eye than other intraocular masses. It is by far the most common intraocular tumor in adults, and reams have been written concerning its differential diagnosis from lesions not requiring removal of the eye. Even though the domed contour or mushroom configuration of malignant choroidal melanoma is quite typical, the first ophthalmologist who sees the patient usually is hesitant to recommend enucleation without a second opinion and consultation regarding alternate choices of treatment. Thus, many more ophthalmologists are required to study this single problem than is the case with most other intraocular lesions. Actually choroidal melanoma is considered a rare disease. Its incidence has been estimated to range from 0.02% to 0.06%, or approximately 2 to 6 patients per 10,000. No other ocular tumor of similar or even more frequent incidence can lay claim to such favored attention.

Third, in the academic field, the neoplasm also evokes much interest. The first-year resident soon recognizes the tumor among tissue slides from the laboratory of pathology and quickly learns to associate prognosis with factors such as tumor size and cellular configuration. Malignant melanoma also has been the subject of special study by laboratories of pathology that collect a large number of cases. Of particular note is the continuing study by the Registry of Ophthalmic Pathology of the Armed Forces Institute of Pathology; by 1962 they had doggedly pursued the follow-up details of 3,385 cases with a survival of 5 years or more from the time of enucleation (Paul, Parnell, and Fraker, 1962).

With such a background there seems little need to rewrite the subject in this text except for those features that apply to the orbit. Until recently, the orbital manifestations received only scant study, for the tumor in this locale has been overshadowed by the attention given to intraocular and epibulbar forms of

the neoplasm. And so, in this discussion of the orbital melanoma, we will re-
phrase only those main points that are necessary for a well-rounded concept of
the subject.

TERMINOLOGY

By the term malignant melanoma, we refer to an invasive neoplasm consisting of cells producing a variable amount of pigment and possessing the potential of spread by either direct local extension or blood-borne metastasis.
Either mode of spread may be fatal, but the behavior of this neoplasm is sometimes so capricious as to defy accurate prognostication. Malignant melanoma
replaces earlier terms such as *melanosarcoma* and *melanoepithelioma*. The definition we have given does not state the pathogenesis of the tumor. The orbital
melanoma may be derived from a malignant transformation of a nevus (epi-
theliogenic) of the eyelid or conjunctiva. More often the orbital tumor consists
of uveal melanocytes of neurogenic (in the sense that the optic vesicle is neurogenic) origin. The rarer primary orbital malignant melanoma probably arises
from neurotrophic melanocytes associated with malignant transformations of
congenital cellular blue nevi and diffuse melanosis cells (oculodermal nevus of
Ota). This differentiation may be immaterial in that all these pigment-
producing cells probably have a common embryologic origin in the neural crest.
Furthermore, by the time the tumor becomes malignant it makes little
difference as to its histogenesis, except as this factor may affect its prognosis. So
little is known about the prognosis as it pertains to the orbital form of malignant
melanoma that, for the time being at least, we may omit the debate as to its
cellular genesis.

INCIDENCE

In the time interval of our Mayo Clinic survey there were thirty-one malignant melanomas of the orbit (Table 15). This is an incidence of 4% of the total
of 764 tumors. However, the subtotal contains one rare case of a malignant
melanoma metastatic to the orbit, three cases of primary malignant melanoma,
and nine cases of malignant melanoma that invaded the orbit from a site other
than the usual intraocular source. Such less common sources of malignant
melanoma are seldom surveyed in relation to total orbital malignant
melanomas. More commonly only those intraocular malignant melanomas that
extend or recur in the orbit are tabulated in large surveys of orbital tumors. The
incidence of this type of secondary malignant melanoma in other large tumor
surveys is: Forrest 6 (2.7%) cases among 222, Silva 9 (3.9%) cases among 230,
and Reese 60 (6.8%) cases among 877. Our incidence is 18 (2.3%) cases among
764 tumors.

The age data of our overall group of malignant melanomas is listed in
Table 15 and a cross reference relative to distribution by decades of life is listed
in Table 3, Chapter 3. Orbital malignant melanomas are predominantly tumors
of middle and late adulthood.Sex ratio was approximately 3:2, male to female.

TABLE 15. Site of Origin, Age, and Sex of 31 Orbital Malignant Melanomas at Time of Initial Surgical Diagnosis

(Primary — 3)		
Orbit	13	Male
Orbit	49	Male
Orbit	61	Female
(Secondary — 27)		
Eye	16	Male
Eye	29	Male
Eye	29	Female
Eye	40	Male
Eye	43	Male
Eye	44	Female
Antrum	45	Female
Caruncle	46	Male
Eye	46	Female
Antrum	49	Male
Face	52	Male
Eye	57	Female
Face	58	Male
Nasal cavity	58	Male
Eye	59	Female
Eye	59	Male
Epibulbar surface	61	Male
Ethmoid sinus	62	Male
Eye	63	Female
Eye	64	Male
Conjunctiva	66	Male
Eye	67	Female
Eye	68	Female
Eye	69	Female
Eye	69	Female
Eye	69	Male
Eye	76	Male
(Metastatic — 1)		
Groin	69 (approx.)	Female

SECONDARY ORBITAL MELANOMA, PRIMARY INTRAOCULAR

This is the type of orbital malignant melanoma most frequently discussed in the literature. The intraocular tumor gains access to the orbit by several means. Least frequent is the invasion of the optic nerve (Fig. 207) either by direct spread of a peripapillary melanoma through the end of Bruch's membrane or by a seeding of viable cells along the surface of the optic disk from large necrotic choroidal melanomas that have leaked malignant contents into the vitreous (Spencer 1975). These eyes usually become blind or glaucomatous. As the malignant cells push posteriorly along the optic nerve it behooves the surgeon to keep a sharp lookout for telltale black seedings on the surfaces of the sectioned optic nerve at the time of enucleation.

Another route of escape results from unfortunate surgical tampering with the barrier wall of the eye. Evisceration, instead of enucleation, of a blind painful eye is one means of such dissemination. The unwise and seldom practiced biopsy of an intraocular mass is another. Still another is the unfortunate circumstance of an intraocular neoplasm subjected to retinopexy in the mistaken belief that the cause of a retinal separation is rhegmatogenous rather than neo-

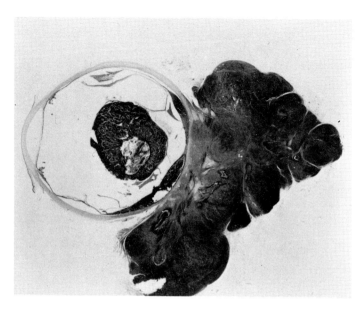

Figure 207. Secondary malignant melanoma: orbital extension occurred along optic nerve. (Hematoxylin and eosin; × 2½.)

plastic. Here the escape of malignant cells is facilitated either by their passage along the penetrating diathermy channels or by release of subretinal fluid. However they escape, the cells assault the orbital tissues in numbers far greater than would be the case if the neoplasm had penetrated the wall of the eye by natural means.

Finally, and most frequently, the tumor escapes by creeping through the wall of the eye along some emissary channel or structure (Fig. 208). In many areas these seedings remain unseen at the time of enucleation. Therefore, the surgeon cannot say positively that enucleation is the final event in the career of the choroidal tumor. In contrast, a lump or nodule on the surface of the eye may be so obvious as to declaim the extraocular neoplasm has made good its effort to escape (Fig. 209).

Because of the tumor's evil reputation, one might assume that only a short time will elapse between enucleation and the first indication of orbital recurrence, if such is going to occur. However, this is not always the case. Several variables make it difficult to be definite on this point. Thus, the interval between enucleation and orbital recurrence might be long (many years) in a hypothetical case wherein the intraocular tumor was discovered early in its growth and the enucleated eye did not show any gross or microscopic signs of extraocular extension. The interval in four of the cases of the Mayo Clinic series was greater than 9 years. Similar or longer intervals have been recorded in the literature; 16 years (Bembridge and McMillen 1953), 28 years (Allen and Jaeschke 1966). In contrast, the interval may be short (a few months or less than a year) in cases wherein the eye had harbored the primary neoplasm for many years before enucleation. In another case from this series the eye was said to have been blind for 11 years before the patient consented to enucleation. In 13

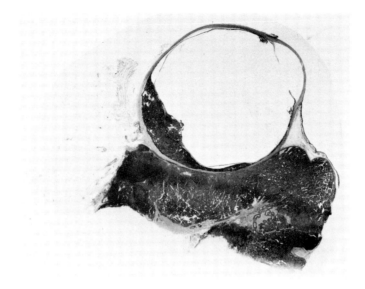

Figure 208. Secondary malignant melanoma: orbital extension through scleral invasion. (Hematoxylin and eosin; × 2½.)

patients of our series in whom orbital involvement was not obvious at time of enucleation, the interval before orbital recurrence averaged 5.5 years, with a range of 5 months to 17 years.

Other factors determining the interval between enucleation and occurrence of tumor are the *cellular morphology* of the initial neoplasm and any *extrascleral extension* at the time the eye is removed. Starr and Zimmerman (1962), from one of the studies of the Armed Forces Institute of Pathology con-

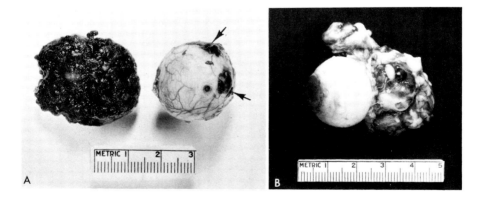

Figure 209. Intraocular malignant melanoma, extrascleral extension: *A*, On posterior surface of enucleated eye (*right*) are two black areas (*arrows*) where malignant melanoma had passed through wall of eyeball. Large black orbital extension of tumor (*left*) measured 3.5 by 2 by 1 cm. The intraocular tumor probably had been present approximately 4 years before enucleation. Immediate exenteration was performed upon discovery of orbital extension. Patient died 9 months later with widespread metastasis.

B, Extrascleral extension of malignant melanoma as large as the enucleated eye to which it is attached; exenteration of orbit was performed but patient died within 4 years from liver metastasis.

cerning 1,842 cases of uveal melanoma, noted 352 (13%) cases with evidence of extrascleral extension. Shammas and Blodi (1977) studied 432 intraocular malignant melanomas and found 45 (10.4%) with histopathologic signs of extraocular extension. However, the fact that extrascleral extension is obvious at the time of enucleation does not necessarily mean orbital extension of the tumor will develop in all such patients. In the Starr and Zimmerman study, 55 (3%) cases had an orbital recurrence. Neither are patients in whom there is no such extension at the time of histopathologic study completely immune from orbital recurrence. The other factor is the histopathology of the neoplasm. The mixed and epithelioid types of malignant melanoma usually recur in the orbit sooner than tumors of spindle B type.

Other variables are *size of the original intraocular tumor* and the *surgical violation of the tissue barrier* that often surrounds the extrascleral extension. The larger the tumor the shorter may be the interval before recurrence. Similarly, the more traumatic the surgical manipulation the sooner will the neoplasm recur. The patient's sex seems to have no bearing on the incidence of these secondary malignant melanomas of the orbit. Neither is one orbit affected more than the other.

The signs and symptoms that herald the onset of orbital invasion by the secondary types of malignant melanomas are relatively constant. The most obvious is the observation of *a black or brown mass nestling in the surface tissues of an orbit that has had a prior enucleation.* When the patient either is a poor observer or does not remove the prosthesis, change in the volume of the orbital contents because of slow growth of the neoplasm causes increasing *difficulty of retention of the prosthesis* in its accustomed position. When buried implants, other than the classic glass spheres, were first recommended several decades ago as a replacement for loss of the eyeball, there was some hesitation in the use of these implants following enucleation for intraocular malignant melanoma on the ground that they would mask a possible recurrence of the neoplasm in the orbit. We believe that insertion of implants may be routine in all enucleations for, in our experience, a recurrence of malignant tumor in such orbits will be more evident and quickly detected than in those orbits that have no implant or contain only a glass ball. There are two reasons for this. First, most of the present-day implants are secured in an approximately constant position by the extraocular muscles that are anchored to their contours. Second, they are relatively large in terms of the volume of tissue displaced. Thus, a small neoplasm will push against the buried implant and cause extrusion of the prosthesis earlier than in an orbit whose volume is not occupied by such an insert.

In orbits containing a glass sphere there also may be some delay in recognizing the presence of the expanding mass, because the glass sphere is not directly anchored by extraocular muscles and may be displaced within the orbit rather than being pushed forward against the back surface of the prosthesis. When it was common to place glass spheres in the orbit following enucleation, it was not uncommon to palpate both the sphere and expanding tumor in cases showing a recurrence. If two masses of different consistency were palpated, the likely diagnosis was malignant melanoma. If only one mass was palpated—and anxious patients who discovered such masses were not infrequent— the likely diagnosis was a glass ball implant that had migrated from its usual position in the center of the orbital cavity. Another symptom that may alert the observer to early growth of a secondary malignant melanoma is *persistent and unexplained edema*, or *swellingof the eyelid* (particularly the lower eyelid) in an otherwise happy and adjusted wearer of a prosthesis.

SECONDARY ORBITAL MELANOMA, PRIMARY EXTRAORBITAL AND EXTRAOCULAR

The other group of secondary melanomas comprised the nine cases (Table 15) in which the primary site of the neoplasm was on the surface of the eye or in one of the cavities or tissue structures adjacent to the orbit. The sample is small and there are too many variables to assess the tumor's incidence and clinical features accurately. All but one case were males and their age range was similar to the patients with secondary melanomas originating within the eye. In spite of measures such as radical excision, irradiation, surgical diathermy, or chemotherapy (singly or in combination at the time of first recurrence) the patients all died from either local spread or metastasis of the neoplasm within 5 years. Little else can be said of this group of melanomas as they affect the orbit.

METASTATIC MELANOMA

As with any neoplasm possessing the potential of metastatic multiplication, the malignant melanoma may sometimes develop in the relatively small orbital space from a systemic source. In so doing, it bypasses its favorite retreat, the liver. As a metastatic intruder it is so scarce as to be of little clinical importance except as a harbinger of doom. For by the time it finds its way to the relatively inaccessible confines of the orbit, dissemination elsewhere, either obvious or hidden, has probably occurred. Orbital metastasis is so unusual that when it occurs it usually is recorded in the literature, particularly if the orbital deposit is the only manifestation of metastasis. Two such reports of particular interest are the ones by Philps (1949) and Foster and associates (1957), referring to two women aged 69 and 56 years in whom the melanoma metastasized to the left orbit from a primary source in the choroid of the right eye. The tumor of Philps' case was encapsulated. The interval between enucleation of one eye and proptosis of the other eye was 4 years in one case and 10 years in the other. The metastasis, of course, may come from any original melanoma; in most cases the primary is in the skin. The series of Font and associates (1967), collected from the files of the Armed Forces Institute of Pathology, seems to be the only one in the literature reporting details of as many as five cases The age range was 32 to 86 years. In this series, three of these patients were blacks. Malignant melanoma in blacks is rare; the odds of an even rarer orbital metastasis would be difficult to compute.

The management of these metastatic quirks is nonsurgical, particularly when other deposits are manifest or known. However, even in such cases, or in patients in whom the orbital station may be the first stopover in travel of the neoplasm, the proptosis may be so great, the expansion of the tumor so rapid, and the neoplasm so deep in the orbit that orbitotomy is necessary either for diagnosis or for relief of pressure on the extruding eye. In such instances, the removal of the tumor usually is incomplete and, we suspect, sometimes hastens the demise of the patient. The one case of metastatic melanoma in the Mayo Clinic series occurred in a woman, aged 69 years. The primary site was a mole in the right groin, which had been treated with cautery.

PRIMARY ORBITAL MELANOMA

This type of melanoma may arise from several possible orbital sources. One source may be scattered melanocytes in the leptomeninges of the optic nerve, the tissues around ciliary nerves, or areas adjacent to scleral emissaria. In two cases in the literature—Jay (1965), a 64-year-old female, Hagler and Brown (1966), a 57-year-old male—the origin was from melanocytes associated with an oculodermal melanosis (nevus of Ota). More commonly the tumor may arise from a hamartomatous rest of a cellular blue nevus. Such an association seemed to be present in the case (a 42-year-old female) reported by Jakobiec and associates (1974), and in two of the three cases from our own survey that will be noted below. The factor responsible for the malignant transformation of a cellular blue nevus is not known.

Several dozen additional reports have either claimed or implied that a particular case is an example of malignant melanoma primary in the orbit. In some the claim is based on the long interval between enucleation of the patient's eye for uveal melanoma and the appearance of a similar neoplasm in the orbit. Even though the interval is 10 years or even 20 years, we do not believe it valid to state that such orbital tumors are primary. Instead, such cases may be variants of the secondary malignant melanoma already discussed. In other reports, surveys of patients have not been so exhaustive as to rule out the possibility that the orbital neoplasm was, in each case, metastatic rather than primary. Then there are still other reports wherein the data are so incomplete, even as to the status of the eye, that it is impossible to classify the orbital tumor according to its true source.

The best documented cases in the literature, in addition to those already mentioned, are those of Rottino and Kelly (a 27-year-old male), Wolter and associates (a 63-year-old female), Drews (a 75-year-old black male), and Coppetto and associates (a 49-year-old female). The age range of these documented cases, plus the three cases we will describe, range from 13 to 75 years with a median age of 53 years. The sex distribution was equal. Additional possible cases of primary orbital malignant melanoma in the literature, but with less supporting data, are those of Walter (48-year-old female), Foster (65-year-old female), Offret (52-year-old female), and Bonnet.

The salient features of the three cases in our Mayo Clinic survey follow.

CASE 1. The father of a boy of 13 years had noted upward displacement of the patient's left eye for 1 month. A nodular mass, palpable in the inferotemporal quadrant of left orbit, seemed to be the reason for limitation in the downward rotation of the left eye.

Exophthalmometry showed that the only difference in measurements of the two eyes was small (2 mm); the left was more forward than the right. There were no other significant findings. The mass was approached through an incision in the inferotemporal conjunctival fornix, supplemented by an external canthotomy. A dark-blue mass (3 by 2 by 1 cm) was removed by blunt dissection (Fig. 210). The tumor specimen was examined by pathologists both at the Mayo Clinic and elsewhere; all agreed the tumor represented a malignant melanoma, epithelioid type (Fig. 211). There was some debate as to whether exenteration should be performed or the patient should be given supplementary irradiation. It was decided to do neither, but to be satisfied with the complete excision of the tumor. The child has been watched closely in the years since orbitotomy; to date, 18 years have passed (1977) without evidence of recurrence of proptosis, palpable masses in the area of the prior neoplasm, or systemic spread.

CASE 2.　A 49-year-old man noticed proptosis of the left eye which progressed so rapidly that about 1 month later an exploratory operation on the left orbit was performed through a transcranial approach. The tumor was incompletely removed because of its proximity to the optic nerve. With some difficulty the pathologist made a diagnosis of hemangioendothelioma. The patient was first seen at the Mayo Clinic 2 weeks after this operation. The findings in the left eye were the following: proptosis, as determined by exophthalmometry, 2 mm; rotation, marked limitation; visual acuity, 20/200; and papilledema, 2 diopters. The orbit again was explored through a transfrontal approach. A pitch-black, nonencapsulated tumor in the posterior, superior, and temporal portion of the orbit was incompletely removed. The position of the mass adjacent to the optic nerve was confirmed. The spread of the tumor was so diffuse that exenteration did not seem worthwhile. The histopathologic diagnosis was malignant melanoma, of mixed spindle and epithelioid type. The patient survived for almost 2 years after the first surgical procedure; death was due to extensive recurrence of neoplasm with involvement of adjacent intracranial structures. Careful search at autopsy for any additional locus or primary source of malignant melanoma was negative.

CASE 3.　A 62-year-old female was seen because of an eight-month history of visual loss, right eye, blepharoptosis, and orbital pain of seven months' duration. An orbital exploration had been performed one month prior to our observation with partial removal of a mass surrounding the optic nerve. Our findings were: light perception in affected eye, very slight proptosis, and striae along the posterior temporal surface of eye. Our histopathologic assessment of the tumor specimen was: multicentric, lightly pigmented, malignant melanoma, epithelioid type, associated with a heavily pigmented fibrous component

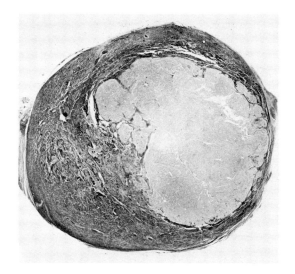

Figure 210.　Primary melanoma of orbit: neoplasm is unusually well circumscribed with pseudocapsule; about one-half the neoplasm is amelanotic. (Hematoxylin and eosin; × 5.)

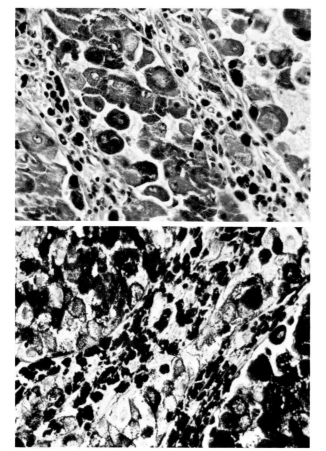

Figure 211. Primary melanoma of the orbit (same specimen
as depicted in Fig. 210): *A*, Neoplasm is epithelioid. Section from
melanotic zone, showing epithelioid features. (Hematoxylin and
eosin; × 285.) *B*, Use of special
technique to impart black color to
melanin. (Fontana silver; ×
225.)

representing a pre-existing cellular blue nevus. An exenteration of the right orbit was performed one week later, elsewhere. The surgeon reported the tumor was extending into the
optic foramen. Histopathologic diagnosis of the exenteration tissue was malignant blue
nevus. The patient died 9 months after exenteration from intracranial spread of tumor.

There were no features common to our cases and those reported in the literature that would establish a standard pattern of clinical onset for primary
orbital melanomas. Those several tumors located in the proximity of the optic
nerve were characterized by visual loss followed by proptosis. Those melanomas
located in the more anterior portion of the orbit were palpable, caused little
ocular dysfunction, and were sometimes visible because of their pigmentation.

PATHOLOGY

Much interest is centered around the correlation between the cytology and
the ultimate course of this tumor. The majority of pathologists now have
accepted a uniform system of classification based on two principal cell types and
variations in their patterns of multiplication. There is close agreement for example, that a growth pattern of spindle cells, designated subtype A, is the least

malignant (but certainly not benign as some writers imply). The spindle cells of this subtype do not possess cell boundaries that stain distinctly in tissue preparations. Instead, the examiner's interest is drawn to the elongated, flattened nuclei that occupy a major portion of the cell. Chromatin frequently is clumped along the long axis of the nuclei and accepts so much stain as to make the nuclei the most prominent feature of the cell (Fig. 212). The cells tend to arrange themselves in columns, so that on longitudinal section the nuclei are closely bunched and parallel to one another; when a bundle of these cells is sectioned at right angles the rod-like nuclei then resemble small round cells. Next in order of malignancy are neoplasms with spindle cells of subtype B (Fig 213). The cells of this subtype are larger and not as closely packed into columns as those of subtype A. The cells of subtype B also have more plump nuclei. The most distinctive feature is the prominent, almost centrally placed nucleoli. If the spindle cells arrange themselves in rows, so as to have the appearance of palisades in longitudinal section, then the neoplasm is considered to be even more malignant than either of the two preceding subtypes and is designated the fascicular type (Fig. 214). With a higher grade of malignancy the spindle cells seem to have evolved into or have been replaced by cells with an epithelioid configuration. The latter are much larger, polygonal cells (Fig. 211). Their cell boundaries usually are much more distinct than those of spindle cells, but size of the cells in relationship to one another is not as uniform as with the precursor spindle cell. The nuclei are oval and relatively hyperchromatic, and conspicuous nucleoli may be spotted here and there in a given tissue sample. In those cells that contain little or no melanin the cytoplasm has a distinctly acidophilic color. The tumor containing a mixture of spindle cells and epithelioid cells is less malignant than the tumor that is composed predominantly of the latter cells. Sometimes the tumor becomes necrotic because the blood supply is interrupted and cell types are then difficult to identify.

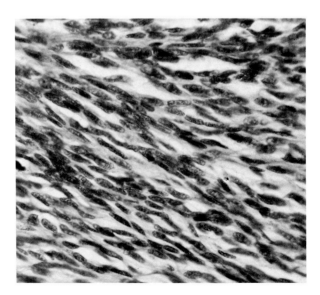

Figure 212. Malignant melanoma, spindle A type: cell boundaries are indistinct and nuclei are elongated and flattened; nucleoli are not prominent and mitoses are scarce. (Hematoxylin and eosin; × 500.)

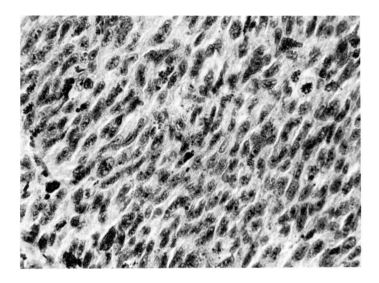

Figure 213. Malignant melanoma, spindle B type: nuclei are plump, with greater variation, and mitoses are plentiful. (Hematoxylin and eosin; × 325.)

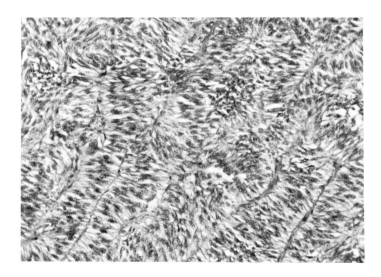

Figure 214. Malignant melanoma, fascicular type: cells are arranged in rows, giving palisaded appearance. (Hematoxylin and eosin; × 200.)

This orderly arrangement with its step-like increase in malignancy has proven useful in the classification and prognosis of the primary intraocular malignant melanoma. However, similar correlations applied to orbital melanomas have not been made. One reason is that the latter tumors are much less frequent than the former and the need for such correlation seems less. Another reason is that the less malignant subtypes (spindle A, spindle B, and fascicular forms) are seldom encountered in the orbit. The majority of orbital melanomas are the mixed, necrotic, and epithelioid types. In those cases wherein the original tumor within the eye was a mixed or epithelioid type, subsequent recurrence in the orbit often shows features matching the histology of the original tumor. However, if the original tumor was predominantly a spindle cell type, the subsequent recurrence usually contains a high proportion of epithelioid cells, indicating a more malignant form. Such tissue sections usually show a greater disparity in size and shape of the cells, and an increase in multinucleated forms of epithelioid cells (Fig. 215). This trend toward a greater degree of malignancy is particularly noticeable in those samples from the metastatic forms of malignant melanoma. The cells in these tissue sections have a "bizarre" or "wild" arrangement. In many of the orbital melanomas, from any source, amelanotic zones of cells are surprisingly frequent. If we assume that the same cytologic-prognostic correlation of intraocular malignant melanomas can be applied to orbital melanomas, then it is justifiable to say the orbital neoplasm is much more malignant than its intraocular counterpart.

TREATMENT AND PROGNOSIS

The management of *orbital* melanoma is quite a different matter from the situation that prevails in a patient with a suspected intraocular melanoma. In the former, the diagnosis is less of a challenge, removal of the eye is not at stake (except for the very rare cases of primary tumor), and the outlook of the patients is more uncertain as soon as the diagnosis is first suspected. The crux of the

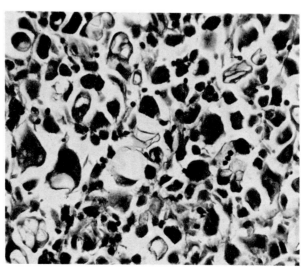

Figure 215. Malignant melanoma, recurrent: neoplasm is epithelioid, but cells are bizarre and variable. (Hematoxylin and eosin; × 325.)

situation is how to treat the neoplasm so as to give the patient the best chance for survival. The dilemma is whether to advise radical removal, such as exenteration, or to be content with a less vigorous approach.

Extrascleral Extension

It has been noted that the larger the intraocular tumor, the more undifferentiated its cytology, and the longer it has remained undetected within the eye the greater will be the tumor's ability to escape the confines of the eye. We recognize the grave implications of these factors when we remove the eye, but if there is neither microscopic nor gross evidence of extrascleral extension or spread along the optic nerve, we must assume that everything possible has been done for the patient up to that point. It is somewhat analogous to the all-or-none law; in other words, one either has or has not cured the patient by enucleating the eye. At present there is no way of assuring the patient that he will be free of tumor forever nor of accurately predicting that he will survive for a limited time. A prognosis specifically suited to an individual patient is not possible. Instead, his survival becomes but a statistical probability modified by some of the factors noted. A less favorable statistic is only of faint encouragement to some, and even a more favorable estimate still is a source of continued worry to others, lest they belong in the minor fraction that does not survive. More variables are added when an extrascleral extension is recognized.

If, upon enucleation, an obvious but well-circumscribed extension still attached to the surface of the eye or optic nerve is found, a conservative approach still is favored, providing the nodule has not been inadvertently incised and tumor is not grossly visible in the surrounding reticular substance of the orbit. Here, we reason that more radical surgical measures will not assure the patient of a greater longevity than the simple excision so far performed. Many observers will disagree with this approach and advise exenteration instead.

If, instead, an additional circumscribed nodule of tumor is found, an extension of tumor along the proximal stump of the optic nerve is observed, or an extraocular nodule has been incised in the course of enucleation, we would proceed with a subtotal exenteration. Also, we think it prudent that a second set of surgical instruments be used for the exenteration procedure to prevent additional tumor seeding.

In their large study of cases with uveal melanomas, Starr and Zimmerman noted a 5-year mortality rate of 66% among 235 patients with extrascleral extension as compared to only a 33% mortality rate among 1,607 cases without extraocular extension.

Delayed Recurrence

The main difference between extrascleral extension and delayed recurrence is a matter of time. In the latter the interval may be very short (a few months) or quite long (17 years in one of our patients). The mass of recurrent tumor may be very small or quite large (Fig. 216). This does not mean the neoplasm is any less malignant than the tumors in the previous group, for all secondary orbital melanomas, regardless of their primary source, closely resemble one another cytologically. Instead, the neoplasm has experienced a greater struggle in estab-

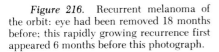

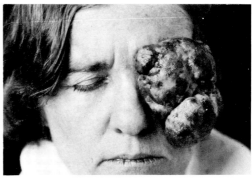

Figure 216. Recurrent melanoma of the orbit; eye had been removed 18 months before; this rapidly growing recurrence first appeared 6 months before this photograph.

lishing a nidus in a new area. This factor of time may have some bearing on the course and management of the orbital recurrence. It is conceivable, for example, that in these cases the body may have more time to build up its defense against onslaught of the cancer through either immunosuppressive factors or cellular barriers.

It is the delayed recurrence for which exenteration of the orbit is most often recommended. Exenteration is the surgical procedure most often recommended as a treatment for orbital malignant melanoma. The rationale for this approach is similar to that advised for malignant neoplasms in other parts of the body; namely, to eradicate the tumor and arrest its spread by widely excising all surrounding tissues. The results in most surgical fields seem to justify the continued use of such radical measures. However, one may be skeptical whether such radical measures are warranted in the problem of orbital malignant melanoma. The difference is partly anatomic.

In the operation for malignant melanoma of an extremity, the leg or arm is severed at a joint some distance proximal to the lesion. This intervening distance may be great enough to contain spread of the neoplasm and permit the surgeon to get beyond the zone of potential seeding. The escape of the neoplasm also is limited, more or less, to one proximal direction, and this pathway must pass through the area of surgical cleavage. In the radical removal of cancer in other organs, such as the breast, the adjacent lymph nodes, which may serve as a temporary residence for the neoplasm, also are removed. Such deterrents are not so easily accomplished when exenterating an orbit.

The vascular channels in and around the orbit are so diffuse that the neoplasm has many different routes to make good its escape: along the vessels passing forward and downward toward the face, through vessels of the superior orbital fissure, or downward by way of the inferior orbital vein and the pterygoid plexus of vessels. Or, it may choose a slower route of egress by creeping along the nerves passing through the optic canals and superior orbital fissure. None of these hatches can be completely sealed by the operation in question. Furthermore, the plane of surgical dissection seldom is more than 2.5 cm (1 inch) from the nearest point of the neoplasm. Thus it is difficult to argue that ramifications of the neoplasm have been completely encompassed.

Such considerations becloud the usefulness of exenteration. By the time exenteration has been performed the neoplasm may already have secured permanent lodging in the body through prior hematogenous dissemination. Still, many ophthalmologists are reluctant to perform any operation other than exenteration because reliance on this operation is so universal among physicians who first see the patient. We have proposed local excision of the orbital nodule in some cases only to find that exenteration already has been suggested by the referring physician. Anything less than exenteration in such situations leaves the implication that all possible surgery has not been performed on the patient's behalf. It seems easier in these situations to follow established opinion than to advocate any other approach, such as local excision to the rare patient who has no preformed opinion or prior advice favoring exenteration.

Also, in some elderly patients with a fairly sizeable recurrent tumor of many months' duration, we will not recommend either excision or exenteration. Here, we suspect that surgery may well break the host–tumor barrier and lessen their interval of survival.

In their review, Starr and Zimmerman mentioned 15 cases treated by exenteration at the time of enucleation because of extraocular spread. One of these patients survived 19 years, but the majority died as a result of metastasis within 13 months. Another 15 patients were treated by exenteration at the time of delayed tumor recurrence. Of these, 11 were dead less than 5 years following surgical removal of orbital recurrences, mostly from metastatic spread. This is a dismal outlook, but Starr and Zimmerman believed exenteration was the treatment of choice if metastasis was not present. Shammas and Blodi (1977) state that patients treated by exenteration have a much better prognosis than those not so treated. They also found that patients treated by early exenteration (performed within two months after enucleation) had a longer survival than patients treated by late exenteration, but their total of patients was rather small for statistical purposes. Eight cases treated by early exenteration had a 5-year survival rate of 87% contrasted to a survival rate of 20% in five patients treated by late exenteration.

The majority of the patients in the Mayo Clinic series with delayed orbital recurrences of an intraocular melanoma were treated by exenteration. Of the ten so managed, all were dead from metastasis within 5 years of the surgical procedure except two patients. One of the latter, who underwent exenteration 1 month after enucleation, was living without recurrence or known metastasis at the end of 4 years. The other survivor, who underwent exenteration 10 years after enucleation, was free of known metastasis and local recurrence when he expired from a heart problem 4 years after orbital surgery. Our series is also too small for statistical meaning, but the high rate of mortality in this group of patients partly explains our disenchantment with exenteration as the therapy of choice for tumor recurrences. Only two of the patients with secondary orbital melanomas were managed by local excision rather than exenteration. One of these patients was still living 3 years later (certainly no worse than the group who underwent exenteration) and the other patient was living 20 years after orbital excision without metastasis or local tumor recurrence.

Primary Orbital Melanoma

The well-circumscribed, bluish-black orbital masses should be completely removed without prior biopsy. Incisional biopsy might well convert the prognosis from tumor-cure to tumor-recurrence. Hogan (1964), also believed that simple excision is adequate because the recurrent tumors often are localized. He referred to two patients who were treated in this manner and were followed for over 20 years. In one of these cases, two excisions of local recurrences were performed. Both patients show no sign of metastasis in this long follow-up period.

On the basis of the above data, we are not convinced that exenteration provides the relief from systemic dissemination that the patient expects nor fulfills its reputation, professionally, of eradicating the evil. If modifying factors such as duration of growth, cytology, size, and extent of the melanoma could be ignored, then management might not be so much a question of excision versus exenteration but of how soon either surgical procedure is performed after the recurrence appears.

Host-Tumor Relationships

Much of the information pertaining to this field is still speculative, but its future application to the problem of malignant melanoma is so likely that it is important to discuss it at this point. Patient survival usually is calculated on the basis of size of the tumor, its duration, and its cytology. In other words, prognosis is tumor-oriented. However, some patients may have innate mechanisms that permit a resistance that is longer than average to the onslaught of the neoplasm. These mechanisms probably include some type of circulatory immunosuppressive cells, as well as fixed tissue elements belonging to the lymphodiscovered in the future as search continues for other host defenses. The more cases of malignant melanoma that we observe the more certain we are of vagaries in its behavior, and it is the host's resistance that probably explains some of these phenomena. For example, we know that malignant melanoma spontaneously regresses. Cases wherein metastatic malignant melanoma is present without an obvious primary site also are known and, in rarer instances, the metastases have persisted but the known primary has disappeared. It seems reasonable to assume the host may sometimes destroy the neoplasm.

Another variable is age of the patient. It is frequently stated that this neoplasm is more malignant in the young; less malignant in the old. In this regard, we have observed a few cases of what appeared to be delayed recurrence of malignant melanoma in persons in the eighth to ninth decades who had refused treatment elsewhere. By reason of their age or threat of exenteration, they had declined treatment and their judgment seemed to be justified by a remarkably slow progression of the tumor nodule. In contrast, there is the belief that host resistance in the aged is less than in the young, and that this accounts for the greater prevalence of cancer in the older group.

Finally there are those cases with survival after removal of the original neoplasm that is so long as to suggest some inherent resistance on the part of the host. Ruedemann (1963) reported a patient with a particularly interesting history: this patient had undergone enucleation of one eye for an intraocular malignant melanoma in 1930, and subsequent excisions and exenterations of the orbital recurrence were performed in 1932, 1933, 1957, and 1960. This patient was still living 33 years after enucleation, without obvious evidence of systemic spread. However, in a study of immune responsiveness in twenty-five patients with choroidal malignant melanoma, Priluck and associates (1979) did not find consistent difference between patients with melanoma and an age-matched control population. Serial immune profiles also failed to identify a change when clinical evidence of metastasis developed.

Radiotherapy

Many radiotherapists in the United States believe that malignant melanomas are radioresistant. Most ophthalmologists were trained to accept this concept but, with time, some become less convinced this dictum should be applied to all malignant melanomas of the orbit. This reputation of radioimmunity is fostered by the tendency to attribute to all malignant melanomas the behavior of the one related to the nevus cell. The latter, such as a malignant melanoma spreading from an eyelid into the orbit, is not radio-sensitive. However, the malignant melanoma derived from the uveal melano-cyte may be less radioresistant. We have been impressed with the beneficial ef-fect from supplementary irradiation in some cases that we have described. Per-haps some of the orbital neoplasms are radiosensitive, but we would hesitate to say they are radiocurable. We do not know of any controlled study using radio-therapy nor have we made sufficient observations of our own to be able to justify our making any positive statements as to the indications for irradiation. Irradiation might be suggested as a palliative measure among the aged with large recurrences who either refuse or might not withstand a radical surgical procedure.

Chemotherapy

The use of these agents to control recurrences and suppress dissemination of malignant melanomas is still in its infancy. Many of these drugs are still under investigation and are not available for widespread trial. We do not know of any cases of orbital melanoma that has been successfully treated with this modality.

In summary, we consider secondary malignant melanoma of the orbit a fatal disease, but the interval between the orbital manifestation and fatal out-come may be so long (many years or several decades) as to make a specific prognosis nearly impossible. Its behavior is so capricious and there are so many variable affecting its management that a universal and successful treatment has not been devised.

References

Allen JC, Jaeschke WH: Recurrence of malignant melanoma in an orbit after 28 years. Arch Ophthal-mol 76:79–81, 1966
Bembridge BA, McMillan J: Malignant melanoma occurring after evisceration. Brit J Ophthalmol 37: 109–113, 1953
Bonnet D: Sur une forme clinique rare de tumeur de l'orbite. Arch Ophtalmol 11:329–333, 1951

Coppetto JR, Jaffe, R, Gillies CG: Primary orbital melanoma. Arch Ophthalmol 96:2255–2258, 1978

Drews RC: Primary malignant melanoma of the orbit in a negro. Arch Ophthalmol 93:335–336, 1975

Font RL, Naumann G, Zimmerman LE: Primary malignant melanoma of the skin metastatic to the eye and orbit: review of ten cases and review of the literature. Am J Ophthalmol 63:738–754, 1967

Forrest AW: Intraorbital tumors. Arch Ophthalmol 41:198–230, 1949

Foster J: An encapsulated orbital melanoma. Brit J Ophthalmol 28:293–296, 1944

Foster J, Henderson W, Cowie JW, et al: Choroidal sarcoma with metastasis in the opposite orbit. Br J Ophthalmol 41:42–47, 1957

Hagler WS, Brown CC: Malignant melanoma of the orbit arising in a nevus of Ota. Trans Am Acad Ophth Oto 70:817–822, 1966

Hogan MJ: Clinical aspects, management, and prognosis of melanomas of the uvea and optic nerve. *In* Ocular and Adnexal Tumors: New and Controversial Aspects. Ed: M Boniuk. St. Louis, CV Mosby Company, 1964, pp 203–302

Jakobiec FA, Jones IS: Neurogenic tumors. *In* Clinical Ophthalmology. Ed: TD Duane, Volume 2, Chapter 41. Hagerstown, Harper & Row Publishers, 1976

Jay B: Malignant melanoma of the orbit in a case of oculodermal melanosis. Brit J Ophthalmol 49: 359–363, 1965

Offret G: *Les Tumeurs Primitives de L'Orbita.* Paris, Masson & Cie, 1951, p 411

Paul EV, Parnell BL, Fraker M: Prognosis of malignant melanomas of the choroid and ciliary body. Int Ophthalmol Clin 2:387–402, 1962

Philps S: Choroidal sacroma with metastasis in the opposite orbit. Br J Ophthalmol 33:732–739, 1949

Priluck IA, Robertson DM, Pritchard DJ, et al: Immune responsiveness in patients with choroidal malignant melanoma. Am J Ophthalmol 87:215–220, 1979

Reese AB: *Tumors of the Eye.* Second edition. New York, Hoeber Medical Division, Harper & Row, Publishers, 1963

Rottino A, Kelly AS: Primary orbital melanoma: case report with review of the literature. Arch Ophthalmol ns 27:934–949, 1942

Ruedemann AD Jr: Malignant melanoma of the orbit: report of a case followed for 31 years which was probably primary in the globe. Am J Ophthalmol 55:363–365, 1963

Shammas HF, Blodi FC: Orbital extension of choroidal and ciliary body melanomas. Arch Ophthalmol 95:2002–2005, 1977

Silva D: Orbital tumors. Am J Ophthalmol 65:318–339, 1968

Spencer WH: Optic nerve extension of intraocular neoplasms. Am J Ophthalmol 80:465–471, 1975

Starr HJ, Zimmerman LE: Extrascleral extension and orbital recurrence of malignant melanomas of the choroid and ciliary body. Int Ophthalmol Clin 2:369–385, 1962

Walter O: Ein Fall von primärem Melanosarkom der Orbita. Klin Monatsbl Augenheilkd 31:357–369, 1893

Wolter JR, Bryson JM, Blackhurst RT: Primary orbital melanoma. Eye Ear Nose Throat Mon 45:64–67, (Aug) 1966

13

Lymphocytic, Plasmacytic, and Granulocytic Neoplasms

The orbital neoplasms discussed in this chapter are derived from several of the principal cellular components of what was once broadly designated the *reticuloendothelial system*. In recent years there has been a uniform trend to designate this system by some term that would be morphologically, more specific and functionally more suitable. *Lymphoreticular system* is one such term that has had widespread acceptance. Many authors think of the latter as including only two principal cell populations, the lymphoid series and the mononuclear (monocyte-macrophage-histiocyte) phagocytic series. Other writers also classify the granulocytic cell series within the meaning of the overall term. For convenience we will consider the extranodal and extramedullary orbital manifestations of the lymphocytic and granulocytic series here, and defer discussion of the tumors of the monocytic-histiocytic family to the next chapter.

No other group of tumors in this text have undergone such an extensive change in classification and terminology in the past decade as the neoplasms associated with the lymphoid cell lineage. All of this is because of new knowledge concerning dissimilar immunologic functions of lymphocytes with similar morphologic features under light microscopy.

IMMUNOLOGICAL PERSPECTIVES

It has been known for some years that patients with various congenital immunodeficiency syndromes differed in their patterns of immune responsiveness and their susceptibility to various infectious diseases. This lead to the recognition of at least two ontogenically different and functionally separate populations of lymphocytes. One group, the B lymphocytes, are derived from bone marrow and are involved in the production of circulating antibodies. These B cells are distributed in the follicles of lymph nodes and spleen, and in the medullary cords of lymph nodes. A second group, the T lymphocytes, also have bone marrow parentage but undergo maturation in the thymus before reaching their principal home in the paracortical portions of lymph nodes and the periarteriolar lymphoid sheaths of the spleen. T cells are involved principally in cell-mediated immunity. A third, undefined, lymphocytic cell system may exist and explain the proliferation of lymphocytes that cannot be identified with immunologic features of either the B or T cells. Also, there is a separate monocytic-histiocytic, M cell, system that, in addition to phagocytosis, plays a supplementary role to the B and T lymphocytes in the processing of antigen.

TABLE 16.   FUNCTIONAL CLASSIFICATION OF ORBITAL LYMPHOID
CELL NEOPLASMS

B Cell Neoplasms	T Cell Neoplasms
Nodular (follicular) lymphocytic lymphoma	Hodgkin's disease
Well-differentiated lymphocytic lymphoma, diffuse	?Poorly differentiated lymphocytic lymphoma; diffuse (children)
Poorly differentiated lymphocytic lymphoma, diffuse (adults)	**Variable Cell Type**
Plasma cell myeloma	Large cell (histiocytic, reticulum cell) lymphoma
Burkitt's lymphoma	Mixed cell lymphoma
Waldenström's macroglobulinemia	

The cells of these several immune systems can be identified by the presence or absence of surface membrane receptors (markers) to differing fractions of immunoglobulin, mitogens, activated complement, antisera, unsensitized sheep erythrocytes, enzymes, and other reagents. The detection of these characteristic markers on the neoplastic proliferation of the cells of the lymphoreticular system has provided new vistas on the cell origin and differing clinicopathologic course of the several tumors that have, morphologically, look-alike features. The functional (surface marker) classification of the several lymphoid neoplasms of the orbit in this chapter is listed in Table 16.

Further work with immunologic criteria has shown that benign reactive lymphoid lesions and inflammatory lymphocytic pseudotumors (pseudolymphomas) contain progeny of B cells and T cells, or a mix of B cell types. In short, such lesions are polyclonal. In contrast, the malignant lymphoid proliferations are almost entirely monoclonal, reproducing the clone of the neoplastic cell. This relatively new information may be helpful in some orbital cases where it is difficult to tell the difference between a lymphoid pseudotumor and a border-line malignant lymphoma on the basis of the light microscopy examination.

Although these exciting investigative techniques are now being applied to the study of nodal and extranodal lymphoid lesions in some immunopathology oriented centers, most pathologists still judge the prognosis of the proliferative process on the degree of differentiation of the neoplastic cell and the growth pattern (that is, nodular or diffuse) in routine fixed tissue sections. The histopathologic classification that we use in the study of our orbital lymphoid neoplasms will be noted shortly.

MALIGNANT LYMPHOMAS

By this term we refer to a group of neoplasms whose principal cellular component is the lymphocyte. In the older literature they were called *lymphosarcoma* and this term, as well as *malignant lymphoma*, are often used interchangeably. Inasmuch as we do not believe there is such a tumor as benign lymphoma, it follows that all lymphomas must be malignant. The adjective, malignant, then becomes redundant and, for this reason, it is often convenient to discuss the neoplasms simply as lymphomas.

They are a very complex group. The lymphocyte may proliferate in a very immature form or grow indolently with a preponderant population of such mature forms as to mimic the morphology of the non-neoplastic circulating lymphocyte. In between these extremes there may be tumors with a mixture of lymphocytes in various stages of cell differentiation. In addition, some lymphomas proliferate in a follicular-like pattern and in others the cell growth is diffuse and sheet-like. Also, the lymphocyte may proliferate as a small cell or a very large cell with, again, a 50–50 mixture of both large and small cells (mixed cell lymphoma). The presence of quite large cells (several diameters larger than a normal lymphocyte) was at one time considered strong evidence that a given neoplasm was not of lymphoid origin. Now it is widely accepted that small, mature-appearing lymphocytes may, under a suitable antigenic stimulus, undergo transformation into a much larger cell. This was an important challenge to the traditional concept that lymphocytes become smaller in the course of cellular differentiation. In addition, the several lymphoma subtypes may vary widely in their biologic aggressiveness, depending in some degree on the functional immunologic factors already noted. Lastly, they are complex because the abnormal proliferation of cells may suddenly appear in anatomic sites (such as the orbit) not normally containing lymphoid tissue. In these extranodal sites the usual architecture of neoplastic nodal invasion is absent and the pathologist must devote more attention to cytologic detail in determining the type and degree of malignancy.

CLASSIFICATION

The classification of Rappaport (1966) currently is most widely used in the study of cytologic detail necessary for clinical evaluation and prognosis. We have abbreviated the usual scheme to make it more applicable to the orbit because many of the systemic lymphomas do not occur in this extranodal site. Also, we have altered some of the original nomenclature, or added optional terms, to incorporate updated terminology. We have made no effort to add a subgroup of lymphomas intermediate between well-differentiated and poorly differentiated lymphocytic types because it would only dilute the significance of an already small sample. Also, our tissue slides were reviewed by an additional pathologist (Peter M. Banks, M.D.) to enhance the accuracy of the histopathologic evaluation and terminology. The histopathologic grouping of the orbital lymphomas in our orbital survey are listed in Table 17.

INCIDENCE

Lymphomas are one of the ten most common orbital tumors (Table 2, Chapter 3). This is a curious fact in view of the absence of lymphoid tissue in the normal orbit. Our 57 cases are approximately 7.5% of our total 764 tumors (primary, secondary, metastatic, and generalized types). An incidence correlation with other large orbital tumor surveys is not very satisfactory because such surveys were published prior to present day concepts of classification and diagnosis, and many include examples of benign reactive lymphoplasia (pseudolymphomas) and other adnexal lymphomas (conjunctiva, caruncle, eyelids). Also, it should be noted that our total of 57 cases includes primary (38

TABLE 17.   HISTOPATHOLOGIC DIAGNOSIS OF ORBITAL
MALIGNANT LYMPHOMAS*

Hodgkin's disease	0
Well-differentiated lymphocytic lymphoma, diffuse	18
Poorly differentiated lymphocytic lymphoma, nodular	6
Poorly differentiated lymphocytic lymphoma, diffuse	21
Mixed cell lymphoma	1
Large cell (reticulum cell, histiocytic) lymphoma, diffuse	10
Total	56†

*Mayo Clinic Series 1948–1974.
†Does not include one unclassified case.

cases), secondary (3 cases), and generalized (16 cases) types of lymphoma. Such a subgrouping would significantly alter other incidence estimates based on anatomic sites. In addition, we use the term, primary orbital lymphoma, very advisedly because it is so difficult to rule out other anatomic foci of lymphoma when the patient presents with only an orbital lesion. Furthermore, the "generalized" subgroup comprises a considerable portion (16 cases, 28%) of our total lymphomas. In these situations the disease was found to be disseminated when the orbital lymphoma was first diagnosed. Some physicians might not include such disseminated cases in a compendium of orbital tumors. The careful study of Rosenberg and associates (1961) is of interest in respect to this involvement of the orbit in the course of lymphoma. In an autopsy study of 1,269 patients with systemic lymphoma, there were 16 (1.3%) with orbital involvement. In the current literature only the series of forty-three lymphomas discussed by Knowles and Jakobiec (1978) might be comparable to our own in respect to scrutiny of clinical features, volume of cases, and histopathologic criteria for diagnosis.

The sex and age distribution of our 57 lymphomas was noted in Table 3 (Chapter 3). Forty-one (72%) of our total lymphomas occurred in the two-decade age period, 51-70 years. Lymphomas are chiefly neoplasms of adults older than 40, with a slight preponderance in males.

HODGKIN'S DISEASE

Ophthalmologists seldom see patients with this disease. Occasionally there will be a call for hospital consultation for nonspecific retinopathy in a patient suffering the terminal throes of the disorder. Or there may be a fortuitous occasion to observe a nodular manifestation of Hodgkin's disease on the surface of the eye or in the substance of the eyelid. But a patient with a true orbital manifestation may never be seen, so rare is Hodgkin's disease in this area. Our experience with the disease, in common with many other ophthalmic surgeons and clinicians, is almost nil. With such sparse beginnings there seems little that would be appropriate to a volume of this type. Still, it has seemed of interest to review briefly the cases purporting to involve the orbit and briefly to note the salient features of its course and histopathology.

INCIDENCE

Orbital involvement by Hodgkin's disease is so unusual that a case report in the literature reporting such an event is immediately perused with considerable anticipation. Alas, efforts to learn more about such a strange clinical association often are marred by the failure of the publication to report all details of the case. What was called an orbital involvement may prove to be a lump in the brow or eyelid upon closer scrutiny of the report. So, the case proves to be one of presumed Hodgkin's disease because no histologic examination of the orbital mass was made. Also, there are cases that may resemble Hodgkin's disease histopathologically, but Reed-Sternberg cells are not found or illustrated in the photomicrographs. Most frustrating are those reports with well-illustrated histologic examples of Hodgkin's disease but in which the author says nothing about the patient's course either before or after the orbital lump is identified. The more complete reports in the recent literature are those of Watillion and associates (1964), Fratkin and associates (1978), Sweeney and associates (1977), and Reese (1976). Five patients are covered in these four reports (three females and two males) with an age range of 39 to 56 years of age at time of orbital involvement.

CLINICAL FEATURES AND COURSE

In patients who develop an orbital mass and have been under treatment for painless swelling of the cervical, axillary, or inguinal lymph nodes — or who have an unexplained mediastinal lymphadenopathy — the ophthalmologist should be on the lookout for a possible Hodgkin's disease. In both documented and presumed cases of Hodgkins's disease, orbital invasion usually appears late in the course of the disease. However, there is no set pattern of orbital involvement. If the tumor is located in the retrobulbar space, visual loss will likely result. In contrast, a mass in the forward portion of the orbit, particularly if it is responsive to chemotherapy and irradiation, seems quite compatible with continued, unimpaired, visual function. Although advances in therapy in the past two decades have significantly improved survival rates, the disease is ultimately fatal.

So, proven examples of Hodgkin's disease with involvement of the orbit are very scarce. It seems there is factual basis for regarding the orbital cavity as a possible lodging point for Hodgkin's tumor in its disseminated form. However, there is some question whether the orbital cavity may serve as the primary locus of the disease such as seems to be the case with the lymphocytic lymphomas.

PATHOLOGY

It is not likely that an ophthalmologist will be called upon to display expertise in the histopathologic diagnosis of Hodgkin's disease. Nevertheless, he should have some acquaintance with the variable cellular patterns of the basic lesion and their correlation with prognosis. In present day classifications the various cytologic phases of the disease are listed in the order of their increasing malignancy. In general, the greater the content of lymphocytes in the tissue sections the more favorable the prognosis; the fewer the lymphocytes the more serious the prognosis. However, the time required to pass through these progressive cellular responses varies widely among affected individuals.

Initially, the lymphocytes proliferate and if a tissue section is examined at this stage, the uniform collections of the cells will resemble the lymphocytic type of malignant lymphoma. Since the Sternberg-Reed giant cells upon which the correct diagnosis is based are scarce at this stage, a careful search must be made for their presence or the diagnosis will not be correct (Fig. 217). Soon abnormal histiocytic cells appear in the affected tissue and these cells may possess such multiple nuclei as to mimic the Sternberg-Reed cell. Next, the host seems to react to this insult by a proliferation of plasma cells and mature granulocytes (both neutrophils and eosinophils) in and around the lymphocytes, Sternberg-Reed cells, and histiocytes already present. This tussle at the tissue level with the noxious agent continues for some months or years until the resistance of the host gradually falters. More and more fibroblasts appear, areas of necrosis become evident in the tissue specimens, and fibrosis finally ensues. The functional capacity of the affected node is compromised and the content of lymphocytes diminishes (Fig. 218). However, the neoplastic elements of the affected site remain and the cytology more and more resembles a poorly differentiated sarcoma. Increasing anemia, weakness, and cachexia of the patient reflect the relentless pursuit by the neoplasm until a fatal termination ensues.

Throughout these different phases the one feature common to all, and the one necessary for unequivocal diagnosis, is the Sternberg-Reed cell. Briefly, it is a large cell (diameter, 15 to 45μ) from two to six times the size of an erythrocyte. The cell is usually irregular in shape and its most distinguishing characteristic is the two (sometimes more) opposing nuclei arranged almost in mirror reflection configuration. The nucleoli are prominent, red staining, and contrast sharply with the finally dispersed and faintly staining nuclear material surrounding them. The cytoplasm of the cell is abundant and amphophilic.

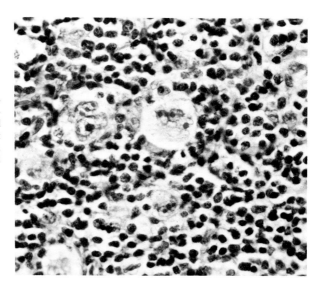

Figure 217. Hodgkin's disease, with lymphocytic predominance: several large, multilobed Sternberg-Reed cells are present against background of small lymphocytes. (Hematoxylin and eosin; × 480.)

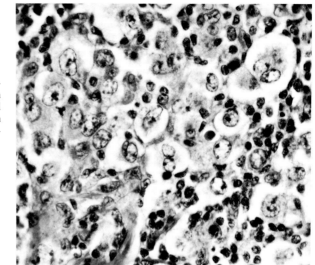

Figure 218. Hodgkin's disease with lymphocytic depletion of background cells, principal cell being Sternberg-Reed cell often arranged in large sheets. (Hematoxylin and eosin; × 440.)

WELL-DIFFERENTIATED LYMPHOMA, DIFFUSE

Although malignant lymphoma is essentially a systemic disease, most cases commence as a localized proliferation of lymphocytes in one lymph node group or one extranodal site. The diffuse, well-differentiated lymphocytic lymphoma is the more common extranodal form of the disease in the orbits of adults. Overall (Table 17), there is a larger number of poorly differentiated orbital lymphocytic lymphomas, but this type affects both children and adults and proliferates in both nodular and diffuse cellular patterns. In the majority of the well-differentiated, diffuse types (15 of 18 cases), the orbit seemed to be the initial or presenting site of the disease. For convenience we have designated such tumors as *primary* orbital lymphomas. We recognize that it is not always possible to be absolutely certain that another locus of the neoplasm is not tucked away in some other anatomic site even though sophisticated investigative procedures such as lymphangiography, bone marrow biopsy, serum evaluation for dysglobulinemia, and inferior vena cavagram are all negative for disseminated disease. Also, in the earlier years of our patient survey many of these diagnostic techniques were not in vogue. We will devote the major portion of our discussion to this primary, diffuse, well-differentiated type because it is the archtype of the orbital lymphomas. The average age of the 15 patients with the primary type was 62.4 years.

CLINICAL FEATURES

For some reason which we cannot explain the disease affected the left orbit of our patients in a ratio of 10:5. This two to one incidence may not be significant considering the small number of total cases. The onset of the disease is insidious and the presenting complaint that brings the patient for consultation usually has been present for a period of 3 to 24 months., with an average of 10 months. All of our patients had observed one or a combination of two of the three predominant symptoms of this type of lymphoma. The most frequent initial sign was *eyelid swelling* or puffiness. Next in frequency was the awareness of some *protrusion or change in position of the eye*. The third most frequent was palpation of a mass or recognition of an enlarging tumor in the conjunctival cul-de-sac. Also, diplopia and epiphora are occasionally noted. In all but two of these patients the tumor could be palpated in the forward portion of the orbit. This accounts for the puffiness of the eyelid and displacement of the eye in the early course of the disease (Fig. 219). We do not have an anatomic or a functional explanation as to why the lymphocytes choose this particular location in the orbit for their proliferation. Their proliferation more anteriorly in the conjunctiva and epibulbar area can be explained, of course, by the normal presence of lymphoid tissue in these areas. In no other major orbital tumor is the ratio of positive palpation to the total number of tumors so high or the tumor so visible except infantile hemangioma.

On palpation these tumors feel somewhat indurated and fixed. However, they are not as hard nor as immobile on palpation as is metastatic carcinoma. The lymphoid tumors are not tender. The comment is frequently made that they have a "shotty," "corded," or "nodular" consistency. The most characteristic, and practically diagnostic, appearance of lymphoma is the reddish pink, flesh-colored, soft mass that protrudes upward through the lower conjunctival cul-de-sac or pushes downward over the upper surface of the eyeball from the superior cul-de-sac (Fig. 220). So characteristic is the appearance of this particular type of lymphoma that an incisional biopsy ordinarily would not be required were it not for the need to convince the radiotherapist that such is the true nature of the tumor before therapy is commenced.

The tumor may grow in any quadrant of the orbit or extend horizontally or vertically into another quadrant (Fig. 221). Of the 15 patients, the tumor was found in the superior orbit in 11, in the inferior orbit in 3 cases. In the remaining case the tumor was found in the posterior portion of the orbit. The statement frequently is made that malignant lymphomas most often occur in the inferior orbit. In our opinion this is not quite true. The well-differentiated lymphoma occurs more frequently in upper portions of the orbit just as do most other neoplasms and cysts. However, if the ratio of neoplasms occurring in the lower orbit to the upper orbit is considered, the lymphomas will have a higher incidence in the lower orbit than almost any other tumor. So frequently is lymphoma a resident of the lower orbit as compared to other primary tumors and pseudotumors that it should be considered first in the differential diagnosis

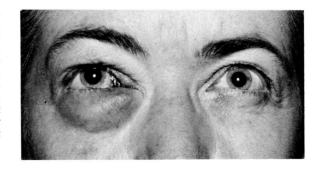

Figure 219. Malignant lymphoma, lymphocytic, well-differentiated type: fullness of right lower eyelid due to slow enlargement of nontender mass in inferior quadrants of right orbit (duration, 7 months), with upward displacement of right eye; mass was firm, somewhat nodular, infiltrative, but not attached to bone. The inferior portion of the orbit is a frequent site for malignant lymphoma.

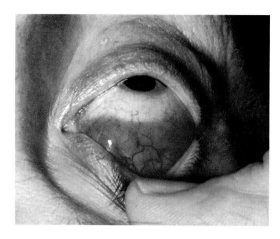

Figure 220.   Malignant lymphoma, lymphocytic type: flesh-colored mass on surface of right eye (forward extension of another mass in superior portion of the orbit) color of mass being typical; prominent blood vessels on surface of mass and tendency of these soft tumors to adapt to the contour of the space in which they are growing are evident.

when a mass is palpated in this neighborhood, unless there is some other obvious clue to the nature of the tumor, such as the color of a hemangioma in this locality or radiographic evidence of bone destruction in the maxillary sinus.

Roentgenograms of the orbit may show increased soft tissue density but this is of little diagnostic value. However, there are occasional reports in the literature of erosion of the roof of the orbit from well-differentiated lymphomas. If the clinical picture suggests lymphoma, but roentgenograms or tomograms indicate bone destruction along the medial wall of the orbit, a lymphoma secondary to an origin in the nasal cavity or paranasal sinuses should be considered. The use of computer tomography and orbital ultrasonography does not seem as necessary with lymphomas as in nonpalpable, posteriorly placed orbital tumors.

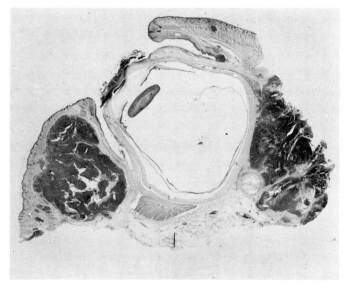

Figure 221.   Malignant lymphoma: extensive neoplasm in both superior and inferior orbit. (Hematoxylin and eosin; × 2½.)

Because of the more forward position of malignant lymphomas primary in the orbit, we seldom observe visual loss, visual field defects, and retinal striae. In the majority of these patients forward proptosis of the eye was neither extreme nor marked. In many of them the upward or downward displacement of the eye from its anteroposterior axis of the orbit was almost as great in amount as the forward proptosis of the eye, measured in millimeters by the exophthalmometer. This is a reflection of the forward position of the majority of the tumors. Also, these lymphomas grow very slowly. As a general rule, increase in proptosis will average 1 to 1.5 mm every two months.

PATHOLOGY

In its favorite haunt, the lymph node, the histopathology of the well-differentiated, lymphocytic type of malignant lymphoma has been well documented, thoroughly discussed, and pictorially delineated in many texts. In the orbit the identification of this subtype is another matter for here the lymph node and the lymphoid follicle do not normally exist. Therefore, many of the histopathologic criteria common to the systemic disease are not found when the questionable orbital mass is first examined microscopically. Interestingly, the usual cytologic manifestations associated with malignancy are not found. In this subtype of malignant lymphoma, for example, anaplasia is not evident. There are no variations in the size and shape of the cell, and the staining reaction of the individual cell does not show the variation so common in malignancy (Fig. 222). Mitosis, though visible, is not a prominent feature in any given field nor does it necessarily signify malignancy. Instead, profuse lymphocytes of mature appearance collect. The cellular unit of this neoplasm resembles the circulating lymphocyte so familiar in normal blood samples. So striking is this cellular uniformity that the descriptive term *monotonous regularity of mature lymphocytes* has been paraphrased by many writers. The simplicity of this pattern of lymphocytes is

Figure 222. Malignant lymphoma, well-differentiated lymphocytic type: diffuse infiltrative sheet of small lymphocytes replaces orbital structures. (Hematoxylin and eosin; × 325.)

quite striking, particularly if the tissue specimen has been removed from the center of the orbital mass. Usually, only two components are noted – the lymphocytes, and either the remaining fibrous framework of the host tissue or the orbital reticular substance. The sample also is generously endowed with fine capillaries. Insinuating itself into every available nook and cranny is the small, seemingly mature lymphocyte with small dark nuclei and no nucleoli. We believe this diffuse, infiltrative feature to be the principal clue to the nonmalignant lymphoid tumors. If the specimen in question contains other cellular components, such as plasma cells, granular leukocytes, or fibrous tissue proliferation, then the diagnosis more likely is pseudotumor than malignant lymphoma. Many times pathologists are handicapped in judging the criteria of pseudotumor versus malignant lymphoma by the sliver of tissue sample submitted for study or excision of just a peripheral portion of tumor at the time of biopsy.

This simple sequence of sameness, so unlike the picture of other neoplasms, has made many pathologists hesitant to designate these tumors as neoplastic. The term *reactive lymphoid hyperplasia* often is applied to this histopathologic situation. These benign reactive lesions will have germinal centers containing a heterogeneous population of lymphocytes with a greater number of mitoses. Another, less appropriate term in our opinion is *benign lymphoma*, which is favored by a minority of authors. In the future, immunochemistry techniques will help differentiate the malignant from the benign lesion by showing the predominantly monoclonal lymphocyte in the former and heterogeneity of the cell markers (polyclonal feature) in the latter. The seriousness of this problem from the patient's standpoint may be illustrated by the following case summary.

A 63-year-old physician was seen because of gradual proptosis of one eye of 6 months' duration. An infiltrative tumor was partially removed from the superior portion of the left orbit. A pathologic diagnosis of malignant lymphoma, lymphocytic type was made. The tissue specimens presented an appearance similar to that described in Figure 223A. The tumor samples also were reviewed at a national meeting of ophthalmic pathologists, many of whom favored the diagnosis of benign lymphoma and reactive lymphoid hyperplasia. Within a few weeks abdominal exploration was required because of an enlarging mass in one flank. Left nephrectomy was done, the tumor being malignant lymphoma, poorly differentiated "lymphoblastic" type (Fig. 223B). Within 2 years the patient died from the spread of malignant lymphoma to the liver.

The gross appearance of these tumors as they are encountered by the surgeon may engender a gamut of descriptive phrases. In color they are predominantly some shade of gray, gray-blue or reddish gray. In consistency they are moist when cut and most are friable; "tapioca-like mass" is an apt description, but they are not necrotic. In the inferior orbit they tend to be lumpy, poorly delineated, nonencapsulated masses. In the superior orbit they are more pancake-shaped and tend to develop a pseudocapsule on their anterior surface as they push against the orbital septum in their forward progress. Posteriorly, the boundaries of such tumors are ill defined.

TREATMENT

All lymphomas are radiosensitive, so much so that their response to this modality of treatment is usually quite dramatic (Fig. 224). It is often stated that all that is required, surgically, is an incisional biopsy to make the diagnosis. Any

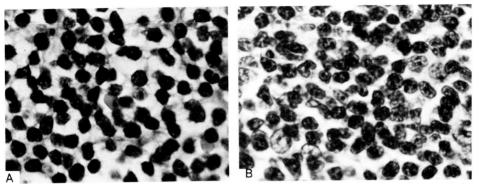

Figure 223. Malignant lymphoma: spectrum of progressive dedifferentiation (immaturity), demonstrated in two illustrations. (In all, hematoxylin and eosin; × 800.) *A*, Well-differentiated lymphocytic type; predominant cell is small lymphocyte with only slight nuclear abnormalities.

B, Malignant lymphoma, poorly differentiated type; nuclei are larger, more variable, and more immature in appearance.

further remarks concerning the tumors' surgical aspects, therefore, may seem superfluous. However, the mechanics of incisional biopsy may be touched upon. The approach to the tumors in the inferior quadrants, of course, is through an incision parallel to and slightly above the inferior orbital rim, and to those tumors in the superior quadrants by an incision parallel to and slightly below the superior orbital rim (see Section III). Such incisions, as they traverse the orbital septum, will usually position the surgeon directly over the tumor. With such easy access to these anteriorly positioned neoplasms, it is strange that so many surgeons take but a sliver of tumor for pathologic study. It is as though once the tumor has been easily uncovered the surgeon becomes bashful to unmask it. In the lower quadrants the tumor is seldom situated where excision of the main mass will do any harm. In the upper quadrants all the tumor that is easily dissected along the plane of its pseudocapsule may be removed. This provides a much more representative sample for pathologic study and such biopsies are (at least grossly) excisional rather than incisional. With samples of such size there should be little doubt as to whether the tumor is a neoplasm or a pseudotumor. It is the picayune samples so frequently submitted that may be responsible for such terms as "reactive lymphoid hyperplasia," or the tendency to diagnose any specimen containing lymphocytes as an example of lymphosarcoma. In the latter situation the pathologist is concerned about misdiagnosing

Figure 224. Malignant lymphomas: response to irradiation. *A*, Swelling of adnexal tissues of left eye due to rapidly enlarging mass in upper nasal quadrant of left orbit for 6 weeks in 59-year-old woman who then had no other systemic evidence of this neoplastic disorder; incisional biopsy revealed malignant lymphoma, reticulum cell type.

B, Same patient 1 week later illustrating responsiveness of neoplasm to irradiation therapy; patient died 4 years later from disseminated form of disease.

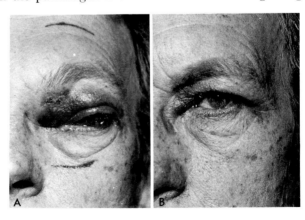

the specimen as inflammatory when it is truly a neoplasm, whereas with larger specimen of a truly non-neoplastic tumor, a greater admixture of cells makes him more confident that the specimen is inflammatory. The present dosimetry of irradiation is in the neighborhood of 4,500–4,600 R (as measured in air). R (as measured in air).

COURSE AND PROGNOSIS

What happens to patients with this type of orbital lymphoma? There are so few long-term studies, based on representative samples, that it is difficult to give a specific answer. It is nearly impossible to obtain follow-up information on some of the series in the literature based only on pathologic specimens. As in all studies involving retrospective data the investigator soon finds that a certain number of patients quickly escape the ken of the attending physician, vanish from the forwarding files of the United States mails, or inconsiderately expire from other causes, before a representative period of follow-up observation has passed. We were fortunate to obtain follow-up information on all our patients with this type of lymphoma primary in the orbit. Some of this interesting data is graphically summarized in Table 18A.

First, we note that only 2 of 15 treated patients died from systemic dissemination of their orbital lymphoma 9 and 13 years after histopathologic diagnosis. All patients received irradiation to the affected orbit after initial diagnosis. Of greater import was the death of five patients from causes other than lymphoma. This is not too surprising in view of the prevalent onset of orbital lymphoma in the sixth and seventh decades. Four of the five deaths were related to heart trouble and one patient died from cancer. It would appear that patients with well-differentiated orbital lymphoma are twice (5:2) as prone to die from some disease other than a systemic dissemination of their neoplasm. A further feature related to survival is that generalized lymphoma of this type is not incompatible with life. The two patients with generalized lymphoma who died from other causes 15 and 26 years after initial diagnosis (Table 18A) had undergone irradiation for their first focus of dissemination 10 and 16 years, respectively, before death. As regards the interval between diagnosis and the first sign of dissemination, there was no set pattern. The longest interval was 10 years in one patient. When dissemination did occur it most often affected some intra-abdominal organ or retroperitoneal node, but there were numerous other ultimate foci of disease in our patients, such as cervical and axillary nodes, scalp, ilium, bladder, stomach, and lung. Of great importance is the fact that only one of the fifteen patients had recurrence of lymphoma in the initially treated orbit. This speaks very favorably for the present methods of treatment of the orbital disease. In the one exception, lymphoma recurred in the orbit 9 years after initial treatment. More cheering is the fact that 5 of the patients are still alive without local or systemic lymphoma 6 or more years after diagnosis. To this favorable group should be added the 1 patient who was free of lymphoma at time of death 15 years after diagnosis.

All this data strongly supports the impression that diffuse, well-differentiated lymphoma is a less malignant form of the neoplasm. An individual with this orbital type of treated lymphoma has a better chance of either living with disseminated disease or dying from some cause other than generalized lymphoma.

TABLE 18A.   GRAPHIC ILLUSTRATION OF CLINICAL COURSE OF 20 PATIENTS WITH
DIFFUSE POORLY DIFFERENTIATED LYMPHOMAS ACCORDING TO SUBTYPES*

TABLE 18B.   GRAPHIC ILLUSTRATION OF CLINICAL COURSE OF 15 PATIENTS WITH
DIFFUSE, PRIMARY, WELL-DIFFERENTIATED ORBITAL LYMPHOMA*

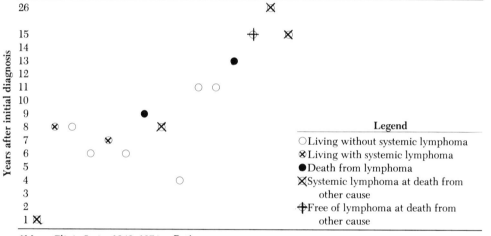

Legend

○ Living without systemic lymphoma
⊗ Living with systemic lymphoma
● Death from lymphoma
✖ Systemic lymphoma at death from
other cause
✛ Free of lymphoma at death from
other cause

*Mayo Clinic Series 1948–1974.   **Patients**

GENERALIZED WELL-DIFFERENTIATED LYMPHOMA

This designation refers to those patients whose well-differentiated orbital lymphoma appeared some time after an initial focus of tumor elsewhere, or who were discovered to have disseminated manifestations of lymphoma at the same time they presented with the orbital neoplasm. There were three patients of this type. Their course was much less encouraging than the group with primary orbital disease. Two of the 3 patients died of lymphoma within 3 years of orbital presentation of the disease. The survivor is living 5 years after orbital involvement with 2 other known tumor deposits that have been responsive to radiotherapy. The group is too small to accurately judge prognosis, but it is our impression that the number of active or treated foci at the time of orbital invasion may be a factor in survival. Thus, an individual with but one known focus of lymphoma, other than the orbit, seems to survive longer than patients with multiple sites of involvement at the time of discovery of the orbital lymphoma.

POORLY DIFFERENTIATED LYMPHOMA, DIFFUSE

These lymphomas, clinically, are a more heterogeneous group than the preceding well-differentiated lymphomas with similar diffuse patterns of cell proliferation. It is likely there are at least two, and perhaps more, separate lymphoma entities within the group. The tendency to divide the poorly differentiated lymphomas into subgroups is based on differing clinical features and age distribution of the patients. This histologic type of lymphoma may be seen in children as well as adults but the course is much different in the two age groups. Among children and young adults the poorly differentiated type is sometimes called *lymphosarcoma of childhood*. The majority of the latter have a T cell origin, whereas the adult lymphomas will have B cell markers similar to well-differentiated lymphomas. The adult poorly differentiated lymphomas probably have a germinal center origin.

In the Mayo Clinic series there were eighteen patients with the adult type of diffuse poorly differentiated lymphoma. The orbit was the presenting site of the disease in nine patients; in seven patients the lymphoma was generalized by the time of orbital involvement; and in one patient the lymphoma was secondary to a paranasal sinus origin. This distribution differs considerably from that noted with the diffuse well-differentiated lymphomas. The average age of the patients with the primary, poorly differentiated lymphomas at time of orbital presentation was 61 years, and 63 years for those with disseminated types. This is almost identical to the 62.4 year average of adults with primary, diffuse, well-differentiated lymphomas. A similar age range, 62 and 65 years, was noted in the 2 patients with orbital lymphoma secondary to a paranasal source. The 3 patients with the childhood-adolescent type of poorly differentiated lymphoma were 1½, 4½, and 18 years of age at time of initial presentation of the disease in the orbit. In the total group the disease affected the left and right orbit in a ratio of 15:6. This two to one predominance of the left orbit also was noted in the group of patients with diffuse, well-differentiated lymphoma.

The onset and early clinical course of adult patients with the primary and generalized subtypes of diffuse, poorly differentiated lymphoma do not differ from the signs and symptoms of the well-differentiated lymphomas already noted. In the childhood and adolescent group of poorly differentiated lymphomas, the early course of the disease progresses more rapidly than in adults. These younger patients are usually brought for orbital consultation several weeks after onset as contrasted to an interval of several months in adults.

PATHOLOGY

These lymphomas also are composed of small to medium-sized lymphocytes but show more variations in cell size and nuclear configuration than diffuse, well-differentiated lymphomas. They are divided into two subgroups on the basis of slightly differing cytologic features between the tumors of children and adults.

In adults, the lymphocytes are more pleomorphic, with nuclei that are elongated, notched, or clefted in shape. Almost all of these lymphomas in the

Mayo Clinic series were composed of neoplastic cells with small cleaved nuclei (Fig. 223*B*). The chromatin is relatively coarse, but a single distinct nucleolus can be seen. Mitotic figures are evident but are not numerous.

In children there is less pleomorphism of the cells but mitotic figures are numerous. The round and oval nuclei have a more diffuse, dust-like distribution of chromatin with from one to three small, inconspicuous nucleoli. The nuclear membrane also may be deeply grooved or creased. This is the subgroup that is believed to have a T cell origin and is so rapidly fatal.

COURSE AND TREATMENT

Although these lymphomas have an onset and early clinical course quite similar to the diffuse, well-differentiated lymphoma, and are treated with radiotherapy in the same manner, the poorly differentiated diffuse lymphomas, as a group, have a more serious prognosis. We have some follow-up information on all but one of the twenty-one patients in the group. In Table 18B we have depicted the course of the patients in the several subgroups of poorly differentiated lymphomas. It is clearly apparent that mortality is much greater in the subgroups of generalized, childhood, and secondary lymphomas than among patients with diffuse, well-differentiated lymphoma (Table 18A). Also, the interval between diagnosis and death in these three subgroups of poorly differentiated lymphomas is quite short in many patients. The survival of the two adult patients with orbital lymphoma secondary to an ethmoid focus was almost as short (a year or less) as in the two children with the childhood type lymphoma. The least malignant tumors of the group were those lymphomas primary in the orbit of adults.

NODULAR LYMPHOMA

One of the important changes in the Rappaport revision (1966) of the older classification of lymphomas was the division into two groups based on the pattern of involvement of the lymph nodes by the neoplastic cells. Those neoplasms growing in a nodular arrangement simulating the germinal follicular centers of normal nodes were separated from the diffuse lymphomas wherein the architecture of the lymph node was completely effaced by the expanding tumor. This division was important because it was found that *nodular lymphomas* have a significantly more favorable prognosis than *diffuse lymphomas*. In an extranodal site such as the orbit, many of the criteria for the diagnosis of germinal center neoplasia are absent, but the tendency of the neoplastic cells to arrange themselves in follicular-like subunits is definitely retained (Fig. 225). In the more common, disseminated, nodal form of nodular lymphoma several cytologic variants are recognized. This subgrouping of nodular lymphomas also has clinical significance in that cell-type population in any given tissue section may tell whether the prognosis is more favorable or less favorable. Those nodular lymphomas composed predominantly of the small cell type have a favorable survival even though the disease is disseminated at time of diagnosis. Those

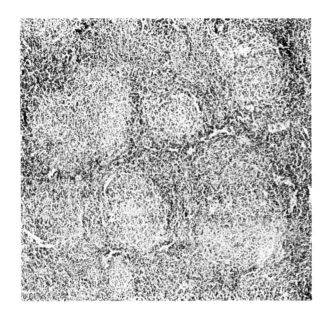

Figure 225. Nodular lymphoma: the nodular aggregates of lymphoid cells create a neoplastic recapitulation of germinal centers. (Hematoxylin and eosin; × 64.)

nodular lymphomas with mixed small and large cell populations have a more labile clinical course and a less favorable survival. Finally, there is the large cell variant which portends the least favorable prognosis. The patient with a nodular lymphoma may progress from the more favorable type to a less favorable pattern during the natural course of the lymphoma, or change to the diffuse form of the disease. These cytologic subtypes ranging from more favorable to less favorable features may be designated poorly differentiated, mixed small and large cell type, and large cell type. All six cases of nodular lymphoma in the Mayo Clinic series were the small cleaved cell (poorly differentiated) subtype.

Nodular lymphomas occur predominantly in older adults, have an equal sex distribution, and are often disseminated at the time of diagnosis. In the orbit they are much less frequent than the several diffuse variants of lymphoma. The six patients in the Mayo Clinic study were in the 53- to 73-year age range with an equal sex incidence. In four of the patients the orbit was the presenting site of the disease. In the remaining two people the lymphoma had already disseminated at the time of orbital diagnosis.

Of the 4 patients with primary orbital nodular lymphoma, 2 died of their disease 2 and 9 years after orbital diagnosis. One patient had no evidence of dissemination nor local orbital recurrence when death occurred from heart disease 5 years after diagnosis. The remaining individual is living without local or systemic lymphoma 14 years after diagnosis. However, in this latter patient, irradiation therapy was necessary for cervical lymphoma in the 9th year of the 14-year interval. This group of four is too small to conclude whether primary orbital nodular lymphoma has or has not a better prognosis than the diffuse, poorly differentiated orbital lymphoma. The two patients with disseminated disease at the time of orbital involvement conformed more closely to the usual course of nodular lymphoma, surviving 13 and 20 years respectively before succumbing to their disease.

MIXED CELL LYMPHOMA

These lymphomas are so named because of nearly equal proportion of small cells (poorly differentiated lymphocytes) and large cells (histiocytic-like lymphocytes) in their makeup. The small cell component has clefted nuclei similar to some cells observed in the normal germinal centers of lymph nodes. The large cells have vesicular nuclei with nucleoli often positioned along the nuclear membrane. It is probable that a continuum exists between the small and large cells in the unfavorable progression of the disease. Most of these mixed cell lymphomas have a nodular pattern, but a separate less common diffuse subtype also is recognized.

One patient with a diffuse mixed cell lymphoma was noted in the Mayo Clinic series. This was a 57-year-old male with slowly progressive proptosis of the left eye over an 8-month period due to a slightly circumscribed lymphoma infiltrating the tissues in the lower anterior inferior orbit. No signs of systemic dissemination were found. The involved orbit was treated with 4,500 rads of cobalt radiotherapy over a 24-day postoperative period. This patient is living without local or systemic manifestations of lymphoma 9 years after diagnosis—an unusually long interval of survival for this type of lymphoma. Strictly on the basis of the histologic appearance of the lymphoma the patient was considered to have an unfavorable prognosis. We explain the paradox of long survival on the basis that the orbital lymphoma was the only locus of the disease at the time of diagnosis, and treatment was given early enough in the course of the disease to effect a significant arrest or possible cure.

LARGE CELL (RETICULUM CELL SARCOMA) LYMPHOMA

This most malignant unit of the family was not identified as early as the others. Roulet (1930), a German pathologist, usually is credited as being the first to consider this group of neoplasms as a separate entity, having proposed the term *retothelsarkom*. But Oberling (Bürki, 1943), a French pathologist, used the term *reticulosarkom* in 1928 for what seems to have been the same neoplasm. Initially, this proved to be a very satisfactory designation for a number of tumors whose cytology was so undifferentiated that other classification was not possible. Furthermore, the reticulum cell was believed to have wide pluripotential facilities as the precursor cell of bone marrow granulocytes, lymphoid cells, mobile and fixed phagocytic monocytes, and vague relationships to plasma cells and endothelial cells. As a result, many of the very immature neoplasias of infants and children were designated reticulum cell sarcoma which in the light of modern histopathologic techniques, would now be reclassified as examples of embryonal rhabdomyosarcoma, neuroblastoma, granulocytic sarcoma, and so on. It was natural, then, to seek a more specific, less generalized term than reticulum cell sarcoma.

When Rappaport (1966) proposed his morphologic classification of lymphomas so widely used today, the term *histiocytic lymphoma* was substituted for reticulum cell sarcoma. This new term was applied because nuclei of these neoplastic cells had features more similar to those of tissue histiocytes than of any other known type of normal lymphoreticular cell. This seemed to be a forward step in the problem of terminology until immunochemistry techniques indicated a very dubious relationship between the reticulum cell and the true histiocyte.

In the past several years a number of limited (five to ten cases) series of reticulum cell sarcomas have been studied with surface markers. These studies agree that reticulum cell sarcomas are a very heterogenous group in reference to cell of origin. As a rule, at least half of the tumors so examined will have B and T cell surface markers indicating their lymphocytic nature. Other cells will be unresponsive to any of the presently known markers; these tumors are of uncertain pathogenesis. A very small minority will have the markers characteristic of the monocytic-histiocytic cell line. So, the term histiocytic lymphoma more often may be wrong than right.

The fact that some reticulum cell sarcomas seem to be a monoclonal proliferation of B cells has suggested a relationship to "transformed" lymphocytes. The latter theory is responsible for the use of the term *large cell* lymphoma. A revised terminology for this group of neoplasms may not be possible until the identity of some of the receptor silent cell populations can be established. For these several reasons the designation, large cell lymphoma, may be replaced by a more suitable term sometime in the future. We have retained the alternate term, reticulum cell sarcoma, in the title of this subchapter for the convenience of those who prefer the older terminology.

INCIDENCE AND CLINICAL FEATURES

In the ten individuals with large cell lymphoma in our Mayo Clinic series, there were five with orbital tumors as the presenting site of the disease, four with other sites of the disease in addition to the orbit, and one patient with secondary invasion of the orbit by tumor from the maxillary antrum. The age range of the patients with large cell lymphoma was 47 to 68 years, with a median age of 57 to 58 years. This data agrees closely with a study of thirteen biopsy-proven cases studied by Jakobiec and associates (1978).

In the clinical evolution of the orbital neoplasm several features differed from those already noted with other lymphomas. *Swelling* and *puffiness* of the eyelid always preceded *proptosis; pain* and *discomfort* around the orbit was quite frequent; and the interval between the initial symptom of the disease and presentation of the patient was much shorter (a matter of a few months). All of this data indicates a more rapidly progressive disease than the prior lymphomas except for the poorly differentiated type occurring in children.

A puzzling feature of large cell lymphoma is its tendency to involve the central nervous system. Such a complication is definitely more frequent than with other lymphomas. The ophthalmologic findings would then include extraocular muscle palsies secondary to cranial nerve involvement, papilledema, visual field defects, and visual loss progressing from one eye to the other.

Another peculiar aspect is the occasional presentation of the lymphoma as an intraocular process resembling an uveitis. Initially, there is blurring of vision in one eye secondary to a clouding and haziness of the vitreous (posterior uveitis). This smoldering uveitis is recalcitrant to the usual medical therapies and vision gradually decreases. Eventually the disease affects the other eye if central nervous system involvement and death have not already intervened.

PATHOLOGY

In the orbit the gross appearance of these tumors is similar to other lymphomas and microscopy is necessary to tell them apart. However, at the cellular level the appearance of the tumor is quite different from other lymphomas. First, the cells are quite large, three to four times the size of lymphocytes. The nuclei stand out in the tissue section because of a heavily marginated nuclear membrane surrounded by a pale, lightly staining amphophilic or eosinophilic cytoplasm. In addition, the nuclei may be folded, cleaved, or kidney shaped. The chromatin is rather coarse, but one to several nucleoli are easily visible. The cytoplasm, which varies in amount, often shows syncytial features suggesting an intracytoplasmic reticulum (Fig. 226). This is responsible for the name reticulum (net-like) cell. Mitotic activity is usually marked. Varying amounts of intercellular reticulin may be seen, but this does not seem to have any bearing on prognosis.

Some pathologists tend to divide the group into subtypes, such as is done with poorly differentiated lymphomas. In one type the cells are quite uniform. In another type the tissue section will show interspersion of phagocytes, which gives the specimen a "starry sky" appearance. In this type, mitoses are abundant. In the third subtype there is marked cellular pleomorphism with multinucleated giant cells.

COURSE AND PROGNOSIS

Most generalizations concerning the prognosis of the orbital forms of reticulum cell sarcoma are based on the mortality rates of the systemic form. It is

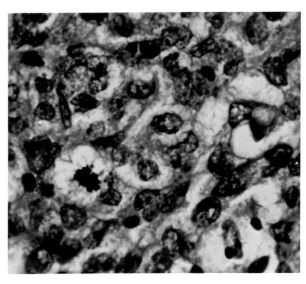

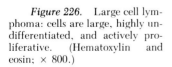

Figure 226. Large cell lymphoma: cells are large, highly undifferentiated, and actively proliferative. (Hematoxylin and eosin; × 800.)

thus believed that the majority of patients will be dead within 2 to 3 years of onset. Any orbital data is also influenced by the likelihood that sarcoma is already multicentric by the time proptosis or lid swelling appears, even though the latter symptoms may be the only apparent manifestations of malignancy. We have some follow-up data on seven patients in whom the orbit was the presenting site of the disease or but one of several multicentric foci of lymphoma. Five of these patients succumbed to their lymphoma, with an average longevity of 2 to 3 years after appearance of the initial focus of tumor. The longest period of survival was 4 years. This average interval is shorter than in adult patients with poorly differentiated lymphoma but longer than in children with childhood lymphoma. Two of our patients with large cell lymphoma are living 2 and 3 years, respectively, from the time of initial diagnosis and treatment. In both of these patients the orbit was the presenting site of the lymphoma, and in one individual, the lymphoma was so circumscribed that it was easily removed intact. However, our series is too small to warrant any statement as to whether prognosis is better among those patients who seem to have only an orbital focus at the time of histologic diagnosis than among those with multicentric lymphoma. All of our patients received radiotherapy in a dosage schedule common to other lymphomas.

BURKITT'S LYMPHOMA

Although we have no cases of *undifferentiated lymphoma, Burkitt's type,* in our Mayo Clinic survey, nor have we seen any cases of orbital involvement other than in West African children, we anticipate that one of our readers will encounter such a case either in the United States or in a predominantly English-speaking country and will want a summary of the salient features of the lymphoma as known up to the present time. This lymphoma is of world wide interest because of its relatively recent recognition as a separate clinicopathologic entity, its rapid progression sometimes associated with a dreadful deformity of the involved orbit, its variable clinical pattern in differing parts of the world, its responsiveness to therapy (in some cases equivalent to a cure), and its possible etiologic association with a virus.

HISTORICAL ASPECTS

Burkitt published his first paper on the subject in 1958. He reviewed the clinical characteristics of an "absurd" type of sarcoma that chiefly affected the jaws of 38 East African children. Most of these children had been seen during a period of 7 years. Subsequently several of his associates (O'Conor et al 1965) also have made contributions to the literature. Chief of these was O'Conor, a pathologist, who seems to have been responsible for associating the neoplasm with the lymphoma family through his study and classification of the pathologic specimens. By 1961 (Burkitt and O'Conor, 1961) the number of cases observed in this part of Africa had increased to 106, among which were 14 with the presenting symptom of exophthalmos. The incidence of this neoplasm among the children of equatorial Africa was so high, the manifestations around the head sometimes so monstrous in appearance, the course so rapidly fatal, and the resemblance to disorders and syndromes previously described so vague that the several publications on this tumor made a great impact. A further point that piqued the curiosity of interested clinicians was the possibility that, because of its distribution in African Negro children living in the malaria belt, the disease might be related to some environmental or social factor or, especially, that it was caused by a virus. This latter possibility was particularly exciting, for the African lymphoma might very well be the key that would reveal the viral etiology of neoplasms for which microbiologists and oncologists had long been searching. Subsequently, high antibody levels to Epstein-Barr virus were found in most African patients with Burkitt's lymphoma.

The publications of Burkitt and others set in motion a scramble to find examples of this disease elsewhere. Physicians soon became aware of similar cases in almost all other continents of the world. In the United States, observers scurried about unlocking files and cabinets of pathologic tissue specimens that might be a reservoir for unsuspected, unrecognized, or unreported examples of the neoplasm. Sure enough, examples of the neoplasm were soon uncovered and reports, prior to the two publications of Burkitt, were rediscovered. All these attempts to establish priority should not detract from Burkitt's efforts. Burkitt was aware that a few others had published observations on these unusual jaw sarcomas. Considering the problems of diagnosis, therapy, and follow-up observation attendant to the care of East African children, we consider that Burkitt's clinical observations were well executed and that his contribution has been a great stimulus for reviewing the subject of lymphoma.

CLINICAL FEATURES AND COURSE

As with other lymphomas of childhood, the neoplasm has a multifocal origin. In most cases the disease commences as a retroperitoneal mass or a nodular involvement of the abdominal viscera. In the tropical zone of Africa, where the disease is most common, such abdominal changes may go unnoticed, but the rapidly growing tumor in the maxilla cannot be ignored. As the tumor expands, the face becomes distorted and the eye protrudes owing to secondary invasion of the orbit. All this occurs in a few weeks. The afflicted child with the swollen abdomen and the bizarre asymmetry of the face has the look of piteous despair. In the nonAfrican case the patient may be spared the hideousness of the facial-orbital involvement because this clinical feature is so much less frequent in these cases. If the disease goes untreated there is soon invasion of bone marrow, dissemination to lungs and central nervous system, and death. The proptosis may be so extreme as to require enucleation of the desiccated, ulcerated eye. Bilateral orbital involvement may occur and the eye may even be invaded by the rapidly growing mass (Feman et al 1969, Karp et al 1971).

The age range of African cases is 2 to 14 years, with maximum susceptibility around 5 to 6 years. The nonAfrican patients may be slightly older, with a median age of 10 to 11 years.

Present treatment protocols utilize parenteral chemotherapy and adjuvant radiotherapy. Cyclophosphamide is the chief chemotherapeutic agent. In general, those patients with localized disease at the time of treatment have a better prognosis than patients with multicentric involvement. According to Ziegler (1977), younger patients (less than 12 years) have better survival periods than older patients with similar sites of lymphoma. Patients with involvement of face and orbit do better than patients with involvement of lung and central nervous system. Arseneau and colleagues (1975) found that serum lactic dehydrogenase levels closely correlated with the extent of the lymphoma, and values were lowest in patients with localized disease. If there is no relapse of the disease within a 12-month period after completion of treatment, remission of the disease may be complete. Great strides have been made in the treatment of this disease in the past decade.

PATHOLOGY

In the gamesmanship of semantics the ophthalmologist should remember the phrase "starry sky," for this is the term used by most observers to describe the configuration of tissue specimens as they appear under lower magnifications (Fig. 227 A). The contrast between the masses of closely packed lymphocytes

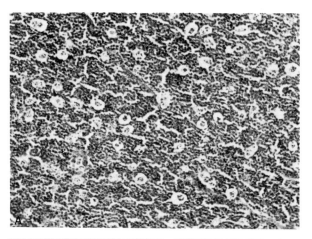

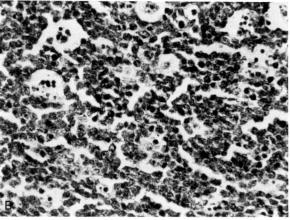

Figure 227. Burkitt's lymphoma. *A*, "Starry sky" appearance is due to histiocytic cells scattered among closely packed lymphocytes. (Hematoxylin and eosin; × 110.)

B, Phagocytosed nuclear material is present within histiocytes; lymphocytes are immature. (Hematoxylin and eosin; × 285.)

and the single histiocytic cells is responsible for this print-like pattern. However, the "starry sky" pattern is not pathognomonic of Burkitt's lymphoma. In tissue sections the lymphoma cells are quite uniform, about 15 to 25μ in diameter, with round or oval nuclei that approximate the nuclei of the interspersed macrophages (Fig. 227 B). Each nucleus may have from one to four nucleoli and mitotic figures are frequent. Each cell has a narrow rim of amphophilic cytoplasm with a number of clear, vacuole-like spaces that may stain positively for neutral fat. The macrophages have a clear, abundant cytoplasm and contain cellular debris. The intercellular reticulin network is delicate and rather sparse.

PLASMA CELL MYELOMA

This is a neoplasm of plasma cells. It is but one of a group of plasma cell dyscrasias that have received much attention in the past several decades because of advances in the field of immunobiology. The plasma cell is one of the principal components of the lymphoreticular system, and its functional role is in the field of immunosurveillance. In this role it is closely allied to the B-type lymphocyte noted earlier in this chapter. Indeed, it is believed that B-type lymphocytes, under the stimulus of an increased need for immunoglobulin, convert to plasma cells to perform the immunosecretory function more efficiently. It follows that any overproduction of plasma cells, either normal or abnormal in degree, will be reflected as an increased production of immunoglobulin, recognized as a "peak" on serum or urine electrophoresis. Although this abnormality is common to all plasma cell dyscrasias sometime in their course, the group may differ widely in other respects such as course, clinical features, and prognosis.

TERMINOLOGY

This tumor, like many others that we have reviewed, has been designated by several different names. Terms such as *plasmacytoma, plasmocytoma, plasmoma,* and *plasmacytoid tumor* will be encountered in the literature. Sometimes one of these names may be applied to the tumor under discussion; in other instances a similar term may be used to designate a tumor containing plasma cells but of a different sort. It is important to determine whether the author is discussing a neoplasm of plasma cells or a granuloma containing plasma cells. The former is malignant; the latter is benign. To eliminate confusion, we favor eliminating all these designations for the benign granulomatous tumor, at least in the orbit. Here it might be better to regard the plasmacytoid granuloma as a variant of the nonspecific, but often mixed cellular, pseudotumors. For the neoplasm, the term selected as the title of this subchapter seems most suitable.

A subdivision of this neoplasm into solitary and extramedullary types also is frequently suggested. The term *solitary myeloma* crept into the literature to designate a single focus of tumor in bone, but this was in the years before diagnostic methods such as bone marrow aspiration were practiced. After a latent period of some years, the solitary focus is replaced by multiple sites of myeloma. The *extramedullary* form refers to a soft tissue focus, generally the submucous tissues and mucous membranes of the respiratory and alimentary systems, and particularly the nasal passages and nasopharynx. Occasionally the terms will be combined thus: a *solitary extramedullary tumor.* The implication is the patient has but one soft tissue focus of disease, at least in the beginning. Both forms — solitary and extramedullary, bony and soft tissue — affect the orbit. When the proliferation of malignant plasma cells become widespread, typically involving the bone marrow, the term *multiple myeloma* is used.

INCIDENCE

The orbit may be involved by an extension of myeloma from an adjacent sinus, by spread from one of the diseased bones of the calvarium, or by a metastatic focus of cells lodging in soft tissues of the orbital cavity. An initial focus of tumor may also lodge between the periorbita and one of the orbital bones. However, the incidence of this tumor in the orbit remains low. In most large autopsy surveys of multiple myeloma patients the orbit usually is not mentioned as a site of involvement.

Rodman and Font (1972) reviewed the literature and tabulated thirty cases that seemed to qualify as examples of orbital involvement by multiple myeloma. Later, in the report of Knowles and associates (1978), the total patients with myelomatous involvement of the orbit in the literature had increased to thirty-four. In the 27-year period of our Mayo Clinic study, there were 4 cases (2 males and 2 females). Their age range was 62 to 76 years at the time of orbital diagnosis. In the Rodman and Font study the age of patients ranged from 30 to 89 years, with a median age of 56.5 years. It is unusual to observe the disease in a patient younger than forty.

CLINICAL FEATURES

The importance of plasma cell myeloma (whether it be the solitary, extramedullary, or multiple form of the disease) to ophthalmology is the frequency of the orbit as the presenting site of the disease. In the survey of thirty cases by Rodman and Font, proptosis was the initial manifestation in twenty-three patients. This fact was confirmed by experience with our four cases. In three of the four, orbital involvement was the initial problem that led to the diagnosis of myeloma. In the remaining patient, orbital involvement led to the correct diagnosis of a "blood abnormality" that had been known for one year.

Proptosis, diplopia on upward gaze, and ptosis of the upper eyelid (alone or in combination) are the features that bring these patients to the ophthalmologist's attention. A shotty, sometimes boggy mass will be palpated well forward in the superior orbit, and there will be definite restriction of ocular rotations, particularly in upward gaze. Pain also has been noted frequently among reports of the orbital disease in the literature but was not noted in any of our four cases. The duration of symptoms is usually quite short (less than 4 months), a feature also noted with reticulum cell sarcoma and poorly differentiated lymphoma of the orbit. However, the amount of proptosis or displacement of the eye may be

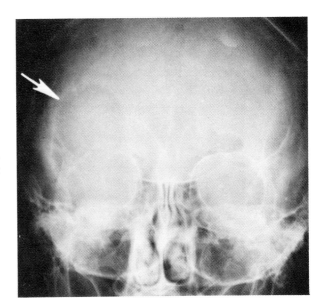

Figure 228. Plasma cell myeloma: large osteolytic defect eroding superior wall of right orbit.

unusually marked (greater than 6 mm) considering the short duration of symptoms. This orbital picture in an elderly individual who also has noted weakness, malaise, or fatigue might well alert the ophthalmologist to the diagnosis of plasma cell myeloma before x-ray examination or biopsy is undertaken.

In many (but not all) cases of orbital involvement, skull x-rays will show single or multiple osteolytic lesions of the frontal bone just above or communicating with the orbital cavity (Fig. 228). In this site the decalcification and moth-eaten appearance of the bone resembles the bony defects seen with metastatic carcinoma. A newly discovered myeloma patient should also have a roentgenographic skeletal survey to uncover the osteolytic defects or areas of impending pathologic fracture.

The patient with initial orbital disease also should have other laboratory examinations to determine the presence or absence of other foci of myeloma or generalized myelomatosis, such as blood hemoglobin (anemia), serum creatinine (renal insufficiency), blood calcium (hypercalcemia), urinalysis (Bence Jones proteinuria), serum electrophoresis (hypergammaglobulinemia), and bone marrow aspiration (plasmacytosis).

PATHOLOGY

In the orbit these neoplasms are soft, rather friable, poorly circumscribed, and have red to blue hues of gray. The tumors have only a scant supporting framework. At the cellular level the tumor may vary considerably in degree of differentiation. In the more mature types the proliferating plasma cells are easily identified by the eccentric position of the cell nucleus and peculiar clumping of chromatin in a cartwheel-like pattern (Fig. 229). In the less differentiated tumors the cells are somewhat larger, nuclear chromatin is more dispersed, and a prominent nucleolus is often seen, but the cells retain the feature of an eccen-

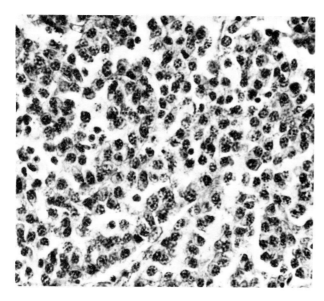

Figure 229. Plasma cell myeloma: this well-differentiated example consists of sheets of plasma cells with characteristic nuclei in which chromatin is clumped in spoke or cartwheel arrangement. (Hematoxylin and eosin; × 250.)

trically placed nucleus (Fig. 230). In both types there is an abundant, basophilic cytoplasm.

TREATMENT AND COURSE

For those cases wherein orbital involvement is the initial manifestation of the disease, irradiation has been most effective. Local excision of the orbital tumor has no effect on subsequent course of the disease and is only useful in reducing the proptosis. As the disease becomes more generalized, chemotherapy seems to be of most value. The course of the disease is entirely unpredictable, although most case surveys emphasize a longevity of only a few years after the disease assumes its multiple form. In a follow-up survey of 866 patients with multiple myeloma, Kyle (1975) found the median survival period was 20

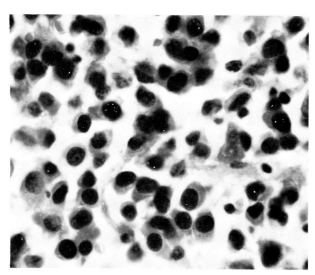

Figure 230. Plasma cell myeloma: plasmacytic nature of this less-differentiated example can be recognized by eccentric nucleus and abundant cytoplasm. (Hematoxylin and eosin; × 800.)

months. Levin and associates (1977) state that if not more than 2 localized plasma cell myelomas are present, the median survival rate is 8 years. Kyle also noted that superimposed infection was the most common cause of death, followed by renal insufficiency. The survival of our 4 patients ranged from 4 to 22 months even though the response of the orbital disease to radiotherapy was encouraging.

MACROGLOBULINEMIA

This interesting disorder combines some of the features of the preceding lymphomas and plasma cell myeloma. It is an abnormal proliferation of lymphoreticular cells which produce increased serum levels of a monoclonal gamma globulin of the IgM class. The elevated electrophoretic values of IgM are not unique to this neoplasia; they also may occur in some lymphomas and lymphocytic leukemias. Also, the increased secretion of IgM may occur as a benign process without the abnormal proliferation of lymphoreticular cells. In fact, it is the latter type of macroglobulinemia that was part of a syndrome first described by Jan Waldenström of Upsala, Sweden. This "essential," nonprogressive macroglobulinemia of Waldenström is associated with an increased viscosity of the blood, oronasal bleeding, anemia, elevated erythrocytic sedimentation rate, lymphadenopathy, sludging of blood in the conjunctival vessels, and a retinopathy suggesting an impending bilateral occlusion of the retinal veins, in addition to abnormal IgM levels. The factor that causes the lymphoreticular transformation, that is, the abnormal proliferation of the plasma cells and lymphocytes that secrete the IgM, is not known.

When neoplasia supervenes, the cells invade the bone marrow, lymph nodes, abdominal viscera, and extramedullary sites, similar to the dissemination of lymphomas. Dissemination into bone, such as was seen in plasma cell myeloma, usually does not occur. A rare extramedullary site of involvement may be the orbit, and this is the reason for our particular interest.

In the orbit the tumors look, behave, and feel like well differentiated orbital lymphomas. However, case reports of orbital macroglobulinemia are very few. Little (1967) reported a 65-year-old male with bilateral painless enlargement of the palpebral and orbital portions of each lacrimal gland which, on biopsy, had the cytologic features of macroglobulinemia. Each orbital mass was treated with irradiation of 3,800 rads with dramatic reduction in size of the tumors. In retrospect, this patient was believed to have had systemic macroglobulinemia for 12 years prior to the orbital deposits. The 58-year-old male of Paufique and associates (1969) also had bilateral orbital masses, but there was a 5-year interval between the involvement of the first and second orbit. The age and sex factors in the two cases agree with the general concept that macroglobulinemia is chiefly a disease of elderly men. We have also seen one orbital case of macroglobulinemia outside the time period of our study but it was associated with a polyclonal gammopathy.

PATHOLOGY

Tissue sections under lower magnifications may closely resemble the picture of diffuse, well-differentiated lymphoma. On higher magnification some of the cells will have slightly larger nuclei that stain less intensely than the average nuclei of the mature appearing lymphocytes. These cells are intermediate between lymphocytes and mature plasma cells and are often referred to as *plasmacytoid lymphocytes*. Many of these cells will have intranuclear inclusions that are PAS positive. These inclusions push the chromatin toward the periphery of the nucleus and are called *Dutcher bodies* (Dutcher and Fahey, 1959). These elements probably represent the increased immunoglobulin secretory functions of the cells. They react positively to the periodic-acid-Schiff (PAS) stain because of the hexose-rich content of the immunoglobulins. Dutcher bodies are not specific for macroglobulinemia but may be seen in other monoclonal as well as polyclonal gammopathies.

GRANULOCYTIC SARCOMA

We have already noted the orbit can serve as an extranodal or extramedullary site for lymphomas sometime during their course from a localized tumor to a disseminated disease. Progression of the disease in some cases was manifested by neoplastic cells invading the bloodstream. In some lymphomas the interval between onset and terminal leukemia was very long (well-differentiated lymphomas) and in others very short (poorly differentiated lymphomas of childhood). A first cousin of the lymphomas, *granulocytic sarcoma* (a member of the granulocytic branch of lymphoreticular neoplasms), has somewhat comparable features. In a localized form, granulocytic sarcoma may precede overt manifestations of a granulocytic leukemia by some months or several years, or the tumor masses may be considered to be but another manifestation of an already established myelocytic leukemia. Currently, an optional term for this neoplasm is *myeloid sarcoma*, but the oldest and most widely used name is *chloroma*.

Chloroma means green tumor and physicians long have known about the tumor because of this color. The first description of a case is frequently attributed to Allan Burns in the period of 1811-1824. The date attributed to his description varies according to which edition of his work is quoted. However, Burns died in 1813, so he could not have described the tumor after the 1811 edition. The case in question in fact was not a patient of Burns' but of his brother (also a surgeon). The patient was a young man (the age was not reported) in whom one eye was enucleated because of rapid protrusion and pain secondary to an expanding mass in the area of the lacrimal gland. The tumor continued to grow, and a similar tumor also appeared in the other orbit. At autopsy the tumors were described as being the size of hen's eggs and possessing a distinctive greenish tinge. Posteriorly in the orbit, as well as in the frontal sinuses, other greenish yellow tumors were found.

Edgerton (1947) has described later events. As time passes, the tumor was named chloroma (1853) and classified with the leukemias (1883). In 1903, it was separated from the lymphoid lineage and placed among the family of myelogenous leukemias. Edgerton annotated 336 cases of chloroma in the literature up to 1947 and described in detail the symptoms of the disease as related to the eye and adnexa. Considering its prevalence at one time, the incidence of chloroma in the United States seems to have decreased. One possible explanation is that in the absence of its green color (a not infrequent occurrence) and obvious leukemia, the tumor cytologically is not easily differentiated from several other undifferentiated sarcomas of children. Until the staining modification of Leder (1964) became widely known these tumors were frequently called undifferentiated lymphoma, reticulum cell sarcoma, or embryonal rhabdomyosarcoma.

Granulocytic sarcoma has a tendency to develop in bones or periosteum, especially those of the skull. Orbital involvement is often seen early in the disease or may even be the presenting problem in an otherwise healthy child. Proptosis is the feature that brings these patients to the ophthalmologist. Although the sarcoma may appear in any age gorup, the incidence is higher in the young. In the Edgerton collection, 202 (60%) of the 336 cases were younger than 15 years. In a review of 33 cases of orbital and ocular involvement (which seems to include 5 cases associated with adnexal structures such as eyelids and paranasal sinus) by Zimmerman and Font, the median age was 7 years with a slight preponderance (3:2) in males. It is noteworthy, in this latter study, that an osseous or soft tissue orbital mass preceded any other sign of the disease in all but four of their cases.

When the expansile, bone-destroying lesion reaches the orbit, proptosis may be quite rapid and alarming, with displacement of the eye in a direction opposite to the usual anterior location of the tumor. If the thinner lateral wall of the orbit is destroyed, the temporal fossa soon fills with tumor and, in bilateral cases, creates a rounded configuration of the head. The latter, associated with the bulging "bug" eyes, gives the patient a very unusual appearance. If the tumor is pigmented, the stretched skin overlying the mass will have a greenish-yellow hue. However, in cases where the tumor is not pigmented, the ecchymosis of the eyelids and progressive proptosis may be not unlike the features of other childhood sarcomas, such as metastatic neuroblastoma, poorly differentiated lymphosarcoma, or even rhabdomyosarcoma (Fig. 231 A). Compare with Fig. 198, Chapter 11, and Fig. 309, Chapter 19). Even though these clinical features are very striking, a clinician may go through a lifetime of practice without seeing a case with initial orbital disease. Only two cases were recorded in the interval of our Mayo Clinic survey and in neither case was the tumor pigmented. These 2 cases, a boy and girl, were 9 and 13 years old, respectively. Roentgenograms will show the destructive lesion of bone similar to those noted with myeloma. In the very young, some separation of the cranial sutures also will be noted.

PATHOLOGY

The cells of this tumor are very undifferentiated and in the earlier stages of proliferation the majority of cells will not yet contain the cytoplasmic granules that are characteristic of more differentiated tumors of the granulocytic family. If the faintly eosinophilic cytoplasm is quite scant, the undifferentiated cells may resemble rhabdomyosarcoma. If the cytoplasm is abundant the tissue specimens are frequently designated reticulum cell sarcoma. The nuclei are round to reniform in configuration. The use of the Leder stain for esterase activity has greatly increased the diagnostic recognition of these primitive cells. This stain, in suitably fixed sections, will bring out the red-brown granules in the cyto-

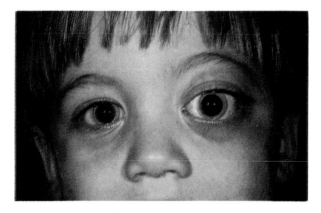

Figure 231. Granulocytic sarcoma: *A,* Proptosis and displacement of left eye with discoloration of eyelid of three weeks' duration in 22-month-old boy. Initial clinical impression was rhabdomyosarcoma.

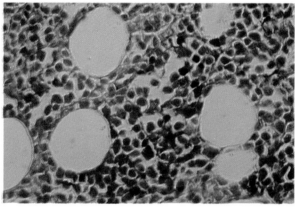

B, The stain for esterase activity reveals cells with dark red cytoplasmic granules indicative of granulocytic differentiation (Leder stain). (Both photographs courtesy of JD Bullock, M.D.)

plasm of these cells that are developing in the myelocytic direction (Fig. 231 *B*). Zimmerman and Font have emphasized that formalin fixed tissue is more suitable for this diagnostic stain than tissue fixed in Bouin's or Zenker's solution. The presence of an enzyme, myeloperoxidase, in the tumor cell is responsible for the green color of some fresh specimens.

COURSE AND TREATMENT

In cases of orbital involvement where there is no other obvious bony mass, anemia, or leukemia, the physician should be suspicious that a latent focus of myelocytic leukemia may already be present or anticipate that such dissemination will occur several months hence. Bone marrow biopsy is the best diagnostic aid in such cases. If all examinations are negative the local orbital involvement may be treated with irradiation and the response, measured in terms of reduction of proptosis, may be quite gratifying. Some clinicians, anticipating forthcoming events, recommend chemotherapy at this stage, but there are no controlled series demonstrating a beneficial effect of this therapeutic shotgun on survival rates. Other clinicians reserve chemotherapy for systemic spread of the disease. In some cases, with an unusually long interval between initial localized onset and terminal leukemic stage, survival has been equated with early treatment but, here again, there is no proof. Whatever the treatment or management, the disease is fatal and life expectancy is rarely longer than one year.

THE LEUKEMIAS

A discussion of the leukemias is but a postscript to the preceding sections of this chapter. Whereas orbital involvement often plays an important role in the diagnostics of some of the lymphoreticular neoplasms, the orbit is only one further link in the chain of complications associated with hematopoietic leukemias. Also, orbital complications may come so late in the course of the disease that their presence is overshadowed by leukemic infiltrates in more important organs or larger anatomic sites elsewhere in the body.

Leukemia continues to be classified as to its course — acute or chronic — in addition to the type of abnormal circulatory leukocyte. With the continued progress in suppressive types of therapy some cases do not run as acute a course as formerly, and the difference between acute and chronic cases is not as meaningful as it once was. In general, the orbit more often is involved by leukemia in the young than in the old, and in acute types more often than chronic types. Proptosis is often sudden in onset and may be quite acute. In such cases, hemorrhage rather than leukemic infiltrates is responsible for the increased orbital bulk. Bilateral orbital involvement is more prevalent with the leukemias than with other tumors in this text. These orbits are seldom biopsied, so there are no firm statistics as to the incidence of leukemic complications in this body site. When hemorrhage or leukemic infiltration of the orbit does occur, we have come to regard it as a harbinger of doom.

Bibliography

Malignant Lymphoma

Aisenberg AC, Long JC: Lymphocyte surface characteristics in malignant lymphoma. Am J Med 300–306, 1975

Arseneau JC, Canellos GP, Banks PM, et al: American Burkitt lymphoma: Clinicopathologic study of 30 cases. Part I. Clinical factors relating to prolonged survival. Am J Med 58:314–321, 1975

Banks PM, Arseneau JC, Gralnick HR, et al: American Burkitt lymphoma. Clinicopathologic study of 30 cases. Part II. Pathologic correlations. Am J Med 58:322–329, 1975

Berard C, O'Conor GT, Thomas LB, et al: Histopathological definition of Burkitt's tumor. Bull WHO 40:601–607, 1969

Braylan RC, Jaffe ES, Berard CW: Malignant lymphomas: current classification and new observations. Path Ann 10:213–270, 1975

Bürki E: Zur Kenntnis des Retothelsarkoms der Orbita. Ophthalmologica 105:253–268, 1943

Burkitt D: A sarcoma involving the jaws in African children. Brit J Surg 46:218–223, 1958

Burkitt D, O'Conor GT: Malignant lymphoma in African Children. I. A clinical syndrome. Cancer 14:258–269, 1961

Feman SS, Niwayana G, Hepler RS, et al: "Burkitt tumor" with intraocular involvement. Surv Ophth 14:106–111, 1969

Fratkin JD, Shammas HF, Miller SD: Disseminated Hodgkin's disease with bilateral orbital involvement. Arch Ophthalmol 96:102–104, 1978

Jaffe ES, Braylan RC, Nanba K, et al: Functional markers: a new perspective in malignant lymphomas. Cancer Treatment Reports 61:953–962, 1977

Jakobiec FA, Williams P, Wolff M: Reticulum cell sarcomas (Histiocytic lymphoma) of the orbit. Surv Ophthalmol 22:255–270, 1978

Karp LA, Zimmerman LE, Payne T: Intraocular involvement in Burkitt's lymphoma. Arch Ophthalmol 85:295–298, 1971

Knowles DM, Jakobiec FA: Orbital lymphoid neoplasms: clinical, pathologic, and immunologic characteristics. *In* Jakobiec FA: *Ocular and Adnexal Tumors.* Birmingham, Ala, Aesculapius Publishing Co, 1978, Chapter 54

Oberling:Cited by Bürki E

O'Conor GT, Rappaport H, Smith EB: Childhood lymphoma resembling "Burkitt tumor" in the United States. Cancer 18:1173–1186, 1974

Patchefsky AS, Brodovsky HS, Menduke H, et al: Non Hodgkin's lymphomas: a clinicopathologic study of 293 cases. Cancer 34:1173–1186, 1974

Rappaport H: Tumors of the hematopoietic system. *In Atlas of Tumor Pathology,* Section 3, Fascicle 8. Washington, D.C., Armed Forces Institute of Pathology, 1966

Roulet F: Das primäre Retothelsarkom der Lymphknoten. Virchows Arch (Pathol Anat) 277:15–47, 1930

Reese AB: *Tumors of the Eye.* Third Ed. Hagerstown, Medical Department, Harper & Row, Publishers, 1976

Rosenberg SA, Diamond HD, Jaslowitz B, et al: Lymphosarcoma. A review of 1269 cases. Medicine 40:31–84, 1961

Sweeney PJ, Hardy RW, Steinberg MC: An unusual case of progressive visual loss. Presented at the Ninth Annual Neuro-ophthalmic Pathology Symposium. St. Louis, February 1977

Watillon M, Prijot E, Farra M: Maladie de Hodgkin localisation lacrymale. Arch Ophtalmol (Paris) 24:153–155, 1964

Yam LT, Tavassoli M, Jacobs P: Differential characterization of the "Reticulum Cell" in lymphoreticular neoplasms. Am J Clin Path 64:171–179, 1975

Ziegler JL: Treatment results of 54 American patients with Burkitt's lymphoma are similar to the African experience. New Engl J Med 297:75–80, 1977

Zimmerman LE: Lymphoid tumors. *In Ocular and Adnexal Tumors: New and Controversial Aspects.* Ed. M Boniuk. St. Louis, C V Mosby Co, 1964, pp 429–446

Plasma Cell Myeloma

Knowles DM, II, Halper JA, Trokel S, et al: Immunofluorescent and immunoperoxidase characteristics of IgDγ myeloma involving the orbit. Am J Ophthalmol 85:485–494, 1978

Kyle RA: Multiple myeloma. Review of 869 cases. Mayo Clin Proc 50:29–40, 1975

Levin SR, Spaulding AG, Wirman JA: Multiple myeloma. Orbital involvement in a youth. Arch Ophthalmol 95:642–644, 1977

Rodman HI, Font RL: Orbital involvement in multiple myeloma. Review of literature and report of three cases. Arch Ophthalmol 87:30–35, 1972

Macroglobulinemia

Bergsagel DE: Lymphoreticular disorders — malignant proliferative response and/or abnormal globulin syntheses — plasma cell dyscrasias. *In Hematology.* Second Ed. Ed: WJ Williams, et al. New York, McGraw-Hill Book Co., 1977, pp 1087–1099

Dutcher TF, Fahey JL: The histopathology of the macroglobulinemia of Waldenström. J Natl Cancer Inst 22:887–917, 1959

Little JM: Waldenström's macroglobulinemia in the lacrimal gland. Trans Am Acad Ophthalmol and Otorhinolaryngol 71:875–879, 1967

Paufique L, Gerard P, Schott B, et al: Pseudolymphome de l'orbite macroglobuline — secretant associé a une méningolymphomatose avec macroglobulinorachie. Ann Ocul 202:1033–1045, 1969

Waldenström J: Incipient myelomatosis or "essential" hyperglobulinemia with fibrinogenopenia — a new syndrome? Acta Med Scand 117:216–247, 1944

Granulocytic Sarcoma

Burns A: *Observations on the Surgical Anatomy of the Head and Neck.* Edinburgh, Thomas Bryce & Co, 1811, pp 364–366

Edgerton AE: Chloroma: report of a case and a review of the literature. Trans Am Ophthalmol Soc 45:376–414, 1947

Leder LD: Über die selektive fermentcytochemische Darstellung von neutrophilen myeloischen Zellen und Gewebsmastzellen im Paraffinschnitt. Klin Wochenschr 42:553, 1964

Zimmerman LE, Font RL: Ophthalmologic manifestations of granulocytic sarcoma (myeloid sarcoma or chloroma). Am J Ophthalmol 80:975–990, 1975

14

Histiocytoses

In this chapter we will discuss three abnormalities *(histiocytosis X, sinus histiocytosis,* and *juvenile xanthogranuloma)* of the fixed tissue component of the monocyte-macrophage branch of the lymphoreticular system, the tissue *histiocyte.* This arrangement is simply one of convenience and we do not mean to imply the three tumors are interrelated. Several other proliferations of tissue histiocytes will not be mentioned because orbital involvement either does not occur during the course of the disease or has not been definitely established.

HISTIOCYTOSIS X

This is a group of diseases of unknown cause characterized by an abnormal proliferation of histiocytes not associated with any known infectious agent or abnormality of lipid metabolism (Porter 1977). The name, histiocytosis X, was proposed by Lichtenstein (1953) to include several entities and syndromes that seemed interrelated but had been originally described as separate diseases and, in so doing, had been burdened with complex eponyms. Lichtenstein's term had no positive meaning in reference to pathogenesis or clinical course, but the letter X did emphasize the many unknowns associated with the several components of the group. A more specific or satisfactory name has not gained widespread acceptance.

HISTORICAL ASPECTS

Hand-Schüller-Christian Disease

In historical perspective, this is the oldest of the several disorders classified as histiocytosis X. It is an interesting quest to discover how this disorder acquired a triple eponym. Many of the orbital tumors in this text either were observed by a European clinician in the 19th century or were described in detail by some pathologist (usually a German) during the latter half of the same century. It is of more than usual interest, then, to find that *Hand* (the first eponym) was an American; even more surprising is that he was only a resident at Children's Hospital in Philadelphia when he made his first report (1893a). Hand had observed an undersized, puny little boy of 3 years during the last 2½ months of the child's life. A striking feature was bilateral exophthalmos, which gave the wizened child a frog-like appearance—a feature subsequently noted in many other patients. The child also passed copious quantities of urine. At autopsy several soft, yellow spots were noted in the calvarium, and somewhat similar infiltrations were found in the abdominal viscera. In presenting these findings to the sage society of Philadelphia pathologists, he postulated that the patient had a form of generalized tuberculosis. The same paper was published later in the same year in a pediatric journal (1893b) with a slight change of title to emphasize the polyuria.

No further cases representing this triad of exophthalmos, bony defects in the calvarium, and diabetic insipidus came to Hand's attention for another 12 years. He then had an opportunity to examine another child with essentially the same clinical triad presented by another Pennsylvanian, Kay, at a medical society meeting in 1905 (Kay, 1906). By this time Hand doubted whether tuberculosis had anything to do with the disseminated disorder. Kay did not venture an opinion as to the nature of the disease except to suspect some lesion in or about the floor of the fourth ventricle, which would easily explain the polydipsia and polyuria. Hand was not to see his third case for another 15 years.

No more was heard about this puzzling and rare disease in the American literature until the report of *Christian* (1920). Christian, of Boston, presented a searching report about a youngster with the symptom complex that has already been described. The distressing polyuria was treated by injections of pituitary extract and Christian implicated a dyspituitarism as the cause of the disorder. Christian also searched the literature and discovered a prior report of *Schüller*, of Vienna (1915). Two of the three cases reported by Schüller seemed to be examples of the same problem; Schüller seemed interested in the intriguing radiologic defects that develop in the skull. But in his perusal of the literature, Christian did not discover the separate reports of Hand and Kay, and after Christian's report the disorder was referred to as Schuller-Christian disease.

Almost before Christian's observations were published, Hand had the good fortune to observe a third case (the sixth known case in the literature). Hand was quite willing to accept Christian's dyspituitarism as a cause of the polyuria but he still wondered as to the basic lesion responsible for the triad. This time he theorized (1921) that the condition was due either to a chronic infectious process or to some benign myxomatous type of neoplasia. Perhaps to emphasize any claim of priority, he incorporated, verbatim, his 1893 paper (by now in its third publication) within the overall survey of the literature and summary that constituted his second case published in 1921.

All of the cases up to this time had exhibited bilateral exophthalmos but not all had been afflicted with the polyuria. None of the observers had made any particular biopsy or dissection of the orbit to ascertain the reason for the exophthalmos but assumed that it was due to defects in the bony orbital plates. After this era, the lipid content of the participating histiocyte was discovered, its nature was identified as chiefly cholesterol, and the disorder was soon classified with the lipoid granulomas and xanthomatoses. By the later 1930's and early 1940's it became suspected that the disorder did not belong to the group associated with disturbances of fat metabolism.

Letterer-Siwe Disease

This was the second of the three components of histiocytosis X to be described. Interest in this syndrome appeared in the literature several decades after descriptions of the one above. Abt and Denenholz (1936), of Chicago, seem to have suggested the eponym of Letterer-Siwe disease. In subsequent articles, Abt's name sometimes also appeared in the eponymous title.

Sture Siwe (1933), of the Children's Clinic at the University of Lund, collected all the prior cases in the literature and outlined the components of the syndrome. The disease seemed to be restricted to infants; the main features were splenomegaly, hepatomegaly, a hemorrhagic tendency characterized by a petechial rash, lymphadenopathy, localized tumors in bone, anemia, fever, and an acute and fatal course. Subsequently it became established that the disease is not invariably fatal. In later publications this disorder came to be discussed as the acute malignant form of histiocytosis X. *Erich Letterer*, of Würzburg, had made an earlier report (1924) but he may not have been the first to describe the syndrome. Letterer made a very detailed report of an apathetic 6-month-old child who showed most of the clinical features described above except for osteolytic lesions. Contrary to some statements appearing in the literature, this feature of the syndrome seems absent as one reads the many details of Letterer's careful observations. There was a "phlegmon" over the child's occiput, but no underlying osteolytic defect was mentioned. However, this small detail is not too pertinent to the story and the reader must remember that all of the characteristic features may not appear in any given case.

Eosinophilic Granuloma of Bone

This was the last of the three disorders constituting the complex of histiocytosis X to be described. It seems to have escaped the eponyms applied to the others. In the first dozen cases or so the lesion seemed solitary and its behavior benign. It was easier, therefore, to apply a descriptive name to the disease than was possible in the preceding disorders with multiple symptoms. Lichtenstein and Jaffe (1940) seem to have been responsible for its name. Otani and Ehrlich (1940), observing this same lesion in their series of patients, designated it *solitary granuloma*. Although both groups were from New York City, they made their observations independently and submitted their material for publication within six days of one another. The latter group had submitted their observations first, but the name submitted by the former group was the one that became accepted. Both groups, however, regarded their descriptions as representative of a separate pathologic entity.

CLASSIFICATION

In the intervening years many observers have considered the three disorders as variants of the same basic disease process, but there have been persistent dissenters to this unitarian concept. A present and popular trend is to classify the histiocytosis X complex into two subgroups, *localized* and *systemic*.

The localized form represents a disease confined to a single organ system. It is essentially a disease of bone and is considered a "reactive" response of differentiated histiocytes to an unknown stimulus. A solitary proliferation of histiocytes would correspond to the component previously described as eosinophilic granuloma of bone. Multifocal lesions of bone would be synonymous with the Hand-Schüller-Christian disease. The soft tissue involvement in the latter condition is considered secondary to the bony lesion rather than a primary predilection of histiocytosis. This "localized" subgroup is considered benign.

The systemic form, in contrast, affects more than one organ system. It, too, may involve bone, but there is widespread visceral involvement in the course of the disease. The cell involved in this more aggressive proliferative disease may be a more immature histiocyte. Because of cytologic similarities to a childhood variant of differentiated reticulum cell sarcoma, the progressive form of systemic histiocytosis has been regarded by some physicians as a borderline neoplasia. This is the subgroup that corresponds to Letterer-Siwe's disease.

Our own experience in ophthalmology is too limited to take a position on either the binary or triune classification. However, because it is easier to write about two rather than three subgroups we will consider the orbital manifestations of histiocytosis X in terms of the former.

INCIDENCE

Ophthalmologists do not often see a patient with histiocytosis, for the condition is uncommon. Most of these cases are seen in general hospital practice. In such situations, the ophthalmologist's interest usually is directed to a unilateral or bilateral proptosis in an infant or small child who has already been studied because of histiocytosis X in some other organ or tissue. The opportunity to observe an infant in whom the initial and presenting symptoms of the disease is proptosis is even less common, and the occasion to observe this initial symptom in an adult is rare. Cheyne (1971) estimated the incidence at one in two million persons per year. Some large surveys of orbital tumors do not mention histiocytosis X as a statistic in their sample.

In our series of orbital tumors there were eight cases (five males, three females). All patients were 2 years old or less except one 17-year-old girl. This girl (Fig. 232) had the localized solitary (eosinophilic granuloma) form of the disease. Two of the children had the systemic (Letterer-Siwe) type involvement. The remaining five were classified as having the localized but multifocal form

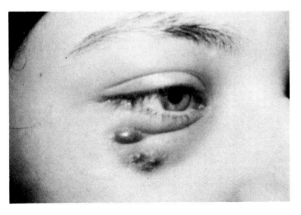

Figure 232. Histiocytosis X: upward and nasal displacement of right eye, and lower eyelid showing reddish discoloration and fluctuant, purple ecchymotic areas in subcutaneous tissue that waxed and waned for 1 month due to recurrent small hemorrhages arising in tumor; this resulted from disease apparently limited to inferolateral wall of orbit but with encroachment of tender and indurated mass into orbital cavity. Initial impression was cellulitis but tomograms revealed lytic defects in bony orbit and, following orbitotomy in this 17-year-old girl, orbit was treated with irradiation. (Courtesy R. W. Neault, M.D.)

(Hand-Schüller-Christian) of bony involvement. These eight patients represent 1% of our total orbital tumors. In the same time interval of the orbital survey, histiocytosis X without orbital involvement was diagnosed in sixty-one patients at the Mayo Clinic. The incidence of orbital involvement in histiocytosis X, therefore, is slightly greater than 1% (8 of 69 patients).

The localized (solitary and multifocal lesions of bone) type of histiocytosis X is primarily a disease of older children and young adults, with an average age of 13.3 years according to Porter. There is no sex predilection. In contrast, the systemic type does have a slight male predominance and occurs most often in the first three years of life.

CLINICAL FEATURES

Table 19 illustrates the presenting complaints among 115 patients observed at the Mayo Clinic during a 35-year period. This compilation reflects the variety of organs, tissues, and anatomic sites affected by histiocytosis X. Table 19 emphasizes the high incidence of masses (either tender, palpable, or visible) overlying the site of an osseous lesion (Fig. 233). In contrast, the incidence of signs such as diabetes insipidus or exophthalmos, as initial manifestations, is low. These data emphasize how frequently a child will see a pediatrician first, or an adult an orthopedist first, rather than an ophthalmologist. The ophthalmologist's role in most of these cases is that of a consultant in cases of proptosis; rarely, his services are required because of intraocular involvement.

When the orbit is affected early in the course of the disease, proptosis usually is unilateral. Ocular protrusion and displacement may be in any direction and there seems to be no set pattern as to the position of the histiocytic masses in the orbit, but the presence of such defects, seen on roentgenograms, does not necessarily mean that the patient always will develop proptosis if this is not already present. Defects in the more forward portions of the bony orbit also may be palpated.

We found that when the orbital disturbance was not the presenting complaint in children, proptosis developed within 6 months of onset of the

TABLE 19. PRESENTING COMPLAINTS IN 115 PATIENTS WITH HISTIOCYTOSIS X*

Complaint	Children (0–14 yr)	Adults (>15 yr)
Palpable or visible mass	27	3
Tenderness	19	24
Rash	8	
Enlarged lymph nodes	5	
Stomatitis	5	1
Otitis	5	
Painful mass	5	
Exophthalmos	3	
Diabetes insipidus	2	3
Fever	1	1
Pain and fever	1	
Headache		2

*From Enrique P, Dahlin DC, Hayles AB, et al: Histiocytosis X: a clinical study. Mayo Clin Proc 42:88–99, 1967

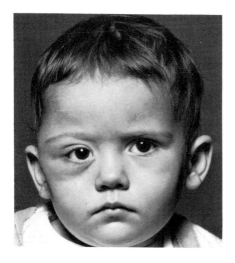

Figure 233. Histiocytosis X: swelling of right upper face, downward and inward displacement of right eye, and forward proptosis (5 mm) were initial signs of histiocytosis involving right zygoma and lateral wall of orbit; this 2-year-old girl eventually died from disseminated disease.

disease in some other anatomic area. The clinical picture of these children with unilateral proptosis associated with unifocal or multifocal bone disease, is not unlike that of children with malignant neoplasms of the orbit. Such children are irritable, they may be feverish and appear ill, but they do not show the pallor, wasting, and listlessness of the systemic type of histiocytosis. When the orbit is involved, frequently there are other nearby signs of trouble, such as draining ears, running noses, swollen jaws, tender lumps in the scalp, ulcerations of the gums, and loose teeth. Bilateral orbital tumors (Fig. 234) seldom are seen except in more advanced stages with some interval between the disease in one orbit and the other. In the more terminal stages with bilateral proptosis, the affected children have a frog-like appearance — a descriptive phrase that was first mentioned by Hand. The flatness of the forehead in these patients seems to accentuate this appearance. Proptosis may become quite marked, but the eyes do

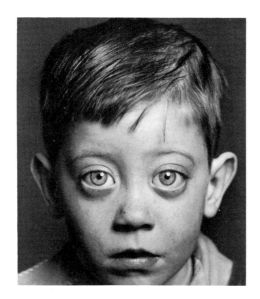

Figure 234. Histiocytosis X: bilateral prominence of eyes was initial sign in 3½-year-old boy of disorder involving the cranium, left zygomatic arch, floor of sella, and one femur.

not pulsate as might be expected from the roentgenographic evidence of such large defects in the surrounding bony orbit. In some children proptosis is not the initial clue to orbital disease; instead, there is some puffiness of the eyelids which suggests allergic soft tissue edema or insect bite.

A smattering of case reports in the literature describe either interesting cases with systemic symptoms and proptosis or cases wherein proptosis was the initial sign of histiocytosis X: the reports of John Wheeler (1931), Gross and Jacox (1942), Straatsma (1958), Chawla and Cullen (1968), Heuer (1972), and Baghdassarian and Shammas (1977) are valuable sources. The report by Wheeler (1931) is interesting because he seems to have been the first to have explored the orbit in a living patient (a 4-year-old child). He found that newly formed, expanding masses rather than defects in the skull were responsible for the proptosis. A report by a namesake (Wheeler, 1946) is even more interesting in that it seems to be the only descriptive protocol in the American ophthalmic literature of an adult patient (age 34) with the presenting sign of proptosis.

ROENTGENOGRAPHIC CHANGES

The defects in the membranous bones of the skull are striking. Most roentgenologists refer to them as circumscribed, sharply delineated, usually round, somewhat punched-out, radiolucent defects in the calvarium (Fig. 235). These defects scattered about the skull may remind one of a handful of radiolucent coins of various sizes distributed over the skull—the so-called geographic skull.

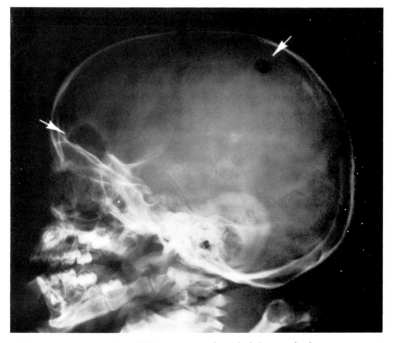

Figure 235. Histiocytosis X: radiolucent, coin-shaped defect with sharp margins in parietal bone (*upper arrow*) and larger defect in roof of orbit (*left arrow*) were initial roentgenographic findings in 2-year-old girl.

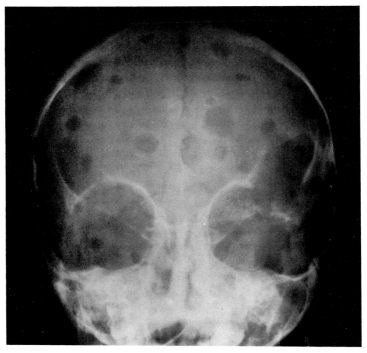

Figure 236.   Histiocytosis X: numerous oval and round bony defects scattered throughout skull; note large destructive lesion in lateral wall of left orbit.

Such defects in the roof of the orbit suggest the configuration of some of the bony defects associated with epidermoid cysts, except that in the latter the edges of the defect are more burnished and sclerotic. When the disease involves the lateral orbital wall, the bony defects are much more irregular and "moth-eaten" than when they appear across the calvarium, and suggest some malignant destructive neoplasm (Fig. 236). It is important to know that the bony defects heal if the child does not succumb to the systemic and visceral manifestations of the disease.

In the healing process the affected bone may undergo sclerosis with ultimate reduction in the overall size of the orbit. This accounts for the residual exophthalmos of some children whose localized disease has been arrested. This sclerosis is not necessarily related to irradiation therapy; it has been observed in patients treated only with chemotherapy. Also, a few patients may show sclerosis of the roof of the orbit at the time of initial x-ray examination. This may simulate the roentgenographic picture of orbital fibrous dysplasia in the same age group of children and adolescents. The hyperostosis of histiocytosis is not as diffuse nor does it extend beyond the frontosphenoidal suture, a feature differentiating the process from fibrous dysplasia.

PATHOLOGY

When encountered in and around the orbit, these tissue masses usually are soft and friable. This feature gives the disease a similarity to some forms of malignant lymphoma. As one attempts to remove or curette this soft tissue, a

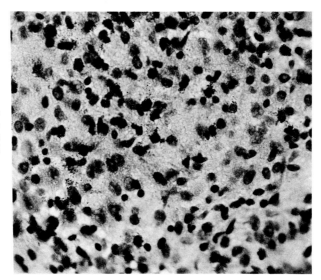

Figure 237. Histiocytosis X: sheets of histiocytes, with finely vacuolated cytoplasm due to lipids, and numerous eosinophilic leukocytes. (Hematoxylin and eosin; × 400.)

gritty sensation, due to a mixture of tiny bone spicules in the granulomatous necrotic mass, is apparent. In this respect, the tissue resembles the lesion of fibrous dysplasia. Hemorrhage or tissue necrosis colors the lesions gray-red, otherwise they may be a yellowish pink.

Microscopically, specimens show sheet-like masses of histiocytes mixed with varying numbers of eosinophils, lymphocytes, and even occasional polymorphonuclear leukocytes (Fig. 237). The histiocytes may vary in size but usually are relatively large (diameter, 15 to 25μ) with abundant vacuolated, eosinophilic cytoplasm. These "foam cells" may contain variable amounts of sudanophilic material in the cytoplasm, which is the result of phagocytosis rather than a function of intracellular synthesis. The nuclei are oval or more typically folded and grooved. The nuclear membrane is distinct. The chromatin is finely dispersed and scanty so the nucleus may not stain densely. The histiocytes rarely show mitosis but do fuse to form multinucleated giant cells of the granulomatous type, with four or five centrally located nuclei (Fig. 238). The histopathologic picture of any given tissue sample at any given time during the course of the disease does not seem to have any prognostic value. The cytology may vary from lesion to lesion and from different sites in the same patient. The histiocytes, on electron microscopy, have distinctive inclusions consisting of tubular structures with saccular dilatation and cross bridges.

TREATMENT

The salutary effect of irradiation has often been remarked, and this form of therapy is one of the oldest of the several approaches that have been devised. Irradiation seems to arrest the progression of the osseous lesion in many patients and thus may hasten healing of the defect. However, irradiation has no effect on the basic nature of the disease process and will not prevent eventual dissemination if this is going to occur. It is most useful in treating the solitary bony lesion or in managing the patient with only a few osseous lesions in scattered

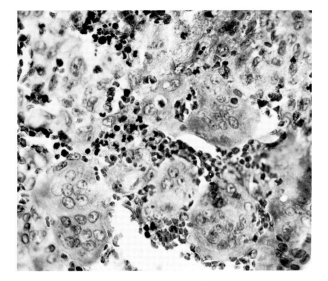

Figure 238. Histiocytosis X: giant cells with several nuclei are common. (Hematoxylin and eosin; × 400.)

areas. The dosage required in these circumstances may approximate 500 to 600 R (not necessarily given all at one time). With irradiation, particularly for infants and children, one must consider how many sites should be treated, for if treatment is continued in new areas, the total body dosage may become excessive. In these cases of progressive multifocal disease of bone we would be inclined to withhold irradiation to the orbit unless proptosis is extreme or visual loss is imminent. In the less severe situations, removal of the bulk of the orbital mass by curettage and suction may reduce proptosis and lessen the need for irradiation. It should be remembered that the localized bony type of histiocytosis is benign and the orbital bony defects may heal without irradiation. The prognosis for the localized form of histiocytosis is good.

We have follow-up data on five of our six patients with localized disease. All are living from 2 to 19 years after onset. Two survivors, 14 and 19 years after onset, are taking medications for diabetes insipidus. It is amazing how complete is the healing of bony orbital lesions in many patients with the passage of time, considering initial size and destructive appearance of the defects.

When the disease becomes more disseminated, particularly if there is involvement of viscera or bone marrow, other modalities of therapy are indicated. Various combinations of antibiotics, antimetabolites, steroids, and cytotoxic agents are used with and without supplemental irradiation. Still, the outlook is guarded. An analysis of sixty-nine patients with the systemic form of the disease collected from three pediatric services (Porter), showed an overall mortality rate of 34%. No patient died who was over age 3 at time of onset.

INFANTILE XANTHOGRANULOMA

This is a reactive disorder of histiocytes associated with a localized, but sometimes multifocal, derangement of lipid material of unknown origin. It most commonly affects the skin of infants and children. Single lesions tend to involve the scalp, face, and neck; multiple lesions tend to distribution over head, trunk, and extremities. It is a benign disorder, but when the eye is affected (the second most frequent site of involvement) the aggressive intraocular growth and attendant hemorrhage may produce glaucoma and loss of vision. At one time it was believed to be a form of histiocytosis X but this association is no longer considered valid.

HISTORICAL ASPECTS

In dermatology the disease was established as a clinical entity early in this century. McDonagh (1912) proposed the name *naevo-xantho-endothelioma* for a benign skin disorder characterized by yellow, tan, or dusky red papules and nodules of variable size chiefly affecting the scalp, face, and neck of children. A pretty colored drawing of the thorax, neck, and head of a child with this affliction illustrated his article. The double hyphen in the name emphasized the three components that McDonagh thought were peculiar to the disorder. He believed the main trouble was an overgrowth of embryonic cells destined to be capillaries, hence the name endothelioma. He placed the disorder in the large class of nevi to explain its appearance in early life, the xanthomatous designation characterizing the fatty change that he noted in the nodules. The hyphenated word gradually disappeared, but the contracted form — nevoxanthoendothelioma — continues in usage to this day.

Helwig and Hackney (1954) proposed the name juvenile xanthogranuloma. They considered this term more descriptive of its pathology and appropriate to its age incidence. Soon there was pathologic proof that xanthogranuloma could occur in the anterior uveal tract and produce hyphema and secondary glaucoma in the eyes of infants. This syndrome of recurrent hyphema associated with an enlarging mass in the iris of an infant's eye is now well known and represents the most important and serious component of the disease.

One of the first orbital examples of the disorder was observed and surgically explored by Ley, of St. Louis, in 1959. Details of this case appeared several years later in the separate publications of Sanders (1966) and Zimmerman (1965). At present, there are now seven cases of orbital involvement, all proved by histologic study. Casual inspection of the American literature indicates that the number of reported cases seems to exceed seven, but several of them are described in more than one publication. (One case was described in four different articles.) Sanders (1966) proposed the term *infantile xanthogranuloma*, because it was more appropriate to the age distribution of the disorder.

If there have been any additional reports of orbital involvement since the above publications we have not found them.

CLINICAL FEATURES

All cases involving the orbit have been in the infant age group — less than 10 months of age at the time of initial examination. The duration of symptoms, such as swelling of the eyelid or proptosis (similar symptoms to those of histiocytosis), has been from 1 week to 2 months. Signs of the disorder sometimes may be observed at birth. The disorder may affect either sex. In the few cases so far observed, the tumor has shown no predilection as to location in the orbit. A tumor may be located forward in the orbit or in the apex; or the tumor may also wrap itself about an extraocular muscle. At least two of the cases, and possibly a third, have been associated with some erosion of the adjacent orbital bone. Only one of the seven children had associated skin lesions in contrast to the high proportion of cutaneous involvement in patients with intraocular lesions.

PATHOLOGY

Histologic examination demonstrates features of a granuloma (Fig. 239). All observers have noted a similarity between tissues removed from the orbit and those obtained from either the surface of the eye or iris. The descriptions of orbital cases have been brief, as the authors assumed the reader was familiar with the histopathology of tissue samples from other sources, particularly the iris. The histiocyte is the main component, and it may appear as a partially lipidized foam cell or in a spindle-cell configuration. There may be a variable number of eosinophils and polymorphonuclear leukocytes in the sample. Capillaries are not as prominent as in the intraocular infiltrate. The most striking feature is the Touton giant cell: this is a moderately large, oval cell with foamy cytoplasm surrounding an orderly circular arrangement of nuclei at the center of the cell.

The gross tissue as encountered in the orbit is soft, somewhat friable, and usually described as some shade of yellow.

COURSE AND TREATMENT

The orbital form of the disease is benign, and all of the tots so far observed evidently have made a reasonable recovery. Even the bony defects in the orbit

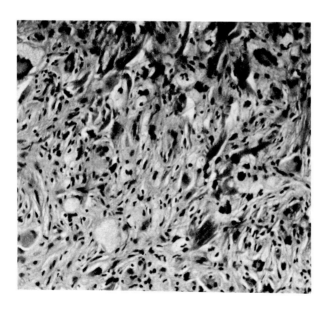

Figure 239. Infantile xanthogranuloma: character of lesion is granulomatous with foamy histiocytic cells and prominent rounded "Touton" giant cells. (Hematoxylin and eosin; × 155.)

seem to heal. All of them have had some tissue removed at the time of exploratory surgery. In some, small doses of irradiation have been effective; in others, prednisone has caused the local symptoms to disappear rapidly. We have had no personal experience of these cases, but our suggested plan would be as follow: All of the visible mass unrelated to adjoining muscle or important nerve would first be excised. The child would then be observed for several weeks. If resolution were unsatisfactory or the condition recurrent, prednisone (30 mg daily, for 3 weeks) would be administered. If this did not effect resolution after an observation period of another several weeks, irradiation (total dosage 250 to 400 R, air measurement) would be considered.

The typical skin lesions might seem to be a ready clue to the nature of the orbital problem but in the majority of cases so far reported they have not been present. Neither, in several cases, did skin nodules develop in the course of the short follow-up periods.

SINUS HISTIOCYTOSIS

This is a puzzling disease of lymph nodes and extranodal structures of unknown pathogenesis which features a rather characteristic infiltration of histiocytes. The disease is benign but may run a protracted course. The frequency and striking nature of orbital involvement heralds the disease as one of the newer members of the family of tumors affecting the orbit.

Almost from the time of the earliest case reports (Azoury and Reed 1966, Destombes 1965, Marie et al 1966, Vincent and Miercourt 1967) up to the present, the names of Rosai and Dorfman have been closely associated with the disorder. In their first report (1969) they described the principal clinical features of the disease in four patients; they suggested the disorder was an entity distinct from other lymphoreticular conditions; and they named the syndrome *sinus histiocytosis with massive lymphadenopathy*. Their review of thirty-four cases (1972) established the disease as a clinicopathologic entity, and in 1979 (Foucar, Rosai and Dorfman) they emphasized the clinical and pathologic features of ophthalmic involvement among 113 cases in the literature. The name they proposed emphasized the prominent cervical lymphadenopathy that was such a striking clinical feature in earlier cases and the propensity of the histiocyte for infiltrating the sinusoidal spaces of the lymph node. Subsequently, many cases have been noted without either massive or even minimal lymphadenopathy. Consequently, several observers have shortened the name to *sinus histiocytosis*. Other publication that have made significant contributions to the subject are those of Lampert and Lennert (1976), Sanchez, Rosai, and Dorfman (1977), and Friendly and associates (1977).

INCIDENCE

The disease principally affects children and young adults. Among the cases in the literature the number of patients of the white race slightly exceeds the number of patients of the black race, but many cases in African children probably are unreported. The sex incidence is approximately equal.

As regards orbital involvement, Friendly and associates analyzed nine cases including four of their own. The age range was 2 to 20 years at time of diagnosis with an average age of 10.1 years. Among a series of 113 patients with microscopically documented disease, Foucar and colleagues found 11 patients with "ophthalmic" disease (orbit, eyelid, or globe). The ages of these patients ranged from 1.7 to 20 years with an average of 8.6 years. The incidence of orbital involvement probably approximates 8 to 10% of all cases of the disease; this figure may be high, because the striking appearance of proptosis favors publication of these cases as compared to cases of nonorbital disease. Bilateral involvement will probably occur in about a third of the orbital cases. No cases of sinus histiocytosis were observed in our Mayo Clinic series.

CLINICAL FEATURES

Orbital involvement may occur as a very early sign of the disease or may appear as a complication in the course of an already established lymphadenopathy. The orbital masses tend to be firm and nodular and seem confined to the medial, superior, or lateral periphery in most cases. Therefore, visual function is not usually compromised to a severe degree unless the proptosis is rapid in onset or reaches an extreme degree. Likewise, oculorotary functions are not seriously impaired. Eyelid masses also may be palpable and are responsible for the puffiness of these tissues in some patients. The duration of proptosis prior to diagnostic biopsy may be as short as several months or as long as 5 to 12 years.

In the earlier descriptions of the disease the principal systemic features were a massive multinodular enlargement of all lymph node systems in the neck, fever, elevated erythrocytic sedimentation, leukocytosis, and hypergammaglobulinemia. Axillary and inguinal lymphadenopathy was less prominent and less frequent. As more patients were observed many variants on this pattern were found. Hilar and mediastinal lymphadenopathy were found in many patients, and involvement of extranodal sites other than the orbit was recognized. Also, it seemed that patients with extranodal disease were less prone to show massive lymphadenopathy, fever, and marked elevation of immunoglobulins than had first been assumed.

PATHOLOGY

Grossly, the orbital nodules are white or yellow-white, discrete, but not encapsulated. Microscopically there is a polymorphous admixture of histiocytes, lymphocytes, and plasma cells. Eosinophils and neutrophils are not usually seen. Mitoses are not present. The histiocytes have round or oval vesicular nuclei with a distinct nucleolus and a vacuolated cytoplasm. A distinctive feature is the phagocytosis of lymphocytes, plasma cells, and erythrocytes in the cytoplasm of some of the histiocytes (Fig. 240). A variable amount of fibrosis also will be seen. In some cases the fibrosis is inconspicuously interspersed between focal accumulations of the polymorphous infiltrate. In other cases the fibrous tissue reaction is quite profuse and dense, segregating and squeezing the histiocytes and lymphocytes into nodules similar to chronic orbital pseudotumor (Fig. 241).

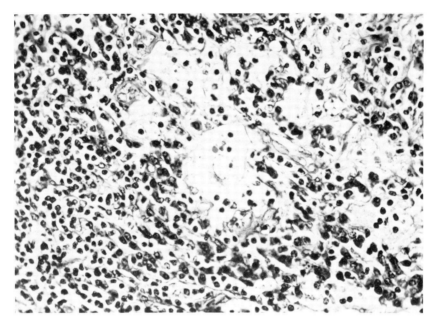

Figure 240. Sinus histiocytosis: orbital tissue showing large histiocytes with pale vesicular nuclei containing mature lymphocytes in their cytoplasm. Lymphoplasmacytic infiltrate surrounds histiocytes. (Hematoxylin and eosin; × 350.) (From Friendly DS, Font RL, Rao NA: Orbital involvement in 'sinus' histiocytosis. Arch Ophthalmol 95:2006–2011, 1977. By permission.)

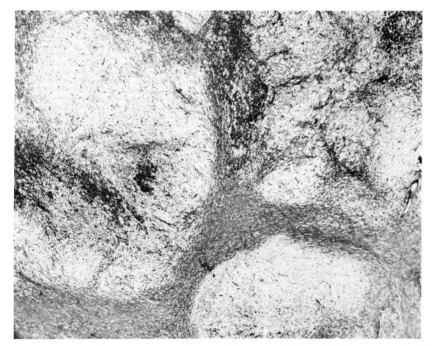

Figure 241. Sinus histiocytosis: orbital mass disclosing well-defined lobules composed of histiocytes and focal collections of lymphocytes separated by broad fibrous septa. (Hematoxylin and eosin; × 25.) (From Friendly DS, Font RL, Rao NA: Orbital involvement in 'sinus' histiocytosis. Arch Ophthalmol 95:2006–2011, 1977. By permission.)

Atypical patterns also may be encountered in some specimens consisting of binucleated or multinucleated histiocytes and giant cells as well as histiocytes with hyperchromatic nuclei and large dark nucleoli.

COURSE AND TREATMENT

This is essentially a self-limited disease, but the course after diagnosis is as variable as the duration of symptoms prior to diagnosis. This makes the effectiveness of treatment uncertain, and there are no controlled studies upon which to base firm conclusions. Antibiotics, chemotherapy, corticosteroids, and irradiation singly or in combinations have been administered without uniform or spectacular effects. Simple excision of the nodules in the orbit may be as helpful as any nonsurgical therapy. The disease eventually recedes, but residual extranodal lumps and matted lymph nodes may be permanent sequelae.

Bibliography

Histiocytoses

References pertaining to the historical aspect of the subject are listed as a group first.

Abt AF, Denenholz EJ: Letterer-Siwe's disease: splenohepatomegaly associated with widespread hyperplasia of nonlipoid-storing macrophages; discussion of the so-called reticulo-endothelioses. Am J Dis Child 51:499–522, 1936

Cheyne C: Prognostic signs of histiocytosis X. Proc Roy Soc Med 64:334–336, 1971

Christian HA: Defects in membranous bones, exophthalmos and diabetes insipidus: an unusual syndrome of dyspituitarism. Med Clin North Am 3:849–871, 1920

Hand A JR: General tuberculosis. Trans Pathol Soc Phila 16:282–284, 1893a

Hand A JR: Polyuria and tuberculosis. Arch Pediatr 10:673–675, 1893b

Hand A [Jr]: Defects of membranous bones, exophthalmos and polyuria in childhood: is it dyspituitarism? Am J Med Sci 162:509–515, 1921

Jaffe HL, Lichtenstein L: Eosinophilic granuloma of bone: a condition affecting one, several or many bones, but apparently limited to the skeleton, and representing the mildest clinical expression of the peculiar inflammatory histiocytosis also underlying Letterer-Siwe disease and Schüller-Christian disease. Arch Pathol 37:99–118, 1944

Kay TW: Acquired hydrocephalus with atrophic bone changes, exophthalmos, and polyuria (with presentation of the patient). Pa Med J 9:520–521, 1906

Letterer E: Aleukämische Retikulose (ein Beitrag zu den proliferativen Erkrankungen des Retikuloendothelialapparates). Frankfurt Z Pathol 30:377–394, 1924

Lichtenstein L, Jaffe HL: Eosinophilic granuloma of bone: with report of a case. Am J Pathol 16:595-604, 1940

Otani S, Ehrlich JC: Solitary granuloma of bone: simulating primary neoplasm. Am J Pathol 16: 479–490, 1940

Schüller A: Über eigenartige Schädeldefekte im Jugendalter. Forschr Geb Roentgenstr 23:12–18, 1915

Siwe SA: Die Reticuloendotheliose — ein neues Krankheitsbild unter den Hapatosplenomegalien. Z Kinderheilkd 55:212–247, 1933

Other references are:

Baghdassarian SA, Shammas HF: Eosinophilic granuloma of orbit. Ann Opthalmol 9:1247–1251, 1977

Chawla HB, Cullen JF: Eosinophilic granuloma of the orbit. J Pediatr Ophthalmol 5:93–95, 1968

Enriquez P, Dahlin DC, Hayles AB, et al: Histiocytosis X: a clinical study. Mayo Clin Proc 42:88–99, 1967

Gross P, Jacox HW: Eosinophilic granuloma and certain other reticulo-endothelial hyperplasias of bone: a comparison of clinical, radiologic, and pathologic features. Am J Med Sci 203:673–687, 1942

Heuer HE: Eosinophilic granuloma of the orbit. Acta Ophth 50:160–165, 1972

Lichtenstein L: Histiocytosis X: integration of eosinophilic granuloma of bone, "Letterer-Siwe disease," and "Schüller-Christian disease" as related manifestations of a single nosologic entity. Arch Pathol 56:84–102, 1953

Oberman HA: Idiopathic histiocytosis: a correlative review of eosinophilic granuloma, Hand-Schüller Christian disease and Letterer-Siwe disease. J Pediatr Ophthalmol 5:86–92, 1968

Porter FS: Lymphoreticular disorders — conditions with abnormal proliferation, possibly malignant. In *Hematology*. Second ed. Ed: WJ Williams et al. New York, McGraw-Hill Book Co, 1977, pp 1141–1147

Straatsma BR: Eosinophilic granuloma of bone. Trans Am Acad Ophthalmol Otolaryngol 62:771–776, 1958

Wheeler JM: Exophthalmos associated with diabetes insipidus and large defects in the bones of the skull. Arch Ophthalmol ns 5:161–174, 193

Wheeler M: Exophthalmos caused by eosinophilic granuloma of bone. Am J Ophthalmol 29:980–984, 1946

Infantile Xanthogranuloma

Helwig EB, Hackney VC: Juvenile xanthogranuloma (nevoxantho-endothelioma) (abstract). Am J Pathol 30:625–626, 1954

McDonagh JER: A contribution to our knowledge of the naevo-xantho-endotheliomata. Br J Dermatol 24:85–99, 1912

Sanders TE: Infantile xanthogranuloma of the orbit: a report of three cases. Am J Ophthalmol 61:1299–1306, 1966

Zimmerman LE: Ocular lesions of juvenile xanthogranuloma: nevoxanthoendothelioma. Trans Am Acad Ophthalmol Otolaryngol 69:412–439, 1965

Sinus Histiocytosis

Azoury FJ, Reed RJ: Histiocytosis. Report of an unusual case. New Engl J Med 274:928–930, 1966

Destombes P: Adénitis avec surcharge lipidique, de l'enfant ou de l'adulte jeune, observées aux Antilles et au Mali (quatre observations). Bull Soc Path Exot 58:1169–1175, 1965

Foucar E, Rosai J, Dorfman RF: The ophthalmologic manifestations of sinus histiocytosis with massive lymphadenopathy. Am Ophthalmol 87:354–367, 1979

Friendly DS, Font RL, Rao NA: Orbital involvement in 'sinus' histiocytosis. Arch Ophthalmol 95:2006–2011, 1977

Lampert F, Lennert K: Sinus histiocytosis with massive lymphadenopathy. Cancer 37:783–789, 1976

Marie J, Bernard J, Nezelof C et al: Adenopathies chroniques avec proliferation reticulohistiocytaire et surcharge lipidique. Ann Pediatr 42:2689–2698, 1966

Rosai J, Dorfman RF: Sinus histiocytosis with massive lymphadenopathy. A newly recognized benign clinicopathologic entity. Arch Pathol 87:63–70, 1969

Rosai J, Dorfman RF: Sinus histiocytosis with massive lymphadenopathy: a pseudo-lymphomatous benign tumor. Cancer 30:1174–1188, 1972

Sanchez R, Rosai J, Dorfman RF: Sinus histiocytosis with massive lymphadenopathy. An analysis of 113 cases with special emphasis on its extranodal manifestations. Quoted by Foucar et al.

Vincent TN, Mierciourt R: Histiocytosis of the eyelid. Penrose Cancer Hosp Bull 3:246–250, 1967

15

Intrinsic Neoplasms of the Lacrimal Gland

From an anatomic standpoint, we have considered the lacrimal gland (see Section I) to be a resident of the orbit and therefore within the perimeter of this survey of orbital tumors. Many authors consider the lacrimal gland and its disorders as a unit separate from other dysfunctions, and sometimes similar afflictions, of neighboring structures. Its large size and specialized function favor such an approach, and similar anatomic and physiologic factors are responsible for treating the eye and its diseases as a subject distinct from lesions of its supporting adnexal appendages. However, this approach would require, for a separate discussion of the lacrimal gland, a recapitulation of the features of some tumors (i.e., malignant lymphoma, histiocytosis, and others) which already have been discussed, and would necessitate inclusion of some granulomas to be discussed in future chapters. But all such tumors may appear anywhere in the orbit and need not be considered as unique to the lacrimal gland itself. Technically, it would be preferable to classify such tumors as occurring in the area of the lacrimal fossa rather than as being simply derived from the gland itself. More properly, tumors of the lacrimal gland should be defined as those whose origin is traced to functional components of the organ. The factor common to these latter growths, then, is a variable degree of proliferation of cellular derivatives of the secretory or ductal epithelium. We have regarded these tumors as being intrinsic to the lacrimal gland; and the benign and malignant neoplasms of this intrinsic type are the subject of this chapter. In addition, we prefer to limit this chapter to those epithelial neoplasms considered primary in the lacrimal gland.

HISTORICAL ASPECTS

Probably because of their conspicuous position in the more forward portion of the superior quadrant of the orbit, neoplasms of this type, as well as other tumors of the lacrimal fossa, have been known since the earlier periods of the printed word. The first description of such a tumor has been attributed to Fabricius von Hilden (Fabricius Hildanus, 1598). It is our belief that this tumor was a granuloma in the area of the lacrimal fossa rather than a tumor of the lacrimal gland proper as it has so often been regarded (see Frontispiece). In the past century, observers have been mostly intrigued by the polymorphism of tissue elements found in many of these neoplasms. This feature more than any other characteristic has been responsible for the diversity of thought as to the relationship of some lacrimal gland tumors to each other, as well as their proper position in the overall classification of neoplasms.

Initially, all these tumors were designated in terms of a *hypertrophic* or *scirrhous* change in the lacrimal gland, and such terms persisted up to the 19th century. Becker (1867) was one of the first to examine these tumors microscopically and he used the term *adenoid*. Becker's tumor seemed to be a combination of an adenoma combined with a *cancroid* of interstitial tissue; it probably was an example of what we now recognize as a mixed tumor. Interest in the microscopic examination of these tumors in the latter part of the 19th century led to several dozen different names, some of which were exceedingly complex in their descriptive phraseology. Warthin (1901), a pathologist at the University of Michigan, reviewed the subject and analyzed some 132 cases in the prior literature. Warthin proposed that they be considered mixed growths, and he related such lacrimal gland tumors to similar growths occurring in the major salivary glands which, at that time, were considered to be of endothelial origin. The term *mixed tumor* (first used by Minssen in 1874) was generally accepted, but the concept of endothelial origin soon was disputed and abandoned. An origin from the epithelial components of the lacrimal gland, next proposed, however, did not explain satisfactorily the origin of the mesodermal-like components of the tumor. Various transformations and metaplasias of the proliferating epithelial cells were proposed to explain this phenomenon. Another more direct explanation proposed a dual origin, that is, the interstitial component from neoplastic mesodermal anlage and the glandular component from similar neoplastic stimuli affecting epithelial cells. Such a theory further popularized the name of mixed tumor for those tumors with a mixed morphology. At present, most observers associate the essential features of these tumors with an epithelial origin of these neoplasms.

MIXED TUMOR

TERMINOLOGY

It is proper, first, to inquire into the meaning of the term *mixed tumor*. Since its first use a century ago (1874), the term has meant different things to different physicians. A student should keep these variables in mind when reviewing the literature because such factors as incidence, course, and prognosis are influenced by the meaning given to this particular designation.

At first, histopathologically, most tumors of the lacrimal fossa were believed to be variants of mixed tumor. The earliest and most important revision was separation of those tumors appearing to be innocent from those with an evil reputation. The latter were designated carcinomas and now are considered as a separate group of neoplasms unrelated to the mixed tumors. The former retained the original generic designation, mixed tumors. Such a division between the good and the bad, based on histopathologic features, helped clinicians because it permitted a more accurate prognosis. A flaw in this arrangement soon was noticed when a few of the apparently benign mixed tumors manifested malignant potential. Such a reversal of behavior was explained on the basis either of a malignant metaplasia of the cells or of a small latent focus of malignant degeneration, overlooked in the microscopic examination of the original tissue sections. Because these malignant mixed tumors were capable of metastasis some pathologists thought it best to include them with the carcinomas, reserving the term *true mixed tumor* for the benign variety. Other observers considered that a second revision in the classification of mixed tumors into benign and malignant types was indicated; this is the prevailing classification.

Correlation between the histopathologic appearance and prognosis of salivary gland tumors also helped to bring about some order in the tumors under discussion (Foote and Frazell 1954). The criteria for separating adenoid cystic carcinoma from benign mixed tumor was established and the tendency of some of the latter neoplasms to undergo a malignant transformation was recognized. At this time the term, *malignant mixed tumor*, came into use (Forrest 1954).

Later, the World Health Organization addressed the problem of terminology (Thackray and Sobin 1972). They proposed *pleomorphic adenoma* as a name for benign mixed tumor and *carcinoma in pleomorphic adenoma* as a substitute for malignant mixed tumor. The latter proposal is somewhat of a contradiction and has not been widely accepted. An optional term, *pleomorphic adenocarcinoma*, also has been used to designate the malignant variety, but this name does not correctly identify the pathology of several of the malignant subtypes of the mixed tumor. From a practical standpoint we prefer to use the traditional terms, benign and malignant mixed tumor, because, in the limited field of orbital pathology, everyone knows what we are talking about.

INCIDENCE

The changing concepts in terminology, noted above, are one of the factors frustrating an accurate assessment of the incidence of mixed tumors based on reports in the literature. In some reports the author does not state whether both benign and malignant variants are included in the designation, mixed tumor. In other reports only a statistical enumeration of benign tumors is noted; the malignant mixed tumors being classified with carcinomas of the lacrimal gland. As a result one survey cannot always be compared with another. The frequency of mixed tumors in our Mayo Clinic survey relative to various classes of orbital tumors is summarized in Table 20. Our figures are considerably lower than

TABLE 20.   FREQUENCY OF MIXED TUMORS IN MAYO CLINIC SURVEY OF ORBITAL TUMORS, 1948–1974

Types	Number of cases	Total orbital tumors (%) n = 764	Total orbital neoplasms (%) n = 552	Primary neoplasms (%) n = 251	Secondary neoplasms (%) n = 227
Benign	13	1.7	2.3	5.1	*
Malignant (primary)	10	1.3	1.8	3.9	*
Malignant (secondary)	5	0.6	0.9	*	2.2
Benign and malignant (primary)	23	3	4.1	9.1	*

*Not applicable.

TABLE 21. INCIDENCE OF PRIMARY EPITHELIAL TUMORS OF LACRIMAL
GLAND FOSSA: RECENT, MAJOR SERIES

Authors	Number of Cases	Type of Neoplasm, Percentage Distribution			
		Benign Mixed	*Malignant Mixed*	*Adenocystic Carcinoma*	*Other Carcinomas*
Font and Gamel	265	136 (51%)	34 (13%)	70 (27%)	25 (9%)
Mayo Clinic (1948–1974)	41	13 (32%)	10 (24%)	12 (29%)	6 (15%)
Ashton (25 years)	54	30 (55%)	2 (4%)	13 (24%)	9 (17%)

other incidence data in the literature because our sample contains a larger number of secondary orbital tumors and more diverse types (cysts, pseudotumors, metastatic neoplasms, orbital involvement with multifocal tumors, and so on) than other surveys.

Data on the incidence of mixed tumors relative to other epithelial tumors in the area of the lacrimal fossa are a little easier to obtain. The recent pertinent information is summarized in Table 21. The largest series, by far, is that of Font and Gamel. Their data is based on cases from the Registry of Ophthalmic Pathology of the Armed Forces Institute of Pathology and is an extension of a similar review of a smaller number of cases by Zimmerman and associates in 1962. This combined review, by reason of its large size, probably is the most complete although it does not represent a consecutive series of cases.

Ophthalmologists are accustomed to the general rule that benign mixed tumors comprise about half of all epithelial neoplasms of the lacrimal gland. The data of Font and Gamel, and Ashton (Table 21) supports this assumption. Our own data shows a lesser ratio of benign tumors to the total number. An explanation of this difference may lie in the very long period of follow-up observation of our patients as compared to most other surveys. In three of our mixed tumor cases (see Fig. 259, patients F29, F23, and M47) and possibly a fourth case (F23), the neoplasm became malignant (and was so classified) during the period of our survey, but, initially, the neoplasms were benign mixed tumors. If data in Table 21 was based on the histologic diagnosis of the original tumor, then our benign mixed tumor group would increase to 16 patients (40%) and malignant mixed tumor group decrease to 7 patients (17%) of the total. This revised data would more nearly compare with the other surveys in Table 21.

As years have passed and experience with mixed tumors has increased, the age range of reported cases has widened. The benign mixed tumor has been reported in children and has been noted as late as the eighth decade. With such a wide age distribution, median and average age data at time of diagnosis is not very relevant. Age span of patients in our survey is noted in Table 3, Chapter 3. About 80% of our benign tumor patients were between the ages of 23 and 55 years at time of initial diagnosis, and a similar age range at diagnosis was noted for the malignant mixed tumor group. About 70% of the patients with benign mixed tumor in the Font and Gamel series were in a similar age range as our own, but their patients with malignant mixed tumor were generally older than our group.

As for the sex distribution, benign mixed tumors occur predominantly in males. In the survey of Font and Gamel the male/female ratio was 1:5:1. The sex distribution of patients with the malignant type was equal. In our series the male/female ratio was 8:5 (benign mixed tumor).

CLINICAL FEATURES

The most noteworthy and constant sign of mixed tumors is *forward proptosis and downward displacement of the eye* in the affected orbit. If the enlarging neoplasm is situated posterior to the lacrimal gland, the amount of forward proptosis will be greater than that of downward displacement. If the tumor is more forward in the lacrimal fossa or adjacent to the superotemporal rim, the reverse is true (Fig. 242). If the tumor is moderate in size there also will be some *inward displacement of the eye*. Other signs are *fullness of the upper lid* or *a palpable mass* in the superotemporal portion of the orbit. These signs — an abnormal position of the eye combined with upper eyelid fullness or a palpable mass — are pathognomonic of tumor in the lacrimal fossa. But these signs are by no means exclusive to mixed tumors, and other tumors common to this area, such as pseudotumor, malignant lymphoma, dermoid cyst, and adenoid cystic carcinoma, may show similar signs. We do not know of any means to differentiate these several tumors by palpation of the enlarging mass and observation of the displaced eye alone. However, other features may differentiate these tumors. In the case of inflammatory pseudotumor, frequent and intermittent episodes of redness of the adjacent portion of the upper eyelid may be observed. With malignant lymphoma the patient may be older than the patient with the mixed tumor. A dermoid or epidermoid cyst of sufficient size to displace the eye in a downward direction usually shows characteristic roentgenographic features. An adenoid cystic carcinoma or related adenocarcinoma that has been present for more than several months usually is painful, whereas benign mixed tumor is painless unless of the recurrent type. Some patients with malignant mixed tumor also will complain of pain but this is not a constant feature unless the tumor is of the recurrent or secondary type. Other symptoms, such as blurred vision, diplopia, retinal striae, edema of the upper eyelid, and papilledema, we consider of minor significance in the overall picture. Diplopia, if present, usually is manifest only when looking toward the affected quadrant. Papilledema and retinal striae are seldom seen unless the tumor is relatively large and lies posterior to the lacrimal gland. We have not observed any patient who has had appreciable alteration of lacrimation, probably because the tumor does not destroy the gland but only compresses it. The lacrimal gland always seems to compensate for the pressure upon it.

Several authors have placed much emphasis on duration of symptoms as a method for clinical differentiation of the two types of mixed tumors. They cite a

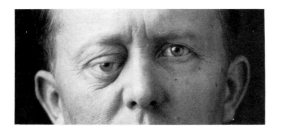

Figure 242. Benign mixed tumor: downward displacement and forward proptosis of right eye, and fullness and slight droop of upper eyelid.

shorter period of symptoms (less than a year) as representative of the malignant mixed tumor and a longer period as characteristic of benign mixed tumors. In our experience the duration of symptoms as a guide to diagnosis is entirely unreliable. In fact, the longest interval of symptomatology (30 years) occurred in one of the malignant mixed tumor patients of our series (Waller et al 1973).

A clinical feature not stressed by clinicians, but important to the planned surgical approach, is the eccentric pattern of growth of some mixed tumors. They commence in the lacrimal gland fossa where they are always palpable, but they may not remain long in this same area in the course of their growth. On many occasions we have palpated what was assumed to be a small mixed tumor only to find, on surgical exploration, a neoplasm much larger in size and extent than anticipated. Almost all mixed tumors will prove to be larger than 2 cm when excised, but only a small area of this total mass may be palpated preoperatively in the superior temporal quadrant of the orbit. Likewise, in the course of expansion, they frequently extend away from their point of origin. We have found them unexpectedly extending well up toward the frontal sinus, growing toward the vertical midline of the orbit behind the orbital rim, sneaking inferiorly below the level of the lateral horizontal palpebral raphe, or filling the posterior-superior temporal quadrant of the orbit well back toward the junction of the eyeball and optic nerve (Fig. 243).

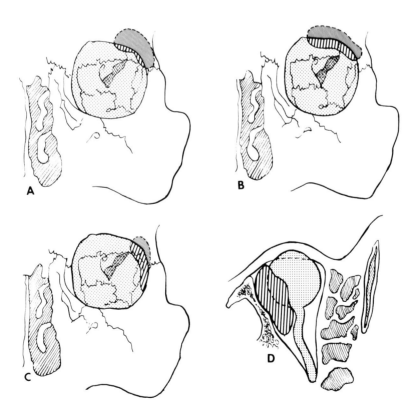

Figure 243. Benign mixed tumor. Diagrammatic representation of eccentric growth pattern in relation to palpable tumor in left orbit. *A*, superior extent; *B*, nasal extent; *C*, inferior extent; *D*, posterior extent. (A, B, C — frontal projections, D — transverse projection.)

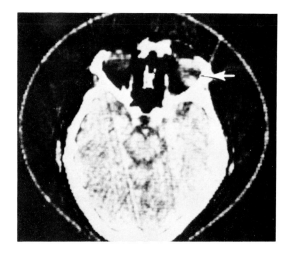

Figure 244. Benign mixed tumor. Computer tomography shows a large (3 × 2.5 × 2 cm) tumor superior and posterior to right eye (*arrow*). The extent of the tumor could not be appreciated by palpation alone. The proptosed eye was displaced inferiorly 7 mm and, therefore, is not visible at this scanning level.

ROENTGENOGRAPHIC CHANGES

The paper by Jones and Pfeiffer (1954) on the roentgenographic diagnosis of lacrimal gland tumors has served as a standard source of information and has been widely quoted in many subsequent articles on this subject. The three bony abnormalities of greatest significance were enlargement of the lacrimal fossa, increased bone density, and bone destruction. Many patients with benign mixed tumor will show enlargement of the lacrimal gland fossa if the growth of the tumor is toward bone. Also, some reactive sclerosis of bone may be present in cases with an interval of symptoms longer than 1 year. If bone destruction is observed the likely diagnosis is one of the malignant neoplasms intrinsic in the lacrimal gland. However, subtle changes in the adjacent bone reflecting the growth of either the benign or malignant tumors are easily missed on standard orbital views. Therefore, we believe it wise to order tomograms (particularly lateral projections) for all tumors in the upper outer quadrant of the orbit. Such tomograms more frequently reveal the bony changes already noted. Even so, a negative tomogram does not necessarily rule out a mixed tumor of either variety. Computer tomography is a valued supplement to show the size of the tumor and, particularly, its medial or posterior extent (Fig. 244).

PATHOLOGY

Benign Mixed Tumor

Perhaps the one distinguishing histopathologic feature common to all benign mixed tumors is their diverse morphologic makeup, which makes it difficult to describe any typical pattern of cellular structure. Grossly, the tumor usually is grayish white, circumscribed, unilobular, and slightly bosselated (Fig. 245). Lacrimal gland tissue of normal appearance often will remain attached to the surface of the tumor during its excision. A definite but thin capsule is present unless the tumor has ruptured during removal or has been partially

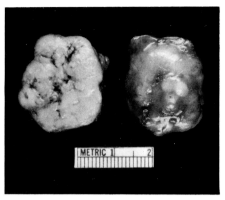

Figure 245. Mixed tumor: Right, surface of tumor is circumscribed and slightly basselated. Left, cut surface is lobulated and variegated in appearance.

stripped away by incisional biopsy. As the tumor continues to grow this thin capsular barrier may lose its identity by fusing with the periorbita and other surrounding soft tissue structures. Such tumors may then be designated as circumscribed rather than encapsulated and, on microscopic study, tumor cells may be found beyond the assumed limits of the pseudocapsule. When sectioned, the specimen may seem less solid than suggested through its intact surface; the tumor consists of lobules of tissue of different density separated by scanty connective tissue septa. Seldom are these tumors entirely homogeneous in make-up.

The variation in structural pattern is evident on the first scan of the tumor under the low power of the microscope (Fig. 246). In some areas a myxoid configuration resembling connective tissue predominates (Fig. 247); in other areas the cellularity suggests a predominantly epithelial nature (Fig. 248). Most of the

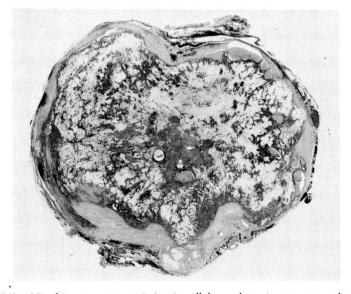

Figure 246. Mixed tumor: great variation in cellular makeup is apparent under low power; clear myxoid areas alternate with cellular epithelial zones, and well-developed capsule is evident. (Hematoxylin and eosin; × 3.)

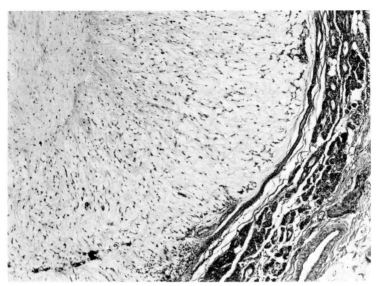

Figure 247. Mixed tumor: myxoid connective tissue component predominates; compressed adjacent lacrimal gland is to right. (Hemotoxylin and eosin; × 50.)

tumors, somewhere in their expanse, show irregularly anastomosing nests of tubular structures resembling the glandular portion of the adjacent lacrimal gland. With the hematoxylin-eosin stain the cellular components of these glandular structures stain purplish blue and the encompassing interstitial matrix appears more reddish. Where these basophilic and eosinophilic elements are roughly equal in proportion they appear distinct from one another under low-

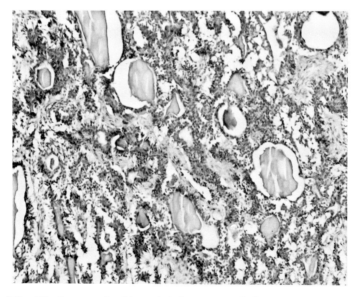

Figure 248. Mixed tumor: in this epithelial zone irregularly anastomosing tubules resemble lacrimal gland. (Hematoxylin and eosin; × 80.)

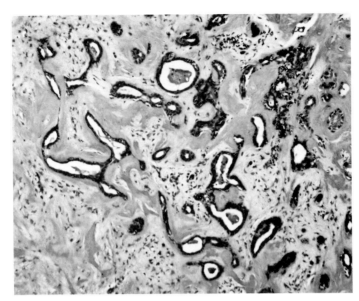

Figure 249. Mixed tumor: tubular epithelial elements are dispersed in hyaline intercellular matrix. (Hematoxylin and eosin; × 80.)

power magnification (Fig. 249). Such a portion of the tumor then resembles a simple adenoma. With greater magnification, this separation of the glandular and interstitial components becomes less real; and on closer inspection, the cells of the former seem to merge gradually with the cells of the latter.

Under still higher magnification the epithelial walls of the interlacing islands of tubular structures show both single- and double-layered profiles. The lumens of some of these tubular structures appear to be empty but most contain a muco-serous, homogeneous, eosinophilic staining material. In areas with a dense and many-layered proliferation of epithelial cells, the lumens are filled with swirls of keratin owing to squamous metaplasia of the lining epithelium (Fig. 250). In the simpler single- or double-layered ducts the epithelial cells are cuboidal. Each nucleus is oval or round, is basophilic, and occupies the major portion of the cell area, and a centrally placed nucleolus occasionally is seen among the finely granular intranuclear chromatin material. The scanty cytoplasm surrounding the nucleus will be faintly eosinophilic. No basement membrane surrounds the epithelial-lined tubes and the cells spiral out almost imperceptibly into surrounding areas, producing cellular patterns which mimic various types of mesodermal tissue. In these transitional zones the epithelial cells may lose their cuboidal shape and become more stellate. In other specimens, cell boundaries become less distinct as the cell is pushed farther from the cords and tubules of proliferating epithelium. The intranuclear material in such cells becomes more coarse and finally disappears, leaving an empty, ghost-like nucleus surrounded by a homogeneous eosinophilic staining matrix. Cases also are described where in this matrix may undergo necrosis or form a hyaline type cartilage (Fig. 251). In large or long-standing tumors the basophilic cells also push into the surrounding capsule in an effort to gain greater freedom for their

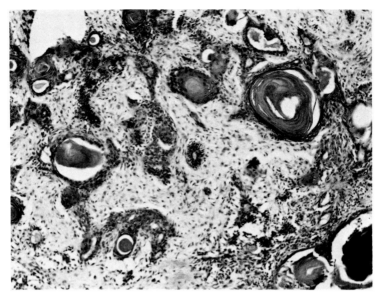

Figure 250.   Mixed tumor: in epithelial zones lumens may be filled with swirls of keratin due to squamous metaplasia of lining epithelium. (Hematoxylin and eosin × 80.)

growth. In some specimens the cellular component may so predominate as to suggest carcinoma, but nowhere are there any mitotic figures or variations in staining characteristics and cell size as in the malignant form. However variable the transition of the epithelial cells may be in some specimens, their proliferation still is orderly.

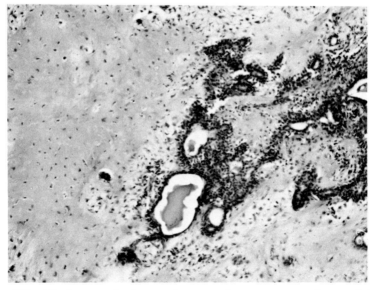

Figure 251.   Mixed tumor: hyaline cartilage may form component of intercellular matrix. (Hematoxylin and eosin; × 80.)

Malignant Mixed Tumor

Our knowledge of this neoplasm is insufficient to allow us to state definitely whether the neoplasm is malignant from its earliest origin or whether it commences as a benign tumor with later malignant change. Among the tumors of the Mayo Clinic series, the malignant alteration seems to have occurred either adjacent to or within an area of benign mixed tumor (Fig. 252). This suggests that the malignant alteration supervened some time after the initial growth of the benign tumor. Most other observers support this concept. When such an alteration occurs, then the degree of malignancy usually is marked though the actual area of malignancy may occupy only a small part of the total area of the tumor.

There are three main forms of malignant alteration. The most common malignant component is adenocarcinoma (Fig. 253). Some of the glandular features of the benign component are retained in the area of the malignancy but the lumens of the acinous structures are irregular in shape and variable in size, and the epithelium surrounding these acinar structures becomes multi-layered. The more oval appearance of similar structures in the benign portion of the tumor vanishes. The predominant feature is the variation in the size and staining characteristics of the individual cells, as compared to similarly positioned cells in the benign section of the tumor. In the area of adenocarcinoma the sizes of nuclei vary; some are large, almost giant size—several diameters larger than non-neoplastic nuclei. Mitotic figures can be seen. Further scanning of the section will reveal some of these malignant cells creeping away from the glandular aggregates to invade and proliferate along the connective tissue separating the lobules of tumor. In these zones of dissemination the nuclei vary even more in size and shape and stain intensely.

Next in frequency is squamous differentiation (Fig. 254). The epithelial cells tend to grow in nests. In some areas the lumen of the glandular element is obliterated by proliferating cells; in other areas a lumen is still visible but the wall of the acinar structure has been irregularly thickened by the unequal growth of adjacent epithelial cells. The nuclei tend to retain their oval or round contours but enlarge to three, or even four, times their usual size. The cytoplasm of these cells retains its eosinophilic properties but is less homogeneous

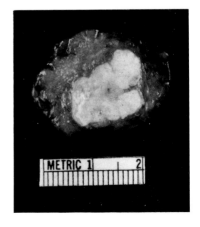

Figure 252. Malignant mixed tumor: outer portion of specimen is highly malignant adenocarcinoma surrounding central benign mixed tumor; clinically, mild proptosis, present for approximately 29 years, suddenly became progressive and severe.

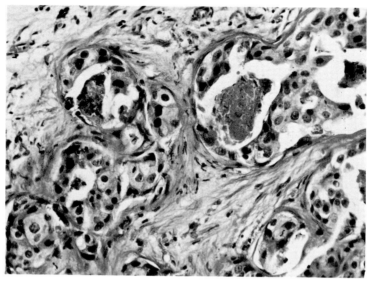

Figure 253.   Malignant mixed tumor: malignant component is adenocarcinoma. (Hematoxylin and eosin; × 400.)

and appears to be more frothy than that of similar cells in benign specimens. An occasional giant cell containing two nuclei may be encountered. The malignant focus gives an overall appearance of disordered, haphazard epithelial proliferation.

The third form of malignant deterioration, the sarcomatous, is the least frequent (Fig. 255). Interlacing bundles of closely packed, deeply staining, spindle-shaped cells can be seen. All of these malignant mixed tumors, regardless of their type, also show some signs of chronic inflammatory reaction. At the time

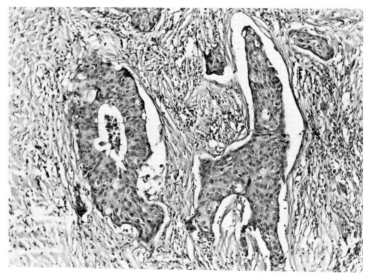

Figure 254.   Malignant mixed tumor: malignant component is squamous cell carcinoma. (Hematoxylin and eosin; × 100.)

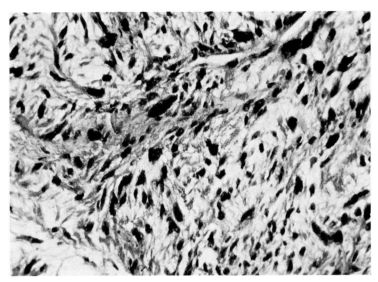

Figure 255. Malignant mixed tumor: malignant component is highly anaplastic spindle cell sarcoma. (Hematoxylin and eosin; × 285.)

of initial excision the benign component of the tumor usually predominates. With each succeeding recurrence the malignant alteration becomes more dominant.

TREATMENT

The management of mixed tumor is surgical. Furthermore, the goal of surgery should be complete removal of the neoplasm. It is likely that all mixed tumors, whether they are benign or malignant, start their careers as circumscribed neoplasms. Unless they are highly malignant or grow quite large, the capsule serves, to some degree, as a barrier to the escape of neoplastic elements. It is true that this capsule may be very thin, and subsequent study may show that cells invade its inner circumference. (Zimmerman and associates [1962] refer to it as a "pseudocapsule"). Still, by careful approach and dissection, the aim of the surgeon should be removal of the tumor with pseudocapsule intact. In addition, some of the surrounding adnexal tissue also should be removed particularly if the tumor is bilobed. A bilobed neoplasm usually is malignant and tumor cells may be found beyond the limits of the apparent capsule when the specimen is examined histologically.

Several older ophthalmic texts advise deep wedge biopsy for situations of this type (Fig. 256). This advice is based on the premise that complete treatment cannot be performed until a correct diagnosis, based on microscopic study, has been made. Still, the recurrence rate of benign mixed tumor will never be lowered nor the mortality rate of malignant mixed tumor decreased until surgeons stop whacking into these dangerous tumors. We believe that the surgeon who makes the initial surgical approach has the best chance of anyone to cure the disease by complete, intact removal of the tumor.

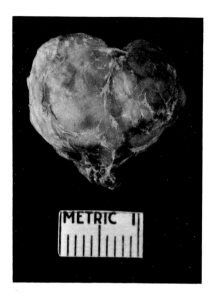

Figure 256. Malignant mixed tumor: large, bilobed, well-circumscribed, adenocarcinoma (grade 3) removed apparently intact; preliminary, deep wedge biopsy of such a tumor would only increase chance of recurrence and may jeopardize patient's life. This patient was followed for 7 years without evidence of local recurrence of malignant tumor.

To attain these objectives we use the anterior-lateral surgical approach (Chapter 25) for all tumors in the lacrimal gland fossa, assuming they will be mixed tumors until proven otherwise by gross inspection or microscopic examination. The unilobular, circumscribed benign mixed tumor is excised intact along with the periorbita attached to its base. The adjacent bone need not be removed unless erosion or destruction is discovered. In the latter event the operation is converted into an en bloc resection (Chapter 25) such as we use for all bilobed tumors or unilobular masses where preoperative assessment has made us suspicious of malignancy.

Some surgeons decry such a vigorous approach to tumors of the lacrimal gland fossa, stating that such surgery is unnecessary for the nonepithelial tumors in this area. Even so, if there is a choice, we believe the patient would rather have a benign condition completely removed by too vigorous means than to have a potentially malignant tumor incompletely treated because of a milquetoast attitude. Still, to quiet these alarums, there is an option for management of those pseudotumors or granulomas that sometimes look like a poorly circumscribed mixed tumor. For these, we recommend the "staged" en bloc resection (Chapter 25) that will permit biopsy away from the surgical field without risk of seeding. If frozen section biopsy shows the lesion to be benign, the operation can be converted into an ordinary orbitotomy at this stage. If frozen tissue study indicates the lesion is malignant the operation is completed as a planned en bloc resection.

The role of exenteration, either as a primary procedure or a supplement to resection with bone removal, in the management of the malignant mixed tumors is debatable. The crux of the matter is that local spread or metastasis of tumor probably is faster or easier through bone than orbital soft tissues. Therefore, extensive removal of bone is more important than extensive removal of soft tissues. If the surgeon can completely excise the soft tissue component of the tumor with its underlying periorbita and bone, then he has probably done all that can be done for the patient, and survival will depend on the extent of bone involvement. Supplementary exenteration in this situation would not increase length of survival in our opinion. However, if removal of the soft tissue component of the tumor is incomplete, subtotal exenteration is necessary even though bone also is removed. The latter approach also is recommended to these patients who are referred for definitive care after a positive incisional biopsy elsewhere.

Exenteration may also be an effective measure for some cases of recurrent malignant mixed tumor of the orbit. In the literature there are some known survivors of surgical management somewhat similar to the case described by Ashton. Recurrent tumor 12 years after local excision was locally excised, another recurrence 7 years later was treated by exenteration, and a third recurrence 2 years later was locally excised. The patient was still living 25 years after the initial operation. In such patients the long interval between initial operation and first recurrence probably indicates that bone was not involved prior to the first excision of the tumor.

In contrast to malignant mixed tumor, the benign variant does not seem to invade bone although it may cause a reactive sclerosis. Recurrent seedings of benign mixed tumor seem to perpetuate themselves along soft tissue planes. Therefore, total exenteration of the orbit would seem to be a more logical treatment for these cases than repeated local excision of recurrent tumor nodules so often performed.

As regards irradiation, we do not believe it is an effective therapy for benign recurrent mixed tumor but it does seem to have some palliative role in the management of malignant mixed tumor that has already spread to bone.

PROGNOSIS

To assess data pertaining to prognosis accurately, the examiner should keep in mind three factors: the date of the publication, the interval of follow-up study, and the type of surgery performed at the initial operation of the tumor. First, most publications prior to those of Foote and Frazell (1954) and of Forrest (1954) included the adenocarcinomas in their definition of mixed tumors. The adenocarcinomas and related neoplasms are now considered in a separate group with a notoriously poor prognosis. Their inclusion with the mixed tumors gave the latter an erroneously poor reputation. More recently, some ophthalmologists have continued to exclude all malignant tumors, even the malignant mixed tumors, from the group designated mixed tumors. This has reversed the prognosis of mixed tumors to the point where it probably is too optimistic. Therefore, it is wise to determine whether the observer is discussing only the benign mixed tumor or whether the malignant type also is included in the prognostications. Next, the period of follow-up also is important. Some of these mixed tumors, particularly the benign type, may not recur for many years after their incomplete removal. Recurrences 15 to 30 years after initial surgery have been reported and we have observed a similar delay before recurrence in some cases. With each recurrence the possibility of malignant metaplasia increases and the prognosis becomes more guarded. Finally, the type of surgery is significant.

In delving through many case reports and surveys (usually in the fine print of the case record), we often find it difficult to know just how much and what type of removal of tumor was accomplished. Some just report that the "tumor was removed" without stating whether the lesion was invasive or encapsulated, or whether delivery was intact or piecemeal. These reports raise the suspicion that much is left unsaid and excision of the neoplasm was not as complete as the surgeon wished it to appear. Other reports indicate a "complete removal" but, again, they do not state whether the capsule was intact or excision was piecemeal. Still others claim "complete removal" after bravely performing an initial deep wedge biopsy with its consequent risk of seeding.

The survey of Font and Gamel is the most extensive and recent in the literature in reference to follow-up information. In regard to benign mixed tumor, follow-up data was available on 113 patients. Those individuals whose tumor had been biopsied prior to excision had a 5-year recurrence rate of 32%, while patients whose tumor was removed with the capsule intact had a 5-year recurrence rate of only 3%. Of the patients who had undergone a surgical procedure for a first recurrence, 70% developed a second recurrence within 15 years. They estimated that at the end of 20 years approximately 10% of patients who had had primary resection of a benign mixed tumor would develop a malignant tumor, while at the end of 30 years approximately 20% would have a malignant transformation. Lastly, they list 4 of their 113 patients as dead of benign mixed tumor. From this data it is evident that benign mixed tumor is not an innocuous tumor, particularly once it has recurred.

In our series we have follow-up information of 10 years or longer on 10 of 13 patients. Six of these 10 patients have had no recurrence in an interval of 10 to 18 years after initial excision. None of these six tumors were biopsied, although in two patients the pseudocapsule ruptured as the tumor was delivered. The other 4 patients were living, 14, 22, 24, and 26 years after initial incomplete removal of their tumor. These four people had had a combined total of twelve operations for recurrences and only one seemed free of recurrent tumor at the time of review. This data also strongly supports the contention that a high recurrence rate is associated with biopsy or incomplete removal of tumor at the initial operation.

The long interval from initial surgery to first recurrence and the malignant potential of recurrent benign mixed tumor is emphasized by the case history of a patient reported by Riley and Henderson (1970).

A 72-year-old woman was seen because of a palpable tumor occupying both temporal quadrants of the left orbit. Displacement of the left eye had been evident for 4 weeks. Past history revealed that 39 years earlier, an orbitotomy had been performed because of a mass in the area of the lacrimal fossa (Fig. 257). The patient had had symptoms of this tumor for approximately 5 years before this initial surgery. At orbitotomy removal of the tumor had been incomplete. A histopathologic diagnosis of benign mixed tumor was made. Tissue slides of this tumor were available for our review and we confirmed the correctness of the original diagnosis. Orbitotomy was indicated, and on this occasion (39 years after the first operation) a huge tumor was removed (Fig. 258). It consisted of two adjacent parts. Tissue in the smaller lobules, attached to the bony rim of the orbit, was benign mixed tumor similar in structure to the tissue sections made 40 years earlier. Tissue in the largest lobe of the tumor, which extended inferiorly and posteriorly into the orbital space, was a highly malignant spindle-cell sarcomatous metaplasia of the original mixed tumor. Five subsequent surgical procedures, including two exenterations, were performed for recurrent tumor, but the patient expired from intracranial spread of tumor 11 months after first recurrence and 40 years after initial surgery.

The prognosis of patients with malignant mixed tumor is much more serious. Again, the data of Font and Gamel is the most complete of any in the

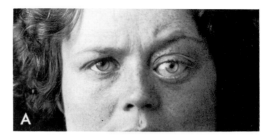

Figure 257. Benign mixed tumor: Preoperative photograph showing displacement of left eye due to benign mixed tumor

literature. Follow-up information was available in 29 of their 34 patients. Twelve patients are dead of tumor and the median survival period approximates 12 years. In our study, follow-up information was available on all ten patients with primary malignant mixed tumor and is summarized in Figure 259. It is evident the mortality rate (eight of ten patients dead of tumor) of our patients is considerably higher than the survey of Font and Gamel. This might be explained on the basis of a longer interval of follow-up study.

Another feature of Figure 259 is the marked variation in survival of the patients after initial surgery. The data suggests this might be related to the histologic character of the neoplasm at time of initial surgery. In the group of four patients at the top of Figure 259, the tumor was considered malignant at the time of surgical diagnosis and their survival was relatively short. Three of these four patients had incomplete removal of neoplasm at the initial operation. The fourth patient of this group had had complete, intact excision of the tumor but without removal of underlying bone.

The survival time of the group of four patients at the bottom of Figure 259 was quite long. The course of patients F-29 and F-23 is similar in respect to a long disease-free interval after incomplete removal of a benign mixed tumor, but only a relatively short survival after the first recurrence of what had become

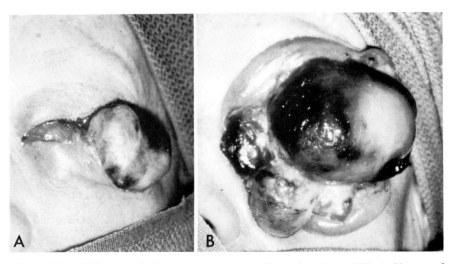

Figure 258. Malignant mixed tumor: same case as depicted in Figure 257. *A,* 39 years after original orbitotomy, with recurrence of tumor, now malignant; tumor was then excised. *B,* Appearance 6 weeks later, showing recurrences of this rapidly growing neoplasm.

PRIMARY MALIGNANT MIXED TUMOR
— ORBIT — CLINICAL COURSE

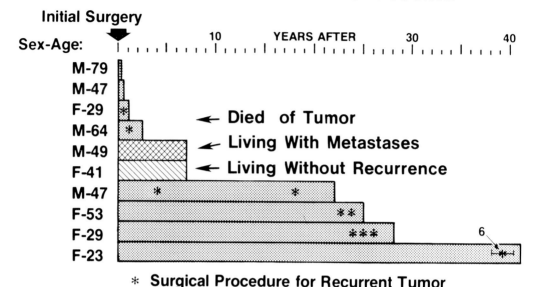

Figure 259.   Clinical course of ten patients with primary malignant mixed tumor of lacrimal gland.

a malignant mixed tumor. The course of patient F-53 also follows this pattern, but we do not know the histologic character nor the method of removal of the initial tumor. The tumor of patient M-47 was initially benign and at the time of first recurrence but was malignant at the time of second recurrence.

ONCOCYTOMA

Two terms—*oncocytoma* and *oxyphil cell adenoma*—are used interchangeably to designate this neoplasm that is very rare in the lacrimal gland. Oncocytoma is the oldest of the two terms and was applied to this type of adenoma by Hamperl (1931). According to Deutsch and Duckworth (1967), Hamperl—at the suggestion of Schaffer—coined the name oncocyte from a Greek term meaning an increase in size. The term *oncocyte* reflects the large size of the cell as compared to the columnar and cuboidal cells usually found in the glandular portions of salivary glands. Oxyphil cell refers to the acidophilic staining properties of these large cells.

Oncocytes also may be found in mucous membranes such as the caruncle and lacrimal sac; in accessory glands of the oral cavity, pharynx, trachea, and esophagus; in the thyroid and parathyroid glands; and along the intestinal tract. Concerning their origin, Hamperl (1962) has claimed that oncocytes develop from a metaplasia and granular degeneration of epithelial cells in the acinar structures of the glandular elements in the above tissues and organs. Oncocytes seem to increase in number with age.

Böck and Schlagenhauff (1938) were the first to discover these cells in the lacrimal gland. They studied 20 specimens of what were believed to be normal lacrimal glands in patients between 48 and 83 years of age; they found oncocytes in 7. Radnót (1939) first discussed oncocytic tumors in the lacrimal gland in an extensive treatise on various pathologic entities affecting this organ. He found small oncocytomas at autopsy in the lacrimal glands of two 69-year-old men. These tumors were clinically asymptomatic.

There are three reports of clinically observed oncocytic tumors of the lacrimal gland in the literature. An oncocytoma was observed in a 39-year-old female by Beskid and Zarzycka (1959). In the other 2 patients, a 59-year-old male (Dorello 1961) and an 81-year-old female (Biggs and Font 1977), the tumors were malignant. This malignant variant is most unusual inasmuch as most of these tumors in their most common site, the caruncle, are benign. No follow-up information was available in the case of Biggs and Font, but Dorello's patient died of intracranial extension 2 years after development of proptosis in spite of orbital exenteration and 3 courses of radiation therapy. Although we have seen an oncocytoma of the caruncle, we have never observed the tumor in the orbit.

In their growth these tumors may retain a glandular pattern or proliferate in nests or sheets of cells. In the glandular pattern the nuclei tend to be displaced toward the lumen of the acinar structure and are comparatively small in relation to the area of granular eosinophilic cytoplasm. In more solid areas the nuclei are relatively larger and occupy a more central position in the cell (Fig. 260). In the benign oncocytoma the cells are polyhedral in shape and uniform in size. Mitoses are infrequent.

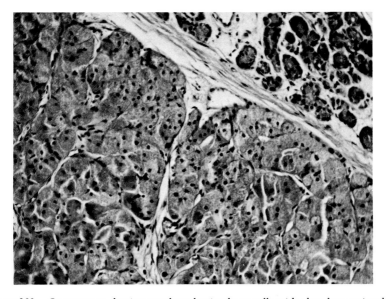

Figure 260. Oncocytoma: benign neoplasm having large cells with abundant eosinophilic cytoplasm; this section is from tumor of parotid gland. (Hematoxylin and eosin; × 155.)

ADENOID CYSTIC CARCINOMA

Because of its distinctive cytologic features, the adenoid cystic carcinoma is known by this name, though it is technically an adenocarcinoma. Earlier ophthalmologists, and many present ophthalmologists, have used its common name, *cylindroma*, which was given to the orbital tumor in 1856 by Billroth, the Berlin surgeon and anatomist. Something more of Billroth's observations on this very malignant tumor and his unhappy patient is worth mentioning.

HISTORICAL ASPECTS

Billroth described a tumor under the name of *Die Cylindergeschwulst* (the cylinder tumor). He regarded it as a most curious, and in many ways an astounding, tumor. The tumor had been described on several occasions, prior to Billroth's description, as "hypertrophy of the lacrimal gland." Mincing the tumor and using the solvents and fixatives of his day, he was intrigued by the system of glass-clear, window-transparent pale cylinders or knobs which appeared in the residue. The compartments of the network formed by these cylinders were long and narrow. The vasculature of the tumor seemed to pass through the center of these amorphous cylinders. Billroth termed these structureless areas *hyaline cylinders* and regarded them as the stroma of the tumor. Unfortunately, he also applied two other terms—cell cylinders and germ cylinders—to the growth pattern of the glandular portion of the tumor, and the overuse of the word cylinder probably accounts for the confusion as to the meaning of the term cylindroma. Some have used *cylindroma* in reference to the acinar and glandular portions of the neoplasm.

Billroth had an unusual opportunity to study the tumor, for a patient of his underwent 7 operations in 2½ years. The patient was a 22-year-old man who had noted progressive downward displacement of the right eye associated with a swelling of the upper orbital rim for 3 years. The movements of the eye were completely restricted and the elevated orbital mass was described as "hard." By the time of the first operation the eye was approximately 2 cm lower than its fellow eye and was so exposed that the patient required treatment in the hospital. With each operation more of the orbital structures were removed: first the tumor, then the eye, next an exenteration, and finally portions of the orbital bones. Even though the bony surfaces were cauterized with a "hot iron" the tumor stubbornly recurred. And throughout, this painful ordeal was unrelieved by the sedatives and analgesics of that period. At the last operation the tumor had extended into the ethmoid bone and the pterygopalatine fossa and filled the adjacent maxillary antrum. In the few weeks before death the patient became insane, probably from intracranial extension. All the salient clinical features of this tumor are found in Billroth's description of this one patient.

The name, cylindroma, now has fallen into disfavor. Its replacement—*adenoid cystic* (or *adenocystic*) *carcinoma*—also designates a particular pattern but refers to the active component rather than the stromal portion of the neoplasm. We do not know who first used the latter term but most pathologists seem to accept the statement of Foote and Frazell (1954) that Ewing, the eminent American pathologist, probably applied this name to the tumor. The adjectives adenoid cystic also designate a type of basal cell epithelioma.

INCIDENCE

Attempts to estimate the frequency of adenoid cystic carcinoma among the entire family of orbital tumors are handicapped by the same factors of confusion relating to classification and nomenclature as noted for the mixed tumors. Twenty-five adenoid cystic carcinomas of the orbit were included in our Mayo Clinic survey, representing an incidence of 3.3% of the total 764 tumors. However, this total included both primary (12 cases) and secondary (13 cases) tumors. The incidence of primary adenoid cystic carcinoma, then, becomes 1.6% of total tumors and 4.8% of all primary orbital neoplasms (251 cases). The incidence of our primary adenoid cystic carcinomas relative to other epithelial neoplasms of the lacrimal gland is 29% (Table 21), a figure closely akin to the values of Font and Gamel, and Ashton.

The age range of our patients with primary tumors at time of diagnosis was 27 to 65 years and the age distribution of patients with secondary adenoid cystic carcinomas was 29 to 82 years. The sex ratio in both groups was nearly equal, 7 males and 5 females in the primary group, and 6 males and 7 females in the secondary group.

In the larger series of primary adenoid cystic carcinomas (70 cases) of Font and Gamel the age range was not unlike our own but there was a slight preponderance of females in a ratio of 1:4:1. As with the benign mixed tumors, the neoplasm is rare in the first decade. But Wolter and Henderson (1969) recently reported a case in a 12-year-old girl and within a month of this observation, another case in a 12-year-old Vietnamese girl came to Wolter's attention (Ley and Wolter, 1969). Adenoid cystic carcinomas of the paranasal sinuses are known to occur even earlier in childhood.

CLINICAL FEATURES

Several of the clinical signs of adenoid cystic carcinoma are similar to those already noted for mixed tumors; namely, *forward and downward displacement of the eye,* a *palpable orbital mass in the superior temporal quadrant,* and *swelling, drooping,* or *fullness of the adjacent upper eyelid.* Lacrimation also may be increased. The mass usually is more firm or "hard" than a mixed tumor. Orbital pain or tenderness on palpation is a common feature of adenoid cystic carcinoma and, when present, should differentiate the mass from benign mixed tumor. Pain and tenderness are caused by spread of the neoplasm into the adjacent periorbita and along nearby nerves, and are ominous because the neoplasm has spread beyond its usual circumscribed border. In recurrent cases, pain may even occur before the multiple seedings become palpable. The pain usually is referred to the eyebrow, forehead, or temple. Mechanical *limitation of eye rotation* on upward and outward gaze on the affected side also is present, but in recurrent cases, or those of long duration, movement of the eye is more severely restricted because of infiltration of the tumor into extraocular muscles. The duration of symptoms prior to initial orbitotomy was 9 months or less in all but three of the twelve patients in our series; this is a significantly shorter period of evolution than that of the average mixed tumor. Adenoid cystic carcinoma grows more sluggishly when it originates in the parotid gland than when in the lacrimal gland.

Roentgenographic Changes

We have not observed any roentgenographic changes that are specific for adenoid cystic carcinoma. For those neoplasms involving the lacrimal gland the frequency and type of bony alteration is similar to those already noted in the malignant mixed tumor group.

Pathology

The predominant patterns are masses and aggregates of closely packed, relatively small cells with indistinct cell boundaries that seem to proliferate around circular and oval acellular spaces (Fig. 261). Both size and number of these spaces may vary. They may be so numerous as to suggest a tissue riddled with holes, an appearance aptly compared to the cut surface of a Swiss cheese; in other areas, these spaces may be so tiny or sparse that the cells seem to proliferate in solid cords. The apparently empty spaces usually contain a material that stains with mucicarmine. The nuclei are easily identified because of their intense staining against the background of scanty pale cytoplasm. The hyperchromatic cell aggregates are surrounded by a hyalinized stroma. The demarcation between cells and supporting stroma is sharp and distinct, a feature that differentiates this neoplasm from the mixed tumor (Fig. 262). Attempts to form a capsule are incomplete. Bone destruction occurs through direct invasion and spread along the haversian canal system. It is dissemination through the latter route that makes this neoplasm so treacherous.

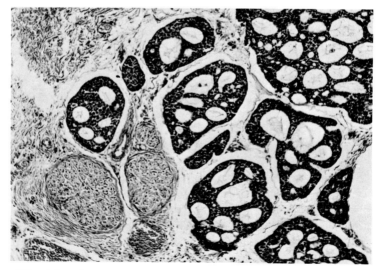

Figure 261.   Adenoid cystic carcinoma: closely packed, small regular cells with prominent ovoid clear spaces, the appearance resembling Swiss cheese; invasion of nerve trunks notable. (Hematoxylin and eosin; × 120.)

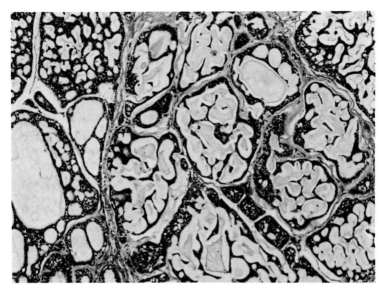

Figure 262. Adenoid cystic carcinoma: spaces may contain prominent hyalinized material, which is resistant to many solvents and accounted for Billroth's original observation. (Hematoxylin and eosin; × 130.)

TREATMENT

The approach to this neoplasm is very similar to the plan already outlined for malignant mixed tumor. A brief recapitulation of the salient features of treatment applicable to adenoid cystic carcinoma follows:

1. Regard all tumors of the lacrimal gland fossa as potentially malignant until proven otherwise either by gross examination or microscopic examination of tumor tissue.

2. Utilize the anterior-lateral surgical route to provide the exposure necessary for complete excision of the tumor and its base.

3. Proceed with surgical dissection as outlined for a planned en bloc resection (Chapter 25).

4. Utilize the "stages" or "interrupted" en bloc resection procedure if, on gross inspection of the mass, biopsy and frozen tissue study seems necessary.

5. If, on frozen tissue study, the poorly circumscribed or infiltrative tumor proves not to be an epithelial neoplasm, replace the bone flap with its attached pedicle and proceed with either excision or closure as indicated by the histologic type of the tumor.

6. Immediate or supplementary exenteration of orbit if surgical dissection has not encompassed tumor.

7. Microscopic examination of decalcified bone flap to evaluate extent of bone invasion by neoplasm.

8. Irradiation therapy if bone tissue is positive for neoplastic cells.

9. Do not operate on lacrimal fossa tumors by the transcranial route.

COURSE AND PROGNOSIS

Of all the orbital neoplasms discussed in this test, a primary adenoid cystic carcinoma is probably the most malignant. We fear it more than malignant melanoma. Not only is the mortality rate high but also the patient may suffer long periods of continuous pain before exhaustion brings about an end to the uneven tussle. Furthermore, in the interval between discovery of the tumor and death, the patient usually is subjected to several radical surgical procedures in an attempt to circumvent the tumor. Also, high doses of radiation may add a burden of malaise to an already miserable patient.

After identification and initial removal of the tumor, the course usually is one of slow relentless spread. In an interval of from one to four years, the patient returns with the first recurrence. Among the 53 patients followed by Font and Gamel, 79% had one or more recurrence. Multiple nodules of tumor now are palpable along the lateral wall or rim of the orbit and the patient will tell of orbital pain radiating to the forehead or temple. Some type of surgery (excision, exenteration, or bone removal) is performed and often combined with postoperative irradiation. After this, survival depends upon the rapidity with which the neoplasm attacks areas outside the orbit. The tumor usually spreads locally by invasion of nerves and blood vessels. Its first choice is the temporal area lateral to the orbit but intracranial intrusion is a close second choice. Less frequently it may travel to an adjacent sinus. If the patient still survives this challenge, the neoplasm eventually obtains its final goal of systemic dissemination.

In the Mayo Clinic study pertinent follow-up data was available on eleven of the twelve patients. Nine of these patients died as the result of spread of neoplasm, one patient with recurrent intracranial tumor died from other causes 8.5 years after initial diagnosis, and one patient is living with locally recurrent tumor and multiple netastases 4.3 years after diagnosis. Among the nine patients who died, the mode of treatment—exenteration alone or combined with bone removal and irradiation—did not seem to affect the outcome, for their fate was the same. Neither did the survival rate seem to be any greater among those who underwent immediate exenteration, as compared to those who had only a simple excision not combined with exenteration as the initial surgical management. The shortest period of survival after initial operation was 18 months; the longest survival was 8.7 years. The average survival period after the initial operation was 3.7 years. The medial survival time in the Font and Gamel series was 4.5 years. This is, indeed, a dismal outlook.

ADENOCARCINOMA

The adenocarcinoma is the basic malignant neoplasm of all glandular structures. Adenoid cystic carcinoma, just discussed, is but a variant of adenocarcinoma that has been accorded a separate designation chiefly on the basis of its prevalence and cytologic pattern. Otherwise the tumors have many clinical features in common. Although the basic adenocarcinoma is not as frequent a primary tumor as adenoid cystic carcinoma, the former comprises the bulk of secondary malignant carcinoma of the orbit. Included in the Mayo Clinic study were 52 cases of adenocarcinoma. Only four of these were primary in the orbit, arising in the area of the lacrimal fossa. The remainder were either secondary or metastatic adenocarcinomas and will be discussed in a later chapter.

The primary adenocarcinomas seldom are discussed as a separate entity. More often they are included with the adenoid cystic carcinomas or "other" carcinomas in the area of the lacrimal fossa. Such is the case with most large tumor surveys. This is understandable considering their infrequency, the clinical signs common to all malignancies in this area, and the difficult task of assembling meaningful data in such situations.

The four patients in the Mayo Clinic survey all were men whose ages ranged from 38 to 51 years. The clinical signs and symptoms were almost the same as those of adenoid cystic carcinoma; indeed, often it is not possible to distinguish them, except on the basis of the histopathologic study. A possible exception is a tendency for adenocarcinoma to grow along the lateral wall of the orbit somewhat lower in position than adenoid cystic carcinoma. If the hard mass is palpated slightly below the lateral palpebral raphe, it is more likely to be adenocarcinoma than adenoid cystic carcinoma. Squamous cell carcinomas primary in the orbit also tend to invade the lower quadrants of the orbit and present below the palpebral raphe. As with adenoid cystic carcinomas, pain was not prominent in the initial clinical course of our patients but was more evident in recurrent cases or those neoplasms of several years' duration. In two of our four patients, definite evidence of destruction of bone was seen on roentgenography.

Three of these four patients have died as a result of the malignancy. None of the three survived longer than 18 months after initial operation in spite of extensive surgery with or without irradiation. The one remaining patient was living 19 years from the time of first operation. Several features of this case are sufficiently interesting as to warrant review of this patient's case history in more detail.

A 51-year-old man was seen because of progressive prominence of the right eye of 1½ months' duration. A hard mass attached to the lateral rim of the orbit was removed through a transconjunctival approach. The histopathologic diagnosis was adenocarcinoma, grade 3. A delay of 1½ months ensued before exenteration was performed. At the time of this second surgical procedure the lateral wall of the orbit, as well as the orbital rim from its midpoint superiorly to its midpoint inferiorly, was removed. In addition, skin and subcutaneous tissue were widely excised lateral to the prior position of the mass. No attempt was made to accomplish a cosmetic type of exenteration. The eyelids were excised; the socket was not grafted. The defect slowly granulated and was finally covered by ingrowth from adjacent skin. Convalescence was considered satisfactory. Within 18 months a mass appeared anterior to the right ear. Excision of the preauricular lymph nodes combined with a total parotidectomy and radical neck dissection was performed. Two lymph nodes from the preauricular area and a nodule in the parotid gland showed adenocarcinoma, grade 3; the type was the same as that formerly removed from the nearby orbit. No further recurrence or systemic manifestation of the adenocarcinoma has been noted. The patient was living 19 years after the initial orbital surgery.

An interesting feature of this case was the absence of any recurrence of the neoplasm in the orbit after exenteration. None was found at the time of parotidectomy and none has been observed since. It is unusual for this neoplasm and related types in this locality not to recur first in the area of the initial mass. Another intriguing feature is the short time required for the neoplasm to seed itself in the preauricular lymph nodes. Did this seeding occur in the 1½ months prior to the initial surgery or did the tumor make its escape in the 1½-month interval between local excision and exenteration? Of interest too is the fact that the patient did not receive irradiation.

In all four adenocarcinomas the degree of anaplasia was considered to be either grade 2 or grade 3. As the degree of malignancy increases, the glandular components of the specimen become more sparse. The proliferating cells, instead, tend to become more compact and grow in closely arranged bundles or solid trabeculae. The connective tissue stroma between these cellular aggregates is scanty. There are much hyperchromatism, nuclear variation, and frequent mitosis, such as would be expected in any carcinoma of such malignancy.

OTHER CARCINOMAS

The least frequent of the intrinsic epithelial tumors of the lacrimal gland are those that probably originate in epithelium of the lacrimal duct system rather than in glandular components, as with the adenocarcinoma and adenoid cystic carcinoma. Two lacrimal system carcinomas should be mentioned: the squamous cell carcinoma and the mucoepidermoid carcinoma. These should be considered not as separate and distinct neoplasms but rather as variants of a squamous metaplasia. Sometimes both types of carcinoma may be seen even in the same tumor, if the entire specimen is examined microscopically. Individual case descriptions of these carcinomas in the literature are sparse and they do not occur in sufficient number in any one survey as to prompt discussion.

SQUAMOUS CELL CARCINOMA

One example of this type of primary lacrimal gland tumor was included in our study; this was the case of a 61-year-old man. The age of patients with this epithelial tumor usually is greater than 50 years. The clinical features are similar to those of the adenocarcinoma of the lacrimal fossa. It is hard, it may present in either upper or lower temporal quadrant, and the duration of symptoms often is 1 year or less. Some tumors may become relatively large during this period (Fig. 263). The tumor tends to grow in a direction away from the bony orbital rim, so that erosion or destruction of bone may not be visible on roentgenography. In contrast, the squamous cell carcinoma that secondarily invades the orbit from some adjacent site almost uniformly produces bony defects.

Histologically, the cellular features are similar to those of the prickle cells of the epidermis. The tumor is infiltrative and shows a variable capacity for keratinization and may show various stages of differentiation (Fig. 264). Grossly, along those surfaces that abut against ocular and adnexal structures, such as the orbital septum and eyeball, the tumor is somewhat circumscribed, but it tends to infiltrate other adnexal tissues.

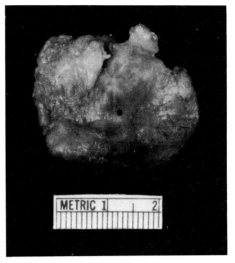

Figure 263. Squamous cell carcinoma: large (3.5 by 2.5 by 1.5 cm) orbital tumor arising from lacrimal gland and occupying major portion of orbital floor: symptoms were only of 6 months' duration.

Squamous cell carcinomas are treacherous no matter what their histologic grading may be. Once the carcinoma has been removed and identified microscopically, the patient should be advised to undergo exenteration. Recurrences may appear locally along the remaining orbital bones, or an enlarged palpable preauricular node may be the first clue to dissemination. In either situation, further radical surgery followed by irradiation may yet offer the patient a chance of survival. For those infrequent situations wherein the tumors metastasize directly to the lung, nothing can be done.

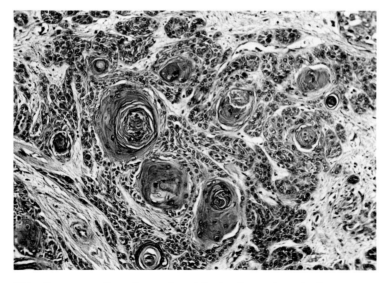

Figure 264. Squamous cell carcinoma: keratinization is prominent in this invasive neoplasm. (Hematoxylin and eosin; × 110.)

MUCOEPIDERMOID CARCINOMA

At one time this neoplasm was classifed with the mixed tumors, which makes information concerning its behavior in this area less accessible than with other carcinomas. Of the several names proposed for the tumor the term *muco-epidermoid*, suggested by Stewart and associates (1945), has been the most widely accepted. This name refers to mixtures of mucus-secreting cells and epidermoid cells that are the main histologic features of the tumor (Fig. 265). Other nonmucus-secreting cells — the so-called intermediate cells as well as the so-called clear cells — also are present. The multimorphic makeup of these tumors and the relative content of one cellular component to another accounts for variations in their histopathologic grading. The more differentiated types have cystic spaces filled with mucus and lined by mixed epidermoid and mucus-producing epithelium. The latter has a special affinity for mucicarmine dye. The former cells are similar to prickle cells and have small regular nuclei. Mitosis is minimal or absent. The cytoplasm of some epidermoid cells does not accept a stain, which accounts for the designation *clear cell*. Neoplasms of intemediate histologic activity show greater cellularity, increased nuclear hyper-chromatism and anaplasia are evident, mucus is less evident, and the epidermoid cellular features are more prominent.

The clinical features of these neoplasms depend a great deal on their histologic makeup. The features of the more differentiated types may be more benign but, in the area of the lacrimal gland, it may be more descriptive to call them less malignant. Thus, in the one case in our Mayo Clinic series, this neoplasm went through an indolent period of 7 years' growth before the patient (a 59-year-old woman) decided upon consultation. In this period proptosis of 7 mm developed in the affected eye. The tumor was thought to have been com-

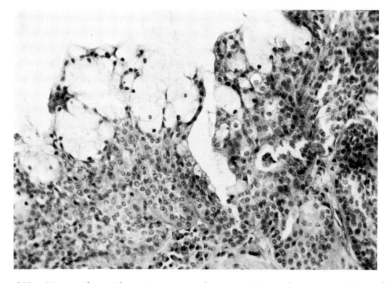

Figure 265. Mucoepidermoid carcinoma: neoplasm is mixture of mucus-secreting goblet cells and epidermoid or squamous cells. (Hematoxylin and eosin; × 200.)

pletely removed at the time of initial orbitotomy through the transcranial approach. Within 6 months the tumor recurred. In this short time the carcinoma had undergone a change in histologic activity from grade 1 to grade 3 malignancy — a common event when neoplasms recur in this area. This tumor was fatal within a year of the second orbitotomy because of intracranial spread. The features of the less differentiated types resemble those of squamous cell carcinomas, that is, a shorter interval of symptoms, more rapid growth, frequent local recurrences, and potential metastasis.

Concerning the management of these neoplasms, rarely, a more differentiated type is so well circumscribed as to permit its complete removal with some chance that it will not recur. However, it probably is prudent not to be misled into the belief that such is the preferred treatment of the majority of these carcinomas regardless of their histopathologic grading or differentiation. Furthermore, in many well-differentiated types, the amount and distribution of mucus-containing spaces may favor easy rupture of their boundary tissues no matter how gently the mass is handled. Escape of this mucus material, even in tumors that seem well resected, is one means by which malignant cells gain access to adjacent tissues. The safest treatment is to advise exenteration after diagnosis has been made at the initial orbitotomy. Irradiation also may be used as palliation for recurrences.

Bibliography

Mixed Tumor

Ashton N: Epithelial tumors of lacrimal gland. Mod Probl Ophthal *14*:306–323, 1975

Becker: Cited by Warthin AS

Fabricius Hildanus [W]: Cited by Warthin AS

Font RL, Gamel JW: Epithelial tumors of the lacrimal gland. An analysis of 265 cases. *In* Jakobiec FA: *Ocular and Adnexal Tumors.* Birmingham, Ala, Aesculapius Publishing Co, 1978, Chapter 53

Foote FW Jr, Frazell EL: Tumors of the major salivary glands. *In Atlas of Tumor Pathology*, Section 4, Fascicle 11. Washington DC, Armed Forces Institute of Pathology, 1954

Forrest AW: Epithelial lacrimal gland tumors: pathology as a guide to prognosis. Trans Am Acad Ophthalmol Otolaryngol *58*:848–865, 1954

Forrest AW: Pathologic criteria for effective management of epithelial lacrimal gland tumors. Am J Ophthalmol *71*:178–192, 1971

Jones IS, Pfeiffer RL: Lacrimal gland tumors: roentgenographic diagnosis. Trans Am Acad Ophthalmol Otolaryngol *58*:841–847, 1954

McPherson SD Jr: Mixed tumor of the lacrimal gland: in a seven-year-old boy. Am J Ophthalmol *61*:561–563, 1966

Minssen H: Cited by Davies WS: Pleomorphic adenoma and adenocarcinoma of the lacrimal gland, with report of thirteen cases. Trans Am Ophthalmol Soc *52*:467–496, 1954

Riley FC, Henderson JW: Report of a case of malignant transformation in benign mixed tumor of the lacrimal gland. Am J Ophthalmol *70*:767–770, 1970

Thackray AC, Sobin LH: Histologic typing of salivary gland tumors. *In International Histologic Classification of Tumors.* No 70 World Health Organization, Geneva, Switzerland, 1972

Waller RR, Riley FC, Henderson JW: Malignant mixed tumors of the lacrimal gland. Arch Ophthalmol *90*:297–299, 1973

Warthin AS: A case of endothelioma of the lachrymal gland (myxo-chondro-endothelioma cylindromatodes), with an analysis of previously reported cases of lachrymal gland tumors. Arch Ophthalmol *30*:601–620, 1901

Zimmerman LE, Sanders TE, Ackerman LV: Epithelial tumors of the lacrimal gland: prognostic and therapeutic significance of histologic types. Int Ophthalmol Clin *2*:337–367, 1962

Oncocytoma

Beskid M, Zarzycka M: A case of onkocytoma of the lacrimal gland. Klin Oczna 29:311–315, 1959
Biggs SL, Font RL: Oncocytic lesions of the caruncle and other ocular adnexa. Arch Ophthalmol
 95:474–478, *1977*
Böck J, Schlagenhauff K: Ueber das Vorkommen von Onkozyten in der menschlìchen. Tränendrüse.
 Z Augenheilkd 94:244–252, 1938
Deutsch AR, Duckworth JK: Onkocytoma (oxyphilic adenoma) of the caruncle. Am J Ophthalmol
 64:458–461, 1967
Dorello U: Carcinoma oncocitario della ghiandola lacrimale. Riv ONO 36:452–461, 1961
Hamperl H: Beiträge zur normalen und pathologischen Histologie menschlicher Speicheldrusen. Z
 Mikrosk Anat Forsch 27:1–55, 1931
Hamperl H: Onkocyten und Onkocytome. Virchows Arch [Pathol Anat] 335:452–483, 1962
Radnót M: Die pathologische Histologie der Tränendrüse. Bibl Ophthalmol Fascicle 28:25–30, 1939

Adenoid Cystic Carcinoma

Billroth T: Untersuchungen über die Entwicklung der Blutgefasse. Berlin, G. Reimer, 1856, pp
 55–69
Font RL, Gamel JW: Epithelial tumors of the lacrimal gland: an analysis of 265 cases. *In* Jakobiec
 FA: *Ocular and Adnexal Tumors.* Birmingham, Ala, Aesculapius Publishing Co, 1978, Chapter 53
Foote FW Jr, Frazell EL: Tumors of the major salivary glands. *In Atlas of Tumor Pathology*, Section
 4, Fascicle 11. Washington DC, Armed Forces Institute of Pathology, 1954
Ley JA, Wolter JR: Adenoid cystic carcinoma: as seen in the orbit of a twelve-year-old Vietnamese
 girl. J Pediatr Ophthalmol 6:162–165, 1969
Wolter JR, Henderson JW: Adenoid cystic carcinoma in the orbit of a child. J Pediatr Ophthalmol
 6:47–49, 1969

Other Carcinomas

Stewart FW, Foote FW, Becker WF: Muco-epidermoid tumors of salivary glands. Ann Surg.
 122:820–844, 1945
Thorvaldsson SE, Beahrs OH, Woolner LB, et al: Mucoepidermoid tumors of the major salivary
 glands. Am J Surg 120:432–438, 1970

16

Secondary Epithelial Neoplasms

The behavior of epithelial tumors primary in the orbit on their favorite stage — the lacrimal gland — has been discussed in the preceding chapter. In this chapter it is appropriate to follow their careers as *secondary* tumors in the orbit. By this we refer to orbital invasion from contiguous anatomic areas, such as the nasal cavity, paranasal sinuses, lacrimal sac, caruncle, parotid gland, surface of the eye, and skin of forehead, eyelid, and temple. Most of the actors previously encountered will appear again; namely, squamous cell carcinoma, mucoepidermoid carcinoma, adenoid cystic carcinoma, adenocarcinoma, and malignant mixed tumor. Two new villians also will appear later in this scene: basal cell carcinoma and meibomian gland carcinoma. Although the former neoplasms will wear the same histologic costumes as described in the preceding chapter, here their portrayal as secondary tumors will be observed and compared to their roles in the previous act. Other soft tissue tumors secondary in the orbit will not be included in the cast, because they either already have been discussed in prior chapters (for example, melanomas, retinoblastomas, and various sarcomas) or wait in the wings for their debut in later chapters, (meningioma).

Some of these secondary neoplasms seldom are discussed as a group in the ophthalmic literature with specific reference to their orbital involvement. Instead, their symptomatology and course in their primary sites are emphasized; and such case discussions usually appear in rhinolaryngologic and oncologic publications dealing with the head and neck. The passage of the neoplasm into the orbit then is mentioned as only one feature of the malignant course or as only another phase in radical surgical management. The ophthalmologist's role is that of an infrequent advisor concerning protection or salvage of the eye in the course of radical surgery or intensive irradiation. As a result, the large number, variety, and seriousness of these neoplasms are not appreciated by the average clinical ophthalmologist. Stanković and associates (1966) have reviewed these secondary orbital tumors with some of these factors in mind.

INCIDENCE

Several factors, other than the infrequent number of surveys, impede assembly of definite incidence data. Chief of these is the variety of types of tumors included in the different surveys. If mucoceles are included among surveys of secondary tumors, the total number relative to primary orbital tumors would be much higher than if neoplasms only are counted. If only neoplasms are surveyed, the total number of secondary neoplasms also might vary according to whether direct extensions of neoplasms from the eye (melanoma and retinoblastoma) are considered secondary tumors. Many surveys exclude these neoplasms of intraocular origin, as well as meningiomas extending into the orbit from an intracranial source. Similarly, some tumor surveys include bony tumors that ostensibly arise in the paranasal sinuses. The difficulty of deciding whether a bony tumor arises on the orbital or paranasal side of an orbital wall already has been mentioned. Most surveys of secondary tumors concentrate on neoplasms arising from areas such as the paranasal sinuses, nasal cavity, and nasopharynx. Unfortunately, the primary source of the tumor and the differing histologic types are not always stated. We should emphasize again that the survey in this chapter chiefly is confined to epithelial neoplasms. The large number of cases, combined with the interesting variety of tumor types in this series, should be representative and serve as a base for pertinent data.

The types and number of secondary epithelial neoplasms in the Mayo series are listed in Table 22). These 107 neoplasms constitute 14% of the total of the orbital tumors. This number is significantly greater than that of any other major survey. Our 107 cases of carcinoma also make up a significant portion of all the secondary orbital tumors listed in table 2 (see Chapter 3). The combined sum of 343 secondary orbital tumors (45% of the total series of 764 cases) may be a surprising and impressive total to those clinicians accustomed to thinking of the orbit in terms of primary and "rare" metastatic tumors.

Table 23 gives details of the probable site of origin of these epithelial neoplasms and the age groups and sex distribution. We realize how difficult it is to determine accurately the source of some of these tumors. Particularly is this true of patients who already have had several surgical procedures on the face and sinuses when first seen; moreover, in some patients, more than one sinus is involved when first observed.

Approximately 77% of the neoplasms in Table 23 arise from the nasal cavity, nasopharynx, maxillary sinus, or the skin in the area of the orbit. Also there is a prevalence of these tumors among patients older than 30 years, with a peak incidence in the sixth or seventh decade. This age distribution has been observed by others. All age data in our series were related to the time of onset of symptoms rather than age of the patient when first observed at the Mayo Clinic.

TABLE 22.   SECONDARY EPITHELIAL NEOPLASMS OF
THE ORBIT, MAYO CLINIC SERIES (1948–1974)*

Histologic Type	Number
Squamous cell carcinoma	58
Basal cell carcinoma	18
Adenoid cystic carcinoma	13
Adenocarcinoma	9
Malignant mixed tumor	5
Meibomian gland carcinoma	3
Mucoepidermoid carcinoma	1
Total	107

*Total number of orbital tumors in series, 764.

TABLE 23. SECONDARY ORBITAL EPITHELIAL NEOPLASMS, MAYO CLINIC SERIES
(1948–1974): PRIMARY SOURCE AND DETAILS OF PATIENTS

Primary Source (No. of Cases)	Male: Female Ratio	Age Distribution, Yr						
		<20	20–29	30–39	40–49	50–59	60–69	>69
Maxillary antrum (37)	21:16	0	1	4	5	11	11	5
Skin of face, nose, forehead, temple, eyelids (29)	23:6	0	2	0	7	5	6	9
Nasopharynx, nasal cavity (16)	13:3	0	1	3	2	7	3	0
Oral cavity (8)	7:1	2	0	2	0	3	0	1
Lacrimal sac (5)	4:1	0	1	1	0	2	1	0
Parotid gland (2)	1:1	0	0	1	0	0	0	1
Ethmoid or frontal sinus (7)	5:2	0	1	1	0	4	0	1
Other areas* (3)	2:1	1	0	0	0	1	1	0
Total (107)	76:31	3	6	12	14	33	22	17

*Single cases of neoplasms arising from surface of eye, conjunctival cul-de-sac and caruncle.

SQUAMOUS CELL CARCINOMA

INCIDENCE

Squamous cell carcinoma is, by far, the most frequent of the secondary epithelial neoplasms discussed in this chapter (Table 22). In our series these carcinomas constituted 54% of our total secondary epithelial tumors and 7.5% of all orbital tumors. They arise most commonly in the maxillary antrum, 28 (48%) of 58 cases. Next in frequency of orbital invasion, 10 cases (17%), were the carcinomas arising in the skin of the eyelid, cheek, and temple. Orbital invasion by squamous cell carcinoma was least frequent from the conjunctiva, caruncle, and surface of the eye; a feature compatible with the more differentiated character of the tumor in these areas. They occur more frequently in males in a ratio of about 2:1 (38:20 male to female ratio). Analysis of our data did not reveal any significant difference in the age of onset among the carcinomas arising from the maxillary antrum, periorbital integumentary areas, or nasal cavity.

CLINICAL FEATURES

A most consistent indication of orbital invasion by this tumor and other epithelial neoplasms of this group is *upward and, often, upward-outward displacement of one eye*. Particularly is this true among those cases that arise in the maxillary antrum, nasal cavity, lacrimal sac and nasopharynx (Fig. 266). In the latter two situations outward displacement of the eye is greater than with neoplasms arising in the antrum. No other orbital neoplasms so consistently appear in the lower two quadrants of the orbit than this group of secondary carcinomas, except for two types: those squamous cell types arising in the ethmoid and sphenoid sinuses and those carcinomas arising in skin structures adjacent to the orbit. The former enter the orbit in a more posteromedial location and the clinical picture resembles that of any other primary or secondary tumor in a similar locality (for example, forward proptosis, loss of vision, papilledema, ophthalmoplegia, pressure on posteromedial aspects of the eyeball); and the latter are associated with a history of previous operations for "skin cancer" and

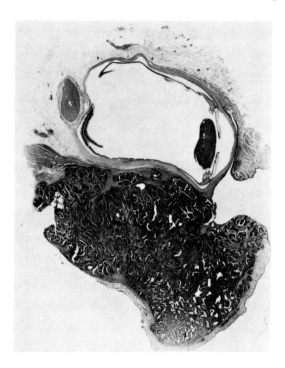

Figure 266. Squamous cell carcinoma: inferior orbit is massively invaded from primary neoplasm in maxillary sinus. (Hematoxylin and eosin; × 2½.)

a more obvious spread of tumor into the orbital cavity (Fig. 267) from the prior operative site.

In the usual case of squamous cell carcinoma arising from the maxillary antrum and nasal cavity the upward displacement of the eye is equal to, or greater than, forward proptosis. This altered position of the eye may be an initial manifestation of the malignant disease for which the patient seeks treatment though, more often, it is but one clue among several that points suspicion toward a primary disease in an adjoining cavity.

Indurated swelling or an obvious *mass in the upper cheek* usually accompanies displacement of the eye. Entry of the neoplasm into the orbital cavity is followed by *increased redness and swelling of adnexal tissues.* The conjunctiva

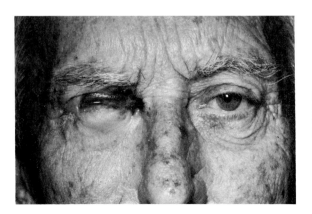

Figure 267. Squamous cell carcinoma: orbital spread from neoplasm of eyelid; this followed several previous excisions and skin grafts.

of the inferior fornix, in particular, may become so chemotic that it begins to prolapse over the margin of the lower eyelid. These clinical signs add an inflammatory perspective to the clinical . picture, but tenderness — diagnostic of cellulitis or orbital inflammation alone — is lacking. *Numbness* along the distribution of the infraorbital nerve may be associated with neoplasms arising in the maxillary antrum. *Pain* along distribution of this nerve branch or, along the upper alveolar ridge also is a common feature. This type of pain is not so common with those neoplasms arising from nasal structures; with these neoplasms, *obstructive respiratory signs* are more obvious and accompanied by *epistaxis.* The patient may even relate that prior operations have been performed for recurrent "polyps." Patients in whom the tumor has arisen from the nasopharynx suffer *dysphagia* and *ulceration of the throat. Epiphora* is an added feature of this clinical pattern among those in whom the tumor has arisen from or is invading the area of the lacrimal sac on its advance toward the orbit. *Ophthalmoplegia* due to fixation of the eye in the orbit by neoplastic invasion of extraocular muscles appears late in the disease or it may follow prior surgery on the adjacent sinuses.

When orbital invasion is a presenting sign in development of the disease, the duration of symptoms may be only a few months for carcinomas arising in the roof or anterior wall of the maxillary antrum, or longer (over 1 year) for those neoplasms originating in the posterior recesses of the sinus cavity. In 18 (64%) of our 28 cases of squamous cell carcinoma arising in the maxillary antrum, histologic evidence of orbital involvement was present at the time of initial surgical diagnosis. In the posterior maxillary antrum the tumor may remain latent for some time and actually be quite extensive by the time orbital symptoms appear. The interval between onset of the carcinoma and its orbital invasion was even longer (several years) in most cases in which the neoplasm commenced in the skin — for example, in the skin of the eyelids and the face. In these cases, the history always included details of several operations, irradiation, and recurrences of tumor. In one case in this subgroup, orbital invasion did not occur until 17 years after treatment of the initial eyelid lesion. This case was an example of a neoplasm that commenced as a basal cell carcinoma but which, after multiple surgical procedures, underwent metaplasia into a squamous cell type.

ROENTGENOGRAPHIC CHANGES

Roentgenography is diagnostic for the group of carcinomas arising in the paranasal sinuses, particularly the maxillary antrum. Here the mucous membrane surface is quite thin and closely applied to bone without intervening strata of tissue. The neoplasm therefore has easy access to bone in the course of its invasive growth. Some thinning of bone occurs early in its growth but at this stage the neoplasm still may be latent. As the neoplasm fills the sinus cavity and exerts greater pressure on the bony walls, the latter structures soon become eroded and destroyed. When secondary orbital invasion occurs, the bony roof and at least one other wall of the antrum usually have been destroyed, and the tumor is large enough to fill the sinus cavity, producing a cloudy, murky, roentgenographic shadow. A cloudy antrum associated with bony destruction was a feature of all cases of neoplasms from this source in our series. Bony destruction of the medial wall of the orbit was present in most of the other cases arising from the nasopharynx or nasal cavity but was not always easily seen on routine views.

PATHOLOGY

In a small zone around the anterior nares, squamous epithelium is normally arranged in a pavement-like pattern similar to that of skin. Elsewhere in the upper respiratory passages squamous epithelium has undergone functional modification into a pseudostratified, sometimes ciliated, epithelium. The histologic pattern of this epithelium is, however, everywhere alike, but it varies according to the functional purposes of the specific anatomic sites. In the mucous membranes of the sinuses and anterior nasal cavity the epithelium is ciliated and less stratified than in skin but it still possesses some characteristics of keratinization of skin. In more posterior recesses of the nasal cavity the epithelium becomes more columnar with little or no keratinization. This histologic pattern frequently is referred to as a transitional type of epithelium. In the nasopharynx the epithelium becomes but a loose and thin layer of squamous cells covering a predominantly lymphocytic-adenoid type of stroma. Such an arrangement usually is termed a lympho-epithelial type of respiratory epithelium. Lower down the respiratory passages, squamous cell surfaces show further changes that make possible their identification with a specific anatomic area when tissue specimens are examined microscopically. The carcinomas, in their growth, reflect these nuances in cellular morphology, but basically, all represent malignant squamous metaplasia.

Squamous cell carcinomas of the maxillary sinus and nasal passages vary significantly in degree of cellular differentiation. In general, the poorly differentiated and anaplastic types are more common than highly keratinizing types (Fig. 268). As the neoplasm becomes more anaplastic, the prickle type cell may take on a spindle shape in some of the higher grade malignancies. The latter cellular patterns resemble the histologic picture of some sarcomas. The cellular boundaries of these proliferating cells also become less distinct, and mitosis and hyperchromatism are observed, as with all malignancies. Foci of degeneration may appear in the highly undifferentiated tumors, giving them a pseudoglandular appearance.

It might be expected that the more malignant types of squamous cell carcinomas would be the ones that would finally reach the orbit. Among the cases in the Mayo Clinic series this was generally true of those neoplasms arising in the maxillary antrum but it was not always so with those tumors from the nasal cavity. Of the 28 carcinomas originating in the maxillary antrum, the malignancy was, in 28, either grade 3 or 4. Of the squamous cell carcinomas arising in the nasal cavity there was a nearly equal distribution among grade 2, grade 3, and grade 4 anaplastic types.

The histopathologic features of the secondary neoplasms arising in the skin of the face, eyelids, temple, and eyebrow were similar to those of squamous cell carcinomas elsewhere in the integument (Fig. 269). They are more differentiated tumors and their course was more prolonged than other carcinomas

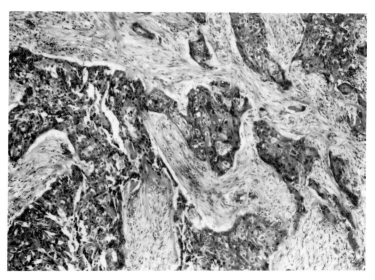

Figure 268. Squamous cell carcinoma: this highly anaplastic neoplasm composed of squamous cells shows little evidence of keratin production. (Hematoxylin and eosin; × 65.)

already noted. Of the ten patients in this category, only one case had malignancy of grade 4 degree.

Two cases among our total of 58 squamous cell carcinomas were examples of low-grade papillary type. These two cases were at the extremes of the age range in our series. One patient was a 75-year-old woman whose eye was enucleated because of the spread of tumor from the maxillary antrum. The other patient was a 7-year-old girl in whom a papillary carcinoma commenced in the region of the caruncle. This is a most unusual location for this type of

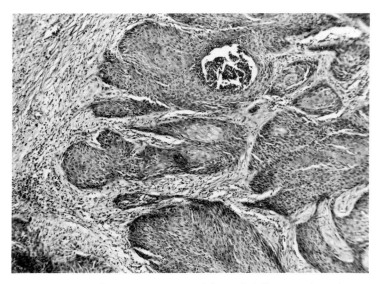

Figure 269. Squamous cell carcinoma: tissues of this well-differentiated neoplasm, primary on eyelid, resemble normal epidermis. (Hematoxylin and eosin; × 85.)

neoplasm. During a period of 14 years the neoplasm in this latter case gradually spread along the conjunctival surfaces at the inner canthus, advanced along the lacrimal canaliculus via the inferior punctum, and then invaded the orbit, in spite of attempted excisions, several treatments with surgical diathermy, and repeated applications of radium. Even after enucleation of the eye and subtotal orbital exenteration, the tumor recurred along the nasal wall of the orbit. Finally it disappeared after another surgical diathermy treatment; and thereafter 7 years passed without recurrence before the patient was lost to follow-up observation at the age of 28.

COURSE AND TREATMENT

The above case exemplifies the behavior of many secondary squamous cell carcinomas in this area; namely, their perversive spread, their refractory response to irradiation, and their final submission only to radical methods of treatment. The outcome in the majority of patients is not as fortunate as this young girl patient. In general, prognosis is related to the degree of malignancy; the more undifferentiated is the tumor, the worse the prognosis. These carcinomas possess potentialities for local invasive growth as well as distant metastatic spread. In many tumors of grade 4 showing a malignant degree of undifferentiation, the prognosis is almost hopeless. Prognosis also is influenced to a lesser extent by other factors. With secondary carcinomas arising from the maxillary antrum, for example, the eventual outcome may be influenced by their size and extent before discovery. Some of these carcinomas are not discovered until they have invaded the orbit and by this time they will be almost beyond the boundaries of a radical dissection. For those carcinomas that invade the orbit from adjacent integumentary structures, prognosis may be altered by completeness of the initial surgical treatment; once the tumor has recurred owing to incomplete excision the opportunity to eradicate the tumor by subsequent treatment is proportionately limited.

Antral Carcinoma

Follow-up data were available on all 28 patients in our series in whom the carcinoma commenced in the maxillary antrum. Eighteen (64%) of these patients are dead of their tumor. The survival period of this group averaged 2.3 years after initial diagnosis, with a range of 4 months to 5 years. One additional patient probably should be placed in this group. The latter is alive 3.5 years from initial diagnosis but has local recurrence in the nasopharynx plus systemic metastasis. The neoplasm is fatal either because of local extension into the brain or systemic metastasis. The lung is one of the favored spots for the latter. Most of these patients were treated for one or more recurrences before the tumor was fatal and the interval between initial treatment and recurrence was seldom longer than two years. A further examination of our data in reference to recurrences suggests that if a patient with this secondary type neoplasm goes 4 years without a recurrence, it is likely the patient will survive the tumor.

All combinations of local surgical excision, subtotal and total maxillectomy, eradication by surgical diathermy, insertion of radium needles, and applications of supravoltage irradiation with or without either enucleation or exenteration were attempted in these fatal cases as the initial or subsequent treatment. If surgical manipulation of the neoplasm in the maxillary antrum was combined with only an enucleation or separated from subsequent orbital exenteration by an interval of time, the chances of cure diminished. Irradiation, either by insertion of radium or from supravoltage machines, seemed only palliative or supplementary in those cases wherein the neoplasm extended beyond the zone of dissection or surgical diathermy.

However, the situation is not hopeless. Two of the total group were living without recurrence or known metastasis 12 and 18 years after the initial surgical procedure. An additional five patients were living without recurrence or metastasis from 4.5 to 19 years after diagnosis when death occurred from other causes. If the total 7 patients can be considered nonfatal cases the cure rate approximates 25%. One additional patient who is living without recurrence 3 years and 10 months from initial diagnosis and one patient who died of pulmonary embolism three days after surgery complete the survey of 28 cases.

In the nonfatal cases, treatment was either en bloc maxillectomy combined with exenteration of orbit or heavy electrocoagulation combined with insertion of radon seeds. The latter method of treatment was an accepted and very popular mode of management 20 to 30 years ago but always was accompanied by a massive slough of devitalized bone.

Nasal and Nasopharyngeal Carcinoma

Follow-up information also was available for our eight patients with carcinoma arising in the nasal cavity and nasopharnyx. In this group the outcome was more dismal than for patients with carcinoma of the maxillary sinus. In 5 patients the neoplasm was fatal within 3 years of initial diagnosis and 2 other patients died within 3 years of initial treatment from uncertain cause. Only one patient of this group is living without recurrence or metastasis 12 years after diagnosis. As in the prior group all modalities and combinations of treatment were employed, except that by the time the neoplasm had reached the orbit, many of the cases seemed to be so hopeless that fewer enucleations and exenterations were elected than in the maxillary sinus group. Furthermore, a common theme among these fatal cases was the interval between the initial symptoms and definitive treatment. These carcinomas did not remain hidden in their early growth as did some of the similar neoplasms in the maxillary antrum. Instead, only an inconclusive biopsy was performed or only a partial excision attempted on what was obviously a recurrent intranasal mass.

Eyelid, Forehead, and Temporal Carcinoma

The course of squamous carcinomas invading the orbit from adjacent areas of the skin is more prolonged than that of similar neoplasms from any other source. In some cases the battle between the tumor and opposing surgeons and hosts lasted over a decade. For this reason our follow-up data is not as complete as for other subgroups of this secondary tumor. Some patients became discouraged, went elsewhere, and were lost to follow-up observation during these prolonged and alternating intervals of treatment and recurrences. Other patients died from other causes while still under observation for recurrent tumor or other related problems. Still, some data common to all eight cases are worth discussing.

All our patients had had several operations or irradiation treatments prior to neoplastic involvement of the orbit. At one extreme was the patient who had had 12 operations on one eyelid in 4 years. In all patients the course of the tumor was virtually relentless after the initial recurrence. Because of the cosmetic importance of this area to the patient, the physician, reinforced by the wishes of the patient, tends to perform as little destructive surgery as possible or to forestall surgical mutilation entirely by repeated irradiation. But once the neoplasm has recurred such attitudes seem to be of little help. Enucleation with or without exenteration usually is performed late in the disease and often fails to halt spread of the neoplasm.

From the information based on these patients we suspect more radical surgical measures should be advised, once the pattern of recurrence is established. Such a bold approach may be the patient's only hope when judged in terms of the tumor's frequent fatal course. If exenteration is done it should be combined with removal of the adjacent and underlying bone unless removal of bone would uncover the intracranial space. Even here, some thought should be given to excision of bone if it is possible to cover the dura by a skin graft.

ADENOID CYSTIC CARCINOMA

Adenoid cystic carcinoma, adenocarcinoma, and malignant mixed tumor already have been discussed in Chapter 15 in reference to their occurrence as primary tumors in the orbit. A discussion of their pathologic features need not be repeated because each neoplasm has basically the same features whether it appears primarily or secondarily in the orbit. Here, we are more interested in any similarities to, or differences in behavior from, other secondary epithelial neoplasms or each other.

Secondary adenoid cystic carcinomas are never mentioned in orbital tumor surveys, and it will be quite a surprise to most ophthalmologists to learn that these orbital invaders are equally as frequent as the carcinomas primary in the lacrimal gland. The site of origin of our group of thirteen (Table 22) was maxillary antrum, ethmoid sinus, and nasal passages (three cases each), oral cavity (two patients), and parotid gland and area of lacrimal sac (each one case). In their anatomic distribution, the tumors resemble the squamous cell carcinoma. The ages of the patients ranged from 29 to 72 years; but 6 of the 10 patients were younger than 37 years of age at the time of onset of the disorder. This distribution includes a greater proportion of young adults than the squamous cell carcinoma, considering the size of the total sample and comparable sites of origin. There were seven women and six men.

CLINICAL COURSE

The symptomatology of the secondary type is as diverse as the symptomatology of the primary type is specific. In those cases where the neoplasm commenced in the oral cavity, lacrimal sac, or parotid gland, some *lump, swelling,* or *chronic ulceration* called attention to the disease and the tumor was diagnosed at this stage. Orbital involvement occurred in these situations at some later time, the interval varying according to the histologic aggressiveness of the tumor. Those adenoid cystic carcinomas originating somewhere along the nasal passages showed a similar course except the initial symptoms were *epistaxis* or *unilateral obstruction of nasal passage.*

The symptomatology of those neoplasms arising in one of the paranasal sinuses (usually the ethmoid or maxillary antrum) was somewhat different. Here, orbital or ocular symptoms were the initial manifestations of the latent malignancy. If the neoplasm was located in the posterior recesses of either the ethmoid or maxillary sunus, *visual loss of one eye, ophthalmoplegia,* and *pain over the distribution of the infraorbital nerve* were the clues to a secondary invasion of the orbit. Tumors arising more forward in these sinus cavities remained occult until an *upward or lateral displacement* of the eye occurred or a mass was palpated along the medial or inferior wall of the orbit.

However, several features differed from those of the preceding squamous cell carcinomas. The adenoid cystic carcinomas did not seem to upset the environmental balance of the orbital and adnexal tissues as did the squamous cell carcinomas (Fig. 270). Orbital tissues seemed much more tolerant to the invasive nature of adenoid cystic carcinomas and did not react significantly by tissue induration or defensive inflammatory signs. Another contrasting point was the slower course of the adenoid cystic carcinomas in many cases. Follow-up data was available in twelve of our thirteen patients. Eleven of these patients died of tumor, but the interval of survival ranged from 7 to 21 years after initial diagnosis in 4 cases. This is considerably longer than the survival period of the fatal cases of squamous cell carcinoma. None of the adenoid cystic

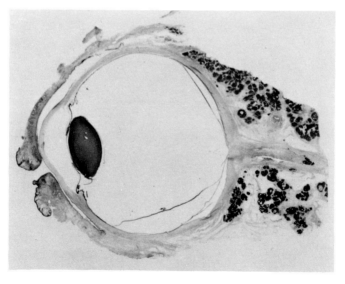

Figure 270. Adenoid cystic carcinoma: primary neoplasm was in adjacent ethmoid sinus; orbital tissues show little reactive inflammation. (Hematoxylin and eosin; × 2½.)

carcinomas in the fatal cases were greater than grade 2 malignancy on histologic grading. This probably explains the slower clinical course of the secondary adenoid cystic carcinomas versus the squamous cell carcinomas. The one nonfatal case was living 32 years after the initial diagnosis and 4.5 years from the last recurrence of tumor, but had had 9 surgically treated recurrences in and around the orbit for a neoplasm originating in the lacrimal sac. The study of our small series leaves the impression that low-grade secondary orbital adenoid cystic carcinomas are just as lethal, or perhaps more lethal, as some higher grade squamous cell carcinomas but that many more years ensue before death terminates their course.

TREATMENT

Surgery, irradiation (radium, radon, and supravoltage techniques), and chemotherapy were used alone and in various combinations in our patients. Extensive surgical dissection was the treatment of first choice. Irradiation of various types often was used in the areas of invasive growth that could not be reached by the surgeon without risk of hemorrhage or interference with vital intracranial function. Chemotherapy was employed when neither of the two other modalities could be given. The slow but stubborn growth of these neoplasms is a challenge to the ingenuity of the surgeon in his attempts to keep ahead of the lesion and yet maintain some protection to the anatomic areas and functional zones that have been seriously compromised by prior surgery or irradiation. Whatever hurdles, barriers, or chasms the tumor must cross, it seems able to survive.

ADENOCARCINOMA

Primary and secondary adenocarcinomas seldom are observed in the orbit. However, they comprise the majority of metastatic orbital tumors that will be discussed in the next chapter. Our series included 9 adenocarcinomas among our total group of 107 secondary epithelial tumors (Table 22). These orbital invaders usually arise in either the maxillary antrum, the ethmoid sinus, or the nasal passages. Often the tumor has invaded two of these anatomic sites by the time of diagnosis. In the Mayo Clinic series two population groups were affected. Three neoplasms occurred in the 37 to 41 year age range; the remaining 6 neoplasms were concentrated in the 54 to 63 age range. The male:female ratio was 7:2. All of the tumors were locally invasive and capable of metastasis.

In their course they combined some clinical features of both secondary adenoid cystic carcinoma and squamous cell carcinoma. In reference to the former they were almost 100% fatal and 1 patient pursued a very indolent course (11 years) before death. In the remaining fatal cases no patient survived longer than 2 years after initial diagnosis, a feature similar to the short survival of patients with secondary squamous cell carcinoma. All 9 neoplasms were histologically grade 2 to grade 4 malignant, but this was of no prognostic significance because, clinically, the course was equally bad in all patients.

MALIGNANT MIXED TUMOR

The secondary malignant mixed tumors invade the orbit from some major or minor sialogenous gland of the head, oral cavity, nose, or paranasal sinus. There were five such patients in our survey, all males. The clinical course varied markedly, depending upon the histological aggressiveness of the tumor at the time of initial diagnosis.

In 4 patients, ages 19, 33, 55, and 56 at the time of diagnosis, the origin of the tumor was a glandular structure in the hard palate, nasal cavity, or parotid gland. The presenting complaint was either recurrent epistaxis, a chronic ulceration of the mouth, or a lump in the cheek. In all four cases the initial pathologic diagnosis was malignant mixed tumor. All 4 individuals were dead in a period of 15 months to 3.5 years after diagnosis either from widespread metastasis or intracranial extension. Orbital involvement occurred about midway in the clinical course and was characterized by proptosis and marked ophthalmoplegia. Radical excision, chemotherapy, and irradiation were of no avail other than whatever palliation they might have provided the patient. The fatal behavior of these malignant mixed tumors was similar to those in the lacrimal gland wherein the malignant change was noted on the initial examination of the incompletely removed tumor.

The remaining patient of the total 5 first underwent removal of a benign mixed tumor of the parotid gland at age 12. Over the subsequent 59 years the patient had approximately 27 surgical procedures as well as irradiation for recurrent tumor that, histologically, appeared more aggressive with each successive excision. At age 71 an orbital exenteration was performed. The mixed tumor became histologically malignant at about age 74 and the patient died from metastasis soon after. The course of this tumor was similar but slower than the lacrimal gland tumors that were initially benign but eventually became malignant.

MUCOEPIDERMOID CARCINOMA

Mucoepidermoid carcinoma, intrinsic in the lacrimal gland, was discussed in Chapter 15. One example of this neoplasm also was found in our series of secondary orbital tumors. This tumor was most unusual because of its slow growth and the ability and will of the patient to withstand multiple disfiguring surgical procedures about the head and neck. The details of this case are these:

A girl, who was 16 years of age when a tumor of 1 year's duration was removed from the soft tissues along the surface of the left hard palate, withstood repeated recurrences, multiple surgical procedures, and various regimens of treatment during a period of 54 years. From the hard palate the tumor extended through bone into the left alveolar ridge and maxillary antrum. Gradually, the neoplasm extended over the midline and involved the right maxilla and maxillary antrum. Spread of the tumor next was into the right orbit, soft palate, and posterior pharynx, and along the chain of lymph nodes on each side of the neck. The carcinoma reached the right orbit about 49 years after it had commenced in the roof of the oral cavity. The patient has had most of the upper face and upper jaws removed on both sides and has been subjected to bilateral neck dissections. She has undergone approximately 18 major surgical procedures for removal of recurrent masses and numerous treatments with irradiation and implantation of radium. This number of operations does not include several skin graft and reconstructive procedures designed to maintain nutritional and respiratory functions. The recurrent mucoepidermoid carcinoma of the orbit extended into the intracranial vault through the sphenoid sinus and the patient died from erosion of the internal carotid artery at age 71.

This case illustrates the unrelenting malignancy of these tumors and the long survival of such patients, until the tumor reaches a vital center or life suddenly is terminated by uncontrolled hemorrhage either from a fungating tumor or during the course of surgery in these areas of the head. It was not until 53 years after the initial histologic study that some of the recurrent nodules of tumor began to change from a differentiated mucoepidermoid carcinoma, grade 1, to a more undifferentiated squamous cell type of neoplasm, grade 3.

BASAL CELL CARCINOMA

The orbital area and upper face are common sites for basal cell carcinomas. Certain features of the skin — its thin texture, its glandular appendages, and its exposure to direct sunlight — make skin peculiarly susceptible to these skin tumors. The orbit may be secondarily affected by these tumors arising along the forehead, eyebrow, side of the nose, upper cheek, and eyelids. The commonest source of orbital invasion is carcinomatous tissue arising in the lower eyelid, particularly in and around the inner canthus (Fig. 271).

Basal cell carcinomas are the most frequent neoplasms of the eyelids and all ophthalmologists encounter these neoplasms in the early stages of their growth. At this early stage, shape and configuration vary. A tumor may be a round, elevated, smooth nodule with a shiny surface or, in the upper eyelid and eyebrow, it may be somewhat warty. Or it may be a sinuous, elongated, superficial, lumpy ulceration along the margin of the lower eyelid. Sometimes a tumor is nodular and elevated but with a scaly center surrounded by a rolled border. But by the time of orbital invasion most of these lesions look similar. In the area of invasion the tissues have become indurated owing to the deep penetration of the neoplasm; and the ulcerated surface, surrounded by an elevated and irregular edge, gives these tumors an ugly, dirty, malignant appearance that seldom is seen with any other slowly growing neoplasm in this area.

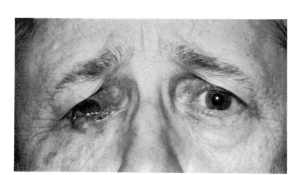

Figure 271. Basal cell carcinoma: lower lid is commonest source for orbital invasion.

INCIDENCE

Basal cell carcinomas occurring on the surface of the eyelids often have been analyzed in terms of their frequency as well as age and sex distribution. However, in reference to orbital invasion, they seldom have been surveyed as a separate subject; instead, they have been included with squamous cell carcinomas in regard to data relating to the general behavior of epitheliomas. This is reasonable in view of their similar age distribution and the many clinical features common to both.

In our series there were 18 secondary basal cell carcinomas (2.3% of the total of 764 orbital tumors). The primary site of all but three of these carcinomas was the eyelid. The three exceptions included sites of origin in the hard palate, side of nose, and cheek. These carcinomas were second in frequency among secondary epithelial tumors from all sources (Table 22) but much fewer in number than squamous cell carcinomas. Squamous cell carcinonas occur in the eyelids much less frequently than do basal cell carcinomas, but a greater proportion of the former reach the orbit because they are so much more aggressive. The less aggressive character of basal cell carcinomas makes it more difficult to determine the age at which the patient's orbital invasion actually occurs. Often the duration of symptoms is so long and the progress of the basal cell carcinoma so gradual that orbital invasion is not especially noticed by the patient. In our 15 patients with a primary site in the eyelid, orbital invasion occurred between the ages of 50 and 80 years in 14. All patients but three were men. The one patient whose basal cell carcinoma started in the hard palate was 33 years of age when symptoms first were noticed. This patient also was a man.

CLINICAL FEATURES

The duration of basal cell carcinomas of the eyelids prior to invasion of the orbit usually is measured in years, a finding that frequently has been confirmed. In our series, the shortest period of evolution was 2 years and the longest, 25 and 32 years, respectively. In one of the latter, the patient (Fig. 272) had had no treatment whatever, and the clinical picture in this case illustrates the natural course of these carcinomas.

Invasion of the orbit is neither clear-cut nor well defined during the slow, progressive course of the usual carcinoma. Symptoms may not be remarkable.

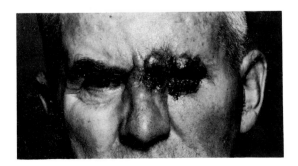

Figure 272. Basal cell epithelioma: typical, indolent, and destructive character of untreated carcinoma, of 25 years' duration, involving left eyelids, eyeball, and orbit; no prior treatment of any kind.

Indeed, the patient scarcely may be aware of the situation except to notice diplopia in extreme gaze nasally, inferiorly, or temporally; upward or horizontal displacement of the eye also may be apparent, but forward proptosis of the eye is not a prominent feature in the anamnesis as it would be with primary orbital tumors. The signs of orbital involvement, however, are more definite. The carcinoma usually has become ulcerated by this time and its surface covered by a smelly, somewhat crusted exudate. The most important clue is a *fixation of the ulcerated lesion to the underlying rim or surface of the bony orbit.* The tissues surrounding this immovable plaque or ulcer also are indurated and show an inflammatory response characterized by redness and swelling of tissues or chemosis of adjacent conjunctivae. However, this inflammatory reaction is not as marked as the reaction usually observed with invasive squamous cell carcinomas. The muscles and soft tissues of the eyelid and the extraocular muscle nearest to the advancing border of the lesion then become incorporated in the invasive process, causing loss of function and fixation of both eyelids and eyeball (Fig. 273). Corneal desiccation from exposure and loss of vision are late sequalea, but orbital invasion should be evident before this. Pain has not been common among our patients, though other authors have mentioned this; perhaps this is because many of our patients were farmers who have a stoic approach to such problems. Pain is due to the involvement of nerves in the periorbita and soft tissues and of muscle bundles.

The common routes for orbital invasion are across the nasal rim and along the medial wall of the bony orbit, just above and along the inferior orbital rim after infiltration of the soft tissues, and along the temporal rim of the orbit with tissue destruction. Of these routes, the first is the most frequent. At the inner canthus, the enlarging ulcer seems to have quicker access to underlying bone than in other areas of the bony orbit. Another possibility is that early basal cell carcinomas are more difficult to eradicate completely in the area of the inner

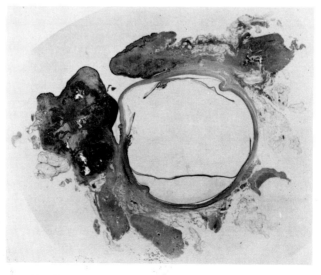

Figure 273. Basal cell carcinoma: invasion of muscles and soft tissues results in loss of function and fixation of eyelid. (Hematoxylin and eosin; × 2½.)

canthus. This is chiefly due to the proximity of the lacrimal excretory channels. A complete excision often is compromised by the surgeon's wish to maintain patency of these channels. The lacrimal drainage passages are easily cicatrized by the slightest surgical trauma and easily occluded even by minimal doses of irradiation. The patient does not understand these hazards and often is unwilling to accept permanent epiphora as a necessary result of complete removal of what seems to be "just a little skin cancer." Consequently, excision is incomplete and the tumor soon is rooted to the soft tissues of both upper and lower eyelids, to underlying tendinous structures, and eventually to periosteum in this area. Once the neoplasm gains access to the periorbita and soft tissues of the orbital cavity, it tends to grow in a circular fashion in preference to a deeper penetration. Thus, all soft tissues of both eyelids and the anterior surface of the eye may be invaded prior to deep passage of the neoplasm into the orbit (Fig. 272). This makes eradication of these carcinomas easier by exenteration than is possible with similar procedures for squamous cell carcinomas.

ROENTGENOGRAPHIC CHANGES

As the carcinoma extends along bony surfaces of the orbit it erodes the bone, and superficial irregularities become roentgenographically apparent. However, such alterations are not of much diagnostic import because the cause of the trouble is obvious. Instead, these roentgenographic changes may be more useful to the surgeon in planning his surgical attack, for it is in the zones of erosion that periorbita must be removed and these area scrutinized for any lingering cells.

PATHOLOGY

The prevailing cells in these carcinomas usually are quite uniform in size and shape and resemble the basal cells of the epidermis (Fig. 274). Their nuclei are ovoid with tiny chromatin particles scattered throughout. The cells tend to grow in tightly packed clusters and the cell boundaries are indistinct. The cytoplasm is relatively scanty and basophilic. Proliferating groups of cells easily are outlined from surrounding stromal tissues of the host by a single layer of more columnar-shaped cells in an orderly palisade-like sequence (Fig. 275). If the cell clusters enlarge, some cells in the center of the clump become necrotic, and cystic spaces form. As the tumors become more aggressive, there is a proportionate increase of mitosis, the cell groups become less uniform and orderly in their arrangement, and growth patterns become more haphazard in contour (Fig. 276). Some basal cell carcinomas may even attempt some keratin formation — an indication of more undifferentiated squamous-like patterns of growth.

TREATMENT

We realize that the question of whether surgery or irradiation is preferred readily stimulates debate. We recognize that each method has merits and drawbacks. There is greater latitude in the selection of either method when the carcinoma is still primary in the eyelid or is still confined to these tissues at the

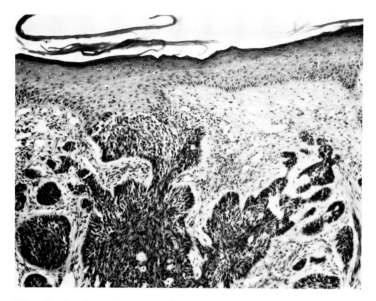

Figure 274. Basal cell carcinoma: small prismatic cells resemble basal layer of epidermis; origin of neoplasm may be traced to this site. (Hematoxylin and eosin; × 100.)

time of first recurrence. Our problem is not the localized, primary lesion but a carcinoma that has become widespread and invasive and already has been treated by these means. All of our patients except one (the individual whose neoplasm progressed 25 years without treatment) had undergone many and various types of surgical removal, irradiation, and combinations of both, prior to the problems involving the orbit. If the extent and recurrence of the

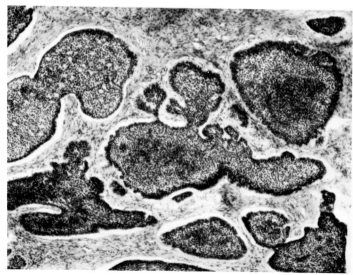

Figure 275. Basal cell carcinoma: cells are arranged in large clusters bounded peripherally by palisade-like layer. (Hematoxylin and eosin; × 65.)

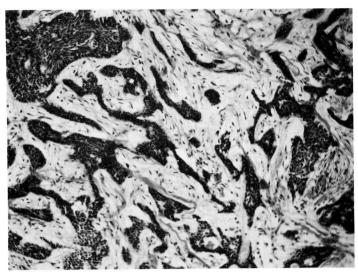

Figure 276. Basal cell carcinoma: in this markedly invasive example the cells are very disorderly in arrangement and there is a pronounced fibrous stromal reaction in the tissues. (Hematoxylin and eosin; × 100.)

neoplasm from its original area in the eyelid are criteria, then it is obvious that one is no better than the other, since recurrences occur with both. With orbital involvement, the choice shifts to that method that will best encompass the carcinoma and, once and for all, eradicate the lesion beyond the zone of possible extent. Either method alone or in combination with one another may have possible application in these situations.

Excision

The first problem is the size of the lesion and its proximity to the precious eye. The diameter of most of these ulcerating carcinomas is between 40 and 60 mm·in at least one meridian. This would be equivalent to the horizintal breadth of the orbit, or it would encompass in an anteroposterior meridian a neoplasm party involving the skin of the face or nose with an extension along one bony orbital surface to approximately one-half the depth of the orbit. Circumvention of a lesion of this size, either by surgery or by irradiation, requires the surgical destruction or irradiation treatment of an area even larger in diameter. Such is scarcely possible without sacrifice of the eye. Indeed, retention of the eye and preservation of its function may have been a factor that prevented adequate treatment of the situation in the first place. To attempt surgical removal of an area of this size without enucleating an eye offers the patient little more than was accomplished by previous treatment. Irradiation sometimes is then proposed in the belief that the neoplasm can be destroyed yet the function of the eye preserved. This belief usually is predicated on the assumption that the eye can be adequately protected by a lead shield. Such protective shielding seldom works out satisfactorily in practice, considering the area irradiated; and most eyes in the orbits so treated still develop a complicated cataract and painful keratitis. Even if it were theoretically possible to protect the eye, the surrounding adnexal tissues are so scarred and their functions so compromised by the dosage of irradiation necessary to destroy the deeply infiltrating tumor that the eye still cannot function for want of protection and support from its adnexal appendages. So, one of the first tenets in treatment is, "the eye must go." If this decision can be accepted by the patient, we then prefer surgery to irradiation, providing that the elderly patient will physically be able to withstand such a procedure as an exenteration, and there has been no prior radical surgery that has required removal of neighboring bone.

In these situations, where the base of the neoplasm has not been disturbed by prior removal of bone, removal en bloc may be performed (Fig. 277). In this approach a wide excision of the ulcerated plaque on the surface of the eyelid, face, or nose is combined with an exenteration of the orbit. Use of the diathermy cutting scalpel for the initial dissection, in preference to the usual incision with the knife, may help destroy any cancerous implants that have wandered peripherally from the visible limits of carcinoma. Frozen section study of fresh tissue removed along the circumference of the lesion also is helpful in revealing unsuspected ramifications of the neoplasm. All periosteum or periorbita in the vicinity of the lesion, of course, is excised. If roentgenography has indicated bony destruction or decalcification, such bone also is completely removed with saws or chisels. If roentgenograms are negative but stripping of the periorbita reveals deeper spread of the tumor, we believe it preferable to remove additional bone. This may result in significant loss of the orbital walls and bony rims and it may even uncover the dura. If the superior wall of the orbit must be sacrificed, the exposed dura may be covered by a skin graft. Such widespread excision of soft tissues and bone may seem unduly destructive, but in our experience this seems the only certain way to forestall later recurrence. Such

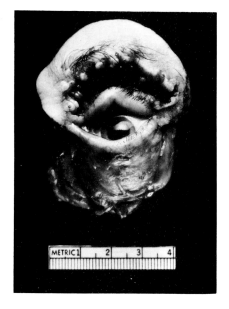

Figure 277.   Basal cell carcinoma: this deeply invasive lesion of the upper eyelid was removed by en bloc exenteration.

a procedure was performed in the patient whose carcinoma had been present for 25 years (Fig. 272). After the operation, it was decided not to add irradiation to the plan of treatment. This patient was followed for 6 years after such surgery and there was no evidence of recurrence.

A somewhat less drastic approach was followed in another patient of our series with a more equivocal result.

This 51-year-old man had had a recurrent basal cell carcinoma of the upper face and eyelids for a period of 6 years, secondary to irradiation for acne. The right upper eyelid already had been removed by the time we saw him. Roentgenography did not show any bone destruction. An en bloc dissection and exenteration was performed, with removal of all periorbita. No bone was removed, but some suspicious areas of erosion along the superior nasal rim of the orbit were treated with surgical diathermy. Local recurrence of the carcinoma in this treated area was observed 3½ years later.

This does not mean that exenteration alone without removal of bone will always be unsuccessful, for we have observed a satisfactory course in some other patients treated by those more conservative means. However, it does illustrate that we cannot take for granted suspicious areas of bone erosion in dealing with this carcinoma. "Bone," sometimes,"also must go."

Reference was made earlier to situations in which the facial bones already had been removed prior to orbital invasion. This type of surgery usually is performed in the management of recurrent basal cell carcinoma arising from a source more distant than the skin of the eyelids. The one case in our series wherein the basal cell carcinoma originated in the hard palate is an example of such an invasive tumor. As a rule some portion of the floor of the orbit may still be intact in such cases. Radical removal of bone and total exenteration of the orbit probably will not reverse the fatal tide in these cases, for the carcinoma, by this time, has filled crevices and foramina beyond the reach of cutting knife. If the eye is hopelessly compromised, the eye and the remaining floor of the orbit may be removed in the manner of a subtotal exenteration. Such an excision may facilitate access to the tumor nodules and colonies deeper in the bony cavities and surfaces.

We have had no experience with the use of cryosurgery for orbital extension.

Radiotherapy

We cannot give any hard and fast rules regarding supplementary irradiation. If we are confident that the lesion has been entirely excised we prefer not to irradiate. If there are suspicious areas beyond the zone of surgical removal, irradiation becomes another important means of trying to eradicate the tumor. These carcinomas are radiosensitive to some degree. Modern techniques with supravoltage machines have a useful palliative effect; it is greater than can be expected with squamous cell carcinomas. Irradiation is beneficial in some elderly patients whose physical infirmities add some risk to extensive surgery. In addition, irradiation is recommended when a patient refuses to lose an eye or will not consent to a disfiguring facial operation.

Some surgeons also recommend that irradiation be administered preliminary to any surgical attack. The rationale of this approach is partly to limit spread of the neoplasm and partly to cause it to shrink to more manageable proportions. The irradiation dose is 3,000 to 4,000 R, given 4 to 6 weeks before operation. With these methods, the area irradiated is larger than it would be if irradation were used only as a postoperative supplement, and delay in healing also may be expected. Frequently, irradiation at this stage is limited by the amount already administered to the carcinoma in an earlier period. One last precaution is that thick bones such as malar bone, are more prone to radionecrosis than other bones in this area.

PROGNOSIS

Prognosis of these carcinomas by the time they reach the orbit is influenced by so many factors that meaningful information on a group basis is nearly impossible to assemble. Many of these patients are in an age group prone to die from disease common to the advancing years. Even so, some of these patients seem quite debilitated from the losing tussle and multiple surgical procedures associated with the spreading carcinoma. In these patients the basal cell carcinoma may be considered an indirect cause of death because the neoplasm may make them more prone to succumb to some of the infectious diseases such as pneumonia. Cure also is possible in some cases but it requires sacrifice of more tissue than some ophthalmologists are willing to admit and many patients willing to accept.

SEBACEOUS CARCINOMA

Sebaceous carcinomas arise from sebaceous appendages of hair follicles of the eyebrow, skin of eyelids, glands of Zeis, and nonciliated glandular structures of the caruncle and meibomian glands. These last glands in the tarsal plate are the commonest origin of sebaceous carcinoma, and this is the principal reason why such a tumor is commonly identified as, and has been given the time-honored name of , *meibomian gland carcinoma* in the ophthalmic literature. Sebaceous glands other than meibomian glands can be the primary site of these neoplasms, and, histologically, it is nearly impossible to differentiate individual specimens from the various sources. As more documented examples of neoplasms from sebaceous structures other than meibomian glands are reported in the future, the more inclusive and proper term *sebaceous carcinoma* will become more widely used. Ginsberg (1965) reviewed the literature on the subject and annotated 142 cases reported through 1963.

INCIDENCE

These are important but, fortunately, infrequent secondary orbital neoplasms. So few cases have involved the orbit that no statistics have been assembled in terms of their proportion of all orbital neoplasms. Incidence of orbital invasion ranges from approximately 6% in the 142 cases reviewed by Ginsberg to 17% (Boniuk and Zimmerman). The latter study encompassed 88 cases from the files of the Armed Forces Institute of Pathology. In the period of the Mayo Clinic survey we encountered three cases with orbital spread. The three patients were men, aged 45, 56, and 76. The age range for the primary tumors in the eyelids at onset is in the 50- to 65-year range. The tumor is somewhat more common in females. It is found twice as often in the upper eyelid as in the lower eyelid.

CLINICAL FEATURES

These carcinomas may present initially in the orbit as a *painless lump* along the superior orbital rim or a mass in the superior conjunctival cul de sac but not necessarily attached to bone (Fig. 278). The primary site then is discovered close by or located in the superior tarsal plate, having been overlooked or disregarded because of lack of symptoms. More commonly, the source of the tumor is known long before orbital invasion, the patient having undergone several surgical procedures for recurrent chalazion. The neoplasm may not reach the orbital cavity until months or several years have elapsed from the time of the initial surgery. With more attention in the present era to histopathologic study of recurrent lesions of the eyelid, the malignant nature of the recurrent nodule may be suspected by the time the patient is referred for additional consultation. The picture then is that of a painless lump with or without surrounding induration depending on the interval of time from the last surgical procedure. Ulceration is not a noteworthy feature as would be the case with basal cell carcinomas. By the time of orbital invasion, masses in the preauricular or submaxillary chain of lymph nodes also may be palpable because lymphatic channels are a favorite means of dissemination for the tumor.

PATHOLOGY

In or near its primary site the tumor retains the acinar configuration of a sebaceous gland. These acinar structures are oval or round masses of variable size (Fig. 279). They are separated from the surrounding supporting tissue by a

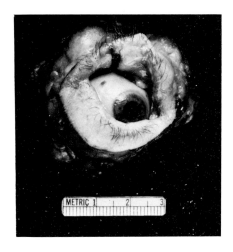

Figure 278. Sebaceous gland carcinoma: neoplasm presented as lump on upper palpebral conjunctiva beneath tarsal plate.

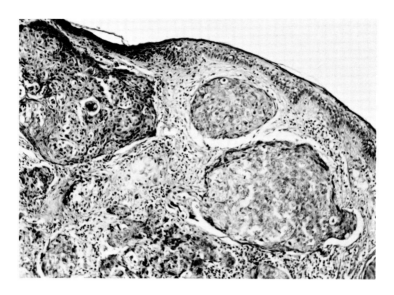

Figure 279.   Sebaceous gland carcinoma: neoplasm is made up of acinar-like masses of malignant cells which resemble sebaceous glands. (Hematoxylin and eosin; × 225.)

basement membrane, and thin septa of connective tissue may subdivide the acinar masses into lobules. Repeated surgical procedures tend to make the carcinoma more malignant so that by the time of orbital invasion the glandular arrangement of cells is replaced by a more undifferentiated pattern of growth. Cords and columns of cells may be seen, suggesting the configuration of a basal cell carcinoma, or, in more malignant forms, the neoplastic cells grow in haphazard clusters and sheets separated only by thin connective tissue septa. Mitotic activity increases as the neoplasm becomes more undifferentiated in its cellular arrangement.

The individual cells are round or polyhedral in the more differentiated forms but become more spindle-shaped with increasing malignancy. The nuclei are oval and vesicular and contain prominent nucleoli. The cytoplasm is scanty and vaculoated. In the faster growing tumors, areas of cystic degeneration occur and the center of some of the acinar lobules contain cell debris and fat. These tumors always have a high content of fat which becomes easily visible, with special dyes, as red-staining splotches and specks.

COURSE AND TREATMENT

Spread of these tumors into deeper tissues of the eyelid, pagetoid sliding along the surface of skin or mucous membranes at their primary site, and lymphatic dissemination all have been observed. Such "triple threat" dissemination favors recurrence of the carcinoma unless it is completely excised. When these neoplasms have reached the orbit, their boundaries usually are such that local excision cannot be done without compromising the function of the eye. Furthermore, a limited resection would not obliterate unseen lymphatic dissemination beyond the periphery of the lesion. For this reason exenteration of the orbit is the preferred treatment.

Lymphatic dissemination from the original tumor is far more frequent than the incidence of orbital invasion. Therefore, it is wise to search for enlarged nodes along the preauricular, submaxillary, parotid, and jugular lymphatic chains when orbital invasion is encountered. If these are found, parotidectomy and block dissection of the lymphatic chain should be performed because the indolent nature of the tumor may not have advanced malignant cells beyond this line of lymphatic defenses. Even this may not check the carcinoma, for death from generalized metastasis (usually to the liver) is not infrequent. The mortality rate among patients with orbital invasion is not known, for there is no long-term follow-up data in the literature. Two of our three patients died from tumor metastasis. The living patient underwent 3 local excisions for rapidly recurring eyelid carcinoma before an exenteration 6 months after onset. He is living without recurrence 12 years after exenteration.

Irradiation usually is recommended for recurrences and nonresectable tumors but the radiosensitivity of this carcinoma after orbital spread seems to be low.

SWEAT GLAND CARCINOMA

To complete this chapter, one additional epithelial neoplasm secondarily affecting the orbit, *carcinoma of a sweat gland*, should be noted. These carcinomas tend to remain quiescent for a period of years before exhibiting infiltrative growth and metastasis. A very detailed case of this type is that of Grizzard and associates (1976). This patient was a 69-year-old male with painful proptosis of the left eye of three weeks' duration when first seen by the authors. Ocular rotations of the affected eye were restricted in all directions of gaze, the conjunctival vessels were injected, and edema and induration of the eyelids were present. A well-healed skin graft was evident in the lower eyelid. A nontender preauricular lymph node was palpable.

Ten years prior to presentation this patient had had a small yellow tumor removed from the left lower eyelid. A recurrence 8 years later was widely excised. On the current admission, multiple biopsy specimens were taken from the orbit, lower eyelid, preauricular lymph node, and parotid gland. All tissue specimens showed a poorly differentiated mucinous secreting adenocarcinoma. The authors concluded the tumor was primary in the eccrine sweat gland of the lower eyelid. The left facial area was treated with 5,600 rads of cobalt irradiation with regression of proptosis and disappearance of the palpable node. There was no recurrence in the 18 months after treatment.

A less typical and more malignant example of orbital involvement was the case reported by Stout and Cooley (1951). A bluish fluctuant tumor about 1.5 cm in size was excised from the lower eyelid of a 44-year-old female. The tumor recurred. Two additional excisions and a course of radiotherapy were followed, after 11 months, by orbital exenteration but the neoplasm had spread to the ethmoid bone. Two additonal excisions were performed, but the tumor continued its growth into the nasal cavity. The patient died 2 years after onset.

These two cases seem to be the only examples in the literature of orbital invasion by sweat gland carcinoma.

Bibliography

Incidence

Stanković I, Litricin O, Stefanović P: Incidence orbitaire des tumeurs du voisinage. Ophthalmololgica *151*:390–404, 1966

Squamous Cell Carcinoma

Batsakis JG: *Tumors of the Head and Neck*. Baltimore, Williams & Wilkins Co, 1974
Jakobiec FA, Rootman J, Jones IS: Secondary and metastatic tumors of the orbit. *In Clinical Ophthalmology*. Volume 2, Chapter 46. Ed: TD Duane. Hagerstown, Harper & Row Publishing Co, 1977

Sebaceous Carcinoma

Boniuk M, Zimmerman LE: Sebaceous carcinoma of the eyelid, eyebrow, caruncle, and orbit. Trans Am Acad Ophthalmol Otolaryngol 72:619–641, 1978
Ginsberg J: Present status of meibomian gland carcinoma. Arch Opthalmol 73:271–277, 1965
Shields JA, Font RL: Meibomian gland carcinoma presenting as a lacrimal gland tumor. Arch Ophthalmol 92:304–306, 1974

Sweat Gland Carcinoma

Grizzard WS, Torczynski E, Edwars AC: Adenocarcinoma of eccrine sweat gland. Arch. Ophthalmol 92:2119–2123, 1976
Stout AP, Cooley SGE: Carcinoma of sweat glands. Cancer 4:521–536, *1951*

17

Metastatic Carcinoma

Among the epithelial tumors that travel to the orbit from distant sources the principal ones are essentially adenocarcinomas. If it were possible to make a thorough search of the ophthalmic literature in all languages, it is likely that we would find examples of orbital metastasis from most organs and tissues whose surfaces or tubular linings are covered by epithelium, except the cornea and lens of the eye. Rather than dwell on many of these unusual cases and reports, we intend in this chapter to discuss the metastatic carcinomas, regardless of their origin, by concentrating on the clinical aspects common to many and the features peculiar to a few. Less attention will be devoted to the histopathologic features of these carcinomas, for by the time they reach the orbit they have become so malignant and undifferentiated that it is sometimes difficult for the pathologist to tell one from another when he does not know the primary source.

INCIDENCE

Ophthalmologists long have been fascinated by metastatic neoplasms lodging in the orbit. Since case reports of such tumors have been numerous, and such publications usually give details of cases believed to be both unusual and rare. Cases of orbital metastasis also are listed in several of the comprehensive reviews of metastatic tumors of the eye and ocular adnexa. More recent surveys of this type which include a significant number of orbital cases are those of Albert and associates (1967), Ferry and Font (1974), and Hutchison and Smith (1979). These surveys relate the types and frequency of metastatic tumors to one another and between the eye and orbit rather than their incidence relative to other orbital lesions. Our Mayo Clinic survey is useful in estimating the incidence of both factors. In Table 24 we have listed their total number and types. The total 56 metastatic tumors comprise 7.3% of our total orbital tumors (764 cases) and 10% of our total orbital neoplasms (552 cases).

Neoplasms such as malignant lymphoma, histiocytosis, and leukemia were not regarded as true metastatic lesions if the orbital invasion appeared some time after the diagnosis of the disease was established by histologic examination of neoplastic foci elsewhere in the body. We regard such orbital tumors as manifestations of a generalized dissemination of the neoplasm, or as pluricentric foci of disease, rather than as metastatic representatives of one another. We conclude from our survey that metastatic orbital neoplasms are not infrequent, and the incidence of this type of tumor has probably increased owing to increased longevity of patients resulting from improved therapeutic measures directed at the primary focus.

TABLE 24. METASTATIC NEOPLASMS OF THE ORBIT
(MAYO CLINIC SERIES, 1948–1974)

Neoplasm	Number
Carcinoma	43
Neuroblastoma	11
Hemangiopericytoma	1
Malignant melanoma	1
Total	56

All surveys emphasize the predominance of carcinomas among the metastatic neoplasms (Table 24) and it is this group with which we are primarily concerned. We have already discussed the second most common metastatic tumor, neuroblastoma, in Chapter 11. The forty-three carcinomas are further analyzed in Table 25 according to their primary source, sex ratio, and age of the patient at the approximate time orbital metastasis occurred. Ferry and Font also have reviewed a sizeable number, twenty-eight cases of metastatic orbital carcinomas, but in ten of these the primary source of the neoplasm was unknown. In perusing Table 25, it is obvious that metastatic carcinomas chiefly develop in adults in the fifth, sixth, and seventh decades. The average age of the patients with primary breast carcinoma at the time of orbital metastasis was 57.6 years. The average age of the patients with lung carcinoma at the time of orbital metastasis was slightly younger, 51 years, but the age range, 39–70 years, was slightly more broad. Metastasis to the right and left orbit was nearly equal, and in two cases both orbits were affected. Bilateral metastases are considered unusual and have been the subject of several case reports (Appelmans et al 1954; Bedford and Daniel 1960, among others).

In the Mayo Clinic series adenocarcinoma from the *breast* (twenty-one in number) was the predominant metastatic tumor (Table 25) and carcinoma from the *lung* (10) and kidney (three) were next in frequency. This incidence is consistent with that of other surveys of this type. Ferry and Font have noted that carcinoma of the gastrointestinal tract is twice as often responsible for cancer deaths as carcinoma of the breast, but the former much less commonly metastasizes to the eye or orbit. Females are predominantly affected by metastatic carcinomas to the orbit chiefly because of the frequency of breast neoplasms. We have not observed any cases of orbital metastasis from the male breast, although two cases of choroidal metastasis from this source have been recorded (Greer 1954). The high incidence of females in this overall group is somewhat offset by the prevalence of metastatic lung cancer among males.

A most intriguing facet of our series was the number of patients in whom the orbital disorder was the presenting symptom of what proved to be a latent primary carcinoma elsewhere; this occurred in 13 patients (approximately 30% of our series). This observation emphasizes the importance of orbital diagnosis in the detection of systemic cancer. Interestingly, both patients with scirrhous carcinomas of the stomach were first recognized in this manner; in seven of the ten patients with lung carcinoma the primary lesion remained hidden until uncovered by orbital diagnosis; and in the four remaining cases, orbital signs were the initial clue in the diagnosis of thyroid, adrenal, renal, and breast carcinoma, respectively. These cases are further discussed later in this chapter. In an additional eight cases the orbit was the first evidence of metastasis and in some

TABLE 25. DATA ON 43 METASTATIC CARCINOMAS OF ORBIT:
MAYO CLINIC SERIES

Primary Source	Histologic Type	Sex and Age	Orbit with Metastasis
Breast (21)	Scirrhous adenocarcinoma	F, 67	R
	Adenocarcinoma	F, 57	L
	Adenocarcinoma	F, 40	L
	Adenocarcinoma	F, 67	L
	Papillary adenocarcinoma	F, 45	R
	Adenocarcinoma	F, 63	R
	Adenocarcinoma	F, 64	L
	Scirrhous adenocarcinoma	F, 62	L
	Adenocarcinoma	F, 68	R
	Adenocarcinoma	F, 60	L
	Adenocarcinoma	F, 53	L
	Adenocarcinoma	F, 45	R
	Adenocarcinoma	F, 59	L
	Scirrhous adenocarcinoma	F, 64	R
	Adenocarcinoma	F, 63	L
	Adenocarcinoma	F, 53	L
	Adenocarcinoma	F, 64	R and L
	Scirrhous adenocarcinoma	F, 50	R
	Adenocarcinoma	F, 48	L
	Adenocarcinoma	F, 50	R
	Adenocarcinoma	F, 67	R
Lung (10)	Scirrhous adenocarcinoma	M, 34	L
	Adenocarcinoma	M, 41	R
	Large cell adenocarcinoma	M, 54	R
	Adenocarcinoma	M, 65	L
	Papillary adenocarcinoma	F, 50	R
	Small cell adenocarcinoma	M, 48	R
	Small cell carcinoma	F, 39	R
	Small cell carcinoma	M, 68	R
	Small cell carcinoma	M, 40	L
	Squamous cell carcinoma	M, 70	L
Stomach (2)	Scirrhous adenocarcinoma	F, 60	R and L
	Scirrhous adenocarcinoma	F, 63	R
Thyroid (2)	Adenocarcinoma	F, 54	L
	Adenocarcinoma	F, 58	R
Kidney (3)	Hypernephroma	M, 56	R
	Hypernephroma	M, 59	R
	Hypernephroma	M, 62	L
Adrenal	Adenocarcinoma	F, 77	R
Prostate	Adenocarcinoma	M, 85	L
Nasopharynx	Squamous cell carcinoma	F, 37	L
Parotid	Squamous cell carcinoma	M, 51	R
Unknown	Squamous cell carcinoma	M, 64	R

cases was the only sign of metastasis for some interval of time in the patient's overall course. All of this latter group except one were women with a prior diagnosis of breast carcinoma. The one exception was a woman with prior thyroid carcinoma.

CLINICAL FEATURES

The symptoms of these metastatic carcinomas depend somewhat on the source of the neoplasm, the site of orbital metastasis, and the histologic type of the carcinoma. A feature common to many is the *suddenness* with which symptoms develop. In contrast to the gradual onset of many primary orbital tumors in adults, patients with metastatic neoplasms often recall within a day or so the sudden events that made them realize something was wrong with their eye. Most often the first symptom is *diplopia*, with or without *eyelid swelling* (upper or lower), and soon followed by *blepharoptosis* if the metastasis had lodged in the superior quadrants of the orbit. These features are due to the frequent lodgment of the itinerant neoplasm in or adjacent to the extraocular muscles. In other words, *muscle involvement with accompanying ophthalmoplegia is both an earlier sign and a more constant manifestation of metastatic carcinoma than of any other type of orbital tumor.* Proptosis also may occur early in the course of the orbital disease but it is not as marked or as obvious as with primary orbital tumors. It tends to be overshadowed by the patient's concern with other manifestations of orbital involvement. If the tumor is lodged posteriorly in the retrobulbar space, sudden *loss of vision* may accompany the diplopia. *Orbital pain* is another early feature that is not observed among other orbital neoplasms. In Chapter 15 it was noted that orbital pain may accompany other malignant carcinomas of the orbit, such as adenoid cystic carcinomas, but in such instances the pain is a later feature of the anamnesis and such tumors usually prove to be primary in the orbit. The pain of metastatic carcinoma is dull and nagging in character.

The further course depends on these various factors. If the neoplasm is located well forward in the orbit, a hard, poorly delimited lump becomes palpable. Such a mass may be palpated in any quadrant, the tumor having no favored space or plan of predilection. Chemosis soon appears, of a degree similar to that observed with secondary carcinomas (Fig. 280). In the meantime, ophthalmoplegia progresses and rotation of the eye is increasingly handicapped. The degree of ophthalmoplegia usually corresponds to the duration of the orbital disease. This clinical picture develops more rapidly with carcinomas metastatic from the lung than with carcinomas from the breast. In the former, the patient usually seeks consultation within a period of 2 to 6 months from onset, but with breast metastasis the evolution of signs takes longer, perhaps 4 to 10 months.

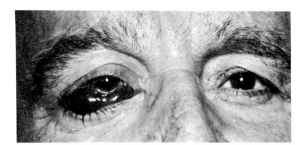

Figure 280. Metastatic carcinoma (hypernephroma): tumor in lower temporal quadrant of right orbit; patient had diplopia, first noted when looking to the right (2 weeks before photograph), soon followed by decrease of vision and steady orbital pain, the latter partially relieved 1 week after onset by appearance of proptosis and chemosis. Orbital tumor was presenting sign of hypernephroma, identified by nephrectomy 1 week after orbitotomy. Orbital manifestations of carcinomas from the lung and kidney are very similar.

Papilledema, continued visual loss, and pressure on the posterior pole of the eye are other features associated with nonpalpable metastasis in the posterior orbit. Whatever the rate of progress, the end picture is one of severe restriction of ocular rotation, much out of proportion to the degree of proptosis or other signs of orbital involvement.

This pattern of orbital involvement may not only be the presenting manifestation of an occult neoplasm elsewhere but may also signal the initial metastasis of a pre-existent neoplasm that was though to have been arrested. The latter is particularly true in some breast carcinomas where the interval between mastectomy and first metastatic focus of tumor is quite long. It will not occur to the patient that a prior surgical procedure may be in any way connected with their present orbital illness. For these reasons it is now routine to ask all patients with proptosis whether any prior surgical procedure was necessary for "tumors" or "growths." A positive reply may, surprisingly, provide the clue to an otherwise puzzling orbital problem.

Another adjunct to clinical diagnosis is the plasma level of *carcinoembryonic antigen.* In some malignant tumors there is an increased production of this antigen proportionate to the amount of tumor and extent of its dissemination. Production of this antigen is fairly high in pancreatic and colorectal adenocarcinomas and less high in breast carcinomas. Plasma levels greater than 10 ng/ml are significant and may be the clue to an occult malignancy, particularly of the gastrointestinal tract. This antigen was first described in 1965 (Gold and Freedman) and received its name because it was present in both extracts of human adenocarcinomas of the colon and in the mucosa of fetal colonic tissue. A nonelevated plasma carcinoembryonic antigen value, however, does not rule out metastatic neoplastic disease. At present, there is no data on the application of this test to a sizeable number of cases of orbital metastatic disease.

Orbital roentgenography also may be a supplement to clinical diagnosis of metastatic disease. Osteolytic defects quite suggestive of metastatic malignancy may occur in the roof or lateral wall of the orbit and accompany the soft tissue metastasis. However, bony involvement is not as common as soft tissue metastasis. As a rule, orbital bone destruction from carcinoma is much more common with secondary tumors than with metastatic tumors.

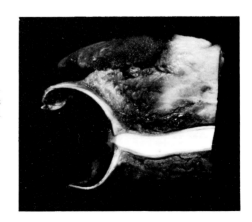

Figure 281. Metastatic scirrhous adenocarcinoma: muscles, nerves, and orbital tissues are encased by tumor and eye is immobilized and may retract posteriorly.

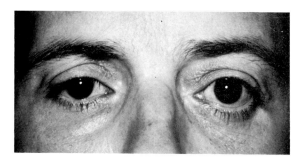

Figure 282. Metastatic adenocarcinoma (breast): a change in appearance of right eye, noticed by this 45-year-old woman 3 months before photograph, marked limitation of upward ocular rotation, blepharoptosis due to partial paralysis of levator palpebrae superioris, and enophthalmos (5 mm) of right eye were features of diffuse adenocarcinoma present in posterior portion of right orbit and were first manifestations of metastasis from carcinoma of breast removed 4 years previously.

Scirrhous Adenocarcinoma

Of greater diagnostic importance is the clinical picture that emerges with the scirrhous type of metastatic adenocarcinoma. The orbital symptoms at onset are similar to those of other adenocarcinomas, but blepharoptosis due to infiltration of the levator palpebrae superioris is more common. However, as the disease progresses, rather than proptosis, chemosis, and tissue reaction characteristic of other adenocarcinomas, the picture is one of the muscles, nerves, and surrounding soft tissues becoming so entwined and infiltrated by the scirrhous tumor that the helpless eye soon is immobilized and pulled posteriorly (Fig. 281). *Enophthalmos* instead of exophthalmos is the rule; the degree of enophthalmos, as measured with the exophthalmometer, usually is 2 to 3 mm as compared to the normal fellow eye, but we have observed a difference of as much as 5 mm (Fig. 282). Six patients of our group showed this diagnostic clue. As the eye becomes more enophthalmic, ophthalmoplegia increases, and the eyes become fixed and "frozen" in forward gaze. Figure 283 illustrates a pronounced, bilateral example of this syndrome of enophthalmos, blepharoptosis, and ocular immobility. In cases of unilateral involvement, the patient, the patient's relatives, and the physician usually are concerned about the fellow eye, which appears proptosed, but the "proptosed" eye really is the normal eye. It is sometimes difficult to convince all concerned that a serious disorder affects the orbit on the side of the enophthalmic eye. *These scirrhous malignancies, regardless of source, are an exception to the almost universal rule that all orbital neoplasms produce proptosis or some displacement, other than in a posterior direction, of the eye.* No other

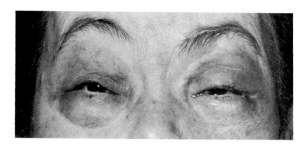

Figure 283. Metastatic carcinoma (stomach, scirrhous type): initial signs of otherwise hidden carcinoma were bilateral enophthalmos, blepharoptosis, and ophthalmoplegia, due to diffuse infiltration of both orbits; no diplopia because eyes were so immobile.

orbital neoplasm, in our experience, produces this clinical picture associated with enophthalmos; and the importance of this clue is further emphasized by the following case.

A 68-year-old woman (the oldest patient in our series with cancer of the breast) complained of pain around the right eye 7 months before our examination and, in the interim, intermittent swelling of the right eyelids. Examination revealed blepharoptosis and an indefinite, firm mass in the lower quadrants of the right orbit. Enophthalmos (2 mm) of the right eye was confirmed by exophthalmometry. Roentgenograms did not reveal any bony defects. Enophthalmos and blepharoptosis were the diagnostic clues to probable metastatic orbital disease. A search for the primary source ensued. An orbitotomy confirmed the presence of metastatic carcinoma, grade 4, which was followed in 1 week by mastectomy for the hitherto silent primary neoplasm.

Bilateral Metastasis

Orbital metastases were bilateral in two patients (Table 25). The primary sources of these metastases were stomach and breast. Some clinical aspects of the patient with bilateral metastasis from the stomach are illustrated in Figure 283. The bilateral or unilateral sites of metastasis, as listed in Table 25, reflect the status of the patient when first under our observation; the data does not reveal the fact that, in an additional three patients, bilateral metastases developed sometime in the subsequent course of the disease. These three all were women with breast metastases. As one patient originally presenting with bilateral breast metastases is listed in Table 25, a total of four of our 21 patients with carcinoma eventually developed bilateral orbital metastases. In the 3 patients who did not have bilateral disease when first seen, an interval of 9 months, 18 months, and 5 years, respectively, elapsed between involvement of one orbit and another.

Two further patients showing an unusual pattern of metastasis were a man with metastasis of a lung carcinoma to the orbit and eye on the same side, and a woman with breast carcinoma metastatic to the right orbit and left eye at the time of our initial examination.

Other clinical aspects of metastatic carcinoma are more oriented toward the source of the neoplasm. These are discussed in the remainder of this chapter. The pertinent information is derived from the literature and from our own survey.

CLINICOPATHOLOGIC FEATURES OF SPECIFIC TUMORS

CARCINOMA OF BREAST

INCIDENCE

The peak incidence for primary breast carcinoma usually is in the fifth decade. The age range in our series (Table 25) was somewhat older than this (average age, 57.6 years; range, from 40 to 68). This difference reflects the interval that passes between discovery of the primary tumor and its metastasis.

In our patients, with one exception, discovery and surgical confirmation of the primary neoplasm in the breast preceded orbital dissemination (Fig. 284). The interval between initial diagnosis and the recognition of orbital metastasis was from 2 to 5 years in the majority of patients. However, in 6 patients there were periods of latency greater than 5 years: specifically, 6 (2 cases), 7, 9, 12, and 27 years. The average latency period among our group was consistent with the findings reported in the literature. In the patient with the 27-year interval, the orbit was only the second site of metastasis, dissemination to one axilla preceding that to the orbit by 13 years. Such long intervals of silence raise the question of whether patients can ever believe they are free from the shadow of this neoplasm.

PATHOLOGY

The histologic structure of adenocarcinomas of the breast varies. Some may be differentiated into papillary-like growths that remain confined to intraductal structures and individual lobules of the breast. Others are highly invasive, anaplastic growths that show little tendency to localize in any glandular or functional components of the breast (Fig. 285). Still others show metaplasia into colloid- and mucus-secreting cells, squamous cells, and signet-ring cells. By the time these neoplasms have reached the orbit through the bloodstream, many of their original characteristics have been lost and they become stubbornly invasive and relentlessly progressive. These carcinomas are well known for their ability to remain latent even after the primary tumor has been discovered and

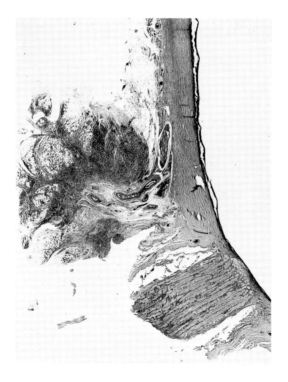

Figure 284. Metastatic breast carcinoma: patient presented with occult primary tumor and symptomatic retro-orbital metastasis. (Hematoxylin and eosin; × 8½.)

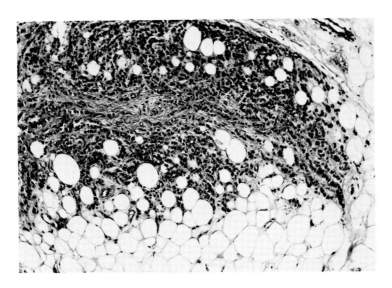

Figure 285. Metastatic breast carcinoma: this highly undifferentiated and invasive neoplasm comprises small dark cells which show characteristic growth pattern of cells in "single file." (Hematoxylin and eosin; × 100.)

removed; and the site they may choose for continued growth, plus the interval that may elapse before metastasis occurs, is unpredictable.

CLINICAL COURSE AND TREATMENT

In most of our patients the orbit was but one locus of metastasis among several that were discovered either at the time of our examination or earlier. However, in five patients the orbit was the initial site of metastasis and, furthermore, the only one that was discovered at the time of our examination. In the latter situation, the ophthalmologist may wonder if radical surgical excision of the orbital metastasis is indicated, on the basis that an orbital focus may be a solitary metastasis. Would removal of such a metastasis, then, prolong the patient's life? Our series is too small to base any conclusions upon it. We were able to obtain follow-up data on four of the five patients in whom the orbit represented the first site of metastasis. The neoplasms of all four patients metastasized to other areas in periods of 3, 6, 12, and 40 months, respectively. Realizing this long latency period and the unpredictable behavior of the neoplasm after removal of the primary tumor, we believe that an orbital metastasis is not a solitary one at the time of observation even though other foci cannot be discovered.

Because we believe that an orbital metastasis is not a solitary metastasis, we have used irradiation for treatment. If surgery were selected as the treatment, exenteration would be required; anything short of exenteration would be useless. In assessing the need for exenteration rather than irradiation as the preferred therapy, the surgeon should keep in mind that women do not readily agree to such cosmetically disfiguring surgery around the face unless assurance can be given that it is virtually curative. We do not believe such assurance is

possible in cases of breast carcinoma and, therefore, irradiation is a logical compromise. However, exenteration may be reserved for those patients in whom
either irradiation is not palliative or the neoplasm is so painful that something
other than irradiation is required. Exenteration was performed in one of our
patients after an initial trial of irradiation had failed to relieve severe orbital
pain; in this case, the neoplasm was eroding into adjacent sinuses and extending
beyond the limits of continued and safe levels of irradiation. Exenteration effectively relieved pain.

Information is available on the progress of nineteen of our twenty-one
women with orbital metastsis. All but 1 died from extension of the neoplasm,
but only 3 of the 18 deceased patients lived longer than 3 years after the presumptive onset of orbital dissemination. The longest survival was 9 years. Seven
years have passed since the onset of orbital metastasis in the 1 living patient but
multiple metastatic foci have been treated in this interval. Orbital metastasis,
then, is an unfavorable prognostic pitfall: a harbinger of doom. We have no
control series, but it is our clinical impression that irradiation treatment does
have some palliative effect in relieving pain; it may provide a few more months
or a year of life, and bolsters the everlasting hopes of the individual. A small
dose of supervoltage irradiation may be given to the affected orbit if the patient
already has had such treatment to other areas of metastasis. Heavier amounts
(2,500 to 3,500 R) might be administered if the orbit is an initial area of spread.
Therapeutic programs are managed by oncologists and the ophthalmologist
plays only a diagnostic and observative role.

CARCINOMA OF LUNG

INCIDENCE AND PATHOLOGY

Metastasis from the lung is second in frequency among carcinomas, both in
our series and in others. Carcinoma of the lung is an inclusive term for several
histologic types regardless of their specific anatomic site of origin. However, the
majority of these carcinomas arise in the main bronchi, tracheal bifurcation, or
lobar bronchi. Microscopically, three principal cytologic types of carcinoma are
recognized: undifferentiated (Fig. 286), adenocarcinoma, and squamous cell
(Fig. 287). Many of these neoplasms have features of several types or combinations of all three. Such combinations are so frequent that some pathologists
include a fourth, "mixed" tumor in their classification. Others recognize the frequency of these mixed types but prefer to catalog such tumors according to their
predominant cellular component. These carcinomas seem to be more common
than was the situation several decades ago. This increase is not entirely attrib-
utable to cigarette smoking. Other factors such as improved recognition by
roentgenography and bronchoscopy and less frequent misdiagnosis by clinicians
and pathologists, may contribute to an increased incidence. There is a definite
preponderance among males (70 to 80%), and the mean age of patients reported in most surveys is between 45 and 60 years. Sex distribution, age of
patients, and histologic types of tumors in our series are given in Table 25.

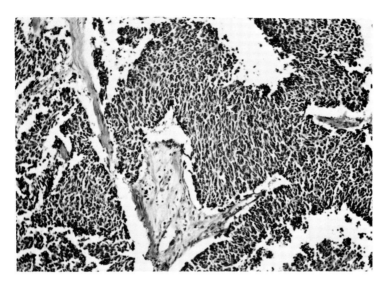

Figure 286.   Metastatic lung carcinoma: undifferentiated neoplasm of small cell (oat cell) type. (Hematoxylin and eosin; × 100.)

CLINICAL COURSE

There seems no positive way of predicting the course of these neoplasms. Some stay close to their point of origin until bronchial obstruction, pneumonia, bronchiectasis, or pleurisy calls attention to the underlying lung disorder. Or, the neoplasm may remain relatively silent until discovered by routine roentgenogram of the lung. Others may disseminate at an early stage while the home colony still is quite small. The undifferentiated types are particularly

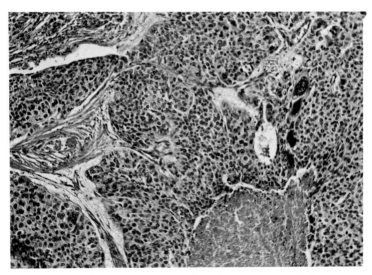

Figure 287.   Metastatic lung carcinoma: neoplasm is squamous cell in type. (Hematoxylin and eosin; × 110.)

prone to early metastasis; and if the primary focus is in a small bronchus in the periphery of the lung, the metastatic deposit may cause symptoms before the primary tumor is discovered (Ferry and Naghdi 1967). This trend to early metastasis certainly is more frequent than with breast carcinoma. Descriptive cases of orbital metastasis from carcinoma of the lung are scarce, but the few available reports, and our own experience, emphasize the latter characteristic. In six of the ten cases in our survey, orbital metastasis was the initial symptom of hidden carcinoma.

In none of the 10 did the duration of orbital symptoms exceed 4 months before consultation was sought. The severity of symptoms, such as orbital pain, ophthalmoplegia, chemosis, visual impairment, and proptosis, seemed to be responsible for early examination. This interval was shorter than in cases of metastasis from neoplasms of the breast. Unilateral proptosis was notable (as much as 10 mm in one case), considering symptoms of only several months' duration. In the case with least proptosis (3 mm) the histologic pattern was scirrhous in type. There were no instances of enophthalmos, such as occurred with breast carcinoma. Neither were orbital tissues fixed and "frozen" as with breast carcinomas, despite consistent ophthalmoplegia. Ophthalmoplegia was the most common and constant feature among all the various signs and symptoms. In one patient metastasis to both the right eye and right orbit appeared to be simultaneous, for symptoms of proptosis and decreased vision were noticed on the same day. In seven patients the metastatic deposit was well forward in the orbit and could be palpated superiorly. In the other three, metastases were posteriorly located.

Life expectancy of these patients is short: a matter of a few months or perhaps as long as 1 year. Administration of systemic steroids supplemented with irradiation usually has some palliative effect.

Bronchial adenoma is an additional neoplasm of the lung that is known to metastasize to the eye, but we have found only one reported example of orbital metastasis (Kulvin and Sawchak). These neoplasms are derived from mucous and mixed glands in the epithelial lining of the air passages, often in a stem or lobar bronchus. Histologically, they are of two types: the carcinoid and the cylindroma. The former is, by far, the more common type and is similar, histologically and clinically, to the carcinoid tumors arising from the enterochromaffin cells of the gastrointestinal tract. They affect a younger age group than do the preceding carcinomas, and the sex distribution is approximately equal. These neoplasms are not as innocent as implied by the name *adenoma*, for they possess the ability to invade surrounding tissues and ultimately metastasize. They grow relatively slowly, so there is a chance of cure if the primary focus is removed early and completely in the course of the disease. Even with complete excision, some years must elapse before it is safe to say the patient has escaped local spread or metastasis. In Kulvin and Sawchak's case—that of a 38-year-old woman with widespread metastasis—the initial orbital deposit was the patient's only subjective concern until she reached a terminal state about 4 months after orbitotomy.

CARCINOMA OF ALIMENTARY TRACT

INCIDENCE AND PATHOLOGY

The principal carcinomas are those of the stomach, colon, and rectum. Only a few instances of orbital metastasis from each regional site have been noted in the past literature, and several of these reports do not record descriptions of the patient. These carcinomas have sufficient characteristics in common to consider them together for purposes of this discussion. Carcinomas of the stomach and large intestine are relatively frequent among the large family of epithelial neoplasms. They are more common among males, and the mean ages at onset from both sources are quite similar — the sixth decade. Carcinomas from the stomach are somewhat more frequent, and occur in patients somewhat younger, than those of the large intestine. All arise from glandular structures lining the alimentary channel, but their histologic types may vary widely, not only from tumor to tumor but within the same tumor. Some may show definite differentiation into acinar structures and papillary patterns with or without mucus-secreting components (Fig. 288). In others, spheroidal cell forms may predominate in carcinomas in which the cell nucleus is pushed to one side, giving rise to the so-called signet-ring cell type. Again, mucus-secreting components may or may not be present. At the most malignant extreme are those undifferentiated neoplasms in which anaplasia is so marked that all glandular orientation is lost. The undifferentiated tumors occur more often in the stomach than in the large intestine.

CLINICAL COURSE

Both patients in our survey were women with metastases from carcinomas of the stomach (Table 25). In each the orbital disorder was a presenting sign of

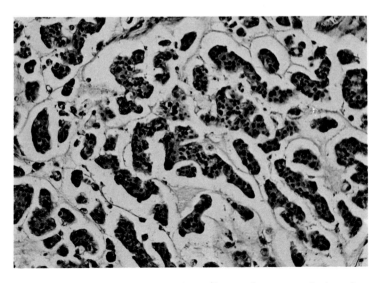

Figure 288. Metastatic stomach carcinoma: papillary and mucus-producing adenocarcinoma. (Hematoxylin and eosin; × 120.)

the latent primary neoplasm. One patient already has been mentioned in connection with the unusual bilateral nature of the metastates (Fig. 283). In the other, the orbital mass and a roentgenographically visible osteolytic lesion of a rib shared attention as signals of possible systemic disease. However, the main subjective concern of this 63-year-old woman was the need for rectal surgery. The patient was also aware of some difference in the appearance of the two eyes. Closer inspection indicated a slight downward displacement and enophthalmos of the right eye. The crux of the ocular problem was a hard nodular mass which was palpable across the floor of the orbit just posterior to the inferior orbital rim. The eye could not be rotated upward because it was fixed to this mass. These findings suggested a scirrhous type of neoplasm. Abdominal exploration revealed a gastric carcinoma with metastases throughout the peritoneal cavity. The patient was treated with cyclophosphamide (Cytoxan) and cobalt irradiation of the involved vertebrae. This palliative therapy permitted the patient 5 additional years of relative freedom from pain before she was overwhelmed by widespread metastasis. The first patient was treated with oral steroids and irradiation. She died 2 years after presumed onset of the orbital metastasis.

Other accounts of orbital metastasis from alimentary tract adenocarcinomas are those also referring to the stomach (Niessen 1956, Chatterjee and Deb 1965) and to the rectum (Richards 1960). Carcinoid tumors of the alimentary tract akin to the carcinoid of the lung noted earlier, also may metastasize to the orbit. Albert and associates (1967), in their statistical survey, refer to metastasis from a carcinoid, and we assume the primary source was somewhere in the gastrointestinal tract. A more detailed case is that of Honrubia and associates (1971). This case occurred in a 71-year-old female with a 13-month history of diplopia and a mass in the inferior portion of the right orbit of 4 months' duration. On examination, palpable masses were also noted in the inferior portion of the other orbit, the posterior triangle of the right neck, and the left breast. Several months prior to presentation, "malignant" tumors had been removed from left neck and scalp. The authors biopsied the tumors in the right neck and left breast and compared the histologic findings to the scalp and left neck specimens previously excised. All specimens were thought to represent the same tumor, argentaffinoma (malignant carcinoid). The patient was living two years later but additional masses had appeared in the right orbit superiorly, right triceps area, and left axilla. Another, unpublished case of metastatic orbital carcinoid tumor has been brought to our attention (Waller 1979). This was a 58-year-old woman who developed 6 mm of proptosis and marked chemosis of the left eye over a period of 10 to 14 days. Vision of affected eye was reduced to 20/40 and marked ophthalmoplegia, particularly in upward gaze, was present. Computer tomography revealed a large mass filling the posterior orbit. Approximately 10 days prior to onset of these orbital symptoms the patient had undergone a resection of a carcinoid tumor of the hepatic flexure of the intestine. On orbitotomy an unencapsulated mass was verified in the posterior orbit which proved to be a metastatic carcinoid tumor. Data on this patient is too recent to have any meaningful follow-up information.

CARCINOMA OF KIDNEY

INCIDENCE AND PATHOLOGY

Examples of orbital metastasis from kidney carcinoma also are few in number. In the statistical summaries of Ferry and Font, and Albert and associates only a total of three cases were listed. One case each were described in the reports of Woody and Geeraets (1966), and Howard and associates (1978). Amdur and Leopold (1959) discovered five prior cases of orbital metastasis, but these may not have all been true examples of direct dissemination to the orbit. In one of these, orbital involvement seemed secondary to metastatic invasion from an adjacent ethmoid sinus. In another report it is not clear whether the orbital mass truly was a separate metastasis or exension of a prior intraocular metastasis through the wall of the eyeball. A third case is an example of Wilms' tumor with metastasis to the orbit, rather than hypernephroma.

In a fourth case the metastasis seemed to be solely to the eye. The remaining single cases of Kalt and Tille (1939), and Amdur and Leopold seem to be true examples of discrete orbital metastasis. We have observed three cases (Table 25). The age (where stated) of all the above cases ranged from 47 to 64 years. Interestingly (where sex is stated), all were males.

Renal carcinoma is a proper term for epithelial neoplasms of the kidney among adults. More often these carcinomas are referred to as *hypernephromas*, a name that reflects earlier concepts of their origin from remnants or rests of adnexal cortex in the kidney. The neoplasm is a type of adenocarcinoma arising either from renal tubules or from islets of nephrogenic tissue which have persisted in the renal cortex. Its histopathologic designation, *clear cell carcinoma*, is based on the clear, vacuolated cytoplasm of large, round individual tumor cells (Fig. 289). These cells may proliferate in sheets or cords,

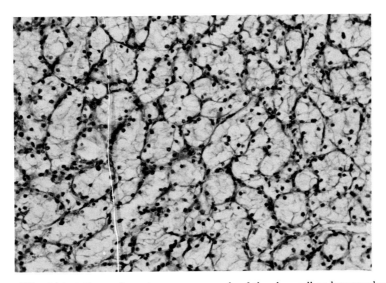

Figure 289. Metastatic renal carcinoma: an example of the clear cell or hypernephroma type. (Hematoxylin and eosin; × 205.)

the latter having some resemblance to tubes and acini. The nuclei are small and may arrange themselves adjacent to the basement membrane of any tubular-like component of the metastatic tissue.

CLINICAL COURSE

Woody and Geeraets state that renal carcinomas are notable for bizarre behavior. They note that cures have been reported following removal of primary tumor and a solitary metastasis, and metastatic lesions have occurred 10 to 20 years after removal of primary tumor. Two of our cases illustrate contrasting clinical courses. In one, unilateral proptosis of 13 mm developed in a period of three weeks associated with severe loss of vision, marked ophthalmoplegia, intense chemosis, and a mass in the inferior orbit. On orbitotomy a gray, friable, necrotic tumor was removed piecemeal. This proved to be the initial manifestation of hypernephroma. The patient of Woody and Geeraets had a similar course before discovery of the primary neoplasm. This short and rapidly progressive course behaves similarly to metastatic small cell carcinomas of the lung. In the case of Kalt and Tillé a period of 18 months elapsed between biopsy of the orbital tumor and discovery of the primary lesion.

In a second case of our series of three, orbital metastasis did not occur until 4 years after excision of the primary tumor. The metastatic nodule was well circumscribed and was removed intact. The tumor in the case of Amdur and Leopold also was of this type. The excision of such a discrete metastatic nodule may be compatible with increased longevity providing other metastatic foci are not present in some more vital area.

Another unusual feature is illustrated by the case reported by Howard and colleagues. In their 47-year-old male a unilateral pulsating proptosis was the presenting sign of the occult hypernephroma. The pulsation was due to a prominent vascular network on the surface of the circumscribed tumor that derived its blood supply from the ophthalmic artery and a branch of the internal maxillary. The authors thought their case was unique among metastatic tumors because of the pulsation, but highly vascular pulsating tumors are known to be associated with other metastatic neoplasms, particularly thyroid carcinoma.

CARCINOMA OF PROSTATE GLAND

INCIDENCE

Adenocarcinomas of the prostate gland are similar to carcinomas of the lung and kidney in that orbital metastasis may be the only clinical clue to a silent and symptomless primary neoplasm. However, carcinomas of the prostate gland differ in their slower rate of growth, so that metastasis probably does not occur as early as with similar tumors from the lung and kidney; another point of difference is that the former carcinomas favor a dissemination to bone (pelvis and vertebrae), whereas the latter neoplasms metastasize more frequently to soft tissues. At the time of their review (1964), Bard and Schulze had located nine other examples in the literature of orbital metastasis from a prostatic carcinoma. They added two cases of their own. Clinical details of a few of these eleven cases were not recorded, and histologic identity of the orbital mass was not proven by orbitotomy in all instances. The latter is not a major defect when the age and debilitated state of some patients in the terminal phases of carcinomatosis are considered. This neoplasm occurs at a later age than other adenocarcinomas among males. Its peak incidence is in the latter part of the seventh decade, which is 10 to 15 years later than the average age of patients with other metastasizing carcinomas.

CLINICAL COURSE

Clinical signs of orbital involvement are similar to those already noted for other carcinomas, that is, early involvement of extraocular muscles manifested by diplopia, progressive proptosis, some degree of pain or paresthesia, edema or drooping of the upper eyelid, visual decrease is metastasis is located posteriorly, and a palpable mass if metastasis is in the anterior orbit. In our 85-year-old patient the involved eye was fixed in position and all vision was extinguished over a 10-month period by a destructive metastatic tumor involving both orbital bone and soft tissues. Two dissimilar features other than age incidence may help to differentiate prostatic carcinoma from other types. First, because of the tendency to metastasize to bone, roentgenograms of the orbit and adjacent bones more frequently are positive than with other carcinomas. Furthermore, the pattern of bony involvement is one of small, fairly circumscribed areas of osteoplasia rather than bony erosion and destruction so typical of other malignancies. This condensation, or sclerosis of bone, suggests stimulation of bone by diffusible substances secreted by the neoplasm. In the case of Schaerer and Whitney (1953), this bony hyperostosis of the sphenoid bone so mimicked meningioma as to prompt a craniotomy despite the patient's age (71 years) and rapid proptosis. Second, this carcinoma also has the peculiar property of secreting acid phosphatase. Increased concentrations of this substance in serum corroborate the suspicious evidence provided by the roentgenogram. Or, in the presence of a suspected orbital metastasis with a negative roentgenogram, increased acid phosphatase values may indicate the need to search further for bony metastasis, particularly in the pelvis or vertebrae.

Life expectancy of these patients is difficult to predict. In some, palliative measures such as orchiectomy and supplementary therapy with diethylstilbestrol seem to exert a definite but temporary beneficial effect. In others, these measures are ineffective and the patient lives for only a few months or less than 1 year after orbital metastasis.

CARCINOMA OF THYROID GLAND

INCIDENCE AND PATHOLOGY

Primary neoplasms of the thyroid gland combine several characteristics already noted as individual traits among other adenocarcinomas that have been discussed. Because of their varied histologic types, thyroid neoplasms resemble adenocarcinomas from the lung. In both organs true carcinomas and benign adenomas may develop, the latter sometimes undergoing malignant change. Some thyroid carcinomas are as indolent and slow in growth as are prostatic carcinomas; others disseminate as rapidly as small cell carcinomas of the lung. These neoplasms also frequently attack bone as do prostatic neoplasms, but their effect is osteolytic rather than osteoblastic. A distinctive feature not shared by prostatic carcinoma is the marked vascularity of some metastatic foci. Thyroid neoplasms occur in an age range (sixth decade) common to many carcinomas in adults but are more common among women.

These are treacherous neoplasms and it is surprising that orbital metastasis is not more common. Histologists recognize problems in separating some apparently benign tumors from those clinically malignant. Furthermore, what may appear histologically benign one day may become clinically malignant the next, or unknowingly may have metastasized some earlier day. Mitosis, anaplasia, and invasive tendencies toward surrounding blood vessels are marks of malignancy. Tumors with predominantly papillary patterns are prone to be, or become, malignant. Some well-differentiated carcinomas may retain secretory characteristics and thereby produce a false hyperthyroidism during metastasis.

CLINICAL COURSE

Some of these challenging features have been noted in a report of an interesting case by Oberman and colleagues (1969). The case was that of a 57-year-old woman who had undergone two craniotomies in a period of several years for what was thought to be, histologically, a chromophobe adenoma. The first operation was a partial resection. At the time of the second operation this unusual tumor had invaded the orbit. Such behavior was most unusual for a chromophobe adenoma with only minimal roentgenographic change. Further inquiry revealed that a subtotal thyroidectomy had been done earlier for a tumor of benign appearance, a moderately well-differentiated medullary carcinoma. When tissues from the orbit and thyroid gland were compared, they were identical and the true diagnosis was metastatic malignant thyroid carcinoma and not chromophobe adenoma. The authors rightly pointed out the difficulty of differentiating benign and malignant tumors of endocrine type.

Knapp (1923) recorded clinical features and histopathologic details of a thyroid tumor metastatic to the orbit in a 66-year-old man; he also reviewed two other cases previously recorded in the literature by Von Eiselsberg and by Jaboulay. We have had an unusual opportunity to review two cases observed during the years of our survey.

CASE 1. A 58-year-old woman complained of orbital symptoms that were the initial indication of an unsuspected thyroid malignancy. Symptoms were drooping of the right upper lid, progressive proptosis of the right eye, and transient diplopia during a period of 8 months. Examination of the right eye confirmed proptosis (7 mm); and a spongy mass was noted in the superior orbit and a destructive lesion of adjacent bone was observed on roentgenograms. The orbital tumor proved to be a highly vascular metastatic thyroid alveolar adenocarcinoma. Thyroidectomy for a "benign" tumor had been performed 29 years before the development of this orbital metastasis. Another thyroidectomy was performed within 10 months after orbitotomy for recurrent multiple thyroid adenomas. Within 4 years a craniotomy became necessary because of recurrent malignancy beneath the temporal lobe. This tumor proved to be similarly vascular and control of bleeding was difficult. The patient died several months later.

CASE 2. A 54-year-old woman complained chiefly of rapid loss of vision in one eye during a period of 5 months. During the month prior to our observations all vision in the left eye was lost. Moderate pallor of the left optic disk was noted on ophthalmoscopy. Roentgenography indicated erosion and decalcification of the clinoid process. A tentative diagnosis of intracranial meningioma was made. Exploratory craniotomy uncovered a soft, expansile, pulsating, apparently vascular mass encroaching on the roof of the orbit, optic canal, and sphenoid ridge. The mass so resembled an aneurysm it was believed wise to defer removal until further study could reveal its source and extent. Subsequent angiograms were negative. Further search then revealed a goiter which had been haphazardly observed and treated for 4 years prior to our observation. A subtotal thyroidectomy was performed and histopathologic study revealed a follicular adenocarcinoma, grade 2, which was invading the adjacent veins. The patient was treated with radioisotopes, supplemented by supervoltage irradiation. Nine months after surgery, metastasis occurred in the left orbit characterized by sudden proptosis and ophthalmoplegia. Further systemic metastases gradually appeared but the patient lingered for another 4 years before death.

CARCINOMA OF ADRENAL GLAND

INCIDENCE

Orbital metastasis from carcinomas of this endocrine gland is most uncommon, but it requires mention because one such case is included among our series of metastatic carcinomas (Table 25). They originate in the adrenal cortex, they are invasive and metastasize easily, and they seem more common in women. We have not found any case reports of orbital metastasis of this type in the literature since the comprehensive review of Burch in 1932. Interestingly, it was his observation of a case of orbital metastasis from bilateral tumors of the adrenal glands that probably prompted Burch to survey the entire literature for examples of other tumors metastatic to the eye and orbit.

CLINICAL COURSE

Burch's case was that of a 33-year-old man with rapid and progressive proptosis, ophthalmoplegia, papilledema, and visual loss for only 5 weeks. The patient died before a definite clinical diagnosis could be made. At autopsy an orbital tumor was found to fill the muscle cone of the involved orbit. This proved to be a metastatic focus of bilateral carcinomas of the adrenal glands.

Our case was very similar except for the sex and age of the patient.

A 77-year-old woman noticed the rapid onset of right blepharoptosis, proptosis, loss of vision, and orbital pain during a period of 2 months. The eye had become blind in a 2-week period prior to our observation. Examination confirmed proptosis (10 mm). The ophthalmoplegia was so marked that the eye was immobile. For several reasons an orbital exploration was not performed. One month later the patient expired. At autopsy, bilateral carcinomas of the adrenal glands were discovered. A metastatic focus was found to fill the inner space of the right orbit with infiltration of the optic nerve and adjacent muscles.

The course of metastatic tumors of the adrenal cortex, therefore, is rapid and the orbital symptoms alarming and severe. There is no satisfactory treatment for these neoplasms.

OTHER CARCINOMAS

Orbital metastases of carcinomas from many other organs are equally as infrequent as those from the adrenal cortex. Information about these carcinomas and their source will be found in the publications of Sniderman (1942) and Van Buskirk (1959), pancreas; Saxena and Darbari (1960), gall bladder; and King (1960), uterus. An unpublished report of carcinoma metastatic from the common bile duct in a 69-year-old male is that of Bullock and Straughen (1978).

TREATMENT

The prognosis of metastatic orbital carcinomas from various sources already has been noted. In general, the outlook is poor; life expectancy of most patients ranges from a few months with the more rapidly progressing types (lung and kidney) to several years with the more slowly growing variants (breast and prostate gland). Radical surgery, such as total orbital exenteration, cannot offer these patients a cure such as is sometimes possible with secondary carcinomas. Neither can the patient be assured that total removal of the orbital carcinoma by exenteration will significantly prolong life, even though the orbital neoplasm is the only known metastatic focus. Therefore, the treatment of patients with orbital metastasis is largely palliative and orbital exenteration is reserved for those patients who may suffer from unbearable pain.

Bibliography

Albert DM, Rubenstein RA, Scheie HG: Tumor metastasis to the eye. I. Incidence in 213 adult patients with generalized malignancy. II. Clinical study in infants and children. Am J Ophthalmol 63:723–732, 1967

Amdur J, Leopold IH: Metastatic hypernephroma to the orbit: report of a case with review of the literature. Am J Ophthalmol 48:386–388, 1959

Appelmans M, Michiels J, Jansen E: Métastases orbitaires bilatérales d'un cancer du sein détection par le phosphore radioactif. Bull Mem Soc Fr Ophtalmol 67:415–426, 1954

Bard LA, Schulze RR: Unilateral proptosis as the presenting sign of metastatic carcinoma of the prostate. Am J Ophthalmol 58:107–110, 1964

Bedford PD, Daniel PM: Discrete carcinomatous metastases in the extrinsic ocular muscles: a case of carcinoma of the breast with exophthalmic ophthalmoplegia. Am J Ophthalmol 49:723–726, 1960

Bullock JD, Straughen AJ: Carcinoma of the common bile duct metastatic to the orbit. Georgiana Dworek Theobald Society, Chicago, Illinois, May 1978

Burch FE: Orbital metastases from malignant tumors of the suprarenal gland. Arch Ophthalmol ns 7:418–431, 1932

Chatterjee BM, Deb M: Metastatic carcinoma of the orbit. Am J Ophthalmol 59:103–105, 1965

Ferry AP, Font RL: Carcinoma metastatic to the eye and orbit: I. A clinicopathologic study of 227 cases. Arch Ophthalmol 92:276–286, 1974

Ferry AP, Naghdi MR: Bronchogenic carcinoma metastatic to the orbit. Arch Ophthalmol 77:214–216, 1967

Gold P, Freedman SO: Demonstration of tumor-specific antigens in human colonic carcinomata by immunological tolerance and absorption techniques. J Exp Med *121*:439–462, 1965

Greer CH: Choroidal carcinoma metastatic from the male breast. Br J Ophthalmol *38*:312–315, 1954

Honrubia FM, Davis WH, Moore MK, et al: Carcinoid syndrome with bilateral orbital metastases. Am J Ophthalmol *72*:1118–1121, 1971

Howard GM, Jakobiec FA, Trokel SL, et al: Pulsating metastatic tumor of the orbit. Am J Ophthalmol *85*:767–771, 1978

Jaboulay: Cited by Knapp A

Kalt M, Tillé H: Metastatic orbital tumor, secondary to a renal epithelioma with late manifestation (abstract). Arch Ophthalmol ns *22*:933–934, 1939

King CM: Metastatic tumor of orbit. J Tenn Med Assoc *53*:143–145, 1960

Knapp A: Metastatic thyroid tumor in the orbit. Arch Ophthalmol *52*:68–74, 1923

Kulvin MM, Sawchak WG: Tumor of orbit: metastatic from malignant bronchial adenoma. Am J Ophthalmol *49*:833–838, 1960

Martin EW, Kibbey WE, Di Vecchia L, et al: Carcinoembryonic antigen clinical and historical aspects. Cancer *37*:62–81, 1976

Niessen V: Orbitametastase eines klinisch-latenten Magenkarzinoms. Klin Monatsbl Augenheilkd *129*:555–559, 1960

Oberman HA, Fayos JV, Lampe I: Pathology-radiation therapy conference: unusual orbital tumor. Univ Mich Med Cent J *35*:36–38, 1969

Richards RD: Unilateral exophthalmos: caused by metastatic carcinoma. Am J Ophthalmol *49*:1034–1037, 1960

Saxena BP, Darbari BS: Metastatic deposits in the orbit from carcinoma of the gall bladder. J All India Ophthalmol Soc *8*:69–71, 1960

Schaerer JP, Whitney RL: Prostatic metastases simulating intracranial meningioma: a case report. J Neurosurg *10*:546–549, 1953

Smiley SS: An orbital metastasis from the urinary bladder. Arch Ophthalmol *74*:809–810, 1965

Sniderman HR: Orbital metastasis from tumor of the pancreas: report of two cases with necropsy findings. Am J Ophthalmol *25*:1215–1221, 1942

Van Buskirk EL: Adenoma of pancreas with orbital metastasis. Am J Ophthalmol *48*:107, 1959

Von Eiselsberg [A]: Cited by Knapp A

Waller RR: Personal communication

Woody JH, Geeraets WJ: Orbital metastasis of renal cell carcinoma. Eye Ear Nose Throat *45*:90–93, 1966

18

Meningioma

The meningioma is a very important tumor in the fields of orbitology and neuro-ophthalmology because of its frequency, its destructive effect on vision, the difficulties associated with its surgical removal, its persistent course, and its sometimes fatal termination.

HISTORICAL ASPECTS

Optic nerve glioma and meningioma once were regarded as the same tumor both by clinicians bold enough to explore the recesses behind the eye and by anatomists at the autopsy table. Thus, it would be difficult to say just who first removed the tumor now designated meningioma. Reference already has been made (see Chapter 11) to the Scottish surgeon, Wishart (1833), who probably removed an optic nerve glioma. Several publications credit Scarpa (1816) as being the first to remove an orbital meningioma. These references usually are traced to Byers (1901), who reviewed the existing literature in his report on optic nerve tumors. Scarpa's description was not available to Byers, but Byers quoted two French physicians who, writing on the subjects of optic nerve tumors and the treatment of orbital tumors at a much earlier date, apparently had read the original. It was said that Scarpa's tumor was removed in pieces and that it was not possible to be certain as to the exact point of origin. It seems that Scarpa removed the tumor without injury to the function of the eye; if this is true it was a most remarkable feat for the early part of the 19th century. Although we have not been able to find the publication in which Scarpa described his operation, we believe that this venturesome surgeon probably was Antonio Scarpa, the renowned Italian anatomist and surgeon who, among his many pursuits, had an interest in the eye. Scarpa did not mention orbital tumors in an earlier (1802) publication on the eye.

This unitarian concept prevailed until the histopathologists, fortified by their microscopes, recognized the difference between the two tumors and further subdivided the neoplasms into histologic types and favored areas of growth. An important study in this period was that of Leber (1877), who differentiated the meningiomas arising within the dural sheath of the optic nerve and those arising in the outer sheath or attached to the latter. Leber also classified them according to their position along the nerve. Byers (1901) proposed that those tumors arising wholly within the nerve sheath be termed intradural and those growths outside the sheath whose origin was more obscure be termed extradural. In the meantime, as observers tried to clarify their histopathologic classification, various descriptive terms were applied to the tumors. The

472

important designation *endothelioma* was suggested by Golgi in 1869. Golgi did not invent this work but applied it to the meningiomas, as opposed to the meaning of the term epithelioma. Soon, the popular and durable name dural endothelioma was applied to this group of tumors because of their suspected origin from the dura. A period of nearly 50 years passed before the chaos of nomenclature finally was resolved by Cushing (1922), who proposed *meningioma*. This was a shortened version of meningothelioma, which had replaced the embryologically and histogenetically correct designation, arachnoidal mesothelioma.

Among the entire gamut of meningiomas we will be chiefly concerned with those that seemingly arise within the orbital cavity or reach the orbit by their expansion from adjacent tissues or structures. Those meningiomas that may affect the visual pathways but remain confined to the intracranial vault are only of supplementary interest. In other words, emphasis will be placed on those meningiomas which by reason of proptosis or the findings uncovered at the time of surgery were known to have encroached upon the orbital cavity.

INCIDENCE

In the central nervous system, gliomas occur much more frequently than meningiomas, but in the orbit the latter are more frequent. Among the 764 total tumors of the Mayo Clinic study series there were 19 orbital gliomas, an incidence of 2.5%. In the same sample there were 68 meningiomas (incidence 8.9%). This prevalence of meningioma over optic nerve glioma has been noted in all other studies of large numbers of orbital tumors. The definite prevalence of meningiomas among females is also generally agreed upon in the literature, though the sex ratio and size of the sample are not always stated. The reason for this high incidence in one sex is not known. Of the 52 cases of orbital meningioma in the Craig and Gogela (1949) series there were 41 females, an incidence of 79%. In our present series of 68 cases the incidence was 76% (52 of the patients were females). Incidence data from other studies are: 21 (84%) females out of 25 primary orbital meningiomas (Karp and Zimmerman), 11 (73%) out of 15 primary optic nerve meningiomas (Wright), and 71% females among 21 orbital meningiomas (Reese). These figures are remarkably close considering the relatively small sample sizes.

A comparison of other incidence factors between the Craig and Gogela study and our own is interesting because both include cases from the files of the Mayo Clinic. The former study was published in 1949 and presumably included all the orbital meningiomas up to that time. A termination point in their study was not stated, but it is likely that it included the tumors at least through 1947 and possibly through 1948 (allowing time for assembly, study, preparation of manuscript, and publication of data). As our own study covered the years 1948 to 1974, inclusively, it is unlikely that there is an overlap of more than 1 year between the two studies. Craig and Gogela classified their 52 orbital meningiomas into two groups: those that seemed to have a primary origin within the orbit and those that extended into the orbit from an intracranial source (secondary meningiomas). The first group included those tumors that seemed to arise from the optic foramen, the sheaths of the optic nerve, and those which lay more or less freely outside the optic nerve or were attached firmly to the peri-

orbita. The diagram of Walsh (Fig 290) illustrates the possible sites of origin of
this group. We agree with Spencer that a site of origin outside the optic sheath
or bony foramen is most unusual and difficult to prove. Nevertheless, we have
rarely encountered, at the time of orbitotomy, meningiomas in the posterior
orbit that seemed entirely separate from the optic nerve. Other cases in the
literature that seem to have proven features of extraoptic or ectopic origin are
Tan and Lim (discrete tumors along the medial wall of the orbit in a 9-year-old
female); Macmichael and Cullen (a circumscribed tumor pushing upward into
the lower conjunctival fornix of a 20-year-old female); and Wolter and Benz
(a firm tumor originating from the superior orbital rim in a 33-year-old
male).

The second group of Craig and Gogela included those secondary
meningiomas whose site of origin probably was the sphenoid ridge, the
basofrontal region, or the area around the sella. Such an anatomic arrangement
was based on the findings at operation or at autopsy. On this basis Craig and
Gogela noted twice as many secondary meningiomas as primary orbital meningiomas (35 to 17). Applying the same criteria to our own series of 68 meningiomas we, too, noted a prevalence of secondary meningiomas in the ratio of 46
to 22. The clinical features of the secondary meningiomas are more subtle than
those of the primary group, so it is important to remember the higher frequency
of the former class when reviewing the symptomatology of the orbital meningiomas.

In bygone years orbital meningioma was almost always considered a
disease of adults, whereas optic nerve glioma was predominantly a tumor of
childhood. This age selectivity always was cited as a convenient differential
among patients who presented with monocular visual loss followed by unilateral
proptosis. In more recent years an increasing number of cases of orbital
meningioma have been recorded in younger people (less than 10 years of age).
Two of the youngest cases on record are the 3-year-old male with a meningioma

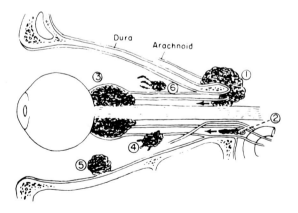

Figure 290. Origins of orbital meningiomas: diagrammatic
representation by Frank B.
Walsh, M.D., personal communication. (Reproduced from Reese
AB: Expanding lesions of the
orbit. Trans Ophthalmol Soc UK
91:85–104, 1971. By permission.)

A. From Arachnoid
  ① - Intracranial
  ② - Around canal
  ③ - Around posterior
       pole of the eye

B. From Ectopic Arachnoid
  ④ - In dura
  ⑤ - In periosteum
  ⑥ - In orbit

confined to the optic papilla (Martin and Scholfield 1957), and a 4-year-old girl with a secondary orbital meningioma arising from the sphenoid bone (Table 26). These and other observations have led to the conclusion that primary orbital meningiomas may be observed at an earlier age than the intracranial variety and are more frequent in children than has been generally assumed. In the series of 25 patients of Karp and associates, 40% were under 25 years of age. We believe this percentage is rather high and may reflect a bias of cases from younger individuals sent to the Armed Forces Institute of Pathology for confirmation of diagnosis because of their unusual age group.

Cooling and Wright (1979) also have commented on the disparity between the age incidence of the series of Karp and colleagues and the data published in the literature. Cooling and Wright suggest that some of the younger cases in Karp's series may, in reality, be examples of optic nerve glioma rather than meningioma. Cooling and Wright cite a case of an 11-year-old girl who underwent a craniotomy for a suspected optic nerve tumor. A gray mass involving the intracanalicular and intracranial portion of the left optic nerve was removed. The histopathologic diagnosis was primary optic nerve meningioma. Three months later, because of marked proptosis, a large tumor involving the intraorbital portion of the left optic nerve was removed through a lateral orbitotomy. The histopathologic diagnosis was astrocytic glioma of the optic nerve. In retrospect, the true clinical and surgical diagnosis was optic nerve glioma, the intracranial tumor representing a collateral hyperplasia of meningothelial cells that so often accompanies an optic nerve glioma. In conclusion, Cooling and Wright believe that diagnosis of optic nerve meningioma in the young should not be made solely on the basis of the histopathologic study of a tissue specimen, because follow-up observation may ultimately reveal an underlying glioma.

Age data relative to our Mayo Clinic survey is listed in Table 26. The salient features of this summary are a broad age distribution (4 to 83 years) of orbital meningiomas, a heavy concentration of the secondary orbital meningiomas in the 30- to 70-year age group, a higher percentage of primary orbital meningiomas in the young, and a differential of 4 years (40 versus 44 years) at time of presentation. Five (7.3%) of the combined total of 68 patients were younger than 20 years of age. Karp and associates also found that in young females the intraorbital meningioma has a predilection for the right orbit (seven of eight patients). The 3 patients of our series younger than 20 years of age with primary orbital meningioma were all males but all had involvement of the right orbit. Among the total 22 patients with primary meningioma the ratio of right to left orbit was 15:7. The laterality ratio among the total 46 patients with secondary orbital meningioma was 22:24, the left orbit predominating. In the combined groups the ratio was 37:31, right to left orbit.

TABLE 26.   AGE DISTRIBUTION OF ORBITAL MENINGIOMAS.*

Group and number (N)	Age range (yrs)	Median age (yrs)	30–70 years of age (%)	Younger than 20 years (%)
Primary N = 22	10–83	40	72.7	13.6
Secondary N = 46	4–75	44	91.3	4.3

*Mayo Clinic Series (1948–1974).

We have not found any statistics in the literature on the incidence of orbital meningiomas relative to total intracranial meningiomas. In the 27-year period of our survey, 486 intracranial meningiomas without orbital invasion were surgically verified. The ratio of intracranial meningiomas to orbital meningiomas, therefore, is 486:68 (roughly 7:1). The grand total of all meningiomas is the sum of these two groups, or 554 cases. The incidence of primary orbital meningiomas (22 cases) relative to total meningiomas then becomes 4%. The incidence of orbital meningiomas (both primary and secondary types) relative to all meningiomas is 12%.

CLINICAL FEATURES

The symptoms caused by a meningioma encroaching on the orbit sometimes may be so diverse that clinical diagnosis may be difficult or impossible, but, on other occasions, the signs of proptosis and loss of vision in a middle-aged woman with roentgenographic signs of hyperostosis are so clear-cut as to make the diagnosis seem simple. Too often the younger ophthalmologist assumes the latter situation to be the most common, encouraged by the retrospective case reviews recorded in the literature, but frequently the former situation prevails, with the diagnosis remaining obscure until the neoplasm is uncovered by the surgeon. The older ophthalmologist, having learned more often from mistaken diagnoses, realizes the wiliness of meningioma and the prevalence of atypical cases. Several basic traits of the meningioma family contribute to this collective clinical caprice.

First, the meningiomas with which we are chiefly concerned are, with but rare exceptions, residents of the posterior orbit. Seldom will they be palpated unless the symptoms have been so ignored by either patient or physician that the tumors have become enormous. Second, their very slow growth, together with their position, may contribute to a greater delay in surgical intervention as compared to other locally destructive tumors in a similar anatomic position. Third, their variable manner of growth makes for difficult diagnosis. Some will grow silently, carpet-like, across the surface of bone (usually designated by the French term *en plaque*), without appreciable reaction in the bone. Others will burrow directly through bony barriers or create such hyperostosis in adjacent bone as to leave telltale signs on roentgenography. Fourth, the location of the growth also contributes to atypical patterns of behavior. Some may select the sheath of the optic nerve in its orbital, canalicular, or intracranial portions. Others may confine themselves to more silent areas along the roof of the orbit or less important portions of the sphenoid ridge.

In contrast, they may insinuate themselves so quickly into important foramina and fissures between the orbital and intracranial cavities as to make their presence quickly known by the neural dysfunction that results. Finally, they may simply grow as a globular lump producing early displacement of the eye so characteristic of other tumors in the posterior orbit (Fig. 291). These variables should be kept in mind in the following discussion of the symptomatology of the orbital meningiomas as a group and of the clinical features of meningiomas in specific locations.

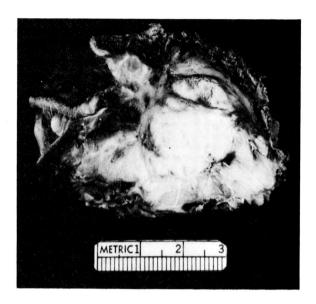

Figure 291. Recurrent meningioma: large tumor removed from left orbit by total exenteration; the patient, a 54-year-old man, had undergone four operations on left orbit, including three subtotal exenterations, one partial resection of tumor, and an enucleation, in the preceding 13 years. Photograph illustrates circumscribed but persistent growth of some intra-orbital meningiomas and difficulties in surgical eradication.

Secondary Meningiomas

Those meningiomas that secondarily invade the orbit almost always involve some portion of the sphenoid bone. Most commonly the wings of the sphenoid bone are the point of origin. Less often, the origin of the secondary orbital meningiomas is the basofrontal area, the tuberculum sella, or the parasagittal-frontal area of the cranium. Whatever the source the meningioma still involves the sphenoid bone in its journey toward the orbit. A possible exception is the meningioma that secondarily invades the orbit from one of the paranasal sinuses, but, even here, the sphenoid sinus is usually involved sometime during the progressive course of the neoplasm. There was one case of the latter type in our own tumor survey.

Although secondary orbital meningiomas of large size and long duration will show a considerable overlap in symptomatology, most of the secondary meningiomas will invade the orbit by one of two routes. The most common pattern of growth is that followed by the meningiomas arising along the lateral portion of the sphenoid ridge. These tumors, either by direct invasion of bone or the reactive hyperostosis they incite, involve the posterior orbital cavity or push laterally into the temporal fossa. The symptomatology of these tumors is more related to their bulk rather than neural, visual, or muscular structures entrapped in their growth. Patients with these meningiomas will present with *proptosis, edema of eyelids,* or *a visible mass in the temporal fossa.* Visual acuity in many of these patients will be normal.

The other pattern of growth is followed by meningiomas arising from the medial portion of the sphenoid ridge, the lesser wing of the sphenoid bone, and those meningiomas from other sources that pass the sphenoid bone en route to the orbit. Here, the tumor gains access to the orbital cavity either through the superior orbital fissure, along the optic canal, or by invasion and hyperostosis of bone at the orbital apex. Consequently, the impact on vision, extraocular muscle function, and optic nerve physiology is severe and overshadows proptosis in the patient's anamnesis.

Proptosis, the most common presenting symptom in this group of me-ningiomas, was present in 71% of cases. As a sign of orbital involvement its incidence was even greater — 88%. When present, the amount of proptosis ranged from 3 to 11 mm. The larger amounts occurred in patients with menin-giomas arising from the greater wing of the sphenoid bone or meningiomas of long duration.

Some degree of *visual blurring* or *visual loss* was the second most common presenting feature, occurring in 47% of the cases. However, when noted, it was severe (less than 20/200 in the affected eye). It was the latter patient who also would have definite defects in the visual fields, marked impairment of ocular motility, or ophthalmoscopically visible changes at the optic papilla (pallor or papilledema). These features reflected the compression of the optic nerve in its intracranial or intraorbital portion as well as entrapment of the nerves passing through the superior orbital fissure. Surprisingly, almost an equal incidence (48%) of patients had a visual acuity of 20/30 or better in the eye of the affected orbit at the time of presentation.

The other symptoms in this group of patients, in order of decreasing fre-quency, were *swelling* or *edema of eyelids*, *headache or orbital discomfort*, *blepharoptosis or diplopia*, and a *palpable mass* either in the orbit or temporal fossa. The duration of all these symptoms was so variable that no distinctive pattern could be stated. One patient, a 68-year-old female, contended that she had had visual loss for 35 years before presentation. The affected eye was blind with 11 mm of proptosis. Among patients who had noted both visual loss and proptosis, the former usually preceded the latter symptom by some time interval and the meningioma was of the type that invaded the orbit at its apex.

The clinician should be alerted to several other clinical manifestations of secondary orbital meningiomas. One of these is impairment of the afferent pupillary light reflex of the eye on the side of the tumor. The pupillary response to an afferent stimulus may be slow and the constriction of the pupil incomplete as compared with the uninvolved eye. Or, in reduced illumination the affected pupil may momentarily dilate in response to light stimulation. This is a subtle manifestation of early compression of the optic nerve by the enlarging meningioma and often precedes the more obvious manifestation of orbital in-volvement noted above. Also, the initial symptomatology may suggest a uni-lateral optic neuritis. Kearns and Wagener (1953) emphasized that, in optic neuritis, the pupil may not react promptly to direct light, yet there may be no impairment of the consensual reflex. However, in meningioma both direct and consensual reflexes may be impaired because of interference with both third nerve fibers as well as the optic nerve.

The visual field defects in this group of meningiomas tend to be prechias-mal in type. In addition to central scotomas and paracentral scotomas the visual fields may show a variety of altitudinal contractions as well as bizarre periph-eral defects. Seldom does an observer need to depend on visual field defects alone to make a diagnosis of orbital meningioma, but these defects are important if there is any suspicion of further intracranial spread of tumor. In the latter situation, visual fields will show bilateral defects or bitemporal char-acteristics of chiasmal involvement by the tumor.

Lastly, there is the frequently forgotten tendency of latent meningiomas to manifest symptoms during pregnancy.

Primary Meningioma

Almost all tumors of this group arise from the sheath of the optic nerve somewhere along its intraorbital course from the back surface of the eye proximal to and including the optic foramen. Although this distance is not great, the anatomic position and pattern of growth of the meningioma along this nerve segment explains the difference in symptomatology from one case to another. If the meningioma arises within the optic canal near the optic foramen, it will quickly compress the nerve because of the limited space for tumor expansion. Such patients will have rather marked loss of central visual acuity in the absence of any other signs of orbital tumor. The presenting picture of these foraminal meningiomas suggests a unilateral retrobulbar neuritis. Although these patients will seek attention early because of their visual loss, the diagnosis of tumor may be long delayed because of efforts to treat the problem as an optic neuritis. These patients also may have temporary obscurations of vision on rotating the eye into extreme fields of gaze.

Meningiomas originating in the sheath of the nerve at its distal juncture with the eyeball may also make their presence known early in their course without proptosis. Here, the mischief may be discovered on ophthalmoscopy by the first physician searching for an explanation of the sudden increase in axial hypermetropia of one eye. Papilledema will be noted and, more important to the diagnosis, an inward bulging or striae of the posterior wall of the eye will be seen; this is due to pressure from the tumor. It is these junctional meningiomas, as well as other long-standing tumors of the optic nerve sheath, which may invade the optic papilla or erode the sclera into the posterior choroid. Cases of this type have been reported by Henderson and Campbell (1977), Coston (1936), Newel and Beaman (1958), and others. Their data suggests that the incidence of intraglobal extension of a meningioma is considerably higher in children than the expected incidence of all types of orbital meningiomas in childhood.

The more common area of origin is somewhere along the sheath of the optic nerve between these proximal and distal points. In this locality the symptomatology is more dependent on the pattern of growth of the tumor. All such tumors commence as intradural tumors. If they remain intradural through a major portion of their course, the symptomatology may resemble the signs and symptoms of primary orbital optic nerve glioma. Visual loss followed by proptosis will usually be the initial sign of the orbital tumor. Pallor of the disk and atrophy of the optic nerve are the eventual consequences of this type of course (Fig. 292).

If, as commonly occurs, the meningioma erodes the dural covering early in its course, its subsequent exuberant growth may resemble that of other extradural tumors in the posterior orbit. In these cases, progressive proptosis, extraocular muscle palsies, edema of the eyelids, and a palpable orbital mass may precede visual impairment by a considerable length of time. In fact, some patients with this type of meningioma may retain a normal visual acuity for a surprisingly long period of time. These patients may not show pallor of the optic disk or have papilledema until late in the growth of the tumor (Fig. 293).

In all twenty-two patients in our survey with primary orbital meningioma *proptosis* was the most common presenting symptoms; this is a feature similar to

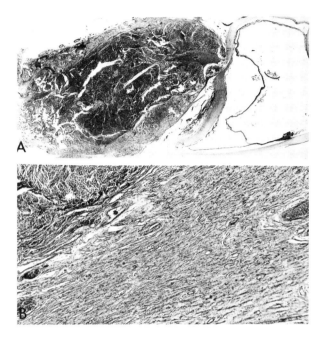

Figure 292. Primary meningioma of optic nerve sheath: *A*, Neoplasm located within optic nerve sheath just posterior to globe. (Hematoxylin and eosin; × 2.) *B*, Neoplasm located internal to dura; optic nerve shows advanced degeneration. (Hematoxylin and eosin; × 30.)

the clinical pattern of secondary orbital meningioma. Also, the pattern of straightforward protrusion with some inferior displacement of the eye in long-standing cases was similar in both groups. The incidence of proptosis in patients with primary meningioma was 77%. This incidence was equal as both a symptom and a sign of tumor. This indicates that patients with primary orbital meningiomas are more aware of their proptosis, or perhaps less concerned with other symptoms of the progressive meningioma, than patients with secondary orbital meningioma. In those patients with proptosis the average amount was 7 mm in the primary group and 6 mm in the secondary group. This does not

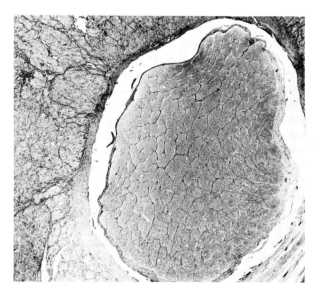

Figure 293. Secondary meningioma of orbit: neoplasm surrounds optic nerve but is entirely external to dura. (Hematoxylin and eosin; × 22.)

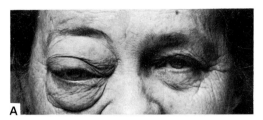
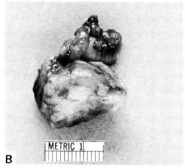

Figure 294. Intra-orbital meningioma: *A,* Slowly progressive proptosis and downward displacement of right eye of 10 years' duration due to tumor attached to back surface of eye; note the boggy edema of eyelids, frequently associated with long-standing intra-orbital meningiomas. *B,* Gross specimen.

agree with statements in the literature that proptosis in the primary group is less great because the patients are seen earlier in the course of their disease.

Some degree of *visual blurring* or *visual loss* was the second most common presenting symptom, occurring in 59% of the patients with primary meningiomas. We did not find that visual disturbance preceded proptosis in the majority of cases in the preoperative phase of the disease. This finding also is contrary to some statements in the literature. Only 26% of the patients in this group retained a visual acuity of 20/30 or better at the time of presentation. This is about half the number of patients with secondary meningiomas who retained nearly normal vision in the course of their disease.

The remaining symptoms in order of decreasing frequency were *edema* or *swelling of eyelids, pallor* or *papilledema of the optic papilla, headache, diplopia,* and a *palpable orbital mass.* The soft tissue edema that is rather peculiar to meningiomas may occur in either the primary or secondary meningiomas. It is pale, somewhat soft and boggy, and resembles the paunchy, bilateral eyelid edema of myxedema seen in women of the same age (Figs. 294 and 295). It occurs with sufficient frequency to suggest the diagnosis of meningioma if it is noted in the initial clinical assessment of the patient. Sometimes the edema is seen as a pale chemosis rather than being confined to the eyelids.

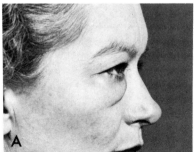
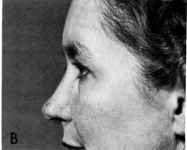

Figure 295. Intra-orbital meningioma; *A,* Right profile and *B,* left profile of face of 39-year-old woman illustrate eyelid swelling and edema sometimes associated with long-standing intra-orbital meningiomas; loss of vision and proptosis of right eye developed gradually over a period of 10 years, but not until swollen eyelids touched back surface of her glasses did she decide to seek consultation.

Another, less common clinical symptom that warrants some comment is the discomfort or headache that was noted by approximately 20% of the patients in the two groups with meningiomas. It was much more frequent in patients with secondary meningiomas. The discomfort was never acute. It was usually dull, not accurately localized, and sometimes difficult for the patient to describe. Inasmuch as orbital pain is not a common feature among orbital tumors, except for tumors in the area of the lacrimal gland fossa and those neoplasms that invade the orbit from a paranasal sinus, the symptom is of some supplementary significance in the preoperative assessment of the patient.

Occasionally, another clue to the diagnosis of meningioma may be seen on ophthalmoscopy. In some cases the meningioma may wrap around the intraorbital portion of the nerve in a cuff-like fashion. If this growth pattern compresses the central retinal vein in the area of its exit from the optic nerve proper, a circulatory shunt will develop between the retinal and choroidal circulation and be manifest as a dilated opticociliary vein (Fig. 27, Chapter 2). This finding is almost pathognomonic of meningioma if observed in a middle-aged female with visual loss, proptosis, and pallor of the disk. In children this finding is less diagnostic because the shunt has also been observed in association with optic nerve glioma.

Lastly, a more than coincidental association between meningioma and neurofibromatosis occurs in the pediatric age group. A child with meningioma is prone to develop a nerve sheath tumor or some manifestation of neurofibromatosis in the central or peripheral nervous system at a later age.

ROENTGENOGRAPHIC CHANGES

Roentgenography is a very important adjunct in the diagnosis of meningioma. A positive x-ray not only confirms the clinical suspicion of meningioma but helps to pinpoint its location and extent. The latter is particularly important if there is a question of whether the neoplasm has invaded the optic canal. Standard orbital views, optic foramen projections, and axial tomography of the optic canals are the studies most recommended.

The principal finding early in the course of most orbital meningiomas is *hyperostosis* of bone. This almost always involves some wing of the sphenoid bone and may gradually spread to the orbital roof, lateral wall of the orbit, posteriorly into the middle fossa, or medially toward the superior orbital fissure. This hyperostosis is a reactive response of bone to the spread of the meningioma along its surface. As the process continues there is more dense *sclerosis* and *osteomatous thickening* of bone (Fig. 296). Finally, the bone may look as eburnated and dense as an osteoma. Less frequently there is actual bone destruction due to invasion by the neoplasm. Such destruction may suggest focal deposits of metastatic carcinoma or the bone destruction of invasive neoplasms from an adjacent paranasal sinus, except that osteolysis of carcinoma has a more moth-eaten appearance, whereas the defects of meningioma have a more clear cut margin. When bone destruction is present it may serve as a warning that a more aggressive or cellular meningioma will be discovered upon surgical exploration. However important the bony changes are to diagnosis, the x-ray findings do not necessarily indicate the size of the soft tissue tumor. For the latter, particularly

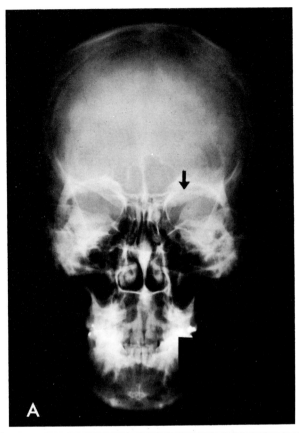

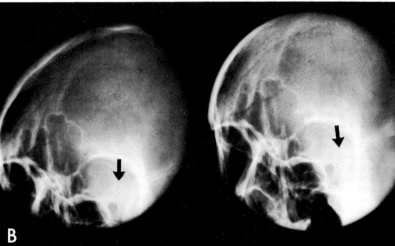

Figure 296.   Sphenoid ridge meningioma: roentgenograms showing thickening of sphenoid ridge (*arrows*) due to meningioma of 2 years' duration. *A*, Standard views; *B*, optic canal views.

the primary orbital meningioma, computer tomography or ultrasonography is a better diagnostic aid. On computer tomography, meningiomas show a more distinct enhancement after intravenous injection of contrast medium than any other orbital tumor except vascular malformations.

The foraminal meningioma may reveal its presence by an enlargement of the optic foramen on standard foramen projections. This enlargement is less round and the margins more irregular than the circular defect seen with optic nerve glioma. Early invasion of the optic canal, either by a canalicular meningioma or tumor from a neighboring bone, may appear on axial tomography as a demineralization and erosion of the bony wall of the canal. Later, hyperostosis and sclerosis may develop along the canal walls to a degree already noted in the sphenoid bone. Calcification, as a rule, is a very late finding.

Perusal of our own series of cases indicate a much higher incidence of positive roentgenograms in the secondary group of meningiomas as contrasted to the primary group. In the latter group, x-rays may show only an enlargement of the orbit, a feature not noted among any of the secondary orbital meningiomas.

PATHOLOGY

Neuropathologists have devoted much thought and study to the histogenesis, classification, and nomenclature of these tumors. The basic cell in these tumors is the meningocyte. Meningocytes are located along the outer surface of the .arachnoid and tend to cluster and clump at the tip of arachnoid villi. Kernohan and Sayre (1952) called the meningocytes *cap cells*, a term frequently quoted in the literature (Fig. 297). These cells are neuroectodermal in origin, but the supporting elements of these tumors — such as collagen, vascular channels, and fibroglia — probably are derived from the mesenchymal primordium of the meninges. The cells of these *meningotheliomatous* meningiomas tend to arrange themselves in solid sheets (Fig. 298). The nuclei of these cells are large,

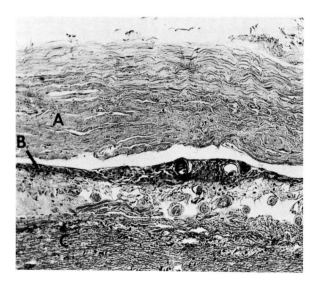

Figure 297. Meningioma: longitudinal section through normal optic nerve and sheath illustrating clumping of arachnoid cells into a "cap." A, Dura; B, arachnoid cluster with psammomas; C, optic nerve; widened subdural space is an artifact. (Hematoxylin and eosin; × 90.) (From Craig WMcK, Gogela LJ: Intraorbital meningiomas: a clinicopathologic study. Am J Ophthalmol 32:1663–1680, 1949. By permission of the Ophthalmic Publishing Company.)

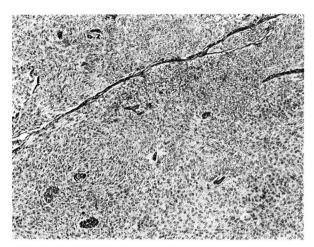

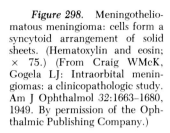

Figure 298. Meningotheliomatous meningioma: cells form a syncytoid arrangement of solid sheets. (Hematoxylin and eosin; × 75.) (From Craig WMcK, Gogela LJ: Intraorbital meningiomas: a clinicopathologic study. Am J Ophthalmol 32:1663–1680, 1949. By permission of the Ophthalmic Publishing Company.)

either round or oval, and vesicular and have a rather uniform distribution. The center of some nuclei have a washed-out appearance. The cytoplasm is finely granular but the cell boundaries are indistinct. Ultrastructurally the cell boundaries show complex interdigitations. Here and there in the tissue specimen pyknotic nuclei, staining darkly, may be seen; these probably represent an intracellular degenerative change. Varying amounts of stroma are interspersed throughout the sheets of cells. Some of this stroma may be exceedingly vascular and in other areas partially hyalinized. Mitotic figures may be miinimal or nearly absent.

Transitional types or mixed cell variants of the meningotheliomatous tumor also may be seen. In one of these variants the tumor cells tend to infiltrate the host tissue in small clumps and lobules. This gives the specimen, when seen under low-power magnification, the appearance of numerous whorl formations (Fig. 299); under higher magnification, these whorls appear to consist of

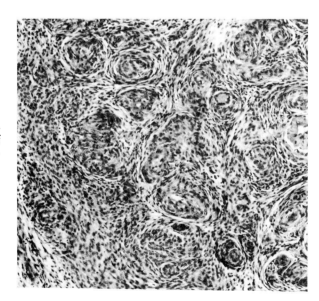

Figure 299. Psammomatous variant: appearance is one of numerous clumps with whorls. (Hematoxylin and eosin; × 100.)

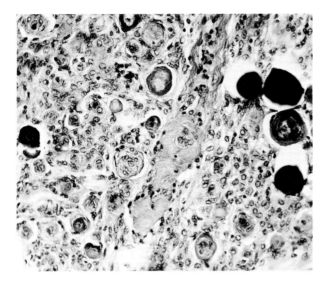

Figure 300. Psammoma bodies: central core of whorl hyalinizes and calcifies to form psammoma body. (Hematoxylin and eosin; × 90.)

concentric layers of cells, with or without a central vascular channel. The central core of the whorl tends to become hyalinized, and finally concretions of calcium salts (*psammoma bodies*) are deposited (Fig. 300). Concomitantly, the more peripheral lamellae of cells become more attenuated and less distinct in their staining qualities. Another tumor variant may incite a fibrous tissue ·response to its growth. Here, the connective tissue may be arranged in dense, almost hyalinized, bundles (Fig. 301) and in others the bundles may appear quite loose. Ensnared within the intertwining connective tissue are the meningocytes, but here the cells are arranged more in streams and strands.

One other, less common, type should be mentioned: the *vascular meningioma*. The features of this type of meningioma (Fig. 302) are closely akin to those of hemangioma. Some have preferred to designate these tumors simply as hemangiomas of the meninges. Others place them in a border zone, histologically, between the two groups. Sugar and associates (1970) have discussed this

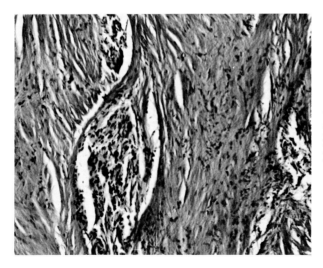

Figure 301. Fibroblastic variant: few meningothelial cells are present in the center, but much of the neoplasm is dense hyalinized fibrous tissue. (Hematoxylin and eosin; × 100.)

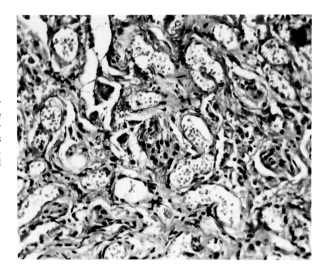

Figure 302. Vascular or angiomatous meningioma: some areas show features of capillary hemangioma, but other areas show features of meningothelial component. (Hematoxylin and eosin; × 205.)

problem. They reported a case in which the tumor finally was called a vascular meningioma because special staining showed that it did not possess the profusion of reticulin usually associated with hemangiopericytoma.

Not infrequently, tissue samples from some tumors will show a more abundant cellular reaction in proportion to surrounding stroma than is observed in the usual meningioma. The cells also may vary in size and shape, and mitotic figures are easily recognized (Fig. 303). These features suggest growth that is more proliferative and aggressive than average. Pathologists, both past and present, have designated these tumors as malignant; but there is some question as to whether such terminology is proper. There is little doubt that such tumors are locally aggressive and that they may cause death from successive recurrences of tumor that finally reach a vital intracranial area. However, they do not metastasize. Perhaps it is preferable to identify these tumors by using the terms *cellular active* or *cellular proliferative* and reserve the term *malignant* for those less frequent types that undergo sarcomatoid metaplasia and seem capable of multiple seeding and metastasis. Four of our meningotheliomatous meningiomas were considered to belong to the *cellular active* class and one case of frank sarcomatous metastasizing meningioma was observed.

TREATMENT

The management of meningioma is surgical. The more complete the removal, the less opportunity for recurrence and the greater chance for cure. The removal of most meningiomas is not easy. Several factors complicate the problem: the *en plaque*, infiltrative growth of most around the orbit (Figs. 304 and 305); and the tendency of meningiomas to envelop important structures passing through the foramina and fissures between the orbit and intracranial vault. Some meningiomas can be removed by the ophthalmic surgeon through a lateral orbital approach but the majority are best handled by the neurosurgeon through transcranial routes.

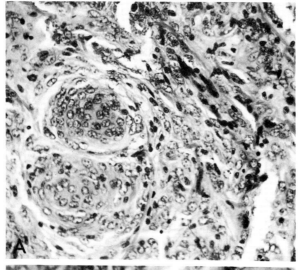

Figure 303. Cellular active meningioma:
A, Tumor is relatively cellular and the nuclei are larger, darker, and more variable. (Hematoxylin and eosin; × 265.)

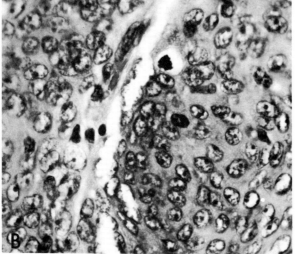

B, Tumor with plentiful mitotic figures. (Hematoxylin and eosin; × 600.)

The primary orbital meningioma that has only a relatively small attachment to the optic nerve is the least difficult to remove. These tumors usually are located on the lateral surface of the nerve sheath, they become quite large, are globular in shape, and finally fill the posterior lateral portion of the orbital cavity. Proptosis may be quite marked and the tumor often is palpable. If no intracranial extension has occurred the roentgenograms are negative except for some enlargement of the orbit. The tumors are easily uncovered through an anterolateral orbitotomy. Most of these large tumors are firm or gristly in consistency, yellow-gray in color, circumscribed, and may not have the vascularity of *en plaque* meningiomas. Rarely, the tumor may be friable and soft in consistency and contain cystic spaces. We also have encountered one well-circumscribed meningioma that grossly resembled a cavernous hemangioma. If the vision of the affected eye has not been seriously impaired, the tumor is resected

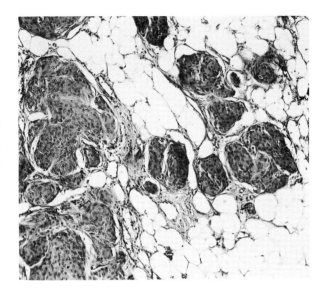

Figure 304. Orbital meningioma: neoplasm, though not considered malignant, is peripherally nonencapsulated and infiltrative. (Hematoxylin and eosin; × 90.)

near its attachment to the optic nerve and delivered. However, if the vision is poor (hand movements or less) and pallor of the optic disk is marked, we suggest removing the optic nerve with the tumor. Occasionally, the proptosis has became so marked or grotesque and the eye has been blind for so long a time, that exenteration of the orbit is proposed to the patient as a primary procedure.

More complicated is the removal of all other orbital meningiomas whether they are the primary or secondary type. Most of these patients will show roentgenologic or neuro-ophthalmologic signs of intracranial involvement, or ophthalmoscopically visible features of pallor of the optic papilla, papilledema, or retinal striae. The latter findings indicate an intimate relationship of the tumor to the optic nerve. The position of the latter tumor is the most difficult to manage surgically.

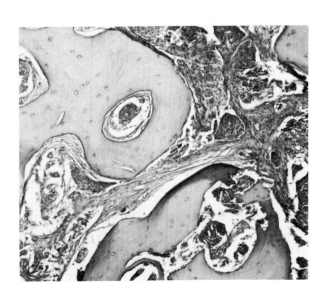

Figure 305. Orbital meningioma: example of extensive infiltration throughout osteomatous bone. (Hematoxylin and eosin; × 64.)

Factors such as the patient's visual status or the patient's ability to cope with a subsequent visual handicap will influence the extent of the surgical excision. If vision in the ipsilateral eye is reduced to recognition of hand movements or less, and if resection would permit more complete excision of the meningioma, there seems little reason to preserve the integrity of the optic nerve anywhere in its course between the eye and optic chiasm. Sacrifice of the optic nerve is more debatable where the vision is relatively good or the defect in the visual field is minimal. Most neurosurgeons tend to work around the nerve in these situations, preferring not to sacrifice the nerve and blind the patient if complete removal of the meningioma is questionable. They reason that the interval before recurrence may be so distant that the patient may continue to have some limited visual function of the homolateral eye, but in practice this caution and good intent are far from satisfactory.

Along the intraorbital portion of the nerve the surgeon may strip the meningioma away from the optic nerve proper inasmuch as a cleavage plane usually is present between these tissues. Or the surgeon may choose to meticulously tease the tumor piecemeal from its optic nerve sheath origin. On the basis of our follow-up data the latter method seems less traumatic than the former in preserving some optic nerve function. If the tumor is foraminal or canalicular in position the surgeon usually unroofs the optic canal. Often, these efforts to preserve vision prove futile. The surgeon also may prefer to electrocoagulate rather than excise portions of the tumor closely attached to blood vessels or the more inaccessible areas at the apex of the orbit. Lastly, some portion of the operation may become more an exercise in the control of hemorrhage rather than the intended removal of the tumor.

Irradiation therapy is used in situations where the basal or chiasmal position of the tumor makes it inoperable.

PROGNOSIS AND COURSE

Factors such as the position of the neoplasm, its size and manner of growth, and its proximity to important structures behind the orbit all influence prognosis. The cellular characteristics of the tumor, however, do not play as important a role in prognosis as compared with other orbital tumors of similar aggressiveness. Nevertheless, a guarded outlook is suggested for those few patients who may have the cellular meningioma and those rare tumors that show pleomorphic sarcomatous features. The latter are as rapidly fatal as other malignant neural tumors. Age of the patient also plays some role in predicting the course of the disease. Meningiomas in children and adolescents seem more rapidly progressive than tumors in the middle-aged adult. In the latter, the slow spread of the tumor may be compatible with a survival of many years.

Neurosurgeons take this well-known trait into consideration when they encounter a meningioma that has infiltrated important structures behind the orbit and prudently are satisfied with only a partial excision.

A study of the course of the patients in the Mayo Clinic series provides more specific data on many of these points. Considering the protracted course of the disease in many patients, the size of the total sample, and the wide geographic distribution of the affected patients, we consider it fortunate to have follow-up information of 5 years or longer (including those that expired from meningioma in less than 5 years) in 60 (88%) of our cases.

Of the sixty patients, fourteen are deceased (twelve patients from the group of secondary meningiomas and two patients from the primary orbital meningioma group). Among the deceased patients, 6 (10%) of the total 60 patients died directly from their meningioma. All meningioma deaths were among those patients with secondary orbital meningioma. Five of these 6 deceased patients were adults (4 males and 1 female), and the interval between diagnosis and death ranged from 3½ to 17 years. Three male adults had the cellular type of meningioma. All of these five patients had had multiple surgical procedures in an effort to stem the spread of the tumor, but to no avail. In each case there was involvement of the basal or midline intracranial structures, or spread of tumor into the middle fossa at the time of initial diagnosis. The nonadult death was a 4-year-old female who died 3 years after diagnosis of a pleomorphic sarcomatous variant of meningioma. The meningioma death could be related to the size, anatomic origin, and cellular aggressiveness of the tumor and confirms the more guarded prognosis of secondary orbital meningiomas. This mortality rate of 10% may be considerably higher than physicians are accustomed to accept on the basis of reviews in the literature of smaller series of cases.

The eight nonmeningioma deaths all occurred in adult females. One of these women committed suicide 15 years after diagnosis of an intraorbital meningioma and one month after an orbital exenteration that was necessary because of continued growth of the tumor. Here, the meningioma was considered an indirect cause of death because of the multiple surgical procedures required for control of tumor growth and orbital pain, and the patient's despondency over the cosmetic consequences of the exenteration. In the other women, survival ranged from 14 to 24 years after initial surgical diagnosis. Interestingly, four of these seven females died from other malignancies (lymphoma, multiple myeloma, and ovarian and thyroid carcinoma). In approximately 50% of the nonmeningiomatous deaths, residual tumor was known to be present in the vicinity of the orbit or adjacent intracranial space. The ipsilateral eye in these situations was usually blind and proptosed.

The follow-up information on the living patients 5 or more years after diagnosis is summarized in Table 27. The clinical course differed in several respects between the patients with primary orbital meningioma (Group A) and secondary orbital meningiomas (Group B). We will discuss Group A first.

The follow-up period of the 17 patients in Group A ranged from 5 to 23 years after surgical diagnosis, with an average of 13.7 years. The number of surgical procedures performed for the relief of the meningioma in this time period averaged 1.76 operations per patient. It is evident that the surgical procedure successfully eradicated the meningioma in the majority of cases, 76% of this group having no residual tumor in the follow-up interval. In terms of visual function or cosmesis, however, the result was dismal. Only one of these tumor-free individuals (patient N.T.) has 20/25 vision, although a visual field defect is present. The visual result in this patient also is remarkable in view of the three surgical procedures required. The patient with cataract (S.W.) also may have useful vision when the opaque lens is removed. These patients without residual tumor underwent a total of twenty-one surgical procedures of which thirteen were by the intracranial route and eight via an orbitotomy. There was a tendency of the ophthalmic surgeon to sacrifice the nerve at the initial orbitotomy and a tendency of the neurosurgeon to preserve the nerve at the time of craniotomy. However, the ultimate visual result was equally poor. It behooves the surgeon undertaking an operation for primary orbital meningioma to warn the patient of the probable crippling visual result. Whether the surgeon does or does not elect to section the optic nerve, we do believe that an effort should be made to preserve the eyeball. We do not suggest enucleation of the eye or exenteration of the orbit unless the cosmetic consequences of the proptosis are extreme, or less radical procedures have not been sufficient to eradicate the persistent, recurrent expansion of the tumor in or beyond the orbit.

The follow-up period on the 29 patients in Group B (Table 27) ranged from 5 to 26 years, with an average of 13.2 years after surgical diagnosis. The number of surgical procedures averaged 1.6 operations per patient. This data does not differ significantly from similar findings in the patients of Group A. However, the number of patients in Group B living without residual tumor is only 45% of the total, a sum much lower than Group A. This emphasizes the difficulty of eradicating a secondary orbital meningioma as compared with a primary orbital meningioma. In spite of this lowered incidence of tumor relief among patients of Group B, their visual result was much better than patients in Group A. Eight (61%) of the 13 patients without residual tumor in Group B have retained 20/60 or better acuity in the affected eye. Also, some of these patients with residual tumor have 20/20 or 20/30 vision. How can this be explained? The answer seems to lie in the anatomic site of the secondary meningioma. In the twelve patients, with or without residual tumor, who still have excellent central acuity, the meningioma involved the lateral portion of the sphenoid wing, the roof and lateral wall of the orbit, the temporal fossa, or combinations of these sites. Although extensive removal of diseased bone was usually necessary, the surgery did not involve direct or indirect manipulation of the optic nerve in its intraorbital, canalicular, or intracranial course. We conclude that operative management of meningiomas of the lateral portion of the sphenoid ridge carries a better outlook for preservation of vision than surgery of meningiomas in any other orbital position. Even so, some residual proptosis (sometimes of considerable degree) is almost always associated with surgical procedures in this particular area of the orbital-intracranial interface. This problem is related to the large amount of bone that is removed in the course of the operation. Most of the patients in the series were operated on in a period of time when cranioplastic procedures were not commonly used to close the bony defect in the roof and walls of the orbit, as they are at the present time. Proptosis, per se, is not an indication of recurrent tumor except when exophthalmometer measurements show a continued, steady increase in displacement of the eye during the postoperative years.

Lest the course of the preceding meningiomas seem unduly bright, another its equivalent) in the majority of patients with residual tumor in Group B. Most of the tumors in these patients arose along either the lesser wing of the sphenoid bone, the basal midline intracranial structures, or the basofrontal area. Some details from our case with the longest follow-up period (26 years) illustrate the relentless course and dismal outlook common to so many of the cases of secondary orbital meningioma.

**TABLE 27. ORBITAL MENINGIOMA: CLINICAL COURSE OF 46 PATIENTS
LIVING 5 OR MORE YEARS AFTER SURGICAL DIAGNOSIS**

Patient	Age at Diagnosis (yr)	Years since Diagnosis	No. of Operations	Residual Tumor	Remarks (Affected eye)
			Group A: Primary Orbital Meningioma		
G.C.	52	23	1	No	Vision 20/60, disk pallor, visual field defect
W.D.	33	13	2	No	Eye blind, proptosis 5 mm but stable
J.F.	10	11	2	No	Vision 20/50, disk pallor, proptosis 10 mm, removal of eye for cosmesis considered
H.H.	51	15	1	No	Nerve sectioned, eye blind
E.H.	41	20	5	No	Exenteration
M.H.	15	5	2	Yes	Ophthalmoplegia, eye useless
E.K.	39	19	1	No	Eye blind
M.K.	51	11	1	Yes	Vision hand movements, proptosis 5 mm and progressing disk pallor
E.L.	47	20	1	No	Vision 20/80, visual field defect, acoustic neuroma
L.M.	29	13	1	No	Ophthalmoplegia, enophthalmos
M.P.	12	9	4	Yes	Vision 20/30, proptosis 12 mm progressing
F.P.	39	7	1	No	Diplopia
D.R.	38	5	1	No	Blind, ophthalmoplegia
C.R.	49	17	1	No	Exenteration
M.S.	34	7	2	Yes	Blind, horrendous proptosis
N.T.	54	20	3	No	Vision 20/25, proptosis 7 mm but stable, visual field defect
S.W.	62	18	1	No	Cataract, proptosis 6 mm stable
			Group B: Secondary Orbital Meningioma		
M.A.	39	12	2	Yes	Vision counts fingers, disk pallor, proptosis 7 mm progressing
B.A.	36	17	3	Yes	Enucleation, head pain
R.A.	40	5	1	?	Optic nerve atrophy, cataract
C.B.	36	20	3	Yes	Nerve sectioned, proptosis 5 mm, orbital recurrence but no intracranial recurrence
V.B.	63	19	1	Yes	Blind, proptosis 12 mm progressing
W.B.	32	8	1	No	Vision 20/20, proptosis 2 mm
C.B.	56	20	1	No	Vision 20/30, some proptosis but stable
J.D.	43	5	1	Yes	Vision 20/20, proptosis 7 mm progressing
S.D.	63	13	1	Yes	Vision counts fingers
R.E.	58	8	2	Yes	Blind, ophthalmoplegia
M.E.	41	17	2	No	Blind, proptosis 9 mm stable
H.H.	58	10	1	?	Vision 20/80, disk pallor, visual field defect
D.H.	44	8	1	No	Vision 20/60, proptosis 4 mm stable
L.H.	66	9	3	Yes	Vision 20/25, disk pallor, proptosis 5 mm
B.H.	45	22	2	No	Blind, proptosis 3 mm stable
G.H.	62	10	1	No	Visual field defeet, disk pallor
K.K.	36	26	3	Yes	Enucleation, proptosis 15 mm in other eye and progressing
M.F.	55	15	1	No	Vision 20/30, proptosis 8 mm stable

(continued on page 494)

TABLE 27.　(Continued)

Patient	Age at Diagnosis (yr)	Years since Diagnosis	No. of Operations	Residual Tumor	Remarks (Affected eye)
C.M.	54	24	1	No	Vision 20/20, disk pallor, proptosis 8 mm stable
G.M.	63	5	1	No	Vision 20/30, proptosis 5 mm stable
R.M.	27	16	2	Yes	Vision 20/30, proptosis 9 mm progressing
D.P.	30	11	3	Yes	Vision hand movements, progressive proptosis, disk pallor
M.R.	62	5	1	No	Vision 20/20, proptosis 4 mm stable
G.S.	68	15	1	No	Optic nerve sectioned
L.S.	49	12	1	No	Neurotrophic keratitis, ophthalmoplegia
O.V.	44	7	2	Yes	Vision counts fingers, disk pallor, proptosis 13 mm progressing
J.W.	64	17	1	Yes	Vision 20/25, proptosis 5 mm slowly progressing
A.W.	68	5	2	Yes	Blind
J.Z.	37	22	2	No	Vision 20/25, proptosis 11 mm stable

Case report (Knudson). A 36-year-old female was first seen in March 1948 because of prominence of the left eye and swelling of left eyelid of one year's duration. Visual acuity and visual fields were normal. The left eye was proptosed 5 mm and mild edema of left eyelid was present. X-rays indicated an osteomatous thickening of the lesser wing of the left sphenoid bone. On transfrontal craniotomy a sessile meningotheliomatous meningioma with considerable surrounding osteomatous bone was removed from the inner portion of the lesser wing of the sphenoid bone. The optic canal was unroofed. Postoperatively, the eye was blind.

Over the next 3-year period, progressive proptosis of the left eye and a palpable mass in the left temporal fossa indicated recurrent meningioma. In October 1951 a radical resection of thickened bone along the roof and lateral wall of the left orbit was performed. Postoperatively, proptosis of the left eye continued to progress, reaching 14 mm in May 1953. At this time an enucleation of the blind unsightly eye was performed and residual meningioma palpated posteriorly in the left orbit. A recheck of the situation in May 1955 revealed continued growth of the meningioma in the left orbit with early spread into the left hard palate. The patient was next seen in May 1969 and, for the first time, involvement of the right orbit was documented. A small mass was palpated in the right lateral orbit, ocular rotations were limited in all directions of gaze, and striae along the posterior wall of the eye were visible by ophthalmoscopy. However, visual acuity of the remaining right eye was still 20/20. In addition, palpable meningioma was now present in the left cheek and the tumors in the left orbit and left hard palate had increased in size.

By June 1974 the swelling of the eyelids and the enlarging tumor of the left orbit began to push against her glasses and interfered with their wear (Fig. 306). A subtotal exenteration of the left orbit was performed removing the meningioma in several large pieces totaling 6 cm in diameter. No malignant change was seen in the histologic examination of the excised tissue but the tumor had become very cellular as compared with tissue first removed in 1948. Also, the proptosis of right eye had increased 16 mm as compared with exophthalmometer measurements in 1953. Still, the vision of the remaining right eye was 20/30 and surgeons were reluctant to remove tumor from the right orbit at the risk of visual loss.

In summary, in the 26-year period of observation, a meningioma of the lesser wing of the sphenoid bone had progressively extended into the left orbit, left hard and soft palate, left cheek, and right orbit.

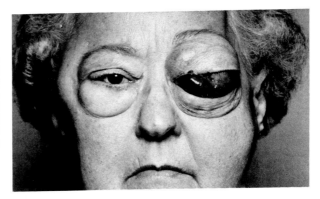

Figure 306. Secondary orbital meningioma. Over a period of 26 years a meningioma of lesser wing of left sphenoid bone has filled left orbit and extended into left cheek, right orbit, and right temporal fossa. An extension into left hard palate is not visible

Another interesting facet of the study of the patients in Group B was a number of instances in which the surgeon believed excision of the tumor was incomplete because some grossly hyperostotic bone remained beyond the area of surgical excision. However, in several such cases a recurrence of meningioma did not develop. This suggests that hyperostotic bone at the periphery of some of these meningiomas represents a reactive response to the tumor growth rather than invasion of bone by tumor cells.

Bibliography

Als E: Intraorbital meningiomas encasing the optic nerve. A report of two cases. Acta Ophthalmol (Kbh) *47*:900–903, 1969

Byers WGM: The primary intradural tumours of the optic nerve: fibromatosis nervi optici. Montreal Stud R Victoria Hosp *1*:1–82, 1901

Coston T: Primary tumor of the optic nerve. Arch Ophthalmol *15*:696–702, 1936

Cooling RJ, Wright JE: Arachnoid hyperplasia in optic nerve glioma: confusion with orbital meningioma. Brit J Ophthalmol *63*:596–599, 1979

Craig WMcK, Gogela LJ: Intraorbital meningiomas: a clinicopathologic study. Am J Ophthalmol *32*:1663–1680, 1949

Cushing H: The meningiomas (dural endotheliomas): their source, and favoured seats of origin. Brain *45*:282–316, 1922

Golgi: Cited by Cushing H

Henderson JW, Campbell RJ: Primary intraorbital meningioma with intraocular extension. Mayo Clin Proc *52*:504–508, 1977

Karp LA, Zimmerman LE, Borit A, et al: Primary intraorbital meningiomas. Arch Ophthalmol *91*:24–28, 1974

Kearns TP, Wagener HP: Ophthalmologic diagnosis of meningiomas of the sphenoidal ridge. Am J Med Sci *226*:221–228, 1953

Kernohan JW, Sayre GP: Tumors of the central nervous system. In *Atlas of Tumor Pathology*, Section 10, Fascicles 35 and 37. Washington DC, Armed Forces Institute of Pathology, 1952

Leber: Cited by Byers WGM

Macmichael IM, Cullen JF: Primary intraorbital meningioma. Brit J Ophthalmol *53*:169–173, 1969

Martin VAF, Schofield PB: Meningioma invading the optic nerve. Brit J Ophthalmol *41*:161–166, 1957

Newell FW, Beaman TC: Ocular signs of meningioma. Trans Am Ophthalmol Soc *55*:297–312, 1957

Reese AB: *Tumors of the Eye*, Second edition. New York, Hoeber Medical Division, Harper & Row, Publishers, 1963

Reese AB: Expanding lesions of the orbit. Trans Ophthalmol Soc UK *91*:85–104, 1971

Scarpa: Cited by Byers WGM

Scarpa A: *Traité Pratique des Maladies des Yeux, ou Expériences et Observations sur les Maladies qui Affectent ces Organes.* (Translated by JBF Léveillé.) 2 vols. Paris, F Buisson, 1802

Sugar HS, Fishman GR, Kobernick S, et al: Orbital hemangiopericytoma or vascular meningioma? Am J Ophthalmol 70:103–109, 1970

Tan KK, Lim SM: Primary extradural intraorbital meningioma in a Chinese girl. Brit J Ophthalmol 49:377–380, 1965

Wishart JH: Case of extirpation of the eye-ball. Edinb Med Surg J 40:274–276, 1833

Wolter JR, Benz SC: Ectopic meningioma of the superior orbital rim. Arch Ophthalmol 94:1920–1922, 1976

Wright JE: Primary optic nerve meningiomas: clinical presentation and management. Trans Am Acad Ophthalmol and Otolaryngol 83: OP 617–625, 1977

19

Neoplasms of Muscle

In this section, rhabdomyoma and rhabdomyosarcoma are discussed, and leiomyoma and leiomyosarcoma are briefly mentioned. The designation of this group of tumors as neoplasms of muscle is in some ways misleading and, in other respects, somewhat inaccurate. There may be some argument whether the rhabdomyomas and leiomyomas actually develop in the orbit, and the infantile form of rhabdomyosarcoma does not arise from muscle per se but from embryonic mesenchymal tissue capable of heteroplastic differentiation into muscle.

RHABDOMYOSARCOMA

HISTORICAL ASPECTS

Rhabdomyosarcoma, a malignant neoplasm related to striated muscle, probably has been known for as long as any other neoplasm discussed in this text. Even so, it has not always been known by this name. In the early literature it was described under such synonyms as *malignant rhabdomyoma, myosarcoma,* and *rhabdomyoblastoma.* Stout made a discerning analysis of the histopathologic descriptions in the literature before 1946. He credited one of the first descriptions to Weber (1854), who observed a localized enlargement of the tongue in a 21-year-old man. One of the first descriptions of the tumor involving the orbit has been credited to Bayer, in 1882. For many years, and certainly in the earlier part of the 20th century, this neoplasm was recognized as a sarcoma arising in striated muscle, usually in adults. Its appearance in the orbit was considered to be rare. The publication of Calhoun and Reese (1942) contains the best summary of the few orbital cases before 1942.

Stout's efforts at classification led to a proposal that some tumors whose cellular detail had some of the characteristics of myoblasts be included with the rhabdomyosarcomas. This proposal was accepted by most observers, which led to the concept that rhabdomyosarcoma need not always arise in muscle; rather it might originate among cells derived from primitive mesenchyme in soft tissues adjacent to muscle. These myoblasts were thought to possess the potential of differentiating into muscle tissue, albeit a distorted neoplastic form. This concept also engendered a means of classifying (with the rhabdomyosarcomas) various neoplasms affecting children which had hitherto been unsatisfactorily designated by terms such as *round cell sarcoma, undifferentiated small cell sarcoma, myosarcoma,* and *spindle cell sarcoma.* By the time of Stobbe and Dargeon's publication (1950), the term *embryonal* had come into usage as a descriptive designation for this more undifferentiated and primitive form of the neoplasm.

Stout's publication (1946) seemed to trigger the explosion of a voluminous literature on rhabdomyosarcoma. In ophthalmology the relevant literature has chiefly emphasized the form of rhabdomyosarcoma occurring in infants and children. What was once regarded as a differentiated neoplasm chiefly of adults is now overshadowed by a more undifferentiated, highly anaplastic, kindred malignancy in children. The 14 orbital cases prior to 1942 have increased by now more than 14-fold.

INCIDENCE

Resurgent interest in this neoplasm has resulted in statistical enumerations of its anatomic distribution in both regions and organs, its frequency in various age groups, and its incidence among other tumor types. The classic rhabdomyosarcoma of adult striated muscle most commonly is observed in the trunk or lower extremities. The more undifferentiated embryonal type is commoner in the head and neck; it particularly is prone to affect the orbit in children. Masson and Soule (1965), reviewing 1,093 sarcomas recorded in the files of the Mayo Clinic between 1910 and 1965, found 88 cases of rhabdomyosarcoma involving the head and neck. About 25% of these arose in the orbit. According to Exelby (1978), between 35 and 50% of all embryonal rhabdomyosarcomas arise in the head and neck, particularly in the orbit. The survey of Knowles and associates (1978) emphasized the preponderance of orbital rhabdomyosarcomas in children and adolescents. They pooled the statistical data from the four clinico-pathologic reviews of Frayer and Enterline (1959), Porterfield and Zimmerman (1962), Ashton and Morgan (1965), and Jones and associates (1966). In this composite of 161 cases, 121 (75%) patients were under 10 years of age and 35 (22%) were in the 11- to 20-year age range. The average age of onset of the cases in the four reviews varied only from 7.2 to 8.2 years. Some of the cases in the survey of Jones and colleagues we would classify as secondary orbital extensions from a primary source in the nasopharynx, nasal cavity, or paranasal sinus, but the age range of patients with primary or secondary orbital embryonal rhabdomyosarcoma is essentially the same. In practice, the medial wall of the orbit is sometimes so eroded that it is difficult to know whether the neoplasm had an orbital or paranasal source.

Data relative to the age range and origin of the neoplasm in the eighteen patients from the Mayo Clinic study is summarized in Table 28. Our youngest patient was 15 months of age at the time of orbital diagnosis. Even younger patients (neonates and infants) were recorded in several of the reviews noted above. The Mayo Clinic study contains a higher incidence of patients over the age of 20 than most surveys. Two of our patients were 39 years old at the time of diagnosis. In one of these patients the origin of the tumor was the nasal cavity. In the other the tumor arose in the soft tissues of the cheek adjacent to the parotid gland. In this patient there was a 3-year-interval between onset and orbital involvement, and this course combined with nearly simultaneous foci of neoplasm in the liver and lungs suggests the orbital tumor may have been metastatic rather than secondary in type. Orbital rhabdomyosarcoma in adults also has been reported by others. The oldest case on record seems to be the 78-year-old male reported by Kassel and associates (1965). In all but two patients of our survey the rhabdomyosarcoma was embryonal in type.

TABLE 28.   AGE DISTRIBUTION AND ORIGIN OF 18 ORBITAL RHABDOMYOSARCOMAS*

Age (yrs)	Orbit	Antrum	Nasal cavity or Nasopharynx	Other	Total
1–5	3	2	1		6
6–10	5	1	1		7
11–15			1		1
16–20					0
Over 20	1	1	1	1	4
	9	4	4	1	18

*Mayo Clinic Series 1948-1974.

The male to female ratio in our survey group was 13:5. In the composite survey of Knowles and colleagues, orbital rhabdomyosarcoma was more common in males in a ratio of approximately 5:3.

CLINICAL FEATURES

The most noteworthy clinical features of this neoplasm are its *sudden onset*, the *rapid evolution of proptosis*, and the *marked adnexal response*. By the time the patient is seen in consultation, only a few weeks to three months may have elapsed from the onset of initial orbital symptoms. This is particularly common in little children, and no other neoplasm affecting this age group except fulminating cases of granulocytic sarcoma, childhood lymphoma, neuroblastoma, teratoma, and histiocytosis X grows so aggressively. Occasionally the period of evolution is longer than 3 months in some adults and in some cases where the origin of the tumor is deep in one of the paranasal sinuses. The rapidity of onset is illustrated by Figure 307.

In children, the orbital onset frequently is attributed to trauma. So often does this occur in the anamnesis that we consider it a possible clue to diagnosis. Actually, on close questioning, the initial orbital manifestation of the tumor is often found to precede the injury. Or the injury is so trivial that it is not etiologically significant. Reference to an injury seems the easiest way for frightened parents to explain the puzzling swelling and proptosis of the affected orbit.

Proptosis, either preceded or quickly followed by *puffiness* and *discoloration* of the eyelids, is almost invariable. Sometimes the degree of puffiness,

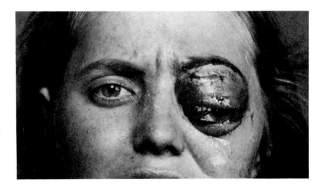

Figure 307. Rhabdomyosarcoma: rapidly enlarging orbital tumor of only 4 weeks' duration, with outward and downward displacement of eye. (From Masson JK, Soule EH: Embryonal rhabdomyosarcoma of the head and neck: report on eighty-eight cases. Am J Surg *11*:585–591, 1965. By permission of the Dun-Donnelley Publishing Corporation.)

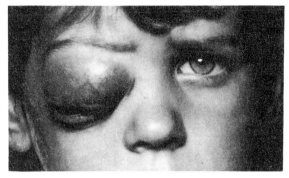

Figure 308. Rhabdomyo-sarcoma: embryonal type. Eye is proptosed downward and outward and there is marked edema of lid.

edema, or ptosis of the eyelid conceals the displaced eye (Fig. 308). In many cases the edematous eyelid has a red or blue color (Fig. 309). A reddish color might suggest the diagnosis of cellulitis, but a differential point is the absence of local heat and systemic fever with rhabdomyosarcoma. A bluish discoloration of the eyelid in an infant might suggest an infantile hemangioma, but, in the latter, the tumor is more soft and compressible than rhabdomyosarcoma and almost always increases in volume with crying. A palpable or visible mass is the next most common presenting feature. In all but one of our nine patients with primary orbital rhabdoymosarcoma, a mass was palpable. The mass may be palpated in any quadrant, and in our series, there was only a slight predilection for the superior orbital quadrant. In contrast, with the secondary orbital rhabdomyosarcomas, the mass most frequently appears medially, inferiorly, or posteriorly in the orbit.

ROENTGENOGRAPHIC CHANGES AND SPECIAL STUDIES

Routine, standard x-ray projections of the orbit are not helpful in either diagnosis or management of rhabdomyosarcoma because they are so often negative. Among the supplementary modalities, such as ultrasonography, computer tomography, and linear tomography, the latter has the most practical value. It will reveal bone destruction not seen by any other means. Orbital bone destruction is always present in secondary rhabdomyosarcomas and may be present in from 25 to 40% of cases of primary rhabdomyosarcoma. Tomograms should be done in both coronal and lateral projections, thereby establishing the extent of the malignant process. This is important in judging the question of threatened intracranial involvement, in planning the best surgical approach, and in determining the field of subsequent radiotherapy. In situations where a mass is not

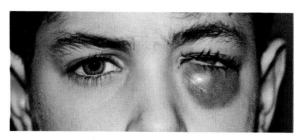

Figure 309. Rhabdomyosar-coma, reddish discoloration and swelling of left lower lid with up-ward displacement of eye of only one month duration in 11-year-old boy. Healed biopsy scar nasally.

palpable, ultrasonography and computer tomography may help visualize the size and position of the orbital mass. However, we think these two modalities are of more value in judging the question of tumor recurrence during the post-diagnostic periods of therapy and observation.

PATHOLOGY

The present trend is to classify these neoplasms into four histopathologic types. The term *pleomorphic* is reserved for those tumors with more differentiated, pleomorphic rhabdomyoblasts. This type is usually seen in the rhabdomyosarcomas of adults. They are very rare in the orbit. The designation *embryonal* is applied to the undifferentiated tumors seen usually in infants and children. *Alveolar* refers to arrangement of tumor cells in clusters resembling a glandular tumor. *Botryoid* is the term for those tumors that grow in a polypoid or grape-like mass from the mucosal coverings of body surfaces and cavities. This botryoid type is not encountered in the orbit except as a secondary invader from paranasal surfaces or the external eye. Both alveolar and botryoid tumors are now considered to be variants of the embryonal type.

Most of the literature on the histologic appearance and clinicopathologic correlates of the embryonal tumor has appeared in the past 20 years. Early in this period some pathologists were reluctant to make a diagnosis of rhabdomyosarcoma in those embryonal tumors where the cells were so undifferentiated that cytoplasmic cross striations had not yet appeared. This led to the designation *embryonal sarcoma* for the undifferentiated, nonstriated tumors and the term *embryonal rhabdomyosarcoma* for undifferentiated tumors with cross striations. The former term still is favored in the European literature but the latter term is increasingly used to designate both subtypes. All of these refinements in nomenclature were suggested at a time when histopathologic structure was believed to have some relation to prognosis. At present, the exact cellular detail of the several subtypes is not regarded as of practical importance in the prognosis of orbital lesions, and all types are treated essentially as the same malignant tumor.

The embryonal rhabdomyosarcoma is the variant most commonly found in the orbit. All but two of eighteen cases in our survey were this type. Grossly, these tumors are some shade of gray, tan, yellow, or white. Usually they are soft, partially circumscribed, lobular growths (Fig. 310) but may be myxoid, jelly-like, and infiltrative with indeterminate boundaries (Fig. 311). Occasionally, we have encountered small (walnut-sized) rhabdomyosarcomas with a pseudocapsule which "shell out" as easily as a benign tumor from the surrounding orbital tissue. Some tumors may have visible patches of red or purplish discoloration secondary to necrosis and hemorrhage.

Histologic descriptions of rhabdomyosarcoma may be quite complex because of the pleomorphism of the rhabdomyoblasts from one specimen to another or even in the same tissue section. The predominant cell in the embryonal type is a spindle cell with an elongated, centrally placed, chromatin-rich nucleus (Fig. 312). The cell is slightly larger in diameter in the area of the nucleus. The cytoplasm is acidophilic and, under higher magnification, may appear granular or vacuolated. These spindle cells may be arranged in parallel

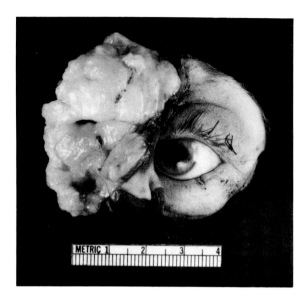

Figure 310. Rhabdomyosarcoma: neoplasm is gray and fleshy. (From same case depicted in Fig 308.)

or interlacing bands. In an adjacent area may be seen the less frequent, small, round cells with central nuclei, surrounded by a narrow rim of pink cytoplasm. These small cells may proliferate in a myxoid or loose syncytial pattern. These embryonal tumors are so undifferentiated that cross striations usually cannot be found, even after diligent search under high magnification. Here, electron microscopy of fresh tissue specimens may reveal the microfilamentary structures that cannot be seen under light microscopy. These microfilamentary bundles or bands are thicker (150A) than the filaments associated with smooth muscle cells. Sometimes a presarcomeric differentiation is indicated by vertical Z band formation.

In the alveolar rhabdomyosarcoma the small cells are arranged in clusters divided by fibrovascular septa (Fig. 313).

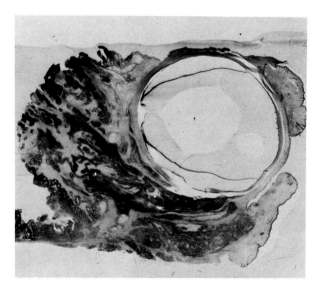

Figure 311. Rhabdomyosarcoma: embryonal type. Neoplasm is invariably extensively invasive. (Hematoxylin and eosin; × 2½.)

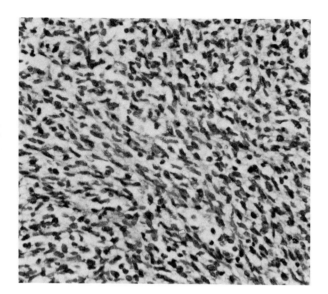

Figure 312. Rhabdomyo-sarcoma: embryonal type. Highly undifferentiated spindle cell sarcoma. (Hematoxylin and eosin; × 285.)

The pleomorphic rhabdomyosarcomas are more solid, circumscribed tumors as compared with the embryonal subtypes. Also, their color varies from pink to reddish-brown. In this subtype the cells are considerable larger but vary markedly in size and shape. Three basic configurations may be seen in the same tumor. The round cell may be five to ten times the diameter of the round cells in the embryonal tumor. The cytoplasm also is more granular. Strap cells or ribbon cells are so named because of their configuration. Some of these cells may have two nuclei arranged in tandem. It is in these cells that cross striations are most easily found (Fig. 314). Other cells of odd configuration are the tadpole or racquet-shaped cells that represent another stage in the differentiation of the rhabdomyoblast. In these cells the nucleus is located at the enlarged end of the cell (Fig. 315). Multinucleated giant cells also may be visible in tissue

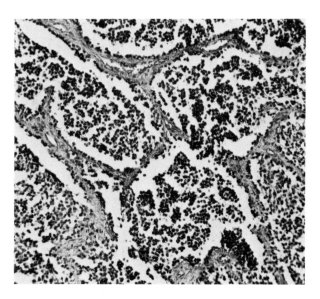

Figure 313. Rhabdomyo-sarcoma: embryonal type. Alveolar arrangement of cells imparts distinctive appearance to this subtype. (Hematoxylin and eosin; × 100.)

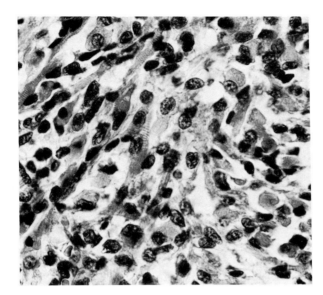

Figure 314. Rhabdomyosarcoma: striated rhabdomyoblasts. (Hematoxylin and eosin; × 700.)

sections of this histologic subtype (Fig. 315). Another giant cell variant is the spider-web cell. In this large round cell, delicate septae radiate peripherally through a vacuolated cytoplasm from a centrally placed nucleus. In the pleomorphic rhabdomyosarcoma, mitoses are present and may be bizarre in configuration.

TREATMENT AND COURSE

No other neoplasm in this text has undergone such a marked change in its therapy in the past 15 years resulting in such an improved prognosis as has rhabdomyosarcoma. Prior to 1965 most cases of orbital rhabdomyosarcoma

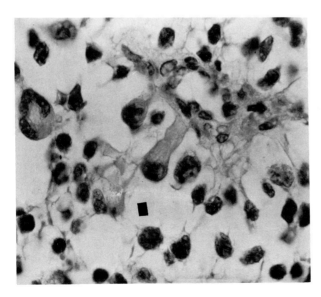

Figure 315. Rhabdomyosarcoma: cells are bizarre and varied, some multinucleated, some tadpole-shaped. (Hematoxylin and eosin; × 600.)

were treated primarily by surgery, and, in the United States, orbital exenteration was the surgical procedure associated with the longest period of survival (Reese 1964, Jones et al 1966). In a series of 44 orbital cases treated by exenteration, Reese noted a 3-year cure rate of 47%, but this survival rate was much higher than any other comparable series of cases reported up to that time.

There followed a period wherein irradiation was used as the major and initial therapy rather than as a supplement to surgical removal (Sagerman et al 1968, Landers 1968, Cassady et al 1968). This mode of therapy had its passionate partisans and its disenchanted detractors.

The next phase in management occurred when surgery and radiotherapy were combined with chemotherapy. The most important event in this phase was initiated in 1972 when members of three cancer treatment groups (Cancer and Leukemia Group B, Children's Cancer Study Group, and Southwest Oncology Group) combined their resources in a multidisciplinary study of the treatment of rhabdomyosarcoma in patients under 21 years of age. This coordinated, prospective study was named Intergroup Rhabdomyosarcoma Study I. Subsequently, most of the major medical centers with facilities to perform the pretreatment evaluations joined the Intergroup Study project.

The Intergroup investigators established certain guidelines for determining the extent (staging) of the disease, standardized the histopathologic diagnosis of the four histologic types of rhabdomyosarcoma, provided the means for record-keeping and statistic recall, established the intervals and frequency of review of the patient's course, and randomized various combinations of treatment for the patients who were entered in the study. All of this was done in an effort to promote some uniformity in the clinical evaluation of the disease, to collect a larger sample of patients for review than would be possible for any individual study subgroup or treatment center, and to minimize bias in the analysis of treatment results. Without such a cooperative effort physicians would still be floundering with the many clinical variables that made management and assessment of prognosis so difficult.

The staging of the disease was a most important concept in evaluating the effect of treatment. Four treatment groups were proposed based on the surgeon's evaluation and extent of surgical excision at the time of diagnosis, confirmed by the pathologist and pediatrician. Basically, all patients with localized disease, completely resected and without regional lymph node involvement, were placed in the most favorable Group I classification. Group II included those patients whose tumor was grossly resectable but in whom microscopic study revealed tumor cells along the margin of resection. Into Group III were placed those patients whose tumor was biopsied or incompletely resected, resulting in gross residual disease. Patients classified as Group IV, the most unfavorable group, had distant metastatic disease at the time of diagnosis.

The radiotherapy guidelines included recommendations for the total dose to be administered to each staging group, the length of treatment, and the variable dosage factors related to the age of the patient and the size of the tumor to be treated. Thus, a patient of any age with an orbital rhabdomyosarcoma in clinical Group II would receive no less than 4,000 rads and no more than 4,500 rads. Patients less than six years of age with a tumor less than 5 cm in staging Group III would receive a similar amount of irradiation, but the dosage would be higher (a minimum of 4,500 rads and a maximum of 5,000 rads) for tumors larger than 5 cm. Children 6 years or older with a tumor less than 5 cm also would receive the recommended 4,500–5,000 rads, but for larger tumors the dosage would be increased to a minimum of 5,000 rads and a maximum of 5,500 rads.

The major thrust of the Intergroup guidelines was to define the type, dosage, and combinations of drugs to be used in the prospective, randomized study. The principal drugs used throughout the study were vincristine, actinomycin D (dactinomycin), cyclophosphamide (cytoxin), and adriamycin. The protocols for the administration of these various drugs in the various clinical groups were quite complex. Thus, an orbital patient age 2 years in clinical Group III might be randomized to a program of vincristine 2 mg/m^2 intravenously on day 0 and 4, dactinomycin 0.015 mg/kg intravenously daily for 5 days, and cytoxan 10 mg/kg intravenously daily for 3 days, with the combination of all three drugs administered as repeated courses every four weeks over a period of two years. Or, the drugs might be given at a more concentrated level for a period of one year. Or, the drug adriamycin might be substituted for the dactinomycin in a randomized patient. In Group III patients, radiotherapy is started 6 weeks after the initiation of chemotherapy and is given in increments of approximately 1,000 rads per weeks until the predetermined total dosage is fulfilled. The protocols also permit initiation of radiotherapy as early as 2 weeks after the beginning of chemotherapy if the disease shows definite signs of progression.

In the course of the Intergroup Study from November 1972 through October 1978, 780 patients were entered in the study and sufficient data was available on 554 for analysis of treatment results (Maurer et al 1978). Fifty-four (10%) patients of the total were classified as orbital cases. Sixty-six percent (36/54) of the orbital cases were Group III, and 28% (15/54) were staged as Group II. The 2-year relapse-free survival rates of the tumors in all anatomic sites in the various staging groups were projected as 83% (Group I), 72% (Group II), 65% (Group III), and 28% (Group IV). No survival rates were separately stated for the orbital cases, but it is evident that these projections promise a brighter future for patients with orbital rhabdomyosarcoma than was noted for nearly the same total of patients undergoing exenteration prior to 1965.

The chemotherapeutic agents administered in the Intergroup study have a potentially high level of toxicity. Children treated under these protocols must be carefully monitored by the pediatric oncologist with regard to blood leucocytes and platelet levels, and a stand-by readiness to treat symptomatically as needed. Also, parents should be counseled regarding the anticipated changes in the child's kinetics and appearance during therapy. In effect, the child may appear worse before appearing better. Figure 316 illustrates the changes that may occur over the first year of therapy. Ophthalmologists also should be aware that an optic neuropathy, a blepharoptosis, partial extra-ocular muscle weakness, and facial nerve paresis may occur during the course of therapy. Those ocular complications have been attributed to the neurotoxicity of vincristine (Albert et al 1967, Sanderson et al 1976).

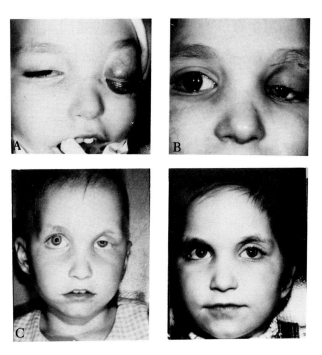

Figure 316. Rhabdomyosarcoma of left orbit in a 3-year-old female. *A*, Preoperative appearance under anesthesia. *B*, One month after incomplete excision of tumor and commencement of chemotherapy. Radiotherapy started 6 weeks after diagnosis. *C*, Five months after diagnosis. *D*, Eleven months after commencement of therapy. (Lekvin 3-312-309.)

The eighteen cases of rhabdomyosarcoma in our survey are small in number compared with the well-controlled Intergroup series, but a striking difference in survival is evident between the patients treated before and after the advent of the combined therapeutic program outlined above. Inasmuch as our survey does not extend beyond the year 1974, only two of our patients were entered in the rhabdomyosarcoma Intergroup study. Both of these patients are living 4 and 4½ years, respectively, from the time of diagnosis. In contrast, only 3 of 15 remaining patients (there was no follow-up on one of the total patients in the series) not treated by chemotherapy were alive 3½, 7, and 16 years after diagnosis. These survivors included two patients with primary orbital rhabdomyosarcoma and one patient with secondary orbital rhabdomyosarcoma. All remaining patients died from the spread of their tumor.

RHABDOMYOMA

Rhabdomyoma is a benign neoplasm composed chiefly of mature striated muscle cells. There is serious doubt whether there exists an unequivocal orbital case. Calhoun and Reese (1942) rejected most of the case reports of purported rhabdomyoma up to the time of their review, classifying them as examples of pseudotumor and neurofibromatosis. Subsequently, one case of rhabdomyoma of the orbit was described among the series of orbital tumors reviewed by Forrest (1949). This involved an 18-year-old man who had had slowly progressive proptosis for a period of 7 years, and a mass was attached to the superior rectus muscle. Diagnosis was based chiefly on the histopathologic finding of irregularly disposed and randomly arranged striated muscle fibers, and absence of an inflammatory component.

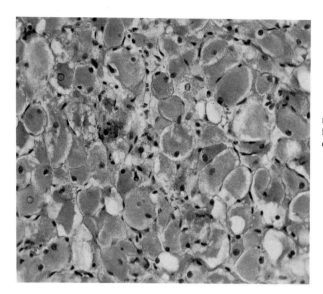

Figure 317. Rhabdomyoma: cross section of specimen from tongue shows striated muscle cells. (Hematoxylin and eosin; × 205.)

Nath and his colleagues (1965) have reported what they believed to be another case. The tumor, in a 35-year-old man, was attached to the inferior rectus muscle. Their diagnosis was based on the presence of a capsule, the absence of a sarcolemma, and striated muscle fibers showing marked anaplasia in their tissue specimen. But the specimen also contained focal aggregations of lymphocytes and plasma cells which would favor a diagnosis of pseudotumor rather than neoplasm. Last, there is the case reported by Knowles and Jakobiec (1975). This was an 8-year-old male with a slowly enlarging mass attached to the left medial rectus muscle extending superiorly and posteriorly into the superonasal quadrant of the orbit. The mass recurred 4 months after partial excision. An exenteration was then performed on the assumption that the case was a recurrent rhabdomyosarcoma. The patient was alive without recurrent tumor 27 years later (1965). In a reexamination of the original tissue sections, the authors concluded that the tumor was a rhabdomyoma, but a reevaluation by another team of pathologists supported a diagnosis of a well-differentiated rhabdomyosarcoma. There were no examples of orbital rhabdomyoma in our Mayo Clinic series.

The histologic appearance of a nonorbital rhabdomyoma is illustrated in Figure 317. The tumor of Knowles and Jakobiec was composed of compactly arranged large, round, or polygonal cells with abundant acidophilic granular cytoplasm occasionally exhibiting cross striations. The cells often displayed peripheral vacuolation because of the presence of large amounts of glycogen. Each cell usually had a single, eccentrically placed, vesicular nucleus with a prominent central basophilic nucleolus.

LEIOMYOMA

Another benign tumor of muscle is leiomyoma, a neoplasm of smooth muscle cells. As with rhabdomyoma, we are skeptical about the occurrence of true leiomyomas in the orbit. Such orbital leiomyomas as have been reported in the literature probably are examples of the venous or vascular leiomyoma, a tumor of blood vessel walls that we classify among the vascular neoplasms of Chapter 5. Except in the walls of blood vessels, smooth muscle fibers in the orbit almost are nonexistent. The orbital muscle of Müller and a peribulbar muscle, or capsular-palpebral muscle of Hesser, are described in some anatomic texts as being the only two smooth muscle bundles in the orbit. The former in humans is but a vestigial remnant of muscular membranes that form the inferior and lateral walls of the orbit in some lower animals; when present, it fans out across the floor of the orbit, having its origin in periorbita bridging over the inferior orbital fissure, and anteriorly it is continuous with the inferior oblique muscle. The peribulbar muscle is a thin band of tissue (width, 5 mm) stretching around the anterior half of the eyeball and is intimately associated with Tenon's capsule. The latter muscle sheath would be a scant source for nutrition of a neoplastic growth, and the former muscle bundle may not always be present. Thus a leiomyoma originating in either of these sources truly would be a curiosity. Another possible source would be the leiomyomatous component of a mesenchymoma, but such a tumor would better be classified in the latter group. Finally, smooth muscle bundles are found in the eyelids but tumors originating in such structures would be secondary rather than primary in the orbit. Terry (1934) has reported a case in which the tumor might have originated in eyelid tissue.

LEIOMYOSARCOMA

The leiomyosarcoma is an uncommon, highly cellular, malignant tumor of smooth muscle involving soft tissues and many viscera. The degree of malignancy varies and hence its course is unpredictable. Some tumors have been partially removed or simply excised and there has been no evidence of recurrence or metastasis after a follow-up period of many years. Other leiomyosarcomas treated by similar methods have been fatal owing to subsequent metastasis.

Leiomyosarcomas are said to occur in the orbit, but well-documented orbital cases are few. No leiomyosarcomas were found in the period of our orbital tumor study. Reese noted 5 among his total series of 877 cases, and Stout and Lattes (1967) referred to 3 orbital cases in a fascicle of the Armed Forces Institute of Pathology. Some duplication in these two surveys is likely because the same material probably was screened. Age, sex, and clinical features of these cases were not recorded.

An equivocal case is that of Bégué and Mawas (1953). Theirs was a case of a 6-hear-old girl with a tumor in the inferior orbit. The tumor was removed but it recurred in several months and exenteration was then performed. The child was followed for 3 years and remained in good health during this period. Bégué and Mawas regarded this neoplasm as an atypical sarcoma, but on the basis of arrangement of the cells, morphology of the nuclei, and the disposition of chromatin material, it was thought to have originated in smooth muscle. No photomicrographs of the tumor were included in their report. Jakobiec and as-

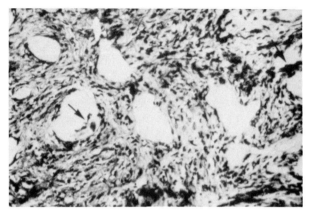

Figure 318. Leiomyosarcoma: the tumor is perforated by ectatic vessels, nuclei are hyperchromatic and irregular. The arrow indicates tumor cells in a vascular space. (Hematoxylin and eosin; × 320.) (From Jakobiec FA, Howard GM, Rosen M, et al: Leiomyoma and leiomyosarcoma of the orbit. Am J Ophthalmol 80:1028–1042, 1975. By permission.)

sociates (1975) thought the histologic description of this tumor was more compatible with the diagnosis of rhabdomyosarcoma.

Two well-studied cases were reported by the latter group. Both were females, aged 58 and 59 years, respectively. In both cases the tumors were located posteriorly in the orbit in the retrobulbar space. The first patient, who was treated by local excision, died of metastatic tumor 15 months after surgery. The second patient developed multiple local recurrences in the orbit. Five surgical procedures were performed including exenteration but the patient died of metastasis approximately 4½ years after diagnosis.

Each of these tumors on histologic examination had pronounced vascular patterns created by ectatic, usually bloodless, spaces. This is a distinctive feature of smooth muscle neoplasms. The tumors were infiltrative, the cell nuclei were irregularly shaped and hyperchromatic, mitoses were frequent, and multinucleated cells were scattered throughout the tissue (Fig. 318). Cytoplasmic filaments (myofibrils) were demonstrated with the trichrome stain.

Future encounters with these tumors in the orbit should be reported.

Bibliography

Rhabdomyosarcoma

Albert DM, Wong VG, Henderson ES: Ocular complications of vincristine therapy. Arch Ophthalmol 78:709–713, 1967

Ashton N, Morgan G: Embryonal sarcoma and embryonal rhabdomyosarcoma of the orbit. J Clin Pathol 18:699–714, 1965

Bayer S: Cited by Calhoun FP, Jr, and Reese AB

Calhoun FP Jr, Reese AB: Rhabdomyosarcoma of the orbit. Arch Ophthalmol ns 27:558–578, 1942

Cassady JR, Sagerman RH, Tretter P, et al: Radiation therapy for rhabdomyosarcoma. Radiology 91:116–120, 1968

Exelby PR: Solid tumors in children: Wilm's tumor, neuroblastoma and soft tissue sarcomas. Ca 28: 146–163, 1978

Frayer WC, Enterline HT: Embryonal rhabdomyosarcoma of the orbit in children and young adults. Arch Ophthalmol 62:203–210, 1959

Green DM, Jaffe N: Progress and controversy in the treatment of childhood rhabdomyosarcoma. Cancer Treat Rev 5:7–27, 1978

Jones IS, Reese AB, Krout J: Orbital rhabdomyosarcoma: an analysis of 62 cases. Am J Ophthalmol 61:721–736, 1966

Kassel SH, Copenhauer R, Areán VM: Orbital rhabdomyosarcoma. Am J Ophthalmol 60:811–818, 1965

Knowles DM, II, Jakobiec FA, Potter GD, et al: The diagnosis and treatment of rhabdomyosarcoma of the orbit. *In: Ocular and Adnexal Tumors.* Ed: FA Jakobiec. Birmingham, AL, Aesculapius Publishing Co, 1978, Chap 49

Landers PH: X-ray treatment of embryonal rhabdomyosarcoma of orbit: case report of a 13-year survival without recurrence. Am J Ophthalmol 66:745–747, 1968

Lederman M: Radiation treatment of primary malignant tumors of the orbit. *In Ocular and Adnexal Tumors: New and Controversial Aspects.* Ed; m Boniuk. St. Louis, CV Mosby Company, 1964, pp 477–490

Masson JK, Soule EH: Embryonal rhabdomyosarcoma of the head and neck: report on eighty-eight cases. Am J Surg *110*:585–591, 1965

Maurer HM, Donaldson M, Gehan EA, et al: The intergroup rhabdomyosarcoma study: update. November 1978. In press

Porterfield JT, Zimmerman LE: Rhabdomyosarcoma of the orbit: a clinicopathologic study of 55 cases. Virchows Arch Pathol Anat *335*:329–344, 1962

Reese AB: Discussion. *In Ocular and Adnexal Tumors: New and Controversial Aspects.* Ed: M Boniuk. St. Louis, CV Mosby Company, 1964, p 447

Sagerman RH, Cassady JR, Tretter P: Radiation therapy for rhabdomyosarcoma of the orbit. Trans Am Acad Ophthalmol Otolaryngol 72:849–854, 1968

Sanderson PA, Kuwabara T, Cogan DG: Optic neuropathy presumably caused by vincristine therapy. Am J Ophthalmol *81*:146–150, 1976

Stobbe GD, Dargeon HW: Embryonal rhabdomyosarcoma of the head and neck in children and adolescents. Cancer 3:826–836, 1950

Stout AP: Rhabdomyosarcoma of the skeletal muscles. Ann Surg *123*:447–472, 1946

Stout AP: Tumors of the soft tissues. *In Atlas of Tumor Pathology*, Section 2, Fascicle 5. Washington DC, Armed Forces Institute of Pathology, 1953, p 89

Weber CO: Anatomische Untersuchung einer hypertrophischen Zunge nebst Bemerkungen über die Neubildung quergestreifter Muskelfasern. Virchows Arch [Pathol Anat] 7:115–125, 1854

Rhabdomyoma

Calhoun FP Jr, Reese AB: Rhabdomyosarcoma of the orbit. Arch Ophthalmol ns 27:558–578, 1942

Forrest AW: Intraorbital tumors. Arch Ophthalmol *41*:198–230, 1949

Knowles DM, II, Jakobiec FA: Rhabdomyoma of the orbit. Am J Ophthalmol *80*:1011–1018, 1975

Nath K, Nema HV, Hameed S, et al: Orbital rhabdomyoma. Am J Ophthalmol *59*:1130–1134, 1965

Leiomyoma

Terry TL: Sarcoma of eyelid: metaplasia of leiomyosarcoma to round cell sarcoma after repeated attempted excisions. Arch Opthalmol ns *12*:689–692, 1934

Leiomyosarcoma

Bégué H, Mawas H: Léiomyosarcom de l'orbite. Bull Soc Ophthalmol Fr 5:490–491, 1953

Jakobiec FA, Howard GM, Rosen M, et al: Leiomyoma and leiomyosarcoma of the orbit. Am J Ophthalmol *80*:1028–1042, 1975

Reese AB: *Tumors of the Eye.* Second edition. New York, Hoeber Medical Division, Harper & Row, 1963

Stout AP, Lattes R: Tumors of the soft tissues. *In Atlas of Tumor Pathology*, Second Series, Fascicle 1. Washington DC, Armed Forces Institute of Pathology, 1967

20

Lymphocytic Inflammatory Pseudotumor

As we are concerned in this text with the various lumps, nodules, masses, and cysts that occupy the orbital space, it is proper to include a discussion of pseudotumor. It is not, however, a true tumor in the sense of persisting and growing independently of surrounding structures. Neither is it a hollow structure, as would be characteristic of a cyst. It is not malignant in the sense of threatening life. Neither is it as entirely innocent as a benign neoplasm, for eyes have been blinded and orbits exenterated because of its growth. Still, it is a definite tumefaction with features that warrant for it a niche of its own.

It is a most puzzling orbital disorder. Its etiology usually is undetermined, and should a cause subsequently be discovered, the tumefaction may no longer qualify as a pseudotumor. It is a self-limited disorder but, in the interval between onset and resolution, the clinical picture may be either so stormy or so mild as to make its course unpredictable. All attempts to treat the disorder may be futile. Therefore, we regard it as one of the most frustrating of the orbital tumors to manage and one that may create more dissatisfaction among patients than any other tumor. The complex nature of the disorder even starts with its definition.

TERMINOLOGY

The term *pseudotumor* seems to have been first úsed by Birch-Hirschfeld (1930) in the period 1905 to 1909. The tumor had been recognized earlier than this under the name of *pseudoplasma*. Pseudotumor, as a name, has only a clinical connotation. Many think it unsuitable because it is nonspecific, it does not give any hint as to etiology, and, more important, it designates nothing in regard to its pathology. In a clinical sense it indicates an orbital process that may simulate or mimic a neoplasm—a phantom neoplasm that upon orbitotomy is never found. In some cases, its masquerade as a neoplasm is so deceptive as to defy diagnosis until orbitotomy. The term *pseudoneoplasm* might be even more appropriate for such situations.

At one time pseudotumor was considered rare, but, as orbital biopsy became more common and less hazardous, an increasing number of nonneoplastic lesions were designated by this term. At one time or another the diagnosis of pseudotumor has included the orbital manifestations of endocrine exophthalmos, retained foreign body, various infections and parasitic diseases, trauma, lethal midline granuloma, adjacent sinusitis, leaking dermoid cyst, involuting lymphangiomas and hemangiomas, polyarteritis nodosa, multifocal fibrosclerosis, sarcoidosis, Wegener's granulomatosis, dysproteinemias, myositis, amyloidosis, and hemorrhage.

If we persist in referring to orbital derangements associated with all these local and systemic disorders as pseudotumor, the term becomes nondescript and practically useless from a diagnostic standpoint. We would prefer that all these pseudotumor-like patterns, instead, be designated by the condition that caused them; thus, gradually, the term would be limited to those pseudotumors of unknown etiology. By this means there will be greater uniformity among publications discussing this entity, and a greater concentration of subsequent observations and research on the chief crux of the problem: the etiology of the majority of pseudotumors. Hopefully, as our diagnostic methods improve, causes can be assigned to more instances of pseudotumor and the nonspecific name of pseudotumor will eventually disappear.

In essence, we are striving to make the definition more restrictive and meaningful. Our concept of orbital pseudotumor is that it is an idiopathic, localized inflammatory disease consisting principally of a lymphocytic infiltration associated with a polymorphous cellular response and a fibrovascular tissue reaction that has a variable but self-limited course. This definition excludes the granulomatous diseases but does include so-called *benign lymphoid hyperplasia*. We consider the latter condition a diffuse form of lymphocytic inflammatory pseudotumor.

INCIDENCE

It is difficult to assess this factor accurately. Most publications that attempt to compare various study series, whether they be large or small, overlook the lack of a universal definition. The incidence data from the Mayo Clinic series is not comparable in many respects to other surveys because our definition is so restrictive. There were thirty-five patients with lymphocytic inflammatory pseudotumor in our study. The sex and age distribution of these patients was noted in Table 3, Chapter 3. Although the disease may occur at any age, 71% of the patients were over 40 years of age at the time of diagnosis. The age of the oldest patient was 88 years and the youngest was 7 years. The left orbit was involved in eighteen cases and the right orbit in seventeen cases. There were no instances of bilateral involvement. The 35 patients represent 4.5% of our total orbital tumors and 10% of primary orbital tumors. These totals are less than the incidence of inflammatory pseudotumor cited in our prior edition because, at the present writing, pseudotumors formerly designated as Type I have been deleted and placed in the separate category of orbital vasculitis (Chapter 21), on the basis of histologic features different from Type II pseudotumors. The pseudotumors formerly designated Type II are the class of lesions we now call lymphocytic inflammatory pseudotumor. This change in classification and terminology in the interval since the 1973 edition reflects our efforts to confine the term to a more homogeneous histopathologic pattern. The high incidence of lymphocytic inflammatory pseudotumor (it was the third most common primary orbital tumor, see Chapter 3) among orbital tumors, combined with difficulties encountered in its diagnosis and management, emphasizes the importance of this condition in clinical practice.

PATHOLOGY

Inasmuch as our concept of lymphocytic inflammatory pseudotumor is so oriented to the histologic picture, a description of its pathology is an appropriate prelude to a discussion of the clinical features of the disease. Some authors have suggested a histopathologic classification of pseudotumors based on the orbital tissue principally affected by the inflammatory process. Thus, if orbital fat is undergoing destruction, necrosis, and replacement, the term *lipogranuloma* often is applied (Fig. 319). However, if muscle is predominantly involved, a subtype of orbital *myositis* is suggested (Fig. 320). In still other cases, an inflammatory invasion of the lacrimal gland is a very common feature

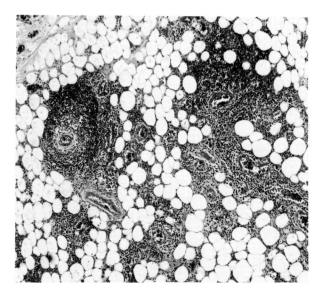

Figure 319. Lymphocytic inflammatory pseudotumor: dense infiltration of lymphocytes into orbital fat with marked vascular proliferation. (Hematoxylin and eosin; × 64.)

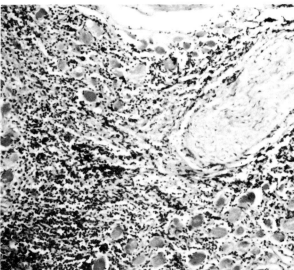

Figure 320. Lymphocytic inflammatory pseudotumor: infiltration of extraocular muscle bundles and nerves. (Hematoxylin and eosin; × 100.)

and the name *idiopathic* or *pseudotumorous dacryoadenitis* is readily applied (Fig. 321). We believe that such classifications founded on tissue selectivity are misleading for several reasons. First, if the biopsy is small, the pathologist has no means of determining the full extent of the disease, and he may gain a false impression that the disorder is limited to a particular orbital tissue. Second, because the lacrimal gland is situated well forward in the orbit, it is easily included in many biopsies and is one reason for the prevalent concept that pseudotumor is a form of dacryoadenitis. Third — at the other extreme — a more cautious approach to muscle biopsy (because of the scar and dysfunction resulting from surgical incision) accounts for the less frequent diagnosis of myositis. Fourth, if large specimens are examined, such as those obtained by exenteration of the orbit, it will be evident that pseudotumor can be a diffuse process involving fat, muscle, nerves, blood vessels, and lacrimal gland in all gradations of extent and severity. In other words, whether the tissue be lacrimal gland or muscle the basic inflammatory process is similar and represents the chance residence of the tumor in that particular tissue. We believe it easiest to think of pseudotumor as having a proclivity to lodge anywhere in the orbit and to grasp any soft tissue structure that stands in the way of its growth.

Other observers are more inclined to propose a classification based on the cellular components of the tumor, but the interpretation and meaning of these cellular patterns vary so much that no one classification has had more than token acceptance. Reese, for example, grouped his cases into five histopathologic categories, whereas Blodi and Gass (1967) grouped theirs into nine histologic types. Such variations from one author to another are understandable when we remember the variety of diseases that have been assigned to the pseudotumor category. The cellular response in any given specimen might consist of lymphocytes, eosinophils, plasma cells, polymorphonuclear leukocytes, and macrophages in differing number and proportion. Furthermore, the architectural arrangement of these cells may vary from one specimen to

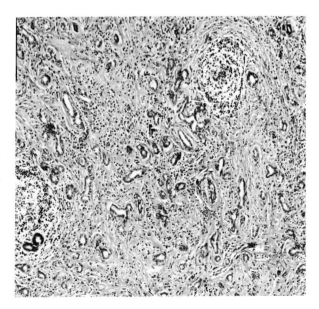

Figure 321. Lymphocytic inflammatory pseudotumor: lacrimal gland practically is replaced by dense fibrous tissue, and focal lymphoid aggregates are present. (Hematoxylin and eosin; × 64.)

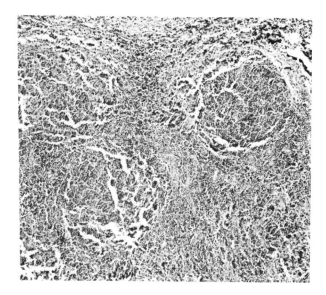

Figure 322. Lymphocytic inflammatory pseudotumor: massive infiltration of orbital tissues by lymphocytes with follicle-like groups of cells. (Hematoxylin and eosin; × 64.)

another. The lymphocytes, in particular, may form a *diffuse*, sheet-like infiltration of mature cells interspersed with oval, follicle-like groups of lymphocytes (Figs. 322 and 323). Some of these follicles will have less dense, paler staining centers composed of larger, more immature "reticulum-like" cells, simulating the germinal centers of lymph nodes. Under higher magnification an admixture of other cells, particularly plasma cells, may be seen scattered haphazardly throughout the specimen. In zones where capillary proliferation is prominent there may be some perivascular cuffs of lymphocytes but there is no true vascu-

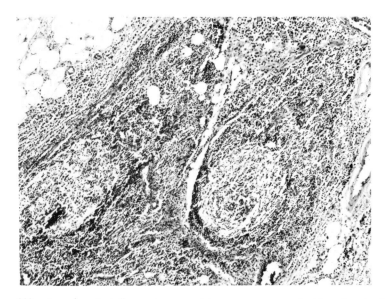

Figure 323.   Lymphocytic inflammatory pseudotumor: arrangement of lymphocytes into follicular structures is characteristic. (Hematoxylin and eosin; × 64.)

litis (Fig. 319). The diffuseness and density of the cellular response may suggest a well-differentiated type of diffuse, lymphoma, but the latter does not have either the follicles, the polymorphous cellular population, or the capillary proliferation of the pseudotumor. Five of our thirty-five cases showed this diffuse lymphocytic histologic pattern.

In other tumor specimens, *fibrosis* is the dominant histologic feature. Here, the lymphocytes are crowded into compact, deeply staining, nodular aggregates by bands of mature fibrocytes (Fig. 324). If the process of fibrosis continues, the nodular collections of lymphocytes are further compressed and isolated, and they stand out prominently as oases of cells amidst a desert of avascular, acellular, collagenized tissue (Fig. 325). The majority of our pseudotumors (eighteen of thirty-five cases) showed the predominant pattern of fibrosis.

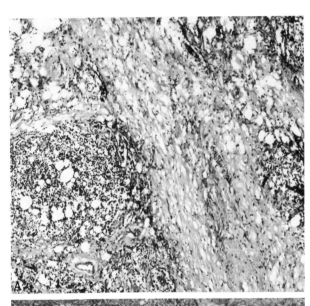

Figure 324. Lymphocytic
A, Lymphoid infiltration is significant but fibrosis is prominent; note follicular arrangement of lymphocytes. (Hematoxylin and eosin; × 40.)

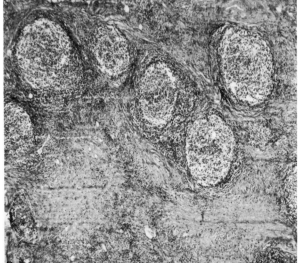

B, Detail of fibrosis. (Hematoxylin and eosin; × 64.)

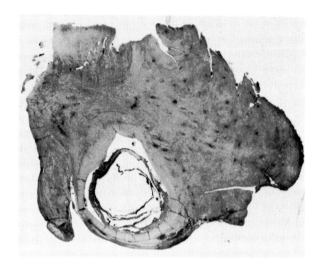

Figure 325. Lymphocytic inflammatory pseudotumor: orbit massively fibrotic and globe trapped in dense connective tissue; small dark spots are lymphoid aggregates. (Hematoxylin and eosin; × 2½.)

A third histologic subtype of lymphocytic inflammatory pseudotumor may show areas of active fibrosis, capillary proliferation, and sheets of lymphocytes. We refer to this subtype as *mixed* (twelve of thirty-five cases). When the tissue specimen is large, such as after an exenteration, all three subtypes may be seen. This suggests a dynamic inflammatory process that commences as a lymphocytic infiltration, continues with a fibrovascular response, and ends as a burned-out, acellular fibrotic residuum (Fig. 326). In the prior edition of our text, these several phases were designated acute, subacute, and chronic, suggesting a continuum of changes related to the duration of the lesion. However, a reexamination of our cases revealed that time was not the only factor that influenced the histologic subtype. For example, several cases with symptoms of short duration (2 months) showed the histologic picture of fairly marked fibrosis. In contrast, one of our cases with the longest duration of symptoms (2 years) showed

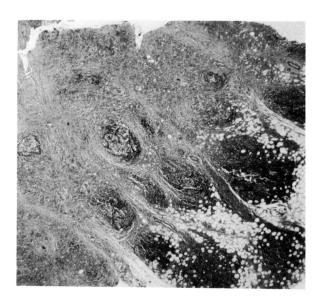

Figure 326. Lymphocytic inflammatory pseudotumor: peripherally, active advancing inflammation; centrally, a chronic fibrotic central zone. (Hematoxylin and eosin; × 16.)

only the features of a profuse lymphocytic infiltration. Therefore, the response of the orbital tissues to the unknown etiologic agent plays some role in the pattern of the cellular response. If the reaction of the orbital tissue to the idiopathic stimulus is intense and acute, the result may be an immediate or accelerated fibrosis. Therefore, our prior designations of acute, subacute, and chronic are not appropriate for these various phases of the inflammatory process in all cases. It seemed appropriate to revise our terminology and use the terms diffuse, mixed, and fibrosis to designate the respective histologic subtypes. We also suspect, on the basis of clinical observation, that the disease may terminate either spontaneously or in response to therapy at any of these several histologic substages.

Although we cannot make a definite correlation between the histologic types of pseudotumor and either the duration of the disease or the clinical features at time of presentation, our data does suggest the diffuse infiltrative type has a better response to therapy than the advanced fibrotic type of pseudotumor.

Descriptions of the gross features of pseudotumor vary. The more common specimen undergoing fibrosis is flavinaceous, firm but somewhat rubbery, nodular, and partially circumscribed. The latter feature is particularly evident in those pseudotumors that grow anteriorly beneath the orbital roof. Also, a cleavage plane may develop where the tumor abuts the tough orbital septum. Sometimes, the surfaces of the tumor and orbital septum fuse. Pseudotumors in these locations tend to be discoid or pancake-shaped with a slight concavity on the surface of the mass adjacent to the underlying eye. Posteriorly, the borders of these tumors are poorly defined. A particularly large, lumpy, fibrous pseudotumor is illustrated in Figure 327.

Those tumors of the diffuse histologic subtype are less firm and have a more reddish-flesh color. This color probably is related to the increased vascularity of this tumor subtype. In contrast is the avascular, hard, gristly character of those pseudotumors that have undergone the end stages of fibrosis. Some of these specimens are grossly fused with the orbital tissues (muscle, lacrimal gland, nerves, periorbita, and so on) that have been entrapped by the growth of the tumor.

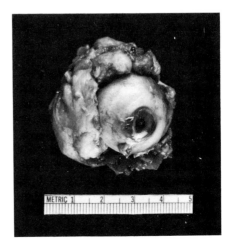

Figure 327. Lymphocytic inflammatory pseudotumor: gross specimen illustrates the lumpy and infiltrative appearance of an orbital pseudotumor almost completely encircling eyeball; tumor was of 3 years' duration, and in this interval orbital decompression, antibiotics and steroids, and irradiation had failed to arrest the inflammatory process and to prevent blindness. Progressive proptosis and pain finally necessitated exenteration.

CLINICAL FEATURES

The four symptoms of lymphocytic inflammatory pseudotumor most commonly noted by the patients were *swelling* or *puffiness of the eyelids, protrusion of the eye, orbital pain,* and *disturbance of ocular motility.* Roughly, one-third of the patients noted three of these four symptoms in their anamnesis, one-third had two of the symptoms, and another third had only one symptom at time of presentation. Only a small minority of patients had noted four or more symptoms in the prediagnostic course of their illness. Swelling and edema of the eyelids with or without some blepharoptosis of the upper eyelid was the chief presenting symptom in about 50% of the patients (Fig. 328). This edema was more firm and more often confined to the upper eyelid as compared with the more baggy edema of the lower eyelids so often seen in patients with meningioma (Chapter 18). Protrusion of the eye was the second most common presenting symptom. It was noted by only twelve of the thirty-five patients, but measurable proptosis was noted by the physician in thirty-two of the thirty-five patients. What is the explanation for this discrepancy? In general, a proptosis of 3 mm or less was usually overlooked by the patient probably because of their concern with other symptoms such as swelling of eyelids, pain, and diplopia. When proptosis was noted by the patient in the course of onset it usually proved to be 4 mm or more at the time of the initial examination. However, there was no specific feature of the proptosis that suggested the diagnosis of pseudotumors.

Orbital pain also was nonspecific. Most often it was described as a dull headache. This clinical feature also was similar to the headache described by patients with secondary orbital meningiomas. Likewise, no specific diagnostic significance could be attached to the disturbance of ocular motility noted in some cases.

Chemosis, redness of the eye or eyelid, a palpable lump, or visual loss was either observed by the patient or noted by the physician in a minority of cases. Of these less frequent symptoms, *redness of the eyelid,* particularly if it is associated with edema, reflects the inflammatory nature of the expanding mass and has some value as a diagnostic clue to pseudotumor. The color hue and edema resemble a cellulitis, but there is no increase in local heat (Fig. 329). This redness and edema of the eyelid may accompany pseudotumors located in the more anterior portions of the orbit but is not observed with pseudotumors in posterior orbital locations unless the process is quite acute.

A palpable mass will be noted either by the patient or by the physician in about 50% of the cases. Pseudotumor is found more often in the superior than the inferior orbit, a feature common to most orbital tumors. In the extreme anterior portion of the orbit, pseudotumors tend to fuse with the periorbita near the superior or inferior orbital rim in a pancake-like configuration. In these cases it will be difficult to palpate the edge of the bone. This clinical feature also is of some diagnostic value. In most all other orbital tumors in a similar position, a discrete depression can be palpated between the tumor and the lip of bone.

Marked visual loss (less than 20/400 in the eye of the affected orbit) may be present in approximately 15% of the patients at the time of initial examination. When present, it indicates a poor visual prognosis no matter what treatment is

Figure 328. Lymphocytic inflammatory pseudotumor: slight downward displacement and 5-mm forward protrusion of left eye (duration, 8 months); marked edema of left upper eyelid is obvious but there was also lack of redness, such as is present in Figure 198. The inflammatory process also was more chronic and less progressive than in the patient illustrated in Figure 329.

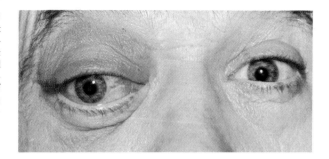

Figure 329. Lymphocytic inflammatory pseudotumor: downward displacement and forward protrusion of right eye with edema and redness of upper eyelid (duration, 3 months) in case of pseudotumor in upper quadrants of orbit; this clinical picture, when present, suggests pseudotumor in the more forward portion of orbit.

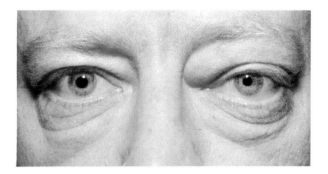

attempted. Some degree of pallor usually develops and eventually these eyes are almost blind. As a rule, the pseudotumor in these cases is large and fills the posterior orbit. In these cases, the affected eye may be almost fixed in position owing to marked involvement of the extraocular muscles. This clinical feature is similar to the extraocular muscle paresis observed in metastatic carcinoma of the orbit.

The interval between onset of symptoms and the initial ophthalmologic evaluation was 6 months or less in 73% of our cases. The longest duration of symptoms was 2 years. As a rule, if symptoms have been present longer than 9 months, it is likely the patient has had some trial of therapy (systemic steroids or radiotherapy) with indifferent results.

Extensive systemic reviews supplemented with a battery of laboratory tests have been unsuccessful in providing a clue to this orbital disease.

ROENTGENOGRAPHY, ULTRASONOGRAPHY, AND COMPUTER TOMOGRAPHY

Although in some cases of pseudotumor the inflammatory process chooses to attack the periorbita, bone erosion and bone destruction do not ordinarily occur with this disease. Therefore, routine orbital roentgenography is usually negative except to show some increased soft tissue density and, rarely, some enlargement of the orbit in pseudotumors of long duration.

Because the pathologic process of pseudotumor is so varied in character (infiltrative, solid, diffuse, circumscribed) and so erratic in its localization in the orbit, neither ultrasonography or computer tomography show a specific and constant diagnostic picture. The diffuse lesions, by ultrasonography, will show irregular borders, heterogeneous acoustic interfaces, and sound attenuation. Such acoustic patterns may resemble other infiltrative orbital processes, such as lymphoma and metastatic carcinoma. The more solid, circumscribed pseudotumor will have more distinct borders but will be difficult to differentiate from some other solid tumors of the orbit, particularly those localized to the lacrimal gland. Should the pseudotumor attach to the periorbita the perimeter of the orbital acoustic shadow may be somewhat scalloped. If the inflammatory process develops adjacent to an extraocular muscle, the muscle bundle will increase in thickness and the resulting shadow will be visible on both computer tomography and ultrasonography. Such a finding might suggest the diagnosis of Graves' disease except that two or more extraocular muscles are usually involved by the latter disorder. Finally, there are those cases that show an inflammatory thickening of the muscle as well as the adjacent sclera (Fig. 42, Chapter 2), a change that probably is more diagnostic of pseudotumor than any other.

In general, neither ultrasonography or computer tomography have been as helpful in the diagnosis of pseudotumor as they have been of value in the diagnosis of most other orbital disorders. The diagnosis of pseudotumor is still a surgical one. We rely chiefly on ultrasonography and computer tomography to outline the extent of the mass as a preliminary to the surgical approach.

COURSE AND TREATMENT

> *There are two horns to my dilemma.*
> *If I don't get hooked on one,*
> *I will on the other.*
> E. S. Gardner, *The D. A. Cooks a Goose* (1942)

This quotation has come to mind on many occasions because of the dilemma associated with a proper choice of management of a patient with pseudotumor. Should the ophthalmologist pursue a nonsurgical, conservative course waiting for the inflammatory process to subside spontaneously? Or should the ophthalmologist undertake a major operation not only to establish diagnosis but also to remove the offending tissue and to relieve proptosis and other attendant symptoms? Those not familiar with the ugly disposition of some pseudotumors when disturbed might well wonder why the conservative, nonsurgical approach to the problem should have any place in treatment. In contrast, those surgeons who have been surprised often by the havoc wrought from their surgical exploration might wonder whether any approach other than the conservative one is justified. On several occasions we have followed the conservative approach with cases believed to be mild examples of orbital pseudotumor but which were never verified histologically. Such situations usually were characterized by a sudden onset of a palpable mass in the more anterior portion of the orbit, some redness and swelling of the eyelid overlying the mass, but little, if any, proptosis, extraocular muscle weakness, or visual disturbance. The mildness of the clinical picture did not make surgical biopsy mandatory and the symptoms resolved in a period of several months, either spontaneously or after a low dosage of systemic steroids.

More often, the ophthalmologist is confronted with a situation in which the clinical features are more severe and progressive, the patients become concerned about a visual disturbance or diplopia, and a possible noninflammatory, infiltrative neoplastic lesion cannot be excluded. Surgical intervention is then necessary to identify the orbital process. These cases are our chief concern in this chapter. How should they be managed and what is the patient's subsequent course? Some answers to these questions were found in the study of the histologically verified cases of lymphocytic inflammatory pseudotumor in the Mayo Clinic series.

Follow-up data of a year or longer was obtained in twenty-nine of the thirty-five cases (Table 29). The orbits of these patients were explored by a variety of surgeons either through an anterior, lateral, or transcranial orbitotomy. The question of supplementary therapy (radiotherapy, systemic steroids) usually was decided by the consulting or supervising ophthalmologist. In other words, this was a very uncontrolled study.

The several forms of management are listed as treatment groups in Table 29. Surgically, the tumor was completely excised, partially resected, or biopsied. Radiotherapy was administered either by orthovoltage or supravoltage techniques in total doses ranging from 350 to 1,350 roentgens. Steroid therapy was administered as prednisone, 40 to 80 mg every other day, for periods of 2 to 3 months. The pre- and postoperative assessment of proptosis, degree of extraocular muscle imbalance, and visual acuity were the three principal clinical features upon which the course and management of the disease were judged. If there was improvement in two or more of the three judging units and no worsening of any of the three preoperative features, the result was considered *good*. If one feature was worse, postoperatively, but the other features were unchanged, the result was considered *fair*. If two or more clinical features were worse in the interval of study the result was considered *poor*.

A review of Table 29 indicates that both good and poor results occurred in each of the three major treatment subgroups. However, a larger proportion of patients in the "complete surgical excision" subgroup had good results as compared with patients receiving other treatment modes. Several factors contributed to this favorable result. First, the pseudotumors were accessible (located in the anterior orbit or lacrimal gland fossa), circumscribed (not as delineated as a benign encapsulated tumor but with a surgical cleavage plane along at least three of the four sides of the tumor), and were not intimately attached to extraocular muscles, nerve, blood vessels, or eyeball. Also, in most patients with this gross type of pseudotumor, the presenting signs and symptoms were usually less severe than in patients in other treatment subgroups. The proptosis was mild (3 mm or less), diplopia was minimal, and visual acuity was normal. In essence, these cases were well suited for surgical management. As a rule, the circumscribed pseudotumors located in the inferior orbit and lacrimal fossa were most suitable for this approach. The largest tumor completely excised measured 2 × 2 × 0.5 cm. Patients in other treatment groups who were judged to have had good results shared one feature in common with the preceding

TABLE 29.   TREATMENT AND COURSE OF 29 PATIENTS WITH
LYMPHOCYTIC INFLAMMATORY PSEUDOTUMOR*

Treatment Group	Patient	Result	Remarks
Surgery			
A. Complete excision	M.S.	Good	7-year follow-up, no recurrence
	C.T.	Good	2-year follow-up, no recurrence
	M.A.	Good	3-year follow-up, no recurrence
	M.D.	Good	5-year follow-up, no recurrence
	E.S.	Poor	10-year follow-up, no recurrence, eye blind
B. Partial excision	H.D.	Poor	14-year follow-up, no recurrence, eye blind
	M.J.	Poor	7-year follow-up, no recurrence, eye blind
	E.M.	Fair	3-year follow-up, no recurrence
	H.S.	Fair	2-year follow-up, slight progression
	E.G.	Fair	1-year follow-up, no recurrence
	P.H.	Fair	5-year follow-up, no recurrence
	K.H.	Poor	3-year follow-up, continued progression, enucleation of eye
	R.K.	Poor	2-year follow-up, no recurrence
	A.M.	Good	28-year follow-up, no recurrence
Partial excision and radiotherapy	G.G.	Good	4-year follow-up, no recurrence
	J.J.	Good	5-year follow-up, no recurrence
	R.T.	Fair	7-year follow-up, no recurrence
	H.L.	Fair	2-year follow-up, no recurrence
	P.M.	Fair	5-year follow-up, no recurrence
	E.R.	Poor	6-year follow-up, continued progression, enucleation of eye
	M.W.	Fair	16-year follow-up, three operations, stable
	C.Z.	Good	5-year follow-up, no recurrence
Biopsy and radiotherapy	G.K.	Fair	1-year follow-up, no recurrence
Partial excision and steroid therapy	C.C.	Poor	3-year follow-up, no recurrence, eye blind
Biopsy and steroid therapy	G.B.	Good	7-year follow-up, one recurrence treated with steroids
	D.H.	Fair	3-year follow-up, no recurrence
Partial excision, radiotherapy, and steroid therapy	R.K.	Fair	3-year follow-up, no recurrence
	G.W.	Fair	3-year follow-up, some progression
Biopsy, radiotherapy, and steroid therapy	G.B.	Fair	21-year follow-up, no recurrence

*Mayo Clinic Series 1948–1974.

subgroup, namely, the disease was not severe to begin with, as judged by the three parameters of proptosis, ocular motility, and visual acuity.

In contrast, the patients with poor results usually had severe disease at the time of presentation, characterized by visual loss, marked impairment of ocular rotations, and long-standing proptosis. The pseudotumors in these cases usually extended over a wide area in the posterior orbit, were infiltrative and fibrotic in type, and were fused to important nerves and muscles. Those patients with optic nerve involvement, as manifested by preoperative decreased vision and fuzzy shadows along the computer tomography display of the orbital portion of the nerve were particularly prone to develop a blind eye in the follow-up period. In other words, many of these patients were in "no win" situations, pre-operatively.

In those patients with a fair result from therapy the character and extent of the pseudotumor were somewhere between the two preceding treatment extremes. Many of these patients had undergone either a partial surgical excision or a biopsy of the mass because the borders of the tumor were still ill-defined for accurate dissection or the tumor was fused to some functionally important orbital structure.

The comparative value of radiotherapy and systemic steroid therapy is less easy to evaluate. It is our clinical impression that radiotherapy is of some benefit to many patients whose pseudotumor cannot be entirely removed. We believe it tends to halt the progress of the inflammatory process and bring about some resolution of the size and extent of the residual tumor in the orbit, except those pseudotumors that show extensive fibrosis on histopathologic examination. The latter tumors may show a poor response to all therapeutic efforts. Our follow-up data also suggests that, in pseudotumors responsive to radiotherapy, small doses of irradiation are probably as effective as large dosage values. We suspect the optimum range of irradiation is from 350 to 600 roentgens. Also, those pseudotumors that have a diffuse histologic configuration seem to respond better to radiotherapy than mixed and fibrotic types of lesions.

The number of patients in our series treated with some combination of systemic steroids is not large, and it is difficult to define its exact role in management. We know that steroid drugs have a salutary effect in many cases but we attribute this to a temporary suppressive effect on the inflammatory process. The drugs (usually prednisone) are easy to give but not so easy to discontinue. Relapses of the inflammatory process are likely to occur when the dosage is decreased, and, in some patients, the disease becomes steroid dependent, with the consequent steroid complications. We are somewhat mistrustful of steroid therapy in lymphocytic inflammatory pseudotumors and prefer a trial of radiotherapy for incompletely excised, progressive lesions. Steroids are reserved for lesions recalcitrant to other treatment modes. Steroids are also useful in those few patients who have recurrent disease. One patient of our series had a recurrence of the pseudotumor five years after initial biopsy and treatment with prednisone. Systemic steroids were again helpful in controlling the recurrent disease.

In judging the effect of any method of treatment, one last factor should be emphasized. Lymphocytic inflammatory pseudotumor in almost all patients is a self-limited disease. If left alone the inflammatory process will run its course, but the duration of the disease is unpredictable. In addition, the severity of the disease at any given time is even more uncertain.

SUMMARY

Several of the salient features of the above discussion, in addition to some conclusions based on our long clinical experience with the disease, are summarized as follows:

1. We would like to encourage a greater uniformity in the terminology of inflammatory pseudotumor and have proposed more restrictive parameters for its diagnosis.

2. The histologic types of lymphocytic inflammatory pseudotumor that we have described do not seem related to the duration or extent of the disease but may have some correlation to the expected response to treatment.

3. The extent of the tumor, its location in the orbit, and the severity of the clinical features at the time of patient presentation are major determinants in the course and prognosis of the disease.

4. Circumscribed pseudotumors in the anterior portion of the orbit are amenable to complete surgical excision.

5. Radiotherapy is often a helpful supplement in the management of the many patients who have had partial resection of the orbital mass.

6. Patients with preoperative visual impairment, or involvement of the optic nerve as manifested by computer tomography, will likely have severe post-operative visual loss.

7. Surgical excision of pseudotumors at the apex of the orbit or adjacent to the orbital portion of the optic nerve is not recommended. Incisional biopsy of such tumors to establish the diagnosis, supplemented with either radiotherapy or systemic administration of corticosteroids, is the treatment of choice for such situations.

8. Lymphocytic inflammatory pseudotumor is almost always a self-limited disease.

Some have said that the prognosis for pseudotumor is excellent. It is excellent if we are talking about its influence on life expectancy or if we compare it to dire diseases such as malignant neoplasm. But if we consider the number of patients who continue indefinitely to have some palpable orbital mass, some permanent displacement of the eye, or some other impairment of ocular function, then the outcome — at least from the patient's viewpoint — leaves much to be desired. There are so many unknowns and uncertainties connected with its etiology and course that pseudotumor continues to be one of the most difficult of all the tumors in this text to manage. Much research needs to be done on all aspects of the problem.

Bibliography

Birch-Hirschfeld A: Die Krankheiten der Orbita. *In Handbuch der gesamten Augenheilkunden.* Vol. 9, Part 1. Ed: A. Graefe, T. Saemisch. Berlin, Julius Springer, 1930

Blodi FC, Gass JDM: Inflammatory pseudotumor of the orbit. Trans Am Acad Ophthalmol Otolaryngol 71:303–322, 1967

Garner A: Pathology of 'pseudotumors' of the orbit: a review. J Clin Path 26:639–648, 1973

Heersink B, Rodrigues MR, Flanagan JC: Inflammatory pseudotumor of the orbit. Ann Ophthalmol 9:17–29, 1977

Reese AB: *Tumors of the Eye.* Second ed. New York, Hoeber Medical Division, Harper & Row, Publishers, 1963

21

Orbital Vasculitis,
Wegener's Granulomatosis, and
Orbital Sarcoid

In this chapter we have elected to discuss three less common disorders that, at present, are lumped together in the broad category of orbital pseudotumors by most ophthalmologists and pathologists. They do share the common trait of forming a tumor that, on clinical grounds, cannot always be differentiated from orbital neoplasms or other pseudoneoplasms without surgical biopsy. Also, it is possible they have a tenuous relationship to one another as localized orbital manifestation of some disturbance of our autoimmune system. Beyond this, they are dissimilar, particularly in their histopathologic features, and we believe, on clinical grounds, that there is sufficient reason to consider them as separate clinical entities. More important, in our crusade to make the term "inflammatory pseudotumor" less generalized and more specific, we have emphasized their dissimilarities from the preceding lymphocytic pseudotumor by placing them in a chapter of their own. One of these conditions is basically an *orbital vasculitis*, another (*orbital sarcoid*) is an orbital granulomatous disease, and the third (*Wegener's granulomatosis*) combines both the features of a granuloma and a vasculitis.

ORBITAL VASCULITIS

In the prior edition of this text, this orbital tumor was described as the Type I histopathologic variant of "inflammatory pseudotumor." We now believe this condition is a clinicopathologic entity separate from the preceding lymphocytic inflammatory pseudotumor. We do not know its cause, but the singular and basic pathologic process is a *vasculitis* or, more specifically, an *angiitis*.

PATHOLOGY

The cellular response in this orbital lesion is a diffuse polymorphic infiltration with eosinophils as the most prominent component. There are also many polymorphonuclear leukocytes and plasma cells, but lymphocytes and macrophages, though present, play a lesser role in this response. There is a striking relationship of the inflammatory infiltrate to small arteries and arterioles (Fig. 330). This picture is similar to an Arthus reaction, or an acute allergic type of vasculitis with necrosis of the vessel wall and resultant fibrinoid changes (Figs.

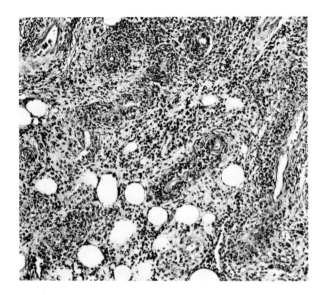

Figure 330. Orbital vasculitis, acute: markedly intense, acute inflammatory reaction of orbital tissue; multifocal vasculitis is apparent at this low power. (Hematoxylin and eosin; × 120.)

331 and 332). The cells tend to concentrate in and around the vessel wall and, here, the eosinophils are particularly striking. Nucleocytoclasis (dissolution of the leukocyte and fragmentation of the nucleus resulting in "nuclear dust"), also can be observed in most specimens. As the affected vessel undergoes dissolution, erythrocytes extravasate into the surrounding tissues, and areas of fibrinoid change and stellate necrosis replace the vessel. Zones of fat destruction and fat necrosis may accompany this acute and diffuse process, but this panniculitis seems to be secondary to the vasculitis rather than a primary process (Fig. 333). Some foreign body granulomatous reaction may be seen in the areas of fat necrosis.

The orbital reticulum responds to this inflammatory process by ingrowth of fibrous connective tissue (Fig. 334). Gradually, the damaged orbital tissue is re-

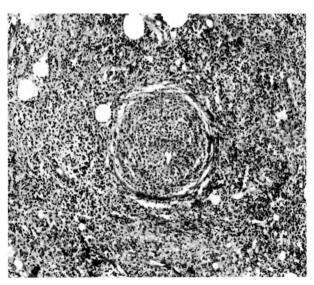

Figure 331. Orbital vasculitis, acute: small artery in center of field shows acute vasculitis in midst of intense inflammation. (Hematoxylin and eosin; × 160.)

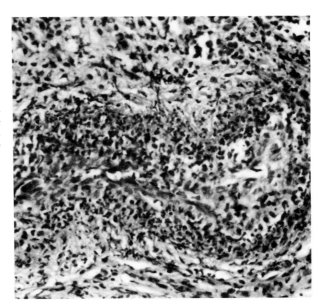

Figure 332. Orbital vasculitis, acute: detail of small artery with intense acute vasculitis; massive infiltration of vessel wall by neutrophils and eosinophils. (Hematoxylin and eosin; × 270.)

placed by a dense fibrosis. However, this does not necessarily imply that the process is entirely healed, because active vasculitis and focal areas of necrosis (often with fibrinoid change) may still be found in scattered parts of the lesion (Fig. 335). Finally, the fibrosis may become quite dense and incorporate all orbital structures. Nerve trunks passing through these areas of vasculitis also may show degenerative changes. If the lacrimal gland is involved, fibrosis and atrophy of the glandular parenchyma may occur. Extraocular muscles also may undergo atrophy and fibrosis.

Thirteen patients from our study series were classified as having orbital vasculitis. Five of these cases showed the acute inflammatory response on histologic exam, another five cases showed some ingrowth of fibrous connective tissue, and the three remaining tumors showed the dense fibrous replacement type of response. There was some correlation between the duration of the disease at the time of diagnosis and the histopathologic subtype. In those cases showing the acute vasculitis and the diffuse polymorphous cellular response, the duration of the disease was only a few months. In contrast, those cases showing advanced fibrosis usually had had symptoms for over a year prior to diagnosis. This correlation between the duration of the disease and the histologic phase of the lesion was not observed among the cases of lymphocytic inflammatory pseudotumor.

CLINICAL FEATURES

The sex distribution and age range of the thirteen patients classifed as having orbital vasculitis are listed in Table 3, Chapter 3. The youngest patient was 12 years of age at the time of diagnosis and the oldest patient was 75 years. This broad age distribution is similar to the age range of patients with lymphocytic inflammatory pseudotumor, except that 60% (8/13) of the patients in the orbital vasculitis group were 30 years old or younger. In the lymphocytic in-

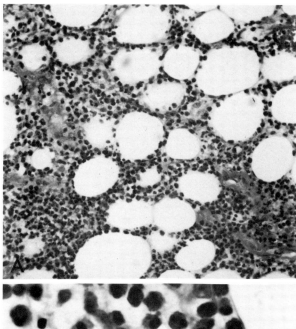

Figure 333. Orbital vasculitis, acute:

A, Acute inflammatory reaction in the fat accompanied by destruction of fat cells. (Hematoxylin and eosin; × 160.)

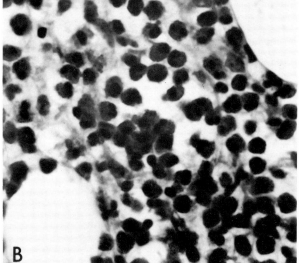

B, Preponderance of eosinophils among the inflammatory cells seen under higher power. (Hematoxylin and eosin; × 400.)

flammatory group, 71% of the patients were over 40 years of age at the time of diagnosis. The disease affected the left orbit in eight patients, the right orbit in four patients, and was bilateral in one patient. The predilection for the left orbit may not be significant considering the small number of total cases. The bilateral case occurred in a female whose right orbit was first affected when she was 18 years old. A partial removal of the tumor resulted in improvement. Two years later a similar problem affected the left orbit and surgical removal of the tumor again brought relief of symptoms, but the process recurred in the left orbit three years later.

The symptomatology of patients with orbital vasculitis and with lymphocytic inflammatory pseudotumor is very much alike. In both conditions a *puffiness, drooping,* or *edema of the upper eyelid* was either the initial symptom or

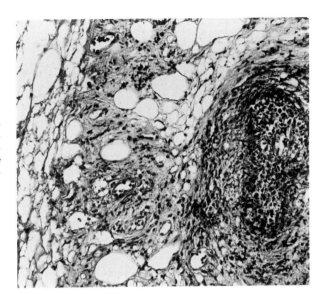

Figure 334. Orbital vasculitis, subacute: vasculitis still apparent, but now fibrous connective tissue is beginning to replace damaged orbital tissues. (Hematoxylin and eosin; × 160.)

the predominant sign of the disease at the time of presentation in the majority of patients. In orbital vasculitis, less frequent symptoms were blurred vision, chemosis, prominence of the eye, redness of the conjunctiva or eyelid, and ocular discomfort, but there was no constant sequence or pattern among these secondary manifestations. Of interest was the notation of measurable proptosis at the time of the initial ophthalmic examination. However, less than half of the patients had noted prominence of the eye in the premonitory stages, because the edematous eyelid either concealed some of the proptosis or was the object of the patient's chief concern. This clinical feature also was noted among patients with lymphocytic inflammatory pseudotumor. This proptosis was quite marked (5 mm or greater) in 6 of the 13 patients. The duration of symptoms at the time of presentation was five months or less in 8 of the 13 patients, but in 2 patients the symptomatology lasted as long as 1½ years. Special studies, such as ultrasonography and computer tomography, were not helpful in differential diagnosis. Preoperative as well as postoperative physical examinations and laboratory surveys did not uncover an explanation for the orbital disease.

TREATMENT AND COURSE

Follow-up data of 6 years or longer was available in 7 of the series of 13 patients. No definite conclusions as to efficacy of therapy can be reached on the basis of so few cases. Neither was therapy administered under any preplanned protocols. Nevertheless, some comment should be made concerning the course and management of some of the patients in the long-interval follow-up group.

Partial surgical excision of the orbital mass was performed in five patients and surgical biopsy was the procedure in two patients. Biopsy, only, was elected in one of the latter patients because of the apical position of the orbital lesion.

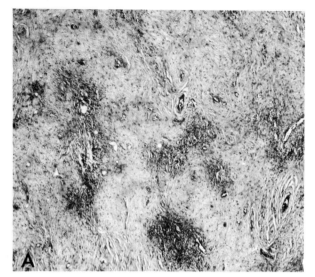

Figure 335.   Orbital vasculitis, chronic:

A, Dense fibrosis predominant but scattered foci of inflammation persist. (Hematoxylin and eosin; × 40.)

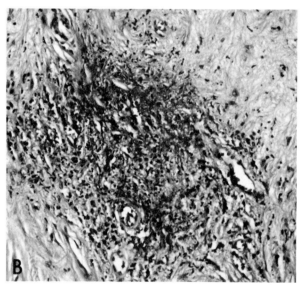

B, Foci of inflammation are situated about necrotic arteries, with nuclear dust and fibrinoid necrosis. (Hematoxylin and eosin; × 160.)

Biopsy also was performed in the one patient with bilateral recurrent disease. In none of the remaining five patients was the lesion completely excised because of lack of encapsulation of the mass and the frequent fusion of the tumor with portions of the extraocular muscles. Nevertheless, some of the tumors were nodular and sufficiently circumscribed that a major portion of the mass could be removed. This "debulking" process reduced the degree of proptosis but, in our opinion, probably did not alter the final functional result. The two patients who had undergone surgical biopsy seemed to have as much improvement over the long term as those patients who had had the major portion of the mass excised. Several of the patients had supplementary orthovoltage radiotherapy and this seemed to hasten the resolution of those cases that seemed destined to improve. None of the patients received irradiation in a dosage greater than 600 roentgens to the affected orbit except one patient who will be noted shortly. In six of the seven patients in the long-term follow-up group, the inflammatory orbital process subsided and there was no recurrence in the 6- to 18-year interval of observation. The seventh patient developed severe pulmonary sarcoidosis 6 years after diagnosis of the orbital tumor. However, in the time interval between the orbital and pulmonary disease there was no recurrence of the orbital vasculitis. In general, the shorter the duration of the disease, the less severe the symptomatology at time of presentation and the more acute the lesion at the time of histologic diagnosis, the more rapid was the response to therapy and the better was the resolution of the disease without serious residuals. In contrast, the more severe and longer the symptomatology, and the more marked the degree of fibrosis at the time of histologic diagnosis, the more severe were the residuals (loss of vision, extraocular muscle palsies, blepharoptosis, and so on) of the orbital process when final resolution occurred. These findings resemble the experience noted in patients with lymphocytic orbital pseudotumor.

Special note should be made of one 44-year-old patient who did not fit the usual but variable pattern of improvement noted above. Rapidly progressive edema of the right eyelids and prominence of the right eye had been present for 2 months when the patient was first examined. A proptosis of 12 mm was present. Vision in the affected eye was 20/80. Nodular masses were palpated in both superior and inferior temporal orbital quadrants. On orbitotomy these masses were partially excised, but an extension of the tumor into the apex of the orbit was left untouched. Histologically, the tumor was classified as a vasculitis (allergic angiitis) of the acute type. The patient received orthovoltage radiotherapy, 590 roentgens, during the first postoperative month. The proptosis continued to progress and, during the fifth postoperative month, an additional 5,000 roentgens of irradiation were given to the affected orbit. At this time, multiple subcutaneous nodules were noted beneath the skin at scattered locations over the body. Biopsy of one of these nodules revealed a histopathologic picture similar to the orbital lesion. The size of the nodules waxed and waned until the patient expired 8 months after the initial orbital diagnosis of what was believed to be a disseminated vasculitis. No autopsy was performed to determine the full extent of the disease.

We hope other cases of orbital vasculitis will be recognized in the future and reported in the ophthalmic literature. Only in this way will we learn more about the disease and its place in the spectrum of orbital inflammatory tumors and necrotizing vascular diseases.

WEGENER'S GRANULOMATOSIS

Historical Aspects

This uncommon disease has been known for over 40 years. However, involvement of the orbit, as one of the anatomic sites of the disease, has been established comparatively recently. Klinger (1931) reported a patient with a strange combination of destructive sinusitis, disseminated vasculitis, splenic granulomas, and nephritis. Later, in two publications (1936 and 1939),

Wegener of Breslau, Germany, described in detail three patients with necrotizing granulomatous vasculitis of the upper and lower respiratory tract as well as glomerulonephritis. Wegener's patients were 38, 36, and 33 years of age (1 male and 2 females). His suggestion that this triad of symptoms was a clinical entity was later confirmed by many others. As further cases were recorded, reports of proptosis of one or both eyes associated with the destructive sinusitis of the disease also appeared. In a summary of the ocular manifestations associated with the syndrome, Straatsma (1957) included six cases with orbital lesions contiguous to nasal and paranasal sinus involvement. The age range of these orbital cases was 21 to 70 years and included 3 instances of bilateral orbital disease. In only three of the total six cases was the orbital disease confirmed by histopathologic study.

In subsequent years other examples of orbital involvement in Wegener's granulomatosis have been suggested by Walton (1958), Harcourt (1964), Blodi and Gass (1968), Faulds and Wear (1960), Cassan and associates (1970), Weiter and Farkas (1972), Henderson (1973), DeRemee and associates (1976), and others. However, on closer scrutiny, not all of these cases would qualify as orbital examples of Wegener's granulomatosis under present standards, either because the patients do not have the signs of organ involvement presently accepted for diagnosis or the histopathologic descriptions of the orbital tumors resemble one of the other orbital necrotizing vascular diseases.

In 1966 Carrington and Liebow introduced the concept that a limited or less diffuse form of the disease exists. Such patient showed lung and upper respiratory lesions but no kidney involvement. These patients also showed a more favorable response to therapy and their survival was longer than in patients with the more diffuse entity described by Wegener. Many others now embrace this concept of a limited Wegener's granulomatosis. Also, it is now known the orbit may be the presenting site of either the limited or diffuse form of the disease.

INCIDENCE AND CLINICAL FEATURES

In our orbital tumor survey we have five cases of Wegener's granulomatosis with histopathologic confirmation of orbital involvement. One of these cases was recorded in detail by Cassan and associates (1970) and the other four patients were noted in the time overlap of the review by DeRemee and colleagues (1976). The male/female ratio was 4:1 and the patient's ages were 15, 39, 39, 58, and 59 years, respectively, at the onset of orbital symptoms. In the 15-year-old patient the orbit was the initial site of the disease; in two patients orbital symptoms developed concomitantly with contiguous but undiagnosed granulomatosis of the nasal passages; and in the remaining two patients orbital disease appeared several weeks after lung involvement. Two of the patients ultimately developed bilateral orbital lesions. This latter feature has been noted by other observers.

As early as 1958 Walton estimated that proptosis occurred in approximately 10% of cases with the systemic disease. More recently (1976) DeRemee and associates noted orbital involvement in 6 (12%) of 50 patients (28 males and 22 females) observed over a period of 10 years. The age range of the patients in the study of DeRemee and his associates was 8 to 75 years. This wide age distribution has been noted by others.

A study of the orbital symptomatology in our group of patients revealed that in four cases swelling or edema of the eyelids was the initial sign of orbital involvement (Fig. 336). This symptom either was so striking or sudden in onset that the patients, with one exception, were not aware of the progressive proptosis. This chain of events was quite similar to the anamnesis of patients in the orbital vasculitis group. Diplopia usually was noted several weeks after onset. One patient noted a combination of frontal headache, blurred vision, and diplopia at the onset of the orbital lesion. One patient was blind in the eye of the involved orbit 4 months after onset and, in a second patient, vision was reduced to 20/400 in one eye 2 weeks after onset. In four of our patients orbital masses could be palpated in two or more quadrants of the orbit at the time of initial examination. In general, the degree of orbital involvement was greater and the size of the orbital masses larger at the time of initial examination than was observed in patients with either orbital vasculitis or lymphocytic inflammatory pseudotumor. The one patient who did not have a palpable mass initially did develop such a tumor as the condition progressed.

Patients with contiguous or concomitnat nasal or paranasal involvement may have severe rhinorrhea, pain and drainage referred to the paranasal sinuses, nasal obstruction, and intranasal ulcerations. In addition, there may be malaise, intermittent pyrexia, migrating arthralgias, and elevated erythrocytic sedimentation rate. Roentgenography in patients with the pulmonary form of the disease usually shows multiple, bilateral, discrete infiltrates, or thin-walled cavities usually greater than 1 cm in diameter with a predilection for the lower lobes.

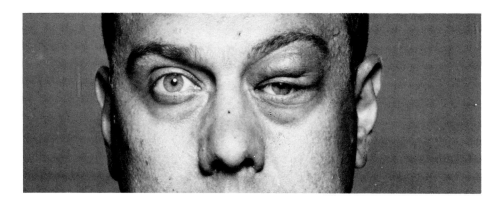

Figure 336. Wegener's granulomatosis: edema of eyelids of six weeks' duration in a 39-year-old male. Diplopia of three weeks' duration. Patient was not aware of proptosis (5mm) and downward displacement of left eye.

PATHOLOGY

The factor that triggers the histopathologic changes characteristic of this disease are not known. Initially, in whatever the target tissue (fat, muscle, sclera, and so on) of the disease, there is an intense focal invasion of inflammatory cells consisting chiefly of lymphocytes, plasma cells, histiocytes, and some polymorphonuclear leukocytes. Eosinophils also may participate in this cellular response in some cases, but these leukocytes are not a prominent feature of this disease in contrast to their role in orbital vasculitis. As the triggering mechanism of the disease persists, the focus of inflammation enlarges, the center of the lesion becomes less cellular and smudged in appearance, and epithelial cells and giant cells with multiple nuclei appear around the periphery of the lesion (Fig. 337). The term *necrotizing granuloma* is applied to this polymorphous cellular mass. If the inflammatory insult continues the center of the granuloma undergoes further necrosis, becomes acellular or hyalinized, and the function of the target tissue is destroyed. Elsewhere, in some adjacent area, a concomitant focal inflammatory reaction involves the smaller arteries and, to some extent, the smaller veins, resulting in a *necrotizing vasculitis* (Fig. 337 *B*). If the etiologic factor subsides or is arrested, the affected tissue undergoes a fibrosis with some attempts toward a functional repair. In cases having a remittent course, the affected tissue may show active necrotizing features in some areas, with fibrosis and repair in other areas.

TREATMENT AND COURSE

Wegener's granulomatosis in its diffuse form (with kidney involvement) is a serious and often fatal disease. The therapeutic use of cytotoxic agents (usually cyclophosphamide), often combined with systemic steroids, in the last decade has increased the frequency of remissions and lengthened survival. The accepted concept that a more localized form of the disease (limited Wegener's granulomatosis) is less virulent and is associated with longer survival also has encouraged a more favorable outlook for the patient.

A review of the course and treatment of the five patients in our survey is not only pertinent to the question of prognosis but emphasizes some of the serious orbital and ocular consequences of the disease. In 2 of the patients an observation period of longer than 20 years was possible. Because of the long course and intricate nature of several of the case histories, only a brief outline of their salient clinical features will be noted.

CASE #1. A portion of this patient's course was recorded in great detail by Cassan and associates in 1970. At the time of their report the patient had been observed and treated over a 16-year period for a surgically verified necrotizing granulomatosis and vasculitis of the Wegener type involving the nasopharynx and both orbits. An interval of 3½ years elapsed between the onset of the disease in the first and second orbit. Lung involvement also appeared 3½ years after orbital onset, and multicentric areas of ulceration of the skin due to necrotizing vasculitis occurred 14 years after initial diagnosis. In the overall interval of their observation one eye had become blind, but the other eye was functionally useful, with vision reduced to 20/40. The chief treatment was prednisone supplemented with orthovoltage irradiation of 480 roentgens to one orbit in 1953 and 900 roentgens to the other orbit in 1960.

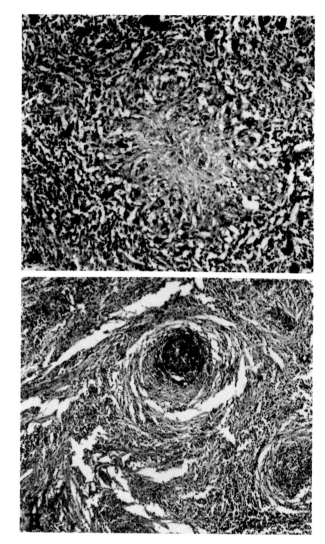

Figure 337. Wegener's granulomatosis of the orbit:

A, Dense infiltrate of inflammatory cells with focal necrotizing granulomas. (Hematoxylin and eosin; ×64.)

B, Subacute vasculitis involving small muscular arteries. (Hematoxylin and eosin; × 100.)

After their report (1970) the patient developed a vascular thrombosis of one segment of the colon. The disease continued quite active in the lung, skin, and one orbit. The patient expired from vascular complications of the disease at age 62, 23 years after onset. An autopsy confirmed the presence of the disease in the lungs but no kidney involvement was found. At time of death, patient was almost blind (recognition of hand movements) in the second eye.

CASE #2. A 23-year period of observation also was possible in this patient. Initially, at age 15, one orbit was affected by a surgically verified inflammatory pseudotumor. At this time (1956) a diagnosis of necrotizing granulomatosis and vasculitis probably was not . entertained because orbital pseudotumors were still such a hodgepodge of histopathologic patterns. The orbit was treated with orthovoltage irradiation of 3,000 rads but the eye became blind and was eventually enucleated.

Fourteen years after onset a surgically verified necrotizing granulomatosis and vasculitis of the Wegener's type occurred in the second orbit. In addition, there was some rhinorrhea and recurrent sinusitis, but multiple biopsies from the nasal passages did not show any disease other than a chronic inflammatory reaction. The patient also developed a subglottic lesion that eventually healed with a partial tracheal stricture. The orbital, nasal, and laryngeal symptoms were stabilized on a treatment program of prednisone and Cytoxan. The Cytoxan was discontinued after one year but the patient was continued on prednisone. At last examination the vision in the remaining eye was 20/20 but palpable masses were still present in the surrounding orbit. At no time did the patient have any clinical evidence of lung or kidney disease.

CASE #3. The initial manifestation of the disease in this 39-year-old patient was surgically verified in the lower lobe of the left lung in 1967. Postoperatively, the patient developed bilateral nasal disease and a left orbital tumor. Biopsies from the nose and orbit were compared with the specimen from the lung and all were considered examples of a necrotizing granulomatosis and vasculitis of the Wegener's type.

Therapy combining isoniazide, prednisone, and Imuran in various doses was administered. The nasal and lung lesions improved but the orbital disease progressed. The left eye became blind before remission of the orbital disease occurred. At the end of the 10-year period of observation the second orbit remains free of disease, there is no clinical evidence of kidney involvement and the patient has been off all systemic medications for 6 years.

CASE #4. This 59-year-old patient developed a flu-like syndrome in 1971 followed by edema of the right upper eyelid, diplopia, and proptosis of the right eye. Clinically, there was evidence of a glomerulonephritis and an orbital tumor. Surgical biopsy showed lesions in both the kidney and orbit consistent with a diagnosis of Wegener's granulomatosis. The patient was treated with prednisone and Cytoxan. Four months later nodular infiltrates appeared in the left lung. Isoniazid was added to the treatment program. All clinical manifestations of the disease improved and the prednisone and isoniazid medications were successively discontinued. Cytoxan was discontinued after a period of 5 years. At the end of a 7-year observation period, the vision of the right eye is 20/25, no orbital masses are palpable, proptosis has disappeared, the kidney disease is inactive, and the infiltrates in the lung fields have undergone fibrosis.

CASE #5. Another 59-year-old patient was first seen in 1972 with a 1-year history of nasal obstruction, malaise, and swelling of the right eyelids. Examination revealed displacement of right eye, an orbital mass, and intranasal granulation tissue. A diagnosis of necrotizing granulomatosis and vasculitis of the Wegener's type was made from the biopsy of the nasal tissue. Treatment with prednisone was started. One year later there was marked exacerbation of the orbital symptoms, opacification of right maxillary sinus, and destructive changes in the nasoantral wall. A maxillotomy was performed and the inflammatory-granulomatous disease was found to extend into right ethmoid and right orbital areas. Leukeran was added to the treatment program. A remission of symptoms then occurred which lasted for 7 years. Both drugs were discontinued in 1977, but 2 months after all cessation of treatment the patient suffered a cerebral infarct. Prednisone and leukeran were restarted and Coumadin was added to the treatment regimen. The patient's course slowly deteriorated and he died from an extension of the central nervous system disease 5 years after initial diagnosis.

Of these five patients with orbital manifestations, two patients have died from the progression of the systemic disease. The other 3 patients are in remission 23, 10 and 7 years after diagnosis. Only one of the patients had the kidney involvement of classical Wegener's granulomatosis. The other four cases could be classified as the limited form of the disease. However, both fatal cases were in the latter category. Bilateral orbital involvement was present in two cases. Blindness or loss of the eye occurred in four eyes of the ten affected orbits. The course of the disease in all five patients was characterized by remissions and recurrences of the disease. The effectiveness of any given therapy at any given time in the course of the disease was uncertain, inasmuch as progression of symptoms in one site and remission of disease in another site were simultaneously noted in several cases.

From the standpoint of the eye and orbit, this can be a most serious disease. Even among the patients who are in a remission phase, we would advise a cautious prognosis.

ORBITAL SARCOID

At the outset it is important to point out the shades of meaning between the words sarcoidosis and sarcoid. In the ophthalmic literature, in particular, authors are prone to apply the word sarcoidosis to what is really an example of sarcoid. *Sarcoidosis* is a multisystem and multicentric disease that may affect an orbital structure sometime in its course. *Sarcoid* is an isolated focal lesion that may never disseminate beyond its original locus. The characteristic granulomatous lesion of the two conditions looks basically the same under the microscope. Some observers use this fact to support the belief that sarcoid may be a mild, early, and almost asymptomatic form of sarcoidosis. The latter may never develop, either because the antigenic stimulus that produces the disease is not sufficiently severe or prolonged, or because host factors arrest the disease early in its course. Thus, patients with the bilateral hilar adenopathy so characteristic of sarcoidosis may never develop any further signs of the disease. Likewise, an orbital sarcoid tumor may never disseminate into a sarcoidosis.

Other observers do not believe sarcoid and sarcoidosis are related, even though, histopathologically, they look alike. These observers prefer the term *sarcoid-like*, rather than sarcoid, to emphasize a probable etiologic difference. Also, there is some clinical evidence to support this viewpoint.

In this discussion we will touch upon both conditions in relation to the orbit but place most emphasis on *orbital sarcoid*, because this is the lesion that, most often, must be differentiated from other orbital tumors.

HISTORICAL ASPECTS

In the course of its evolution to its present status as a systemic disease, sarcoidosis has had more than an average share of eponymous designations. Eponyms such as *Boeck's disease, Besnier's disease, Schaumann's disease, Besnier-Boeck-Schaumann's disease, Hutchinson-Boeck's disease,* and *Mortimer's malady* frequently have appeared in the literature. There is some difference of opinion as to who first described what is now considered the cutaneous form of sarcoid. Both Hunter (1936) and, more recently, Scadding (1967) have published interesting and informative reviews on the historical aspects of the subject. Hunter believed that the Englishman Jonathan Hutchinson probably described the first case in a publication of 1875. This was the Hutchinson who noted the notched teeth associated with congenital syphilis. Apparently, illustrations of the same patient appeared in another of Hutchinson's publications 2 years later (1877) and this is the reference quoted by Scadding. The patient, a man in the sixth decade, had purplish, smooth, nontender elevations on the fingers and dorsum of one hand, and on the front of one leg. Hutchinson referred to it as a papillary psoriasis. The patient also had gout. This description seems compatible with the present concept of cutaneous sarcoid, but strangely, Hutchinson (1898) did not associate this case with the one he described as Mortimer's malady some 20 years later. (Scadding [1967] attributes this discrepancy to Hutchinson's belief that the skin lesions of the first case were associated with the gout.) Who was Mortimer? This was the last name of a woman, aged 64 at the time of onset, who had cutaneous lesions on the cheeks and upper arms. All subsequent observers seem to agree that the illustrations of these cutaneous lesions depict the disease that subsequently would be called sarcoid. Hutchinson proposed to Mrs. Mortimer that one of the lesions be biopsied, but this so frightened her that she disappeared from follow-up observation for 2 years. Hutchinson thus lost the opportunity to be the first to make a histopathologic study of the disease.

If Hutchinson's first case is not accepted as an example of cutaneous sarcoid, then priority should go to Besnier (1889). Besnier, of France, observed a 34-year-old man in whom, over a period of 10 years, purplish red elevated lesions had involved the ears, nose, and fingers. Besnier named the disorder *lupus pernio*, or chilblain lupus. The first histopathologic study of similar lesions in another patient was the privilege of Caesar Boeck (not to be confused with his uncle Carl Boeck), of Norway, in 1899. Boeck thought the disorder was a benign form of sarcoma and named the skin disease *multiple benign sarkoid*. Boeck's patient also had lymphadenopathy.

In the next two decades, the subcutaneous nodules were noted, the roentgenographic changes in the long bones were associated with the disorder, and the systemic potentialities of the disease were recognized. However, it was not until about 40 years after the report of Boeck that a histopathologic study of an orbital nodule was performed; the manifestations of sarcoid in the eyelids, the conjunctiva, and within the eye, in contrast, were well known. Merrill King (1939), at a meeting of the American Ophthalmological Society, presented what he thought was the first case of orbital sarcoid, but he probably was unaware of a similar case that Holm (1937) of Denmark had described 2 years earlier. Holm had described a mobile, bean-shaped nodule on the orbital rim of a 63-year-old man, but it is not clear from the details of the biopsy on which side of the orbital septum the nodule was located—whether it was located on the eyelid or in the orbit.

An even earlier example of possible orbital sarcoidosis was the case of Reis and Rothfeld (1931). Their patient was a girl who died at the age of 17 years. For a period of 2 years, there had been sarcoid infiltration of the skin, bilateral exophthalmos, involvement of one eye and both temporal lobes, and radiographic changes of the metacarpals and phalanges. Although autopsy was performed, the cause of the exophthalmos was not discussed nor was a histopathologic examination of the orbital tissues performed.

Before leaving the brief historical aspects of this tumor, one additional eponym, *Mikulicz's syndrome* or *disease*, should be mentioned. Mikulicz was a Polish surgeon who described a bilateral enlargement of the lacrimal and salivary glands. Mikulicz (1892) thought that the bilateral disorder was due to some external infection. This disorder now is believed to have several different causes, one of which is sarcoidosis. Painless, bilateral enlargements of the lacrimal glands, particularly in blacks, might very well be but another manifestation of the tumor under discussion.

INCIDENCE

An estimate of incidence will depend on whether sarcoidosis and sarcoid are regarded as separate conditions or lumped together as manifestations of the same disease. First to be considered are those few cases in the literature in which a tumor is removed from an orbit and which, on histopathologic examination, shows a picture like that of sarcoid similar in all respects to tissue from a disseminated case of the disease. After long-term observation, however, such patients do not develop obvious sarcoid lesions in other tissues of the body. The five (four females and one male) cases of orbital sarcoid included in the Mayo Clinic study were of this type. The female patients were 53, 57, 62, and 72 years of age at the time of orbital diagnosis. They were followed 9, 8, 13, and 14 years, respectively, without signs of systemic involvement. The male patient was 85 years old at the time of diagnosis, but in a period of 6 months he developed a diffuse, poorly differentiated lymphoma and survived only another month. The presence of the sarcoid lesion soon followed by the malignant lymphoma may not be simply fortuitous. In this situation the sarcoid reaction in the orbit may have been the result of an altered immunologic reaction secondary to a silently evolving malignant lymphoma. The female cases with their long follow-up cannot be called examples of sarcoidosis as the word is applied to the disseminated form of the disorder. In another sense, however, can they be regarded as examples of benign isolated sarcoidosis — or is the appearance of the tumor just a nonspecific tissue response to some local but unknown etiologic factor? Some cases reported in the literature are similar to these cases in that the unilateral orbital tumor is the one symptom that brings them to the attention of the physician. The tumor is removed and duly examined, but more extensive study reveals such roentgenographic features as bilateral hilar adenopathy or radiolucent areas in some of the long bones. Such cases may be presumptive examples of sarcoidosis because the systemic manifestations eventually disappear without being subject to histopathologic study. It is never known in these cases whether the orbital lesion was the primary manifestation or just another phase in the dissemination of the disorder. Rarer still are those cases in which both the presenting orbital tumor and a lymphadenopathy occurring later are found to have similar cellular patterns; the case of Melmon and Goldberg (1962) is an example. These cases more nearly fulfill the criteria of orbital sarcoid developing into sarcoidosis.

Next to be considered are those cases in which bilateral enlargement of the lacrimal glands develops during the course of sarcoidosis. In many of these cases orbital involvement was only presumptive because a biopsy of the mass was not performed. Last are those instances in which the location of the mass is loosely referred to the orbit but is actually in the eyelid.

Considering these variables in terminology and histopathologic verification, an estimate of the orbital incidence of either sarcoid or sarcoidosis is very difficult. Jensen (1957) counted eleven cases of what he regarded as orbital sarcoid up to the time of his report.

The one factor upon which there is general agreement is the higher prevalence of sarcoidosis among blacks in North America. As regards sex incidence, the disorder seems slightly more common among females. The ophthalmic literature gives the impression the orbital sarcoid is more frequent among the elderly. People with the unilateral isolated sarcoid-like tumors usually are older than 45 years. However, patients with proven sarcoidosis who develop bilateral enlargement of the lacrimal glands or a tumor in one orbit usually are younger than 45 years. The age range, then, for the broad group of cases having a similar histopathologic appearance is from adolescence onward.

CLINICAL FEATURES

There are several well-documented cases in the literature in which orbital sarcoid was found in the rear of the orbit. In the majority of unilateral cases, however, the tumor is well forward in the orbit, associated with some puffiness or drooping of the upper eyelid, and can be palpated as a firm, painless, nontender mass in any quadrant of the orbit. From this position it may grow forward and become attached to the skin, it may extend posteriorly toward the apex of the orbit, or it may spread from one quadrant of the orbit to another. It may even remain as a relatively discrete, isolated lump near the lacrimal gland.

If the clinician has the unusual opportunity to uncover a sarcoid-like tumor ‚in one orbit of a patient whose only complaint is proptosis, a further search should be made for additional manifestations of sarcoidosis. Such systemic manifestations may be evident at the same time as the orbital disease, but rarely they may not be known to the patient, or they may develop later (i.e., several weeks or months). The most important examination is a routine roentgenographic search for bilateral hilar lymphadenopathy. This enlargement of lymph nodes (particularly those in the cervical and axillary chains), plaques or nodular swellings of the skin, chilblain-like swellings of the face and phalanges, nodules in the eyelids or epibulbar masses, uveitis or retinal periphlebitis, and facial nerve palsy. The small bones of the hands and feet and the long bones of the forearms and lower legs should be examined roentgenographically. Results of certain special studies also may be helpful: the serum calcium concentration (increased in sarcodosis); the plasma protein concentration (hyperproteinemia and hyperglobulinemia); the response to intradermal injection of tuberculin (anergy); and the response (a nodular reaction or positive Kveim reaction), to the intradermal injection of a heated suspension of tissue particles from a lymph node in cases of sarcoidosis. The Kveim test is so complicated a procedure, and is so often negative in atypical cases, that it is not considered a very reliable diagnostic test by many clinicians. Should follicle-like, granulomatous lesions appear in the inferior conjunctival cul-de-sac in a patient under observation for possible sarcoidosis, these tumors may be biopsied and obviate the need for a scalene node biopsy to establish the diagnosis. Such conjunctival biopsies will be positive in from 25 to 33% of cases with the systemic disease. Conjunctival biopsies are not positive in patients with localized orbital sarcoid.

One additional clinical feature should be noted. Sarcoid tumors may occur anywhere along the length of the optic nerve and simulate an optic nerve glioma or optic nerve involvement by meningioma.

PATHOLOGY

The essential lesion in sarcoid is the noncaseating epithelioid cell granuloma. In the older literature this often was called the hard tubercle, in order to distinguish the lesion from the soft caseating tubercle of tuberculosis. The word *tubercle* refers to a well-delineated, oval or round group of epithelioid cells. The sarcoid tubercles vary in size and number but usually are scattered diffusely throughout the tissue specimen (Fig. 338). Within the tubercle (granuloma),

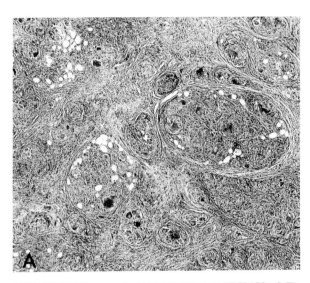

Figure 338. Sarcoidosis:
A, Numerous small noncaseating granulomas replace the orbital tissue, and much associated fibrosis develops between granulomas. (Hematoxylin and eosin; × 35.)

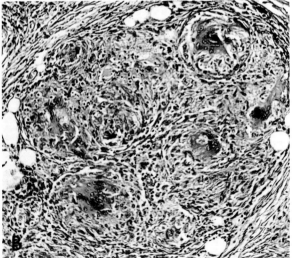

B, Detail of granuloma. (Hematoxylin and eosin; × 130.)

giant cells also will be found and the whole is surrounded by lymphocytes. The lymphocytic infiltration never is as marked as in the granuloma of tuberculosis nor are the lymphocytes concentrated into follicles or groups of heavily staining cells as in lymphocytic inflammatory pseudotumor. The term *epithelioid cell* may mislead the clinician. The cell has no histogenous relationship with epithelium but the pictorial similarity has given origin to this well-established but unfortunate usage of the term. This polyhedral cell is really a large mono-nuclear phagocyte that traces its origin to the tissue histiocyte or its close cousin, the mobile blood monocyte. The oval nuclei of these cells are pale-staining, owing to the sparseness of chromatin material. More striking are the giant cells. The most common giant cell is the one designated the Langhans type. In this type, the nuclei are arranged in an arc or an incomplete circle around the periphery of the cell surrounding an eosinophilic, central, granular cytoplasm. Less frequently an even larger type of giant cell may be seen in which 12 to 18 nuclei are scattered throughout the cytoplasm or clumped together in a heap at one end of the cell. There may be an acellular zone in the center of some of these tubercles; this may be referred to as an area of fibrinoid necrosis but it does not represent actual caseation. Sometimes inclusion bodies also may be seen; such, however, may not be easily seen except by a pathologist who is familiar with the configuration of the various types. Three types usually are described and all occur within the giant cells.

One type of inclusion body is lamellated structure that resembles the con-figuration of a seashell. The smallest is about the size of a leukocyte but, as successive layers of calcium salts are deposited, the inclusion body may increase to 10 or more times its original diameter. It stains deeply with hematoxylin. It frequently is called the Schaumann conchoid body. Another type of inclusion body is an almost colorless, doubly refractile vesicle near the center of the giant cell (diameter, 1 to 5 μ). A third type of inclusion body is the asteroid body. This is a stellate, spider-like object (diameter, 5 to 20 μ) that is found inside a vacuole within the giant cell, staining pink with hematoxylin and eosin.

The clinician should not assume that the inclusion bodies, the noncaseating tubercles, and the giant cells are specifically diagnostic of sarcoid. The inclusions may be found in other types of granulomatous reactions as well as some infectious diseases. In isolated specimens from the orbit, a search should be made for the acid-fast staining bacillus of tuberculosis. A more conclusive diagnosis of orbital sarcoid is possible if tissue cultures for tuberculosis are negative. In most cases reported in the literature, such cultures were never performed, so diagnosis remains largely presumptive. A granulomatous reaction to a foreign body also should be ruled out.

TREATMENT

In three of the four female patients in the Mayo Clinic study, the sarcoid-like masses were located in the more forward portion of the orbit. They were easily uncovered through an anterior orbitotomy and the unencapsulated tumors were partially excised. In a follow-up period of 8 to 14 years these patients seemed to do well. The remaining portion of the tumor gradually disappeared without visual impairment. In the remaining female patient the course has been quite different. Over a period of twenty years this patient has undergone six orbitotomies for recurrent left orbital tumor. At each operation a fairly extensive removal of a nonencapsulated mass was performed but, at the end of 25 years of observation, recurrent tumor is again palpable. Culture and acid-fast stains of the granulomas have always been negative. Neither has the patient ever developed any similar process in the other orbit or any systemic signs of disease that might suggest sarcoidosis. The microscopic appearance of the successive tissue specimens look the same except for an increasing degree of fibrosis. At the present time we do not have an explanation for this recurrent and most atypical behavior of orbital sarcoid.

In these patients in whom the orbital mass is but one additional manifestation of an already established sarcoidosis, or in whom the tumor is diffuse or occupies the posterior recesses of the orbit, we would favor administration of prednisone. Inasmuch as prolonged (months or several years) therapy is usually required, supervision of an internist is mandatory. During the course of therapy, ophthalmologists should watch for any ocular side effects. Fortunately, the symptomatology of the disease usually can be controlled on a fairly low maintenance dose of steroids, thus minimizing drug-induced sequelae. Unfortunately, remissions of the disease often recur when the drug is discontinued.

Bibliography

Orbital Vasculitis and Wegener's Granulomatosis

Blodi FC, Gass JDM: Inflammatory pseudotumor of the orbit. Brit J Ophthalmol 52:79–93, 1968
Carrington CB, Liebow AA: Limited forms of angiitis and granulomatosis of Wegener's type. Am J Med 41:497–527, 1966
Cassan SM, Divertie MB, Hollenhorst RW, et al: Pseudotumor of the orbit and limited Wegener's granulomatosis. Ann Int Med 72:687–693, 1970
DeRemee RA, McDonald TJ, Harrison EG, Jr, et al: Wegener's granulomatosis. Anatomic correlates, a proposed classification. Mayo Clinic Proc 51:777–781, 1976
Faulds JS, Wear AR: Pseudtumor of the orbit and Wegener's granuloma. Lancet 2:955–957, 1960
Harcourt RB: Orbital granulomata associated with widespread angiitis. Brit J Ophthalmol 48:673–677, 1964
Henderson JW: *Orbital Tumors.* Philadelphia, WB Saunders and Co, 1973
Klinger H: Grenzform der periarteritis nodosa. Frankfurt Z Path 42:455–480, 1931
Straatsma BR: Ocular manifestations of Wegener's granulomatosis. Am J Ophthalmol 44:789–799, 1957
Walton EW: Giant cell granuloma of the respiratory tract. Brit Med J 2:265–270, 1958
Wegener F: Über generalsierts, septische Gefásserkrankungen. Verh Dtsch Ges Pathol 29:202–208, 1936
Wegener F: Über eine eigenartige rhinogene Granulomatose mit besonderere Beteiligung des Arteri ensystems und der Nieren. Beitr Pathol Anat 102:36–38, 1939
Weiter J, Farkas TG: Pseudotumor of the orbit as a presenting sign in Wegener's granulomatosis. Surv Ophthalmol 17:106–119, 1972

Orbital Sarcoid

In the following list of references the publications of Hunter, Longcope and Pierson, and Scadding contain extensive bibliographies.

Besnier E: Lupus pernio de la face: synovites fongueuses (scrofulotuberculeuses) symetriques des extrémités supérieures. Ann Dermatol Syphilol 10:333–336, 1889

Boeck C: Multiple benign sarkoid of the skin. J Cutaneous Genitourin Dis *17*:543–550, 1899

Holm E: A case of sarcoid of Boeck. Acta Ophthalmol (Kbh) *15*:235–238, 1937

Hunter FT: Hutchinson-Boeck's disease ("generalized sarcoidosis"): historical note and report of a case with apparent cure. N Engl J Med *214*:346–352, 1936

Hutchinson J: Cases of Mortimer's malady (lupus vulgaris multiplex non-ulcerans et non-serpiginosus). Arch Surg (Lond) *9*:307–311, 1898

Jensen VJ: Sarcoidosis of the orbit. Acta Ophthalmol (Kbh) *35*:416–419, 1957

Khan F, Wessely Z, Chazin SR, et al: Conjunctival biopsy in sarcoidosis. Ann Ophthalmol *9*:671–676, 1977

King MJ: Ocular lesions of Boeck's sarcoid. Trans Am Ophthalmol Soc *37*:422–458, 1939

Longcope WT, Pierson JW: Boeck's sarcoid (sarcoidosis). Bull Johns Hopkins Hosp *60*:223–296, 1937

Melmon KL, Goldberg JS: Sarcoidosis with bilateral exophthalmos as the initial symptom. Am J Med *33*:158–160, 1962

Mikulicz J: Ueber eine eigenartige symmetrische Erkrankung der Thränen- und Mundspeicheldrüsen. *In Beiträge zur Chirurgie Festschrift Gewidmet.* Ed T Billroth. Stuttgart, F Enke, 1892, pp 610–630

Nichols CW, Mishkin M, Yanoff M: Presumed orbital sarcoidosis: report of a case followed by computerized axial tomography and conjunctival biopsy. Trans Am Ophthaolmol Soc *76*:67–75, 1978

Papo I, Beltrami CA, Salvoline U, et al: Sarcoidosis simulating a glioma of the optic nerve. Surg Neurol *8*:353–355, 1977

Reis W, Rothfeld J: Tuberkulide des Sehnerven als Komplikation von Hautsarkoiden vom Typus Darier-Roussy. Arch Ophtalmol (Paris) *126*:357–366, 1931

Scadding JG: *Sarcoidosis.* London, Eyre & Spottiswoode, 1967

22

Miscellaneous Orbital Tumors

Most of us prefer to so arrange medical diagnostics as to facilitate appropriate treatment, if such is possible. Some of the human ills, however, are so complex or so unusual that a classification is not easily arranged, and in most medical texts some space is reserved for a discussion of these lesions that do not quite fit the accepted norm. Such discussions often are relegated to the end of the text, which implies that authors regard such nonconforming entities as being less important, or avoid until the last a discussion of a little-known entity, or hope that the problem will conveniently vanish during the interval of procrastination. Our text is no exception. To designate some of these orbital mavericks and orphans we have used the familiar cliché *miscellaneous, and we will discuss here the orbital lesions of amyloidosis, ectopic lacrimal gland, Mickulicz's disease and Wilms' tumor.*

AMYLOIDOSIS

This puzzling disorder has been known for well over a century, yet there are still many unknowns. In the past two decades much attention, stimulated by an increasing recognition of the widespread clinical manifestations of amyloid deposition, has been given to a possible solution of these problems. In the recent literature several fine reviews of both ocular and sytemic amyloidosis have been published (Cohen 1967, Doughman 1968, Brownstein, Elliott, and Helwig 1970, Glenner et al 1972, Isobe and Osserman 1974, and Knowles et al 1975). The orbit is but one of several anatomic sites that recently have been added to the long list of potential sites for amyloid deposition. Just why there are so few reports of orbital amyloidosis in the older literature is something of an enigma. Because amyloid deposits may simulate other orbital tumors and because the incidence of orbital amyloidosis may increase in the future, it is proper that some space be given to a discussion of this curious derangement.

HISTORICAL ASPECTS

In the medical literature of the 19th century, this unique disorder first was classified with other waxy or lardaceous degenerations of organs and tissues observed at autopsy. The designation *waxy* now seems as appropriate as the

547

term amyloid that was subsequently applied to the disorder. Virchow (1855a,b) noted this waxy material had tinctorial characteristics similar to those of starch (amylose). Both substances stain blue-violet with iodine and sulfuric acid. It was but a natural sequence to designate the starch-resembling substance *amyloid*.

The earliest reference to this amyloid material affecting ocular structures seems to be that of Coats (1915). He reported a 42-year-old man who, over a period of 17 years, had been observed by several physicians because of a slowly progressive, disabling, infiltrating process involving adnexal tissues surrounding one eye. The disease commenced as a growth on the bulbar surface of the eye, gradually extended around the circumference of the eye, and infiltrated the sheaths of the optic nerve. Histologically, the picture was chiefly that of an amyloid degeneration, but a marked fibrocytic response, with lymphocytic reaction and some giant cells of foreign-body type, also was apparent.

Many cases of a more localized form of amyloidosis affecting the conjunctiva have since been recorded, but cases of *orbital* amyloidosis with or without associated subconjunctival deposits or eyelid amyloidosis remain sparse. One example of localized orbital amyloid in a 42-year-old woman was recorded by Pollems (1920), but there was then a long hiatus before amyloid disease in the orbit again was reported.

CLASSIFICATION

Amyloidosis, basically, is an extracellular deposition of insoluble protein that may either be localized or ubiquitous in distribution. The size of the abnormal deposit, the organs involved, and the degree of progressiveness of the metabolic abnormality determines the disability that is produced. It has been known for many years that amyloid deposition is a common complication of many chronic debilitating infections and inflammatory diseases. Such amyloidosis with an antecedent cause has been classified as the *secondary* type. Later, in the clinical evolution of the disease, a *heredofamilial* form of amyloidosis was recognized which, in the field of ophthalmology, may produce perivascular retinal deposits and characteristic vitreous opacities. Also, an amyloidosis associated with *myeloma* and other plasmacytoid dyscrasias was soon recognized. A *primary* (not associated with any known cause or antecedent disease) localized type of amyloid is the lesion most commonly encountered in the orbit, and it is this form of amyloidosis that is our concern in this chapter.

However, this long-used classification is undergoing considerable revision because of more intensive study of the immunochemistry, biochemistry, and ultrastructural features of the abnormal protein. At present, several major classes of proteins have been identified with the ultrastructural configuration and physicochemical properties of amyloid (Kaiser-Kupfer, 1977). One class is related to immunoglobulin- (light chain) producing cells; another class is a synthesis of a nonantibody protein. The source of the amyloid from an isolated orbital nodule has not yet been subject to these investigative techniques. In the future, classifications may be based on the biochemical abnormality or precursor cell of origin of the amyloid, rather than its distribution in various tissues and organs with or without known clinical antecedents.

INCIDENCE AND CLINICAL FEATURES

The sex and age distribution of localized orbital amyloidosis can be summarized quickly by reviewing the few proven cases recorded in the literature. Nehen (1979), Handousa (1954), Kassman and Sundmark (1967), Schubert (1972), Easton and Smith (1961), Radnot and colleagues (1971), Savino and colleagues (1976) and Howard (1966) show unilateral examples of the disease. Knowles and colleagues (1975), Pollems (1920), and Jensen (1976) reported bilateral cases of the localized type of orbital amyloid. These eleven patients ranged in age from 27 to 78 years with a female:male ratio of 7:4. Another case of Howard (1966), and the case of Raab (1970), suggest an orbital amyloidosis associated with some systemic manifestations of the disorder. These were both male patients, ages 60 and 55 years, respectively. The two patients (one male and one female) observed in the time period of our study were 57 and 64 years of age, respectively. Both cases were considered examples of localized orbital disease at the time of initial surgical diagnosis, inasmuch as a general physical and laboratory survey did not uncover any other manifestations of amyloidosis. The status of the disease in the female patient remained localized to one orbit through a follow-up period of seven years. The male patient developed severe systemic dissemination of the disease four years later and expired from the disease eight years after diagnosis. These two cases are too few for meaningful incidence data.

Assessment of the clinical features and course of the orbital disease also is restricted by the small total cases. In the six cases of localized orbital disease (including our female patient) the duration of the disease (where stated) was as short as 1 year and as long as 12 years before presentation. A palpable but painless mass, some proptosis or displacement of the eye, and some restriction of extraocular motility, was present in the majority of cases. The restriction of extraocular motility was rather mild in one case, but in another the eye was immobile. This reflects the variable degree of infiltration of the extraocular muscles as well as the severity of the disease from one case to another. Recurrent subconjunctival hemorrhage and ecchymosis of the eyelids were not a prominent feature in the clinical course of these orbital cases as they are in amyloidosis of the eyelids and surface of the eye. Of the seven orbits affected by the localized disease the mass of amyloid was palpable in the superior temporal quadrant (three cases), superior nasal quadrant (three cases), and inferior orbit (one case).

In the even fewer cases of orbital amyloidosis associated with some positive systemic manifestations, the prediagnostic duration of the disease was longer, the orbital masses larger, the proptosis greater, and the extraocular muscle involvement more severe than the cases with localized orbital disease.

Several published reports have stated that strictly localized amyloidosis does not become systemic. Perhaps these ophthalmologists have not followed some of their cases long enough to be positive on this point. We regarded our male patient as an example of primary localized orbital amyloid only to find, in time, that the disease became systemic. Because of the rarity of this situation in the literature we include a summary of the clinical features of our case.

A 57-year-old man noticed progressive downward displacement of the left eye and painless swelling of the left upper eyelid for nearly 2 years. He made the interesting observation that rubbing the affected eyelid made it bleed intermittently. This feature — minor episodes of intermittent bleeding into subcutaneous tissues — is characteristic of amyloidosis around the orbit and eyelids, but it has not been noted in all reported cases. A mass with indefinite borders extended across the two upper quadrants of the orbit. Systemic review revealed neither obvious diseases nor any clues as to the nature of the orbital process. No bony changes were apparent on the roentgenogram. At anterosuperior orbitotomy the mass was removed incompletely. The tissue was friable and bled easily; it was yellow-red and felt stringy and waxy. The mass had no capsule, and the tumor so infiltrated surrounding structures as to negate complete excision. There was no obvious fibrous tissue reaction. This operation did little to relieve the patient's symptoms.

The first indications of generalized amyloidosis appeared approximately 4 years after the initial orbital manifestations. The patient subsequently required treatment of pleural effusions and congestive heart failure on several occasions. He died 8 years after initial orbitotomy. At autopsy, amyloid deposits were seen in the myocardium, lungs, liver, kidneys, spleen, pancreas, esophagus, stomach, adrenals, skeletal muscle, and eyelid of the other eye.

When orbital amyloidosis is discovered, other systemic signs of amyloidosis and disorders commonly associated with amyloid deposition should be sought. One of the latter disorders is plasma cell myeloma, and a bone marrow biopsy might help to exclude this. Latent dysgammaglobulinemia might be uncovered by urinary and blood immunoelectrophoresis and examination of the urine for Bence Jones protein. Elevation of the erythrocytic sedimentation rate might be a clue to disorders associated with amyloidosis but which are not yet manifest. Of particular interest to ophthalmologists is examination of the eyes for unusual numbers and types of vitreous opacities. The vitreous opacities that have proved to be amyloid deposits may be so numerous and thick as to resemble "glass wool." They are thought to be almost diagnostic of the familial hereditary type of amyloidosis.

PATHOLOGY

Amyloid material is an amorphous substance that often can be identified grossly by its yellow color, its waxy or glassy character, and its tendency to bleed easily. By touching the material during an orbitotomy the diagnosis may be possible even before histopathologic examination confirms the eosinophilic, acellular infiltrative character of amyloidosis (Fig. 339). If there is any doubt after gross examination, a host of available dyes can be used to help identify amyloid deposits. Probably no other orbital tumor has been subject to so many tinctorial tests and treatments as have amyloid deposits. With the standard hematoxylin and eosin stain, amyloid looks pink. With the classic iodine and dilute sulfuric acid stain (used by Virchow), the amyloid material stains a blue-purple; but the reaction is inconstant and not as dependable as those in other staining methods. The dye most widely used is Congo red, which imparts an orange-pink tint to amyloid deposits. The diagnostic value of this test, however, is the unique green birefringence that is visible under the polarizing microscope. Other dyes, such as periodic acid-Schiff (reddish purple), Masson's trichrome (bluish purple), and crystal violet (metachromatically purple) may be used to confirm the diagnosis. Amyloid also fluoresces with some of the fluorochrome substances, but the reaction is not as specific nor as reliable as the birefringence

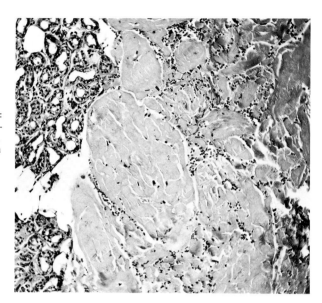

Figure 339. Amyloidosis: orbital tissues are massively infiltrated by eosinophilic, hyaline, acellular material. (Hematoxylin and eosin; × 100.)

with Congo red (Fig. 340). Perivascular deposition of amyloid also occurs and is responsible for the increased capillary fragility and easy bleeding.

Under light microscopy amyloid has an amorphous appearance but with electronmicroscopy it has a definite fibrillary pattern. The fibrils are fine, rigid, and nonbranching, giving the lobule of amyloid a pleated appearance.

TREATMENT

Except for surgical removal of as much as possible of the offending substance, there seems to be little else to offer patients with orbital amyloidosis. Excision is useful in patients in whom the amyloid deposit is well circumscribed, as it was in one of Howard's (1966) cases. This case of localized amyloid had not shown any recurrence of the tumor in a 4-year period of observation. But in some cases, including our own, the infiltration of amyloid is beyond the bounds of reasonable resection. If all amyloid were removed from some orbits so affected, the resultant scar and disability of ocular function would equal or be worse than the original disability. Our own patients derived little benefit from orbitotomy, which proved to be more diagnostic than therapeutic. The female patient, whose orbital disease has remained localized over a 7-year period, has had an additional orbitotomy for recurrence of the orbital amyloid since the original diagnosis. The eye in the affected orbit is still proptosed, the mobility is severely restricted, pallor of the optic disk is present, and vision is reduced to finger counting. The final outcome of a case of localized orbital amyloid may depend on the size of the tumor, its location in the orbit, and the presence or absence of progression. These variables also were noted with the inflammatory tumors of the two preceding chapters and contribute to the unpredictable course of the disease.

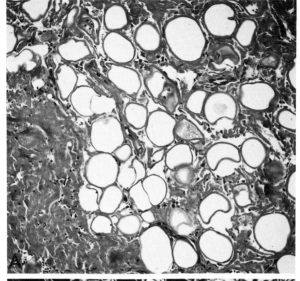

Figure 340. Amyloidosis:

A, A distinctive feature is the formation of "amyloid rings" as the material surrounds fat cells. (Hematoxylin and eosin; × 100.)

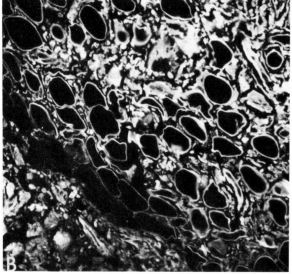

B, When treated with thioflavin T, amyloid deposits bind this fluorochrome substance and show bright fluorescence in ultraviolet light. (Magnification, × 100.)

ECTOPIC LACRIMAL GLAND

The word *ectopic*, from a pathologic standpoint, is applied to the displacement of some tissue or organ from its usual or normal anatomic position. This term does not necessarily imply that function in the malposed tissue is abnormal, nor is it usually applied to some abnormality in configuration or function of a tissue or organ in its normal anatomic site. For the latter situation, the word *aberrant* more often is used as a descriptive designation. The nuances of these words are mentioned because both have been applied to orbital masses. However, both terms are alike in the sense that some congenital factor is believed to be responsible for the abnormality in question.

Lacrimal gland tissue of true ectopic type has been observed on the epibulbar surface of the eye, at the corneal-scleral limbus, around the extraocular muscles, and even within the eye. Although such misplaced glandular tissue may not have a normal secretory function, some of these ectopic lobules may undergo a physiologic enlargement proportionate to the growth of the child. Those congenital nests of tissue on the surface of the eye are in the most conspicuous location, and any nodular or lobular hypertrophy there is usually noticed in infancy or early childhood. Even so, hypertrophy of ectopic tissue more deeply placed around an extraocular muscle or within the eye may not be evident until strabismus or visual disability develops in later childhood. It would be reasonable to assume that glandular rests located still deeper within the orbit might not become manifest until late childhood or adolescence; in this way the situation is similar in age distribution to another developmental abnormality, the dermoid cyst, which sometimes is encountered in the deeper areas of the orbit.

That such ectopic glandular tissue should or could occur in the orbit does not seem to have been the subject of any comment in the literature until recently. Green and Zimmerman (1967) reviewed the subject of ectopic lacrimal gland tissue, and included what they thought were eight cases with orbital involvement. They also noted two earlier French references. According to one of the latter articles (that of Boudet and Bertezéne), unilateral exophthalmos was the result of a lacrimal gland adenoma in an ectopic position within the orbit. We have reservations as to whether the majority of cases described by Green and Zimmerman are true examples of ectopic lacrimal gland tissue in the orbit.

Most of their tissue samples were removed either from the superotemporal quadrant of the orbit or from an area posterior to the lacrimal gland. We are hesitant to designate tumors involving lacrimal gland tissue in such areas as ectopic. Instead, we wonder if such tissue rather is an alteration of lacrimal gland tissue secondary to some orbital inflammation or granulomatous process. It is not uncommon for pseudotumor to infiltrate and distort the lacrimal gland in the course of its undisciplined advance. When the orbit has been subjected to prior biopsy, as were some of the cases of Green and Zimmerman, the function of the lacrimal gland also may be altered. This would account for fibrosis, acinar atrophy, cellular infiltration, and cystic degeneration that have been observed in some specimens. Other distortions of the lacrimal gland may occur in association with endocrine exophthalmos. In one case among the series under discussion there was a history of bilateral proptosis, though diagnosis of an ectopic gland was made on the basis of surgical exploration of only one orbit. Finally, in the course of orbitotomies for tumors unrelated to the lacrimal gland, we have observed apparently normal glandular tissue located posterior to the eye. Four of the eight patients recorded by Green and Zimmerman were in the fifth decade of life, which is difficult to reconcile with the view that the origin of the disorder rests in a supposedly congenital abnormality such as ectopic lacrimal gland.

Another report bearing on the problem is that of Baldridge (1970). His case was that of an 18-year-old man with unilateral proptosis of at least 3 years' duration. A flattened mass of lacrimal gland tissue (dimensions, 30 × 10 mm) was removed at a lateral orbitotomy. The tumor did not seem to have any

direct connection with an apparently normal underlying lacrimal gland. Histologic examination confirmed the acinar structure of normal lacrimal gland
tissue. Baldridge referred to this accessory tumor as an aberrant lacrimal gland.

A more recent report is that of Jacobs and colleagues (1977). This case was
a 69-year-old female who developed 6 mm of proptosis of one eye over a period
of 9 months associated with a decrease in vision. Vision was reduced to counting
fingers. Papilledema also was noted. A fleshy, pink, soft, encapsulated mass 15
× 12 × 2 mm, without any discernible connection to a normally appearing
lacrimal gland, was removed from the posterior-inferior orbit. The orbital mass
was not visible on standard computer tomography but became visible after contrast. It is strange that this glandular enlargement occurred so late in life and
created such a marked visual disturbance.

When these developmental anomalies of the lacrimal gland occur in the
orbit, total excision of the enlarging mass would seem to be more appropriate
than biopsy or piecemeal resection.

This place in our text is as appropriate as any to note another strange
ectopic orbital mass. This was a nontender, movable lump under the right
eyebrow of a 47-year-old female reported by Wolter and Roosenburg (1977).
The lump had been present for some 20 years and simulated a lacrimal gland
tumor. It measured 24 × 15 × 10 mm in size and proved to have the structure
of a lymph node on histopathologic examination. The authors assumed it was
congenital.

MIKULICZ'S DISEASE

In Chapter 21 the possible relationship between sarcoidosis and a disorder
associated with the name of Johann Mikulicz, of Breslau, was mentioned.
Because Mikulicz's disease usually involves some bilateral tumefactions of the
lacrimal glands and because, in this text, these secretory organs are considered a
part of the orbit, some discussion of Mikulicz's disease seems proper.

Mikulicz's first observation of a patient with bilateral enlargement of the
lacrimal and salivary glands was briefly noted in the résumé of a medical meeting held in Königsberg in 1888. A more detailed report of this case (a 42-year-
old male) with a review of several additional cases clinically resembling his
own, but reported by others both before and after 1888, was made later by
Mikulicz in 1892. In brief, Mikulicz had partially resected these tumors on
several occasions, had studied their histologic makeup, and presented several
drawings of the salient clinical features of this strange case. His observation of
this patient extended over a period of only a few years because the patient died
from an abdominal disorder that seemed to be unrelated to the recurrent tumors
of the lacrimal and salivary glands. Mikulicz believed that this bilateral, symmetric disorder was benign; but, as further cases came to his attention, he concluded that some cases resembled a similar tumefaction associated with what
was then called lymphosarcoma.

Mikulicz's observations stimulated a host of case reports from other observers. In less than 20 years, some 80 to 90 examples of Mikulicz's disease then
were recorded in the literature. By this time it became evident that bilateral en-

largement of the lacrimal, parotid, and submaxillary glands was not always a benign, self-limited, pathologic entity, but was often a secondary manifestation of some generalized systemic disorder that sometimes was fatal. In addition to lymphosarcoma, these tumors were also attributed to leukemia, sarcoidosis, tuberculosis, and syphilis. With each succeeding decade in the present century, Mikulicz's tumors were associated with further clinical and orbital complexes, such as pseudotumor, Sjögren's syndrome, macroglobinemia, and endocrine ophthalmopathy. Attempts by Schaffer and Jacobsen in 1927 to classify this hodgepodge into two major entities — Mikulicz's disease proper (reserved for cases believed to be benign and without obvious cause) and Mikulicz's syndrome (all cases caused by a variety of systemic disorders) only led to more confusion because some cases of Mikulicz's disease later proved to be examples of Mikulicz's syndrome. In time, many clinicians confused the "disease" with the "syndrome," the pathologic parameters of the various cases were not yet so standardized as to provide guidelines for accurate classification, and the terminology of the "syndrome" sometimes was shifted to cases with only bilateral enlargement of the parotid gland.

In recent times, the histopathologic interpretation of these strange tumors of the lacrimal and salivary glands has made great strides, and it is now possible to make a more specific clinical diagnosis. Thus, tumors secondary to malignant lymphoma, sarcoidosis, and leukemia can be differentiated from one another. Similarly, it is also possible to classify some swellings of the lacrimal gland as examples of inflammatory pseudotumor on the basis of the polymorphic changes noted in Chapter 20. One new entity has emerged from these careful pathologic evaluations: the so-called *benign lymphoepithelial lesion* (Godwin 1952, Font, Yanoff, and Zimmerman 1967, Meyer, Yanoff and Hanno 1971, and others). This term gradually is replacing the older, less specific eponym.

The histologic hallmark of this disorder is a proliferation of the intraductal epithelium forming so-called epimyoepithelial islands (Fig. 341). These cellular conglomerates are a mixture of the proliferating inner layer of epithelium as

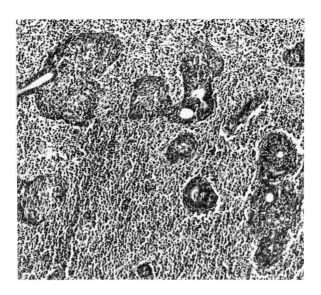

Figure 341. Benign lymphoproliferative lesion: proliferating epithelium and myoepithelium form intraductal cellular aggregates surrounded by a sea of lymphocytes. (Hematoxylin and eosin: × 120.)

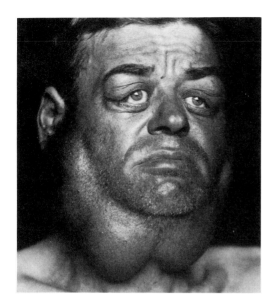

Figure 342. Mikulicz's disease: biopsy revealed the benign lymphoepithelial lesion; note symmetric involvement of the lacrimal, parotid, and submaxillary glands.

well as the outer myoepithelial layer of cells with preservation of the basement membrane. In long-standing cases the epimyoepithelial islands may undergo a squamous metaplasia or hyalinization, but the process remains benign. The other principal histologic feature is a diffuse lymphocytic infiltration of the stroma which may invade the acinar and ductal structures and ultimately compromise their function.

Figure 342 illustrates the clinical appearance of a case that was observed outside the time period of our study. Treatment has not been very satisfactory, although some remission of the glandular enlargement may temporarily occur with administration of systemic corticosteroids.

WILMS' TUMOR

This is essentially a neoplasm of embryonic renal cells, a *nephroblastoma*. This cellular, undifferentiated sarcoma may rarely metastasize to the orbit. This clinical feature is the principal reason for including a short discussion of this tumor in this chapter. Nephroblastoma has never been a popular term, possibly because of confusion with neuroblastoma. As a consequence, the nephroblastoma continues to be associated with the name of Max Wilms, a German surgeon, who published a monograph on the subject in 1899.

Although nephroblastoma and neuroblastoma are both common neoplasms of early life, the neuroblastoma more commonly metastasizes to the orbit (Chapter 11). The nephroblastoma also metastasizes readily but its favorite routes of escape are first the lung, next the liver, and rarely the bones. It usually occurs in children between one and five years of age (Exelby 1978) but may be seen in young infants and the newborn. It is extremely rare after age 8. The sex incidence is equal.

The best documented examples of orbital metastasis are the single cases of Apple (1968), Fratkin and associates (1977), and Goulding (1947). Other probable cases are those reported by Algan and associates (1955), Crawford (1967), and Mortada (1968). Two of the total six cases had bilateral orbital involvement. Like neuroblastoma, the orbital metastasis may be the presenting site of the disease but, more often, orbital involvement appears sometime after the abdominal primary is discovered and treated.

Of greater importance to diagnosis is the peculiar association of Wilms' tumor with congenital aniridia. Thus, in a given case of congenital aniridia, an ophthalmologist may have the unique role of predicting an undiscovered neoplasm of the kidney (Di George and Harley 1965). This genetic misdirection was first noted by Miller and colleagues (1964). Their review of 440 patients with Wilms' tumor uncovered 6 patients with congenital sporadic aniridia. This association was confirmed in another way by Fraumeni and Glass (1968), who found 6 patients with Wilms' tumor among 28 children under 4 years of age with congenital bilateral aniridia.

Microscopically, the tumor is composed of three elements: primitive renal parenchyma cells known as blastoma cells, mesenchymal stromal tissue which resembles embryonal rhabdomyosarcoma, and epithelial cells in different stages of differentiation.

NASAL – ORBITAL POLYPOSIS

In chapter 3 we emphasized the high frequency of secondary orbital tumors relative to total orbital tumors from all sources in a large consecutive series of patients. The majority of these secondary tumors come from next-door neighbors of the orbit, such as the nasal cavity and paranasal sinuses. This fact is not generally appreciated by either ophthalmologists or rhinologists who may have little contact with each others' surgical fields. It is a constant surprise as to just what may "turn up" in the orbit from one of these sources. Two almost simultaneous reports in the ophthalmic literature (Jakobiec et al 1979, and Rawlings et al 1979) of polyposis again emphasize this point.

Polyposis is neither a cyst (Chapter 4) nor a neoplasm (Chapter 16); hence, the reason for placing the subject in this chapter. In both of the reported cases (a 70-year-old female and a 15-year-old male) there was a long history of prior nasal or sinus inflammatory disease, associated with surgical efforts to eradicate the problem. Finally, proptosis (bilateral in one case) occurred because of erosion of the thin ethmoid plate by the inflammatory process. In both cases the eroded bone as well as the orbital masses were visible by suitable radiographic studies, but orbitotomy was necessary to establish the diagnosis and relieve the proptosis.

Bibliography

Amyloidosis

Brownstein MH, Elliott R, Helwig EB: Ophthalmologic aspects of amyloidosis. Am J Ophthalmol 69:423–430, 1970
Coats G: Diseases of the sclera: hyperplasia, with colloid and amyloid degeneration, of the episcleral and circumdural fibrous tissue. Trans Ophthalmol Soc UK 35:257–274, 1915

Cohen AS: Amyloidosis. N Engl J Med 277:522–530; 574–583; 628–638, 1967

Doughman DJ: Ocular amyloidosis. Survey Ophthalmol *13*:133–142, 1968

Glenner GG, Ein D, Terry WD: The immunoglobulin nature of amyloid. Am J Med 52:141–147, 1972

Easton JA, Smith TH: Nonspecific granuloma of orbit ("orbital pseudotumor"). J Path Bact 82:345–354, 1961

Handousa A: Localized intra-orbital amyloid disease. Brit J Ophthalmol 38:510–511, 1954

Howard GM: Amyloid tumors of the orbit. Brit J Ophthal 50:421–425, 1966

Isobe T, Osserman EF: Pattens of amyloidosis and their association with plasma cell dyscrazia, monoclonal immunoglobulins and Bence-Jones proteins. New Engl J Med 290:473–477, 1974

Kaiser-Kupfer MI, McAdams KPWJ, Kuwabara T: Localized amyloidosis of the orbit and upper respiratory tract. Am J Ophthalmol 84:721–728, 1977

Kassman T, Sundmark E: Orbital pseudo-tumors with amyloid. Acta Opthalmol 45:220–228, 1967

Knowles D, Jakobiec F, Rosen M, et al: Amyloidosis of the orbit and adnexa. Surv Ophthalmol *19*:367–384, 1975

Nehen JH: Primary localized orbital amyloidosis. Acta Ophthalmol 57:287–295, 1979

Pollems W: Über tumorförmige lokale Amyloidosis in der Orbita. Arch Ophthalmol (Berlin) *101*:346–361, 1920

Raab EL: Intraorbital amyloid. Brit J Ophthalmol 54:445–449, 1970

Radnót M, Lapis K, Fehér J: Amyloid tumor in the lacrimal gland. Ann Ophthalmol 3:727–742, 1971

Savino PJ, Schatz NJ, Rodrigues MM: Orbital amyloidosis. Can J Ophthalmol *11*:252–255, 1976

Schubert E: Amyloid tumor der Orbita. Klin Mbl Angenheilk 160:467–468, 1972

Virchow R: Ueber den Gang der amyloiden Degeneration. Virchows Arch [Pathol Anat] 8:364–368, 1855a

Virchow R: Zur Cellulose-Frage. Virchows Arch [Pathol Anat] 8:140–144, 1855b

Ectopic Lacrimal Gland

Baldridge M: Aberrant lacrimal gland in the orbit. Arch Ophthalmol 84:758–759, 1970

Boudet, Bertezéne: Cited by Green WR, Zimmerman LE

Green WR, Zimmerman LE: Ectopic lacrimal gland tissue: report of eight cases with orbital involvement. Arch Ophthamol 78:318–327, 1967

Jacobs L, Sirkin S, Kinkel W: Ectopic lacrimal gland in the orbit identified by computerized axial transverse tomography. Ann Ophthalmol 9:591–593, 1977

Wolter JR, Roosenberg, RJ: Ectopic lymph node of the orbit simulating a lacrimal gland tumor. Am J Ophthalmol 83:908–914, 1977

Mikulicz's Disease

Font RL, Yanoff M, Zimmerman LE: Benign lymphoepithelial lesion of the lacrimal gland and its relationship to Sjogren's syndrome. Am J Clin Pathol 48:365–376, 1967

Godwin JT: Benign lymphoepithelial lesion of the parotid gland (adenolymphoma, chronic inflammation, lymphoepithelioma, lymphocytic tumor, Mikulicz disease): report of eleven cases. Cancer 5:1089–1103, 1952

Meyer D, Yanoff M, Hanno H: Differential diagnosis in Mikulicz's syndrome, Mikulicz's disease, and similar disease entities. Am J Ophthalmol 71:516–524, 1971

Mikulicz [J]: Discussion. Berl Klin Wochenscchr 25:759, 1888

Mikulicz J: Ueber Beiträge zur Chirurgie Festschrift Gewidmet. Edited by T Billroth. Stuttgart, F Enke, 1892, pp 610–630

Schaffer AJ, Jacobsen AW: Mikulicz's syndrome: a report of ten cases. Am J Dis Child 34:327–346, 1927

Wilms' Tumor

Algan B, Vitte G, Defines M: Metastase orbitaire d'un nephroblastome. Bull Soc Ophtalmol France 5:323–324, 1955

Apple DJ: Wilms' tumor metastatic to the orbit. Arch Ophthalmol 80:480–483, 1968

Crawford JS: Diseases of the orbit in the ophthalmologic staff of the hospital for sick children. *In The Eye In Childhood.* Chicago, Year Book Medical Publishers, Inc, 1967, Chapter 15

Exelby PR: Solid tumors in children: Wilms' tumor, neuroblastoma, and soft tissue sarcomas. Ca 28:146–163, 1978

Fratkin JD, Purcell JJ, Krachmer JH, et al: Wilms' tumor metastatic to the orbit. JAMA *238*: 1841–1842, 1977

Fraumeni JF, Jr, Glass AG: Wilms' tumor and congenital aniridia. JAMA *206*:825–828, 1968

DiGeorge AM, Harley RD: The association of aniridia, Wilms' tumor and genital abnormalities. Trans Am Ophthalmol Soc *63*:64–69, 1965

Goulding HB: Orbital metastasis from Wilms' tumor. Trans Ophthalmol Soc U Kingd *67*:491–492, 1947

Mortada A: Roentgenography in orbital metastasis with exophthalmos. Am J Ophthalmol *65*:48–53, 1968

Wilms M: Die Mischgeschwültse der Niers. Heft I. Berlin and Leipzig, A Georgi, 1899

Nasal-Orbital Polyposis

Jakobiec FA, Trokel S, Iwamota T: Sino-orbital polyposis. Arch Ophthalmol *97*: 2353-2357, 1979

Rawlings EF, Olson RJ, Kaufman ME: Polypoid sinusitis mimicking orbital malignancy. Am J Ophthalmol *87*: 694-697, 1979

Radnót M, Lapis K, Fehér J: Amyloid tumor in the lacrimal gland. Ann Ophthalmol *3*: 727-742, 1971

Savino PJ, Schatz NJ, Rodrigues MM: Orbital amyloidosis. Can J Ophthalmol *11*: 252-255, 1976

Schubert E: Amyloidtumor der Orbita. Klin Mbl Angenheilk *160*: 467-468, 1972

23

Tumors of Uncertain Origin

GRANULAR CELL MYOBLASTOMA

The term *granular cell myoblastoma* reflects a formerly well-rooted belief that these tumors were derived from striated muscle. In earlier years the tumor was most closely associated with Abrikossoff (Moscow), who published two papers (1926 and 1931) on the subject. The majority of the tumors are found in the oral cavity, particularly the tongue, but the ubiquitous distribution of the tumor in many other body tissues and anatomic sites makes its origin from striated muscle highly unlikely.

In the course of time other cell systems were considered as possible sites of origin. One of these was the histiocyte, and the term *granular cell histiocytoma* reflected this belief. A more popular and current concept supports a neural genesis, reflected in the term *granular cell schwannoma*. Other clinicians believe the tumor arises from a primitive undifferentiated fibroblast, a precursor of both the schwannoma and myoblastoma lineage. This uncertain origin is the reason for discussing the tumor in a separate chapter.

CLINICAL FEATURES

Although the cell genesis of the tumor is unsettled and the question of a malignant variant is equally in dispute, most observers visualize the neoplasm in its common, benign encapsulated form. This solitary, nontender mass generally affects patients between 30 and 50 years of age (Morgan). In the orbit the tumor may be attached to any structure. Orbital examples of the tumor will be found in the reports of Dunnington (1948), Sakamaki (1963), Morgan and Fryer (1969), Timm and Trimmel (1966), Chaves and associates (1972), Obayashi and associates (1969), Gonzalez-Almaraz and associates (1975), Drummond and associates (1979) and Morgan (1976). The ages of these patients ranged from 8 to 55 years, with an equal sex ratio. The treatment is excision.

PATHOLOGY

The tumor is made up of cords and clusters of cells separated by fibrous septa (Fig. 343). The cells are somewhat polygonal and vary somewhat in size. The nuclei are round or oval, usually central, stain darkly, and are small in

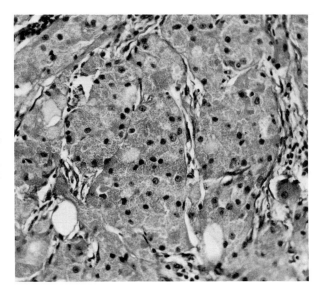

Figure 343. Granular cell myoblastoma: neoplasm is composed of regular, polygonal cells with abundant finely granular cytoplasm (Hematoxylin and eosin; × 245.)

proportion to the expanse of the surrounding cytoplasm. The cytoplasm contains numerous acidophilic granules that probably comprise a glycoprotein-lipid complex. The overall appearance of the cell has been described as being foamy, but there are no vacuoles, and special staining reveals no fat within the cell. Neither irregularity of cell type nor nuclear mitosis nor giant cells can be found in a manner to suggest malignancy. Striations such as might be found in other myogenic tumors are absent.

ALVEOLAR SOFT PART SARCOMA

This descriptive term was first applied by Christopherson and colleages (1952) to a group of 12 tumors of the extremities collected over a period of 17 years. These tumors had distinctive histopathologic patterns, were believed to be of mesenchymal origin, and had not been satisfactorily assigned to any other group of neoplasms. They noted some histologic resemblance of these sarcomas to paragangliomas but did not consider their tumors to be paragangliomas because such tissue was not known to occur in the extremities. In retrospect, they probably were not aware of a review of seventeen cases of malignant tumors of nonchromaffin paraganglia by Smetana and Scott a year earlier. The tumors of Smetana and Scott had many of the clinical features described by Christopherson and colleagues as *alveolar soft-part sarcomas*. To explain the presence of *malignant nonchromaffin paragangliomas* in the extremities, Smetana and Scott hypothesized that the tumors arose from cells of paraganglia, similar to carotid body tumors, that were attached to vessels traversing skeletal muscles. Also, at about the same time period, a possible relationship between an organoid type of *malignant granular cell myoblastoma* and alveolar soft part sarcoma was considered. Gradually there emerged the concept that these tumors were variants of the same neoplasm, but the name, alveolar soft part sarcoma, seems to have survived as the preferred designation. In addition, the tumor is now believed by many to have a neural genesis and to be related to paraganglia. However, this theory of histogenesis is not universally accepted and this is the reason for also discussing the neoplasm in this chapter.

CLINICAL FEATURES

The age range of the patients of Christopherson and his colleagues was 3 to 38 years, but only 1 of the 12 patients was older than 30 years. The age range of patients with malignant nonchromaffin paraganglioma is quite similar. The tumor is most common in the thigh, is circumscribed, usually painless, and is associated with skeletal muscle or musculofascial planes. Although in many cases these neoplasms have seemingly been adequately excised, local recurrences and metastases are frequent. This gives the neoplasm a very treacherous reputation.

Orbital examples of these neoplasms, however they may be named, are very few. A brief resumé of some of these interesting but rare cases seems worthwhile.

Dunnington (1948) recorded a 40-year-old male with a tense, red mass in the nasal portion of the lower eyelid. The orbit was exenterated but the tumor recurred locally 1½ months later. This was excised but generalized metastasis soon followed.

Altamirano-Dimas and associates (1966) reported the neoplasm in two children. One was a 10-month-old male with a deviated eye and a slowly growing mass in the inferior orbit of eight months' duration. A yellowish-white, circumscribed mass attached to the inferior oblique muscle was widely excised. The patient expired 11 months later with local recurrence and probable intracranial extension of neoplasm. The other child was a 3-year-old female with a mass in the lateral portion of the orbit of one year's duration who died of cardiac arrest during orbitotomy. The tumor was round, pale yellow, multilobulated and surrounded the optic nerve but did not invade the nerve structure.

Nirankari and his associates (1963) noted a 38-year-old male with redness and nasal displacement of the eye of five months' duration owing to a vascular mass overlying the lateral rectus muscle. The tumor was locally excised, but an extensive local recurrence 15 months later necessitated an exenteration. Radium therapy was administered but another recurrence of the tumor appeared in the remnant of the lower eyelid in 6 months.

Varghese and colleagues (1968) observed a 13-year-old female with proptosis and impairment of vision of three months' duration due to a vascular growth in the lateral orbit and lateral conjunctival fornices. A circumscribed mass was found infiltrating the lateral rectus muscle. An exenteration was performed but the tumor recurred a few months later.

Abraham and colleagues (1968) reported a 55-year-old male with a 3-week history of red eye and 6 mm of proptosis associated with a mass in the inferior orbit. Although this white rubbery tumor involved the entire insertion of the inferior rectus muscle, it was totally excised. One month later an exenteration was performed. The patient was living without recurrence one year later.

Grant and associates (1979) described an 18-year-old female with a dilated epibulbar vessel on the temporal aspect of the right eye and 3 mm of proptosis that developed over a 2-week period. A diffuse noncohesive tumor in the retrobulbar space was subtotally removed through a lateral orbitotomy. Radiotherapy (6,000 rads) was administered to the affected orbit postoperatively over a 6-week period with regression of proptosis. No further follow-up data was stated.

Also, we have had the privilege to examine the tissue specimen from an unreported case of Dr. R. N. Serros and Dr. W. H. Schrader of Orlando, Florida. A mass of 3 months' duration was observed on the medial aspect of the equator of the eye in a 31-year-old female. The tumor was yellow-tan in color, slightly lobular, and was partially attached to the medial rectus tendon. The mass was removed but the surgeon was not positive that excision was complete. There was no recurrence of the tumor in the 8-month period of postoperative observation.

From these cases it is evident that these neoplasms usually involve the more anterior structures of the orbit, particularly the extraocular muscles. The duration of the orbital tumor prior to presentation is reasonably short and the tumor either is visible or easily palpated. Also, the tumors occurred over a wide age range. Only 1 patient was still free of tumor 1 year after diagnosis.

PATHOLOGY

These neoplasms tend to be circumscribed. Histologically, the cell groups are arranged in an alveolar-like pattern which gives the tumor an organoid appearance (Fig. 344). The alveolar clusters are delineated from one another by a fine connective tissue network that is easily outlined by reticulin stains. Fibrous septae containing vascular channels course through the tumor, subdividing the individual alveolar clusters into larger, pseudolobular collections of cells. The nuclei are moderately large, basophilic, eccentrically placed,

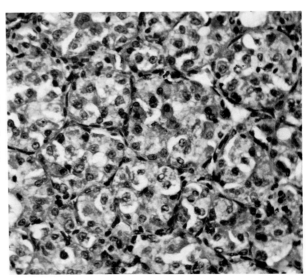

Figure 344. Alveolar soft part sarcoma: clusters of cells separated by fine fibrous septae give organoid appearance to the neoplasm. This example is from the thigh. (Hematoxylin and eosin: × 245.)

vesicular, and may contain more than one nucleolus. The granular cytoplasm is not as coarse as noted in the granular cell myoblastoma and is less eosinophilic than the cytoplasm of rhabdomyosarcoma cells. The cytoplasm of some cells contain rod-like granules that are PAS positive, the stain not removed by diastase. The ultrastructure of these neoplasms has been the subject of several reports: Welsh and colleagues (1972), Unni and Soule (1975).

Bibliography

Granular Cell Myoblastoma

Abrikossoff A: Über Myome, ausgehend von der quergestreifen willkürlichen Muskulatur. Virchows Arch (Pathol Anat) *260*:215–233, 1926

Abrikossoff AI: Weitere Untersuchungen über Myoblastenmyome. Virchows Arch (Pathol Anat) *280*: 723–740, 1931

Chaves E, Oliveria AM, Arnaud AC: Retrobulbar granular cell myoblastoma. Brit J Ophthalmol *56*:854–856, 1972

Drummond JW, Hall DL, Steen WH, Jr., et al: Granular cell tumor (myoblastoma) of the orbit. Arch Ophthalmol 97:1492–1494, 1979

Dunnington JH: Granular cell myoblastoma of the orbit. Arch Ophthalmol *40*:14–22, 1948

González-Almaraz G, de Buen S, Tsutsumi V: Granular cell tumor (myoblastoma) of the orbit. Am J Ophthalmol 79:606–612, 1975

Morgan G: Granular cell myoblastoma of the orbit. Arch Ophthalmol 94:2135–2142, 1976

Morgan LR, Fryer MP: Granular cell myoblastoma of the eye. Case report. Plast Reconstr Surg *43*:315–317, 1969

Obayashi K, Yamada Y, Kozaki M: Granular cell myoblastoma in the orbit. Folio Ophthalmol Jap *20*:566–574, 1969

Sakamaki Y: A case of intraorbital myoblastoma. J Clin Ophthalmol (Tokyo) *17*:883–884, 1963

Timm G, Timmel H: Zum myoblastenmyom am Auge. Klin Monatsbl Augenheilkd *148*:665–671, 1966

Alveolar Soft Part Sarcoma

Abrahams IW, Fendon RH, Vidone R: Alveolar soft-part sarcoma of the orbit. Arch Ophthalmol 79:185–188, 1968

Altamirano-Dimas M, Albores-Saavedra J: Alveolar soft part sarcoma of the orbit. Arch Ophthalmol 75:496–499, 1966

Christopherson WM, Foote FW, Jr, Stewart FW: Alveolar soft-part sarcomas: structurally characteristic tumors of uncertain histogenesis. Cancer 5:100–111, 1952

Dunnington JH: Granular cell myoblastoma of the orbit. Arch Ophthalmol ns *40*:14–22, 1948

Grant GD, Shields JA, Flanagan JC, et al: The ultrasonographic and radiologic features of a histologically proven case of alveolar soft-part sarcoma of the orbit. Am J Opththalmol 87:773–777, 1979

Nirankari MS, Greer CH, Chaddah MR: Malignant nonchromaffin paraganglioma in the orbit. Brit J Ophthalmol 47:357–363, 1963

Serros RN, Schrader WH: Personal communication

Smetana HF, Scott WF, Jr: Malignant tumors of nonchromaffin paraganglia. Milit Surg *109*:330–349, 1951

Unni KK, Soule EH: Alveolar soft part sarcoma. An electron microscopic study. Mayo Clin Proc *50*:591–598, 1975

Varghese S, Nair B, Joseph TA: Orbital malignant nonchromaffin paragnaglioma. Alveolar soft tissue sarcoma. Brit J Ophthalmol 52:713–715, 1968

Welsh RA, Bray DM, Shipkey FH et al: Histogenesis of alveolar soft part sarcoma. Cancer *29*: 191–204, 1972

SECTION III

The Surgical Approaches
to Orbital Tumors

24

The Anterior Surgical Approaches

In the ophthalmic literature, the surgical approach to orbital tumors often is discussed by a surgeon, usually an ophthalmologist or neurosurgeon, who is skilled in this particular surgical field. The surgeon advances the concept that most, if not all, orbital tumors are located within the boundaries of the author's surgical specialty, and that successful management is achieved less often if the orbit is approached by some other route or by surgeons of other specialties. Most of the conflicts revolve around the proper means for removing primary and secondary tumors located in the posterior portion of the orbit. Often overlooked are the many neoplasms (noted in Chapter 3) originating in the paranasal sinuses and periorbital spaces that require more extensive surgical manipulation than can be skillfully and completely accomplished by either the ophthalmologist or the neurosurgeon. Thus, the management of orbital tumors interests two additional specialty groups: rhinologists and maxillofacial surgeons who have experience in this field. We do not believe the orbit is the exclusive domain of any of these surgical specialties. We do believe the interests of the patient are best served by directing them to the surgical specialist who has had the most experience in grappling with tumors in a given location. In this and the following chapter we will discuss those several approaches that have served us well either as the primary surgeon or as a collaborator with a surgeon of another special field.

HISTORICAL ASPECTS

The first attempt to extricate a tumor from the orbit probably was made through an incision somewhere on the anterior surface of the eyelids or through the medial or lateral conjunctival fornices. Details of the "who, when, and where" of such a procedure are lost in antiquity; but it was not likely to have been a notable event when first accomplished. Instead, the resection of tumorous protrusions, which competed with the eye for the limited space of the orbital cavity, probably evolved naturally from the surgical incision that had long been used for the drainage of septic pockets and hematomas in this area. Most of these first surgical ventures probably involved the inferior orbit, because this was the most dependent portion of the orbital space and the orbital septum was less resistant to the pressures of inflammatory and neoplastic masses than the corresponding fascia of the upper eyelid. Furthermore, in these earlier years orbital tumors probably were not removed unless they were large and easily accessible in the more forward portions of the orbital cavity. The deeper tumors were left untouched, but if the unilateral proptosis became too severe the eye instead of the tumor was removed.

The next step in the surgical management of orbital tumors was the bold extirpation of both the eye and the tumor, such as was performed by Bartisch (1583) (Fig. 345). The first successful effort to remove a deeply situated orbital tumor through an incision in the lower eyelid — without sacrifice of the eye — probably was made in Europe during the early part of the 18th century, but such an innovative proccedure did not become popular for another century because of the high mortality from meningitis and sepsis. In the 19th century, general surgeons, who then performed the major share of orbital operations, added many refinements to the basic antero-inferior orbitotomy and other anterior surgical approaches. In the 20th century, orbitotomies were increasingly performed by ophthalmologists whose names soon were associated with the various anterior incisions that previously had been described by general surgeons.

INCISIONS

Figure 346 illustrates the position of the numerous incisions now available for an anterior approach to orbital tumors. Commencing at the lateral aspect of the right eye and proceeding clockwise, the incisions may be identified as, and correlated with, the *anterior temporal*, the *superior (brow)*, the *superior nasal*, the *superior temporal*, and the *inferior* approaches. The last may be approached either by an incision parallel to the inferior orbital rim or by an incision parallel

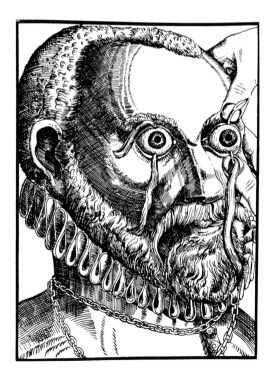

Figure 345. This illustration has appeared in several publications recounting the early history of ophthalmology. It illustrates two stages in Bartisch's operation. A strong needle and thread have been thrust through the substance of the left eye, while in the right the thread is positioned for maintenance of traction on the eyeball during orbital manipulation. (From Snyder C: Our Ophthalmic Heritage. Boston, Little, Brown & Company, 1967, p 136. By permission.)

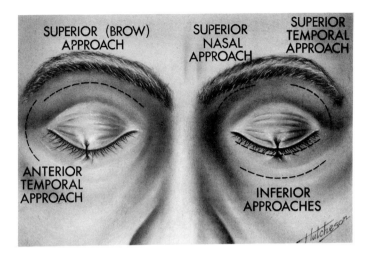

Figure 346.   Diagrams of various incisions (*dashed lines*) for anterior orbitotomy.

to and just inferior to the margin of the lower eyelid. All but the last are curvilinear, and, topographically, they approximate the bony rim of the orbit. The configuration of these incisions follows the contour lines of the surface tissues in this area of the face, which helps to minimize unsightly scar in the course of healing. Keeping the incisions closely approximated to the bony orbital rim seems to provide more direct access to the majority of orbital tumors and less surgical trauma to the soft tissue structures and appendages of the eyelid than incisions elsewhere. A continuous incision across the upper and lower nasal quadrants, comparable to the anterior temporal incision depicted in Figure 346, has not been recommended because it would necessitate cutting across the functionally important lacrimal excretory passages. Furthermore, there is little need for an incision combining exposure of both inferior and superior nasal quadrants because primary orbital tumors rarely grow in the area directly posterior to the medial canthal tendon. This zone, however, is a favorite lodging place for serious secondary tumors originating in the skin, nasal passages, or maxillary antrum; in such cases, the lacrimal passages must be sacrificed if an extensive excision will save the patient from further growth of tumor. The temporal and nasal transconjunctival approaches are supplementary anterior routes with incisions that follow the contour of the nasal and temporal conjunctival fornices. Occasionally, a transconjunctival approach is necessary to remove a visible mass attached to one of the extraocular muscles anterior to the equator of the eye.

Some surgeons have suggested that the lateral transconjunctival approach be used for palpating the orbital contents. If an encapsulated tumor is palpated, the incision can be extended into one of those to be described for the lateral orbitotomy, and the tumor so removed. If the tumor is not encapsulated, a biopsy only is performed. On the basis of those diagnostic clues outlined in Section I, it would not seem necessary to subject the patient to a surgical procedure simply to provide adequate palpation of the mass. If more accurate assessment of the orbital contents by palpation is required, it would seem preferable to provide better visualization, as well as improved tactile evaluation of the orbital lesion, by using one of the standard approaches through the skin. The goal of an operation on the orbit should be the removal, not the palpation, of the orbital tumor if at all possible.

Superior Nasal Incision

For the upper nasal approach, the line of the incision is first outlined on the skin with an indelible marking pencil. This preliminary topographic mapping is suggested for all the skin incisions discussed in this and the following chapter. The incision may be made with a Bard-Parker knife directly over, just superior, or slightly inferior to the bony orbital rim. Most surgeons prefer the incision to follow the contour of the bony orbit in this quadrant, though in some texts these incisions are illustrated as ascending into the eyebrow on a less acute arc. Most rhinologists who approach a suspected orbital mucocele in the frontal sinus favor an incision above the edge of the orbital rim. Our standard incision extends from just above the underlying medial palpebral tendon almost to the midpoint of the superior orbital rim (roughly equal to one-fourth the circumference of the orbital rim); it will be 25 to 30 mm long. Whether this incision is made above, directly over, or slightly inferior to the orbital rim, the objective is to reach the junction of the periosteum, the periorbita, and the orbital septum. Tiny bleeding points in the skin can be clamped with mosquito hemostats and, after a minute or so, the hemostat usually can be released without further bleeding. The coagulating diathermy should be used carefully at this point because it so readily produces scar in the thin skin of this area. This reluctance to use the coagulating type of surgical diathermy extends to other skin incisions along other areas of the orbital rim. A preliminary injection of a local anesthetic agent containing epinephrine or phenylephrine also is used by some surgeons to staunch the hemorrhage at this early stage of the orbitotomy. After the skin has been passed, the subcutaneous tissues and bundles of the orbicularis muscle may be separated with the knife or the cutting current of the Bovie unit. The latter is another means for diminishing bleeding but, again, diathermy should not be used on the skin itself. Once the junction of the periorbita, periosteum, and orbital septum has been uncovered, the incision is complete.

Superior (Brow) Incision

There is more latitude in the position of the incision for the superior (or brow) approach as to whether it is placed above the eyebrow, in the eyebrow, or slightly inferior to the lip of the bony rim. An incision placed along the superior edge of the eyebrow is approximately 5 to 10 mm above the entrance to the orbit. General surgeons once favored an incision in this location; they dissected inferiorly beneath the eyebrow and along the surface of the galea aponeurotica to reach the orbit proper. All ophthalmologists who have performed "sling" operations for blepharoptosis agree that this area is extremely vascular and that bleeding can be troublesome. An incision more directly through the eyebrow was popularized by ophthalmologists who subsequently became interested in this surgical field; this approach is most often associated with the name of Benedict (1949). Benedict's incision is described as being placed 5 mm above the rim of the orbit and within the hairline of the eyebrow. By placing the incision in this area, it was assumed that the cosmetic blemish would be minimized; but dimpling still may occur. Bleeding from an incision within the hairline also can be troublesome owing to the vascular tissue surrounding the hair follicles. As a rule, bleeding is less profuse with incisions inferior to the eyebrow. The latter incisions also may heal somewhat irregularly, but they blend smoothly with the crescentic folds in the skin of the eyelids and are less noticeable than the more rigid and fixed scar running through the eyebrow. However, the final appearance of an incision may depend not so much on the position of the incision in relation to the orbit as on the attention given to wound closure and suturing.

Whatever the variation among surgeons in the position of this mid-superior incision, there is less variation in its curvature and length. Most surgeons make the incision parallel to the superior orbital margin. In length, the incision should extend across the middle two-thirds of the orbital margin (approximately one-third the circumference of the orbit). This brow incision should be longer than the superior nasal and superior temporal incisions illustrated in Figure 337 because it is used more often when the exact position of the tumor in the upper orbital quadrants is neither known nor can be definitely palpated. On the other hand, the shorter superior nasal and superior temporal incisions are preferred when the tumor is more definitely confined to one of the upper quadrants of the orbit. Such quadrantic tumors more frequently are palpable, and are situated more forward in the orbit. In general, the more posterior the tumor the greater the length of the incision.

Superior Temporal and Anterior Temporal Incisions

In curvature and length, the superior temporal incision is similar to the superior nasal incision. The former may commence in the eyebrow and then curve laterally and inferiorly to the area just above the lateral palpebral tendon (often designated the lateral palpebral ligament and sometimes referred to as the lateral canthal tendon) or it may be positioned in the skin of the upper eyelid just inferior to the hairline of the eyebrow. There are fewer blood vessels — and consequently less bleeding — in the subcutaneous tissues of this temporal area than in the comparable zones of an incision in the superior nasal quadrant. In former years the superior temporal approach was commonly used for almost all palpable masses in the lacrimal gland fossa. We believe this incision is inadequate for these tumors because their size is often larger than anticipated and because there is a 40 to 55% chance the tumor is malignant. The latter requires more generous surgical exposure to ensure a more complete removal. We now approach all such tumors through an anterolateral incision (Chapter 25).

The anterior temporal incision is longer than the preceding one for it is designed to permit exploration of both temporal quadrants. Its extent is approximately equidistant above and below the lateral palpebral raphe. It may be combined with a horizontal incision across the lateral side of the orbit if the need for lateral orbitotomy also becomes apparent. At one time, an incision of this length was not recommended because paresis of the orbicularis oculi muscle was feared; but the nerve supply to this muscle of the eyelid is so profuse and so devious that any postoperative weakness of the orbicularis oculi resulting from an incision in this area will be minimal. The skin is thin and delicate along the temporal margin of the bony orbit and should be handled judiciously to prevent postoperative scarring.

Inferior Incisions

For inferior orbitotomy, the surgeon has the choice of an incision through the skin either across and parallel to the middle two-thirds of the inferior bony orbital rim or a more linear incision 5 mm inferior and parallel to the row of eyelashes along the margin of the lower eyelid. Of the two, the former is the older and the most widely used. The objective in making this incision is to gain access to the junction of the periosteum on the anterior surface of the maxillary bone with the periorbita covering the floor of the orbit, and also to the fascia separating the tissues of the eyelid from the reticulum of the orbit. This fascial divider in the lower eyelid corresponds in function and position with the orbital septum in the upper eyelid but is much thinner. The skin overlying the inferior bony rim of the orbit also is extremely thin and this feature, combined with the tendency of the healing skin to adhere directly to the underlying periosteum, creates a more visible scar than would occur with incisions elsewhere along the bony rim. The prominent position of the inferior orbital rim in the topography of the face tends to accentuate any postoperative scarring.

This problem may be solved in several ways. Some surgeons close incisions in this area with subcuticular stitches rather then with the usual interrupted, running, or lock sutures. Another possibility is to offset the incision from the insertion of the orbital fascia into bone, so that skin can unite with an underlying layer of subcutaneous tissue rather than directly with the incision line in the orbital fascia. This can be done by placing the curvilinear incision several millimeters above the bony rim so that the surgical wound will lie more properly in the lower eyelid. The more linear incision which extends across the length of the lower eyelid just inferior to the eyelid margin is an extension of this idea. In this approach, the inferior rim of the orbit is reached by tunneling between the skin and the surface of the orbicularis oculi — a cleavage plane that is easy to find and to follow. For a tumor of any given size, however, the incision in this area must be longer than a standard incision overlying the bony rim. The inferior orbitotomy incision, wherever it is made, is adequate for most tumors in the inferior orbital quadrants.

INTRA-ORBITAL TECHNIQUES

Having incised the skin, subcutaneous tissue, and orbicularis oculi muscle, the surgeon with his scalpel somewhere along the orbital rim is ready to enter the orbit proper. Two choices are available for this next step. Either the surgeon may enter the orbital cavity directly by an incision through the orbital septum or he may attain the same goal indirectly by making an incision through the periorbita after it has been separated from bone. By taking the former route, the surgeon directly enters the orbital space; by taking the latter route he opens the peripheral orbital space.

Direct Approach to the Orbital Space (Fig. 347 A)

This seems a logical route to expose tumors in the *superior quadrants* that originate in the anterior portion of the orbit and push against the orbital septum as they expand forward. In the superior quadrants, bulging of the orbital septum just inferior to the bony orbital rim usually means that the tumor will be found immediately beneath this fascial septum. Among the orbital tumors that often behave in this manner are occasional hemangiomas (in children of school age) that push forward in the superior nasal quadrant; malignant lymphomas that infiltrate the posterior surface of the orbital septum in the area of either the trochlea or the lacrimal gland; many pseudotumors that conform to the arch of the orbital roof in the course of their spread; dermoid cysts; and many of the intrinsic tumors of the lacrimal gland.

The incision through the orbital septum should be made slowly and carefully, either with Stevens scissors or the cutting diathermy current, taking precautions not to cut open the tumor capsule, should such be present. Circumscribed and encapsulated tumors in this area tend to fuse with the orbital septum because the former push relentlessly against the unyielding resistance of the latter. These precautions in the initial dissection, however, are not so pertinent if the tumor is frankly infiltrative, as is a lymphoma, for example. The incision through the orbital septum also should be made <u>close to the orbital rim</u>

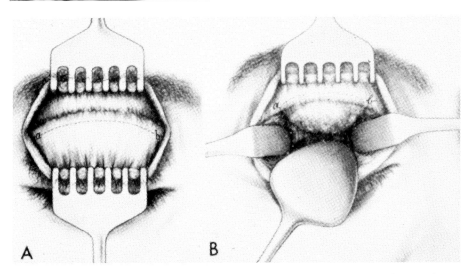

A   **B**

Figure 347. Superior approach to anterior orbitotomy: *A*, Incision *a-b* is made just inferior to superior orbital rim for entry indirectly into the orbital space. *B*, Incision *a-b* is made just superior to orbital rim for entry into peripheral orbital space. (From Elschnig A: Operations for tumors of the orbit. Surg Gynecol Obstet 45:65–73, 1927. By permission of Surgery, Gynecology and Obstetrics.)

so as to ensure entry into the triangular space bounded inferiorly by the superior surface of the tendon of the levator palpebrae superioris, superiorly by the check ligament of the levator muscle and bony orbital rim, and anteriorly by the back surface of the orbital septum.

If the division of the orbital septum is made more inferiorly than this point, the tendon of the levator muscle is more likely to be damaged because this broad flat structure tends to fuse with the orbital septum as these adjacent tissues pass inferiorly toward the margin of the upper eyelid. In all manipulations in the central two-thirds of the superior orbital quadrants, the surgeon should be careful not to injure the levator palpebrae superioris muscle and tendon, regardless of whether entry is through the orbital septum or through the periorbita. Once the orbital septum is broached, the fused surfaces of the tumor and the orbital septum may be separated with the blunt tips of the Stevens scissors. Where the tissues are less fused and a cleavage plane exists, the lacrimal sac elevator can be substituted for the scissors as a dissecting instrument.

When opening the orbital septum in the *superior nasal quadrant* just inferior to the superior orbital notch, a descending branch of the superior orbital artery occasionally may be seen or accidentally severed. If the vessel is intact, small ties should be placed on its proximal and distal segments before it is cut, because bleeding may be quite brisk from either segment of the severed vessel. Once this vessel is severed, the proximal stump may be difficult to tie or to clamp because of the tendency of these vessels to retract. Similar problems arise with terminal branches of the frontal and dorsal nasal arteries in and around the trochlea, particularly in highly vascular tumors. Bleeding from small arteries is commoner in this quadrant than in the other quadrants of the orbit. If one of the vascular malformations (see Chapter 6) should be encountered, a tie should immediately be placed around the dorsal nasal artery as it merges with the angular artery, the latter representing the terminal portion of the facial artery. Venous bleeding from any source in this zone may be handled with the surgical coagulating current.

While working in this quadrant, the surgeon may or may not choose to separate the trochlea from its attachment to the periorbita along the orbital rim. This maneuver may be done by a sharp rap with the hammer and chisel along the base of the trochlea, or its base may be cut with sturdy medium or large curved scissors. As the surgeon gains experience in working in the orbit, he will find that he tends to work around the trochlea rather than sever it from its attachment.

We have more reservations, however, about using this direct approach across the *superior temporal quadrant* and through the orbital septum unless there is an obvious, well-encapsulated tumor, such as a dermoid cyst. Our hesitancy is based on the frequency with which tumors with serious malignant potential are found in this area. Most such tumors, usually one of the neoplasms intrinsic in the lacrimal gland (see Chapter 15), either become fused to periorbita as they expand or quickly seed themselves into periorbita if their pseudocapsule is incised, such as readily occurs if the orbital septum is opened directly over the bulging mass. Each situation is, of course, different; in general, in the case of these tumors, we combined the superior temporal incision with the lateral orbitotomy (the anterolateral appoach, Chapter 25).

Entry into the orbital space in the *inferior quadrants* poses no particular problems. The incision through the thin musculofascial tissue that is analogous to the orbital septum of the upper eyelid may be made directly over or within several millimeters of the orbital rim. No particular precautions are necessary with incisions in this area, as is the case with the upper eyelid, which contains the levator palpebrae superioris. In the inferior quadrants, the incision into the orbital cavity should be set off from the lines of the skin incision. Except for the malignant lymphoma, most primary tumors in the inferior orbital quadrants are located more posteriorly and do not tend to fuse with the tissue structure of the eyelid, as occurs in the superior quadrants. The nodular masses of some lymphomas may push upward into the inferior cul-de-sac rather than move forward into the eyelid. We still prefer to approach suspected lymphomas in the inferior cul-de-sac through the standard approach rather than through the inferior conjunctival route, which is associated with more bleeding and a greater tendency for scarring to bind the conjunctival cul-de-sac to the orbital rim.

Primary tumors located in the inferior nasal quadrant may be more difficult to manipulate than similar tumors in the corresponding temporal quadrant owing to the origin of the inferior oblique muscle. In practice, however, we tend to work around the obstruction rather than to detach the muscle origin. Relatively greater latitude is possible in the dissection and removal of primary tumors located in the inferior orbit than in any other orbital area because it is more spacious, the visibility is better, and there are fewer important nerves, blood vessels, and muscles (the ciliary ganglion is one exception).

Approach to the Peripheral Orbital Space (Fig. 347 B)

An alternative route into the orbital cavity is through the space between the periorbita and bone: the peripheral space. This is the preferred approach to those tumors that originate in bone and expand into the peripheral space. These tumors usually are evident on routine roentgenography or orbital tomography. Mucoceles, malignant neoplasms arising in the ethmoid and maxillary sinuses, osteomas, fibrous dysplasia, chondromas, aneurysmal bone cysts, histiocytosis X, plasma cell myelomas, epidermoid cysts, and some cavernous hemangiomas in adults are examples of such growths. If the roentgenographic findings suggest a meningioma, we usually prefer to approach it by the transfrontal route, because it tends to be located in the posterior orbit and to spread within the cranium.

When the approach to the peripheral space is used in cases of tumors in the *superior quadrants*, the incision is made through the periosteum overlying the frontal bone approximately 1 mm above the conjoined attachments of periorbita, orbital septum, and periosteum. Using a curved and sturdy periosteal elevator, the surgeon gradually passes proximally along the orbital rim remaining in the cleavage plane immediately adjacent to the bone. As the true orbit is entered, the periorbita falls away from its union with bone along the nasal, superior, and temporal walls. This plane is followed across the arc of the upper orbital walls except around the nerves and blood vessels passing through the notch; trauma to the supraorbital nerve is carefully minimized. With blunt manipulation, the surgeon keeps the vessels and nerves on the bony side of the cleavage plane, but often, in order to obtain better exposure of the peripheral space, he must ligate some branches from the main artery bridging into the tissues of the eyelid. This dissection with the periosteal elevator around the supraorbital notch may leave a small dehiscence in the periorbital surface, but this is of no consequence. In the superior nasal quadrant, the trochlea falls inferiorly as the periorbita is separated from the bone in this area. When the surgeon has separated periorbita from bone either in one quadrant or across the roof of the orbit, he is ready to dissect the tumor that adheres to bone, occupies a major portion of the peripheral space, or lies in the midportion of the orbit just inferior to the periorbita.

If the tumor is a bony one — such as an osteoma, a fibrous dysplasia, or an aneurysmal bone cyst — the portion of the tumor extending into the orbital cavity may be removed with hammer and chisel or biting rongeurs. With these benign tumors, the object is to remove that portion of the growth that will provide decompression of the orbital space and relief of the proptosis. Such benign tumors need not be completely removed if dissection entails a risk of injury to the dura or intracranial contents. Along the thin roof of the orbit there is more likelihood of entry into the intracranial vault than along the nasal or temporal wall. If, in spite of careful dissection, the dura is nicked it can be closed with a fine, silk suture, but if the tear is more uneven it may be plugged with a small piece of fascia or muscle. Bleeding from tumors usually comes from pieces of periorbita or mucous membrane which still adhere to the mass on one of its surfaces. Further retraction of these covering tissues or compression of the bleeding vessel with a hemostat usually stops the bleeding. For the more malignant tumors, such as chondrosarcoma, sinusectomy will be required in an effort to remove the lesion as completely as possible.

A soft tissue tumor, such as a cavernous hemangioma, occasionally develops in the peripheral space, and complete removal offers no particular problem, except in the ligation or coagulation of the feeder vessels.

A more cystic tumor, such as an epidermoid cyst or a mucocele, may not lend itself to complete dissection. The walls may be so thin that the tumor may rupture easily during manipulation, or the wall of the tumor that has pushed against the periorbita is so fused to the latter tissue or to the superior surface of the levator palpebrae superioris as to make it unwise to attempt refined dissection along this side of the mass. Instead, it seems more practical to incise such a cystic tumor on the surface nearest the surgeon. The contents of a cystic mass then may be removed with an appropriate instrument (sucker tip, spoon, or curette). Once the liquid or soft contents of the mass have been evacuated, the lining should be carefully teased away with fine-toothed forceps or scraped away with curettes. The remaining fibrous wall then may be lightly touched with a desiccating type of diathermy along the interior surface, so as to eradicate any tags of secreting membrane that were missed with the forceps or curettes. The desiccating diathermy usually controls oozing of blood from the cavity of the cyst. In cases of mucocele, a drainage passage from the affected sinus into the nasal cavity also should be provided. A small wick of Silastic may be inserted along the drainage passage to keep this open until the wick is removed through the nasal cavity in the postoperative period.

A tumor associated with histiocytosis X usually contains a pulpy material

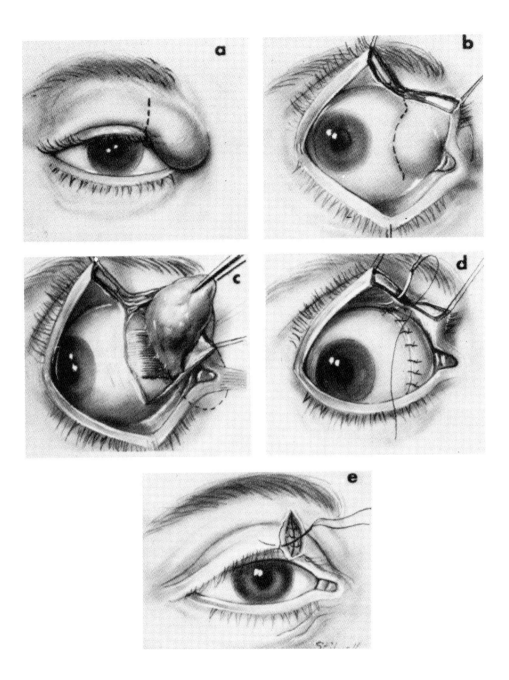

Figure 348. Technique of transmarginal incision for exposure of anterior orbital tumor: *a*, Direction of vertical transmarginal full-thickness incision (*dashed line*), temporal to tumor. *b*, Incision (*dashed line*) extended to upper fornix; conjunctival extension of wound is parallel to fibers of levator muscle. *c*, Dissection and extirpation of tumor; note wide exposure of mass. *d*, Closure of conjunctiva. *e*, Closure of eyelid wound in layers by direct approximation, with 6–0 silk interrupted sutures. (From Smith B: The anterior surgical approach to orbital tumors. Trans Am Acad Ophthalmol Otolaryngol 70:607–611, 1966. By permission of the American Academy of Ophthalmology and Otolaryngology.)

that bleeds easily when disturbed. Such portions of the tumor as are adequate for frozen-section histopathologic study may be removed, but the major portion of the lesion need not be excised. The response to irradiation is likely to provide as much relief of proptosis as would total surgical resection.

An approach through the peripheral space less often is required for tumors located in the *inferior quadrants.* The incision through the soft tissues overlying the inferior orbital rim may be made near the junction of the periosteum of the facial bones and the periorbital covering of the orbital bones. The periorbita across the inferior quadrants is lifted easily with a Freer elevator. Usually there is no bleeding from the infraorbital artery as it passes along its bone channel, unless dissection is carried posteriorly beyond the midpoint of the anteropos-terior axis of the orbit. For tumors beyond this point, a lateral orbitotomy or a partial maxillectomy probably is necessary. Tumors at this depth along the peripheral orbital space likely will be of the malignant type.

Transmarginal Approach

An innovation in the anterior orbital approach is the transmarginal route proposed by Smith (1966). His method is represented diagrammatically in Figure 348. These illustrations suggest this operation is most suitable for tumors situated well forward in the orbit that have extended into the eyelid. Many surgeons would assume that such tumors could be exposed adequately by either a transcutaneous incision directly over the tumor or the standard transcon-junctival route. Smith's incision permits a wider exposure of the surgical field than would be possible by a transconjunctival incision confined to the superior fornix. Smith believes that improved instruments and sutures eliminate the notching and deformity of the margin of the eyelid that so often are residuals of full-thickness, vertical incisions in these tissues.

CLOSURE AND POSTOPERATIVE CARE

During closure, attention should be given to the union of two principal layers, the fascia and skin. Careful suturing of the fascia, whether it be orbital septum or periorbita, will discourage adhesions between the undersurface of the skin and the bone, and minimize scar formation. As a rule, the incisions required for anterior orbitotomies do not have to withstand unusual pressure or swelling in the postoperative period; plain catgut sutures (4-0 or 5-0) seem to be sufficient for the fascial layers. Whether the fascia is reunited by a running stitch or by interrupted sutures is immaterial, though we prefer the interrupted type of sutures. In the upper quadrant and brow incisions, interrupted catgut sutures also may be used to unite the layers of orbicularis oculi muscle.

For skin closure of upper quadrant and brow incisions, 5-0 silk sutures are practical and may be inserted in an interrupted pattern or as a running suture. Our preference is the use of a subcuticular stitch (Fig. 349) for skin closure of both superior and inferior orbitotomies because of the minimal postoperative blemish. Skin incisions made directly over the inferior orbital rim neither heal as well nor blend into the contour lines of the surrounding skin as do incisions that are set off more superiorly into the elastic portions of the lower eyelid.

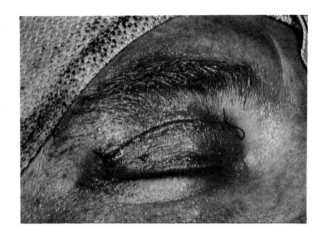

Figure 349. Superior orbitomy: skin closure with a black silk, subcuticular stitch.

The preplaced traction suture holding the eyelids together during the course of the orbitotomy now is removed, and the eye and eyelids are covered with an eye patch or a two-layered gauze strip. This cover is secured with adhesive skin strips. There should be no need to apply the head bandage or to insert rubber drains into the depths of the orbital cavity, as were so common in the yesteryears of orbital surgery.

In the immediate postoperative period, most surgeons favor some antibiotic therapy, chiefly because of the prevalence of staphylococcal infections among hospital populations. Administration of these antibiotics is tapered off over a period of 5 to 10 days. In general, there seems to be little reason to restrict bathroom privileges, and the patients may walk as soon as they wish. The eye patch or dressing may be removed on the second or third postoperative day, and most patients can be released from the hospital on the third or fourth postoperative day.

Bibliography

Bartisch G: Augendienst. Dresden, M Stöckel, 1583

Benedict WL: Surgical treatment of tumors and cysts of the orbit. Am J Ophthalmol 32:763–773, 1949

Elschnig A: Operations for tumors of the orbit. Surg Gynecol Ostet 45:65–73, 1927

Iliff CE: Primary orbital tumors: therapy. In *Proceedings of the Second International Symposium on Plastic and Reconstructive Surgery of the Eye and Adnexa.* Ed: B Smith, JM Converse. St Louis, CV Mosby Company, 1967, pp 116–120

Smith B: The anterior surgical approach to orbital tumors. Trans Am Acad Ophthalmol Otolaryngol 70:607–611, 1966

Stallard HB: Surgery of the orbit. Ann R Coll Surg Engl 43:125–140, 1968

25

The Lateral
Surgical Approaches

Over a period of several decades, the lateral (temporal) orbitotomy has displaced the anterior orbitotomy as the favored route for the removal of many orbital tumors. Interest in this approach to orbital tumors has paralleled the surgical advances and modifications that have been made in this procedure in the past 75 years. In general, we use the lateral orbitotomy or some modification for all suspected primary orbital tumors that are beyond the perimeters of palpation, except in those cases of proptosis in which loss of vision, papilledema, or roentgenographic alterations of the optic canal, the sphenoid bone, or bony orbit suggest the diagnosis of a meningioma, an optic nerve glioma, or some bony tumor that extends into the intracranial vault. For tumors that can be palpated through the eyelids or conjunctival fornices we still favor an anterior orbitotomy, except for tumors that seem to be intrinsic in the lacrimal gland. For these latter tumors, we tend to use a combined anterior and lateral approach more frequently. In short, the lateral orbitotomy has passed from being a new, radical, and controversial approach to being an accepted and almost standard alternative to anterior orbitotomy.

HISTORICAL ASPECTS

The lateral orbitotomy was an important advance in the evolution of orbital surgery. It provided the surgeon with a new and improved approach to the retro-ocular space and made possible, through exposure of the posterior aspects of the tumor, the complete removal of some orbital masses that formerly had been excised through anterior orbitotomies only partially because of limits of space and visibility. Some of the first major efforts to reach the retrobulbar space by removing the lateral bony rim and wall of the orbit were those of Passavant (France), Wagner (Germany), and Krönlein (Switzerland), and each made his contribution independently. Passavant utilized this approach chiefly for the exploration of an orbit containing a vascular malformation. Wagner (1886) advocated nibbling away a wedge-shaped piece of orbital rim and the adjoining bone of the face to provide more room in the search for foreign bodies associated with skull fractures. Two years later, Krönlein (1888) described his new operation for removal of orbital dermoid cysts.

Krönlein's osteoplastic resection of the exterior orbital wall (1888) was a daring and innovative procedure for his era. The crux of this operation was the manipulation of a hinged flap of bone to provide improved access to the rear of the orbit; the bone flap subsequently was replaced in its original position. The bone flap was fashioned into a "wedge" with a hammer and chisel. The wedge included the "entire outer margin of the orbit and the portion of the outer orbital wall which is between this margin and the inferior orbital fissure." The margin of the orbital rim was the base of the bony wedge. The chisel cuts were made superiorly in the zygomatic process of the frontal bone just above the zygomaticofrontal suture and, inferiorly, at the base of the frontal process of the zygomatic bone just above its arch. The chisel cuts were directed posteriorly toward the inferior orbital fissure and, when completed, permitted outward and dorsalward rotation of the bone as a flap toward the ear. The bone remained hinged to the "skin-fascia-muscle flap" of the temporal area, which provided nutrition of the bone when the flap was replaced and sutured. Figure 350 illustrates the size and shape of the bony opening described by Krönlein.

The subsequent history of the lateral orbitotomy has been concerned chiefly with modifications of the skin incision and the size and manipulation of the bone flap, but the basic approach through the lateral orbital wall remains the same.

INCISIONS

Several incisions are applicable to lateral orbitotomy. Various alterations in the position, length, and shape in these incisions have been proposed to provide an easier access to the bony wall, to permit a more extensive removal of bone, or to assure a less disfiguring scar.

Standard Krönlein Incision. This incision (Fig. 351) was crescentic, its convexity being directed anteriorly. The superior and inferior ends of the

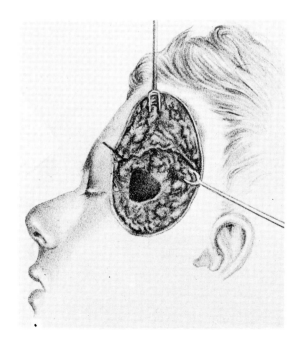

Figure 350. Reproduction of the illustration appearing in Krönlein's original publication of 1888 depicting a "view of the operative field" during the course of "osteoplastic resection of the exterior orbital wall." The hole in the bony lateral wall is easily seen; Krönlein did not report the dimensions of this bony aperture. (From Krönlein RU: Zur Pathologic und operativen Behandlung der Dermoidcysten der Orbita. Beitr Klin Chir 4:149–163, 1888.)

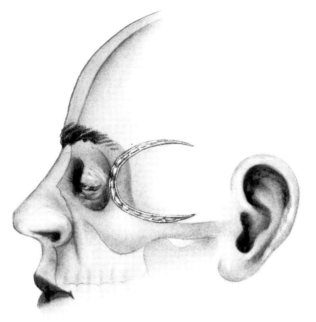

Figure 351. Crescentic incision of Krönlein.

incision were approximately 3 cm anterior to the ear. The curved inferior arm
of the incision corresponded to the superior border of the zygomatic arch; the
superior arm of the incision commenced in the temporal fossa along the semi-
circular ridge of the lateral face of the frontal bone and continued on a line
slightly above an imaginary dorsal projection of the superior orbital margin.
The apogee of the curved, forward portion of the incision was located over the
area of the zygomatic tubercle. The incision was made through the skin, subcutaneous tissue, temporalis fascia, and temporalis muscle so as to permit all
these tissue layers to remain attached to the bone flap, when this was fractured
posteriorly. Contrary to most present surgical procedures, Krönlein did not
make any special effort to separate skin from the underlying fascial tissues
during the initial dissection.

Modified Krönlein Incisions.   Shortening of the Krönlein incision resulted
in proportionately less scarring, but, even with better suture techniques, some
residual blemish almost always developed because the curve of the incision ran
counter to the surface topography of the temporal area. However, by
lengthening the radius of curvature and reversing the direction of its convexity,
a surgeon could make an incision of nearly equal length parallel to the lateral
orbital rim. Such incisions, though as dimpled as the classical Krönlein wound,
blended better with the contours of the skin and were less noticeable when
healed.

The transition to an incision with a dorsalward convexity lessened the
amount of skin included as part of the combined soft tissue-bone flap that continued to be hinged posteriorly, and established the precedent of making the
skin incision along cleavage planes separate from those cuts made in the underlying temporalis fascia and bone. It was, however, difficult to fashion a large
flap consisting of both bone and temporalis muscle through such incisions, and
further modifications soon appeared. Chief among these was the addition of a

horizontal arm that bisected the vertical crescent of the initial incision at its midpoint. The resulting incision resembled somewhat a letter *T* that had been rotated 90°; superior and inferior triangular-shaped skin flaps were formed (Fig. 352). Such skin flaps could be dissected from the underlying subcutaneous tissue in superior and inferior directions to such a width as to permit easier formation of the bone flap. The horizontal arm of these *T*-incisions could be made any length appropriate to the surgeon's plan. The vertical crescentic portion of the incision tended to be more constant and it usually extended from just above the zygomaticofrontal suture line to just below the origin of the zygomatic arch, a distance that seldom exceeded 40 mm. These incisions are still used today, but some surgeons find it difficult to obtain a good cosmetic closure of the skin at the junction of the vertical and horizontal cuts.

Berke-Reese Incision. The next transition was the elimination of the curved vertical arm of the incision. With this incision the skin was opened with a straight horizontal cut, extending from the lateral canthus toward the ear and passing over the midpoint of the lateral orbital rim at about the level of the insertion of the lateral palpebral raphe (Fig. 353). Such an incision currently is referred to by the name Berke or Berke-Reese, owing to the widely circulated descriptions of the orbitotomy procedure between 1951 and 1953 by Berke (1953) and Reese (1956). Such incisions had been proposed earlier but they had not received much attention. Swift (1935), for example, used a horizontal incision that was 7 cm long for his approach to orbital decompression.

Berke described his incision as being 30 to 40 mm long and extending horizontally from the lateral canthus toward the ear. A lateral canthotomy made

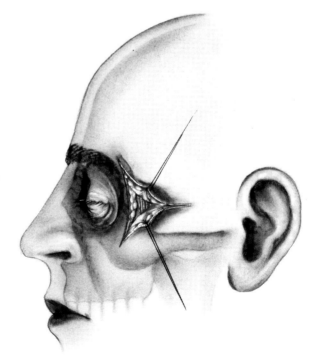

Figure 352. Lateral orbitotomy: curved *T*-incision.

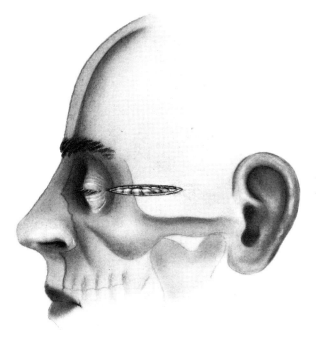

Figure 353. Lateral orbitotomy: horizontal incision (Berke approach).

with scissors was included at the ocular end of the incision. This feature permits wider retraction of the skin flaps and provides better exposure for the preparation of the bone flap, but a careful reconstruction of the lateral canthus is necessary at the end of the operation (Fig. 354). The problems connected with this reconstruction have, however, made some surgeons eliminate the lateral canthotomy of Berke's incision. If the lateral canthus is not well restored to its original anatomic configuration, tears may dribble from the lateral conjunctival cul-de-sac when fibrosis and contracture of the incision occur in the postoperative period.

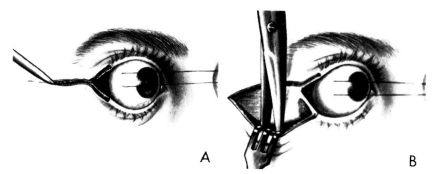

A   **B**

Figure 354.   Lateral orbitotomy: Berke incision combined with a lateral canthotomy. *A,* Traction suture inserted into tendon of lateral rectus muscle. *B,* Lower skin flap is undermined with heavy scissors and separated from underlying temporalis fascia and lateral orbital margin. (From Berke RN: A modified Krönlein operation. Trans Am Ophthalmol Soc *51:*193–226, 1953. By permission of the University of Toronto Press.)

We found this incision (without the lateral canthotomy quite adequate for the removal of the lateral wall of the orbit in cases of malignant endocrine exophthalmos requiring orbital decompression, but the incision did not provide sufficient space for the hinging of a large bone flap such as would be required for the approach to large tumors in the posterior orbit. Orbital decompressions for Graves' ophthalmopathy are now done by another route, and we, as well as other surgeons, either have returned to the T incision or one of the anterolateral approaches for the majority of orbital tumor cases. Thus, the Berke-Reese incision no longer is used as routinely as was once the case.

Hairline Incision. To eliminate completely the visible blemish of any incision in the area of the temporal orbit, so-called hairline incisions have been proposed as an alternate approach for lateral orbitotomy. One of these, the *Guyton incision* (Guyton 1946), is illustrated in Figure 355. Guyton originally advocated the incision for cases of orbital decompression. His incision was made just within the hairline anterior to the ear. The incision was approximately 7 cm long, with a slight concavity forward, but it did not extend inferiorly beyond the middle tragus of the ear. However, Guyton noted that the length, curvature, and exact position of the incision in relation to the ear could be varied to make certain that any resulting scar would be entirely covered by hair. Such an incision, wherever placed in the hairline, is 6 cm or more from the lateral orbital rim, which is the goal of the initial approach. The incision, therefore, requires a relatively large skin flap and an extended dissection as compared to some of the other incisions that are more directly related to the orbital rim. In recent years this incision is seldom used, at least for entry into the orbit through the lateral orbital wall.

Anterolateral Incision. An incision having the horizontal component of the Berke approach and the curved arm of the superior temporal incision (see Chapter 24) also should be noted (Fig. 356). This continuous but right-angled incision has a somewhat L shape configuration. According to de Takáts (1932), one of the first to advocate such an incision was a Swiss contemporary of Krönlein, Theodor Kocher. Kocher's incision was a sweeping, curved cut

Figure 355. Lateral orbitotomy: Guyton's hairline incision for lateral orbital approach. (From Guyton JS: Decompression of the orbit. Surgery *19*:790–809, 1946. By permission of the CV Mosby Company.)

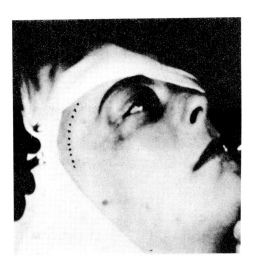

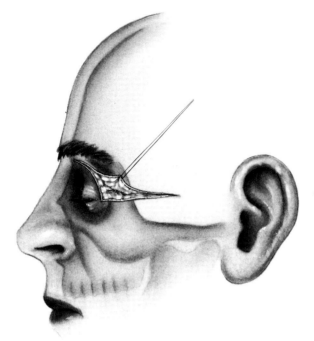

Figure 356. Anterolateral orbitotomy: L-shape incision.

parallel to and slightly above the eyebrow, extending from the midpoint of the latter to the level to the zygomatic arch. The incision was completed along a horizontal arm just above the zygomatic arch.

Stallard (1968) modified the incision by introducing a gentle curve in place of the acute angle between the vertical and horizontal arms. This not only facilitated closure but reduced the puckering of the skin that often occurred at the apex of the acute angle. In recent years we have used this curved anterolateral incision almost exclusively for our approach to retrobulbar lesions and tumors of the lacrimal gland fossa. Other surgeons have subsequently proposed additional modifications, shifting either the curved vertical arm or the horizontal arm superiorly or inferiorly to encompass the planned removal of bone.

All the incisions discussed take in both the skin and subcutaneous tissue. When the superficial bleeding vessels have been secured, the dissection between subcutaneous tissue and temporalis fascia has been completed, and the skin flaps retracted, the initial stage of approach is complete. The surgeon is now ready to perform those maneuvers that will remove the bony barrier to the orbital cavity.

THE BONY ORBITOTOMY

In the original Krönlein operation, the skin and the subcutaneous tissue and the temporalis muscle with its fascia were included with the bone flap when this was removed temporarily from the lateral wall of the orbit. Today, all incisions are designed to keep the skin and subcutaneous tissue separate from the underlying tissues; and, after the incisions have been completed and the skin flaps retracted, the soft tissues attached to the bony rim and lateral orbital wall will be uncovered. Our discussion will proceed on the assumption that one of the more recent approaches to the lateral orbital wall has been selected by the surgeon.

The initial dissection usually is directed toward the exposure of the lateral bony rim. A curved vertical incision is made through the thin but tough, almost avascular tissue covering the lateral bony rim. This covering tissue comprises the fused layers of orbital septum, temporalis fascia, and periosteum. The incision should commence near the mid-vertical plane of the superior orbital rim and extend slightly below the level of the zygomatic arch. This incision may be made directly over the flat surface of the anterolateral face of the bony rim or it may run parallel to the anterolateral edge of the bone. We prefer the former because, once the knife cut has been completed, it is easier to enter the cleavage plane between periosteum and bone with a periosteal elevator. The most important tissue structure along this bony rim is the lateral palpebral tendon. Tagging this bundle of tissue with an identifying suture tie as it is released from its attachment to bone enables the surgeon to replace it properly later in the operation.

Next, the anterior lip of the incision through the periosteum is peeled away from bone by blunt dissection with a sturdy periosteal elevator. The periosteum is firmly attached to bone along the anterior lip of the bony rim and directly over the zygomaticofrontal suture. In the latter position the periosteum may fray as attempts are made to lift it away from the irregular surface of the suture. The periosteum should be elevated along the entire course of the incision overlying the anterolateral bony rim. Once the dissection has been carried around the anterior lip of the bony rim, the cleavage plane between periorbita and bone (peripheral orbital space) is easily entered with the dissector.

The periosteal elevator may be used for some distance superiorly, far posteriorly (approximately 25 mm), and inferiorly along the inner aspect of the lateral orbital wall. At this point, the zygomatic artery, as it crosses the peripheral space to continue its course through bone, may tear and bleed briskly. The bleeding usually subsides spontaneously but it may have to be touched with the coagulating diathermy electrode, either at this time or later, when the bone flap is hinged. This wide manipulation within the peripheral orbital space makes the bone saw easier to use subsequently and permits removal of a greater vertical length of bone than would be possible if elevation of the periorbita was discontinued as soon as the anterior lip of the bony rim had been passed.

At this point, the surgeon may cut the bony rim either right away or after he has removed additional soft tissue from the outer face of the lateral orbital wall. We have used both methods but we tend to favor the latter choice, even though it takes longer. In this alternative, the posterior lip of the knife incision in the periosteum is peeled and pushed dorsalward with a periosteal elevator until the anterolateral bony rim is uncovered. The surgeon also may continue blunt dissection around and behind the posterior edge of the lateral bony rim for some distance down into the temporal fossa. This portion of the blunt dissection may take time because the fibers of the temporalis fascia and periosteum are attached tightly to bone. The periosteum, temporalis fascia, and the temporalis muscle gradually are rolled posteriorly to a point just anterior to the vertical zygomaticosphenoid suture. After the bone flap has been fractured along this suture line, the roll of muscle and fascia will remain attached to the posterior lip of the fractured bony wall and serve as its soft tissue hinge. Short, parallel, horizontal cuts also may be made in the free anterior lip of this tissue roll superiorly and inferiorly to facilitate the rotation of the bony flap after its fracture.

Figures 357 and 358 illustrate several of the anatomic features concerned with the fashioning of the bone flap. The minimal resection of bone depicted in Figure 357 a-a' is seldom used nowadays. The superior extension of the bone incision was advocated by Stallard (Fig. 357) to provide wider access to the orbital cavity. We frequently use this modification for our approach to tumors of the lacrimal gland fossa, although we tend to curve the bone cut in the superior orbital rim in preference to the right angle cut depicted by Stallard. The still wider exposure provided by the modification of Jones (Fig. 357 y') requires a division of the zygomatic arch posterior to the zygomaticotemporal suture, a division of the zygomatic bone in the cheek, and a hinging of the flap on the masseter muscle. We have not found that such a large flap of bone is necessary for the removal of the average retrobulbar tumor. A bone flap such as depicted in Figure 358 (also Fig. 357 b-b') has provided an adequate window for our usual lateral approach.

The Stryker saw is the favored tool for the bone incision. Soft tissues are protected from the oscillating blade of the saw by inserting a ribbon retractor or periosteal elevator into the peripheral space along the inner surface of the lateral orbital wall. When the cuts into the bone are sufficiently deep (approximately 1 cm), the free edge of the lateral orbital rim may be grasped with a double-action forceps or a rongeur; the bone then may be fractured outward and posteriorly on its hinge of soft tissue. When completed, the vertical length of the bone flap will approximate 28 mm in women and 30 mm in men. Its width will measure about 14 mm. The hinged bone flap may be wrapped in a

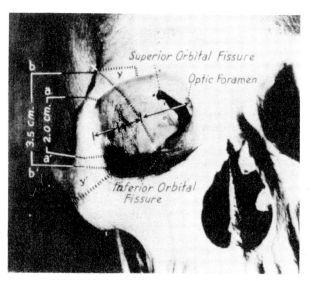

Figure 357. Relevant landmarks of the bony orbit: a-a'— minimal resection of the lateral orbital wall; b-b'—full resection of the orbital wall; y—extended orbitotomy of Stallard; y'—extended orbitotomy of Jones; x-x'—junction of the orbital and cranial cavities. (From Reese AB: Expanding lesions of the orbit. Trans Ophthalmol Soc UK *91*:85–104, 1971. By permission.)

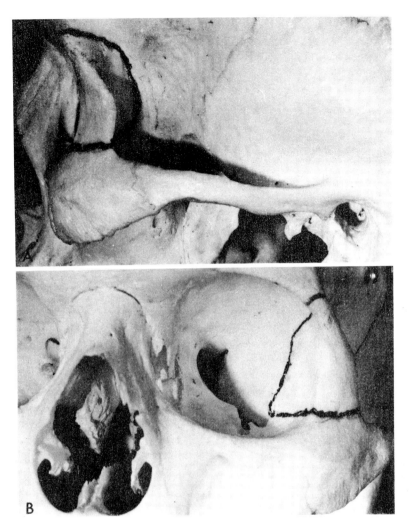

Figure 358. Details of lateral orbitotomy: size and shape of reflected piece of bone outlined by ink (cadaver skull). *A,* Side view. Shape of flap is quadrilateral (almost rectangular); upper edge of incision is roughly parallel and 1 cm superior to zygomaticofrontal suture; lower edge of orbitotomy is at base of frontal process of zygomatic bone, on level with upper border of the zygomatic arch; and fracture line corresponds to zygomaticosphenoid suture, which is covered by vertical arm of ink outline.

B. Oblique frontal view. Posteroinferior corner of bone incision is near junction of zygomaticosphenoid suture with lateral extension of infraorbital fissure.

layer of warm, moist gauze and retracted posteriorly so as to lie peripheral to the direct surgical field.

At the margin of the fracture line (the zygomaticosphenoid suture), the surgeon will be about half the distance to the middle fossa and about one-third the distance to the orbital apex and positioned on a horizontal axis that would pass just behind the eyeball. Many surgeons recommend additional removal of sphenoid bone posterior to the fracture line of the zygomaticosphenoid suture in order to increase the surgical working space. If such is deemed necessary, the periorbita covering the posterior half of the lateral orbital wall should be separated from bone with a narrow periosteal elevator for a short distance; otherwise the vascular periorbita will be nipped or nicked with the biting rongeurs and become a source of annoying and persistent oozing of blood throughout the operation. On the other hand, the surgeon should not be too bold in the posterior extent of this separation of periorbita because of the danger of trauma to the orbital branch of the middle meningeal artery. This arterial branch sometimes is relatively large, and bleeding from it may be severe and difficult to manage. Consequently, surgeons must be wary of this vessel. If further removal of bone is elected, a sturdy rongeur is necessary to bite away the exposed edge of the sphenoid bone because this structure widens perceptibly as it passes posteriorly. The spongy makeup of this wedge of bone may be another source of hemorrhage before the surgeon enters the intra-orbital spaces. The potential problems resulting from separation of periorbita and the difficulties of removing pieces of the sphenoid bone in this area detract from the advantages of the additional working space. We find that we use this supplementary osteotomy less and less; we are content to work in the orbital cavity through the space provided by the initial bone flap.

When the bone flap of the usual lateral orbitotomy has been retracted to one side and the bony defect enlarged with rongeurs to its final size, the shiny lateral surface of the periorbita (the capsule of the orbit) comes into full view. A depression or dimpling of the fascia may bisect the field horizontally. The lateral rectus muscle is immediately beneath this area and roughly divides the field into superior and inferior halves. Identification of the lateral rectus at this stage and upon subsequent entry into the orbit is made easier by insertion of a traction suture into its tendon early in the operation, in the manner illustrated in Figure 354. Tugging on this traction suture from time to time will help to keep this important muscle in full view throughout the subsequent intra-orbital manipulations. Before opening the orbital capsule, the surgeon should inspect the operative field to assure himself that all major bleeding has been stopped, and that most minor oozing has been discouraged from structures such as the bone edges, temporalis muscle and fascia, and skin. Once the intra-orbital work commences, visibility should not be obstructed by bleeding from these sources.

En Bloc Resection.   This procedure requires some modification in the orbitotomy just described. We favor an en bloc resection if we suspect the presence of an intrinsic neoplasm of the lacrimal gland. In this approach the neoplasm, its periorbital base, and surrounding bone are removed en bloc in a one-stage procedure. This will minimize seeding of the neoplasm should it prove to be a benign mixed tumor, and circumvent neoplastic contamination of adjacent structures should the tumor prove to be one of the infiltrative malignant lesions of the lacrimal gland.

The first modification of the standard lateral orbitotomy occurs after the periosteum has been incised along the superior and lateral rim of the orbit to expose the bone. Instead of introducing a periosteal elevator into the peripheral orbital space along the inner aspect of the lateral orbital wall, appropriate incisions are made in the periorbita and orbital septum to uncover the anterior and medial surfaces of the tumor and to delineate the superior and inferior margins of the mass (Henderson and Neault 1976). The osteotomies are then made to encompass the tumor and its periorbital base. As a rule, the superior osteotomy is made at a higher level along the anterolateral rim (Fig. 357 y) than is used for the standard lateral orbitotomy. The bone cuts are directed posteriorly such that bone will fracture along the customary line of the zygo-maticosphenoid suture but remain hinged to a tongue of temporalis fascia and muscle. The tumor and its attached bone may then be moved forward and laterally away from the orbital cavity and isolated from the surrounding surgical field by wrapping a narrow strip of gauze around the fascicle pedicle. This gauze collar provides support should the surgeon suspect the tumor is not a lacrimal gland neoplasm and wish to identify the tissue by an incisional biopsy and frozen tissue study. Should frozen tissue study confirm the non-neoplastic nature of the mass (as in the case of an inflammatory pseudotumor), the tumor may be stripped from its periorbital base and the hinged bone flap replaced in its original bed. If the frozen tissue study proves the tumor to be a nonradio-sensitive neoplasm, the fascial pedicle below or beneath the gauze collar is severed and the pathologic tissue is removed withour further contact with the margins of the operative site. The bone flap and its attached tumor need not be subjected to incisional biopsy if the gross appearance of the tumor suggests an intrinsic neoplasm of the lacrimal gland.

INTRA-ORBITAL TECHNIQUES

Various methods of opening the "capsule" of the orbital contents have been suggested, but most of these have not been associated with eponymous designa-tions, as have the skin incisions. Cruciate, horizontal, vertical, and flap-like in-cisions have been proposed. If, on the basis of palpation through the periorbita or the preoperative clinical assessment, the tumor is primarily quadrantic in position, we prefer a *horizontal incision* through the periorbita above or below the position of the lateral rectus muscle corresponding to the quadrant to be ex-plored. The anterior extent of the horizontal incision above the line of the lateral rectus muscle may be restricted somewhat by the closer approximation of the periorbita to the lacrimal gland than elsewhere. Below the lateral rectus muscle, the periorbita may be opened across the entire length of the operative field. If the tumor is not quadrantic in position but is located more centrally immediately behind the eye, we make horizontal incisions through the peri-orbita across both upper and lower quadrants, and join the incisions near their posterior terminus by a supplementary vertical arm. This forms a flap of peri-orbita that can be reflected anteriorly to give an approach to the retro-ocular tumor either above or below the plane of the lateral rectus muscle, as the ensuing dissection may dictate. We prefer to work around this muscle rather than to sever its belly or detach its tendinous insertion. If necessary, this muscle may be retracted by a narrow linen surgical tape or a gauze strip. Such cloth retractors are much less traumatic to this muscle than any of the metal devices.

Once the capsule of the orbit has been opened, the retro-ocular tumor should be either visible or palpable. If the tumor is not visible but is palpable, further separation and deeper penetration of the orbital reticular tissue should bring the lesion into view. In separating the lobules of the reticular tissue, we try to minimize the use of the cutting instruments and rely instead on cotton-tipped applicators. This will materially reduce bleeding—an important consideration at this stage of the orbitotomy. As the presenting surface of the tumor is uncovered, further palpation usually allows one to determine the position of the mass in relation to the optic nerve, the superior orbital fissure, and the back surface of the eyeball. The configuration of the tumor—whether it is infiltrative, circumscribed, or encapsulated—also should be evident by this time.

Infiltrative Tumors. A positive identification of most infiltrative tumors cannot be made on the basis of their color or configuration. Therefore, an incisional biopsy usually is the first major intraorbital procedure. The superotemporal surface of the mass is probably the preferred site for biopsy in most cases because it is the side of the tumor nearest the surgeon, it is less prone to encompass important nerves or vessels, and it is usually less vascular. While awaiting the frozen tissue examination any bleeding from the biopsy site or any capillary oozing resulting from palpation of the mass should be staunched.

The next step in the intraorbital manipulation will depend on the histopathologic diagnosis. If frozen tissue study indicates a malignant neoplasm, the extent of further dissection may well depend on the nature of the neoplasm. Some neoplasms, such as rhabdomyosarcomas, may be "debulked" as extensively as possible without injury to the eye, optic nerve, or extraocular muscles in anticipation of postoperative chemotherapy and radiotherapy. Other neoplasms, such as malignant lymphoma, can be left alone in view of their favorable response to postoperative irradiation. However, most malignant neoplasms in the retrobulbar space are not amenable to further surgical manipulation at this time. Instead, the surgeon usually terminates the orbitotomy, closes the incision, and awaits the result of fixed tissue diagnosis before discussing with the patient alternate therapies, such as exenteration or radiotherapy.

If the frozen tissue study indicates a benign process, the extent of further surgical dissection will depend on such factors as the size and extent of the mass, the configuration of the mass (diffuse or partially circumscribed), and the amount of preoperative proptosis. A diffusely infiltrative process, such as a plexiform neurofibroma, the fibrotic stage of one of the tumors belonging to the family of inflammatory pseudotumors, or an extensive fibromatosis, might well be left alone because surgical excision is of limited help to the patient. Other benign infiltrative lesions may be partially circumscribed. Here we make an effort to partially remove the mass if it can be accomplished without harm to the levator palpebrae superioris, the extraocular muscles, or the optic nerve; keeping in mind that the patient probably consented to orbitotomy in the hope of reducing a unilateral proptosis.

Noninfiltrative Tumors. A benign, noninfiltrative tumor, of course, is more favorable for complete excision. Such a tumor usually is truly encapsulated or possesses such a pseudocapsule that it can be removed completely. We do not recommend incisional biopsy in these cases and are content to defer histopathologic examination until the entire mass is removed. Instead, a careful dissection is carried along the surface of the mass, either under direct vision or by guiding the dissecting instrument along the proper cleavage plane with the finger of the surgeon's nondominant hand. The forefinger of the surgeon's dominant hand or cotton-tipped applicator is excellent for this type of dissection. As dissection proceeds, traction and mobilization of the tumor is improved by applying one of the cryoprobe tips ordinarily used for either retinal detachment or cataract surgery (Henderson and Neault 1976). The freezing bond between tumor and cryoprobe is quite strong, and the forces of traction seem more evenly distributed over the surface and through the interior of the mass than would be possible with the conventional fixation instruments. The use of the cryoprobe also will reduce the shredding or tearing of the tumor's capsule and lessen the risk of rupturing the wall of a cystic tumor. The cryoprobe may be repetitively defrosted and shifted to other areas on the surface of the mass where traction will most efficiently uncover the masked side of the mass.

Tumors Involving Orbital Portion of Optic Nerve. For a tumor such as a *meningioma* or an *optic nerve glioma* intrinsic in the orbital portion of the optic nerve, we usually recommend the transcranial approach owing to the possibility of extension of the tumor along the optic canal or through the superior orbital fissure toward the intracranial vault. Preoperatively, diagnosis of such a tumor is usually possible by computer tomography of the orbit plus those features already discussed in Chapters 11 and 18. Occasionally, a mass is uncovered in the posterior orbit whose surface either is fused to a portion of the optic nerve sheath or attached to it by a pedicle not visible on computer tomography. Such would be the case with most primary intraorbital meningiomas, some epidermoid cysts encroaching on the posterior orbit, or hemangiomas and lymphangiomas located at the orbital apex of children. In these cases we try to peel away the tumor from the periphery of the optic nerve sheath, but this can seldom be done without some risk to vision. Inasmuch as these cases usually do not have a serious preoperative visual impairment, the surgeon must be content with only a partial excision. Otherwise, the visual loss attendant on complete removal of the orbital mass may outweigh the putative benefits of the orbitotomy from the viewpoint of the patient.

Manipulations around the intra-orbital portion of the optic nerve constitute the most difficult challenge encountered by the surgeon who works through a lateral orbitotomy. The nerve is about 2.5 cm (1 inch), from the surgeon's position along the plane of the bone flap. Even with good illumination, visibility of this portion of the optic nerve is not ideal and the available space is easily diminished by bleeding. To overcome some of these inherent problems, several ophthalmologists supplement the lateral orbitotomy with some approach along the medial orbit. These combined approaches will be noted in the following chapter.

Importance of Hemostasis. The goal of the lateral orbitotomy has been accomplished once the tumor has been identified and removed. The next step is hemostasis of all major bleeding points and arrest of oozing. The need to staunch hemorrhage and to prevent formation of a hematoma in the postoperative period deserves special emphasis. Too often, a surgeon may close the orbitotomy without proper regard to hemostasis or assume that insertion of drains will compensate for the frustrations of trying to arrest unseen bleeders in the depths of the orbit. We have observed instances of unilateral visual loss associated with pallor of the optic disk, postoperatively, after lateral orbitotomies for pseudotumors, intra-orbital meningiomas, and plexiform neurofibromas. All of these tumors are notoriously vascular, and the pseudotumor and the plexiform neurofibroma are nearly impossible to excise completely. Incomplete excision, of course, leaves cut surfaces that tend to bleed unless extra precautions are taken to arrest all bleeding points. We believe that *increased intra-orbital pressure secondary to inadequate hemostasis at the completion of the orbitotomy, combined with continued seepage of blood into the retro-ocular space in the postoperative period, was a major factor in the ultimate blindness of such patients.* Any bleeding points that can be seen should be clasped with the bipolar cautery. If bleeding is too brisk for the effective use of the bipolar device, the Anthony-Fisher suction cautery is helpful to the surgeon in evacuating the blood and cauterizing the bleeding point simultaneously. Seldom is there room in the posterior orbit for direct sutures or ties to provide more permanent hemostasis.

Other factors, either alone or combined with retro-ocular hematoma, may contribute to visual loss and ultimate pallor of the optic disk after operation. Trauma to the optic nerve by the surgical instruments or by prolonged digital examination of the retro-ocular space is an obvious reason for this unfortunate complication. We believe there is a more common but unrecognized reason: *the final application of a bandage or dressing that exerts excessive pressure on the eye in the immediate postoperative period when the stage of reactive tissue edema is at its climax.* The old-fashioned elastic head bandage, which is snugged tightly over the orbitotomy incision and adjacent eye, is a common culprit in this respect. Fortunately, this kind of bandage is now being used less frequently. External pressure probably compromises the flow through the central retinal artery, and affected patients usually are totally blind when the pressure dressing subsequently is removed after a period of several days. The ocular fundus of such patients may or may not show the classical cherry-red spot in the macular area.

Failure to remove the intermarginal lid suture at the completion of the operation is another factor causing undue counterpressure on an eye that is being proptosed forward by postoperative hemorrhage and edema in the posterior orbit. Another factor causing visual loss is associated with a decompression operation performed as a treatment for endocrine exophthalmos. The surgical procedure itself may superimpose such a reaction on an already edematous, hypertrophied, orbital reticular tissue that the blood supply to the retina is obstructed, in spite of the additional decompression space. Long and Ellis (1971) have reviewed this problem from the standpoint of their own as well as other surgeons' experience in this field.

CLOSURE AND OPERATIVE CARE

Our objective during closure is to restore the lateral bony wall to its approximate preoperative status. A loose closure of the periorbita with a running plain catgut suture is first attempted, but such a closure is usually incomplete because of shredding of the periorbita consequent to the surgical manipulations necessary for the delivery of the orbital mass. A number of surgeons believe that closure of the periorbita is optional, and we have no strong opinion for or against this belief. Next, the hinged bone flap is rotated back to its normal axis unless it has been removed in the course of an en bloc resection of a neoplasm of the lacrimal gland.

Regardless of the disposition of the bone flap, the soft tissue hinge of temporalis fascia and muscle is repositioned as well as possible and anchored by chromic catgut sutures to the periosteum and fascia of the adjoining untouched bone. Particular attention is given to the replacement of the lateral palpebral tendon and raphe to their junction with the periosteum and temporalis fascia along the restored line of the lateral orbital rim. Chromic catgut also is used for this step. Additional closure of soft tissue structures and subcutaneous tissues is accomplished with either interrupted chromic or plain catgut sutures. No drains are inserted. Next, the skin incision is closed either with interrupted silk sutures or a subcuticular pullout silk thread. Finally, the intermarginal lid suture and the traction suture near the insertion of the lateral rectus muscle are removed and the interior of the eye is inspected by ophthalmoscopy. The intermarginal suture in the eyelid is not replaced.

The orbitotomy incision is covered with two layers of gauze squares, and the closed eyelids and the underlying eye are covered with a gauze strip. These dressings are loosely secured with any of the commercially available adhesive strips or tape. All dressings may be removed the day after surgery. At one time, we kept the eye and the incision covered for several days, on the assumption that such dressings, combined with moderate external pressure, suppressed postoperative tissue edema. In retrospect, however, it seems probable that such prolonged bandaging and pressure do not actually prevent postoperative hemorrhage and edema, if these are going to occur. In view of the consequences of unforeseen or unanticipated rises of intra-orbital pressure in the postoperative interval, we believe that it is wiser to have the eye uncovered, even though the ecchymosis of the eyelids and adnexa may upset the patient.

Antibiotics, in appropriate maintenance doses, also are administered. The administration of tablets containing a proteolytic enzyme for the reduction of inflammation and edema is optional.

Bibliography

Berke RN: A modified Krönlein operation. Trans Am Ophthalmol Soc 51:193–226, 1953

Berke RN: Management of complications of orbital surgery. In *Complications in Eye Surgery*, second edition. Ed: RM Fasanella. Philadelphia, WB Saunders Company, 1965, pp 373–387

De Takáts G: Surgery of the orbit. Arch Ophthalmol ns 8:259–268, 1932

Guyton JS: Decompression of the orbit. Surgery 19:790–809, 1946

Henderson JW, Neault RW: The use of the cryoprobe in the removal of posterior orbital tumors. Ophthalmic Surg 7(2):45–47, 1976

Henderson JW, Neault RW: En bloc removal of intrinsic neoplasms of the lacrimal gland. Am J Ophthalmol 82:905–909, 1976

Jones BR: Surgical approaches to the orbit. Trans Ophthalmol Soc UK 90:269–308, 1970

Kocher [T]: Cited by de Takáts G

Krönlein RU: Zur Pathologie und operativen Behandlung der Dermoidcysten der Orbita. Beitr Klin Chir 4:149–163, 1888

Long JC, Ellis PP: Total unilateral visual loss following orbital surgery. Am J Ophthalmol 71:218–220, 1971

Passavant: Cited by Wecker L

Reese AB: Expanding lesions of the orbit. Trans Ophth Soc UK 91:85–104, 1971

Stallard HB: A plea for lateral orbitotomy with certain modifications. Brit J Ophthalmol *44*:718–723, 1960

Stallard HB: Surgery of the orbit. Ann R Coll Surg Engl *43*:125–140, 1968

Swift GW: Cited by Guyton JS

Wagner W: Die Behandlung der complicirten Schädelfracturen. Sammlung Klin Vorträge Chir *85*: 2405–2510, 1886

Wecker L: *Traitéorique et Pratique des Maladies des Yeux*. Second edition. Volume 1. Paris, Adrien Delahaye, 1866

26

The Combined Surgical Approaches

In this chapter we will note procedures devised either to improve the surgical exposure of the orbital apex or to remove malignant neoplasms not amenable to the surgical approaches described in the two preceding chapters. Each procedure involves more extensive surgical manipulation than either the anterior or lateral orbitotomy alone.

COMBINED LATERAL AND MEDIAL ORBITOTOMY

In Chapter 25 we discussed some of the problems connected with the removal of tumors from the intraorbital portion of the optic nerve. In our own experience the area nasal to this portion of the optic nerve is the most difficult to visualize other than by a transfrontal craniotomy. This least accessible zone is a triangular area (when viewed from a transverse plane), with its base corresponding to an imaginary line from the back surface of the eye to the medial wall of the orbit; its apex at the optic foramen; and its sides formed by the medial wall of the orbit, medially, and the medial surface of the intraorbital optic nerve laterally. Many others have recognized the complexities of a surgical approach to this area.

In the early years of orbital surgery this zone was reached by an incision through the nasal conjunctival cul-de-sac. Later, an approach was proposed through the peripheral orbital space along the medial wall of the orbit, with an incision of periorbita directly over the assumed location of the lesion. Although the anatomic goal of such incisions was reached, the area available for surgical manipulation was very cramped and the zone of visibility was even more narrow. More recently, Smith (1971) and McCord (1978), among others, have described surgical procedures designed to improve the surgeon's approach to the orbital portion of the optic nerve.

These procedures are basically quite similar, in that a medial orbital approach is combined with the standard lateral orbitotomy. In both operations the orbit is explored after reflection of the lateral bone flap. The patient's head is then repositioned and the anteromedial aspects of the operation continued. In the Smith procedure, a 360 degree peritomy is made through conjunctiva, and a black silk traction suture is placed beneath each of the rectus muscle insertions. In the McCord operation a 180 degree peritomy is made in the nasal conjunctiva and the medial rectus muscle temporarily detached from its insertion (Fig. 359). In both procedures the anteromedial approach and the lateral approach are combined in-

597

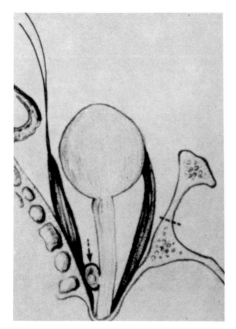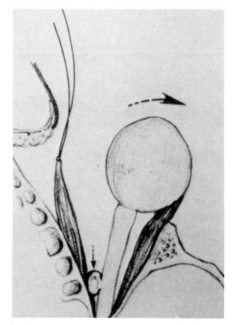

Figure 359.   Combined lateral-medial orbitotomy (diagrammatic representation). Left. Lateral orbital wall is removed along dotted line. Medial rectus muscle is detached from its insertion and tagged with a traction suture. Right. Eye is displaced laterally *(large arrow)* to expose tumor *(small arrow)* along medial aspect of optic nerve. (From McCord CD, Jr: A combined lateral and medial orbitotomy for exposure of the optic nerve and orbital apex. Ophthalmic Surg 9(3):58–66. 1978. By permission.)

to one surgical field by incising and retracting the lateral canthal tendon and raphe. In the Smith procedure the orbital optic nerve is brought into view by displacing the eye anteriorly and laterally into the temporal fossa by traction on the 4 silk sutures beneath the rectus muscle tendons. In the McCord procedure the optic nerve is exposed by retraction of the medial rectus muscle toward the medial orbital wall and lateral displacement of the eye into the space created by hinging the bone flap. We have used modifications of both procedures on infrequent occasions where the anterior orbitotomy alone was not sufficient to remove a tumor either attached to or a part of the orbital portion of the optic nerve. This combined approach provides an improved three-dimensional view of the orbital problem.

In the closure of these extensive dissections it is very important to restore meticulously the lateral canthal tendon and raphe to their preoperative anatomic position.

CRANIOFACIAL-ORBITAL RESECTIONS

These are the newest of the major surgical approaches to the orbit, so recent and so infrequently practiced that a universal descriptive term has not yet evolved. These radical procedures, however named, represent another advance in the medical profession's effort to eradicate malignant neoplasms of the orbit. They are designed principally for those large primary malignant neoplasms that involve orbital bones. They also may be recommended for situations in which less radical surgical procedures have failed to eradicate the orbital neoplasm, or in patients whose orbital disease is considered inoperable by standard means. In short, their scope is one step beyond the long-practiced orbital exenteration and the limited bone resections of the lateral orbitotomy.

One of the descriptions of this operative approach is that of Murray and associates (1972). Actually, their first cranio-orbital resection was performed as long ago as 1957 and was a modification of earlier surgical procedures proposed for the complete extirpation of cancer of the paranasal sinuses involving the orbit. Their interest in a more extensive orbital procedure was initiated by prior failure to cure a single patient with recurrent orbital rhabdomyosarcoma by exenteration. This particular time period was considerably earlier than the present era of combined chemotherapy, radiotherapy, and surgery for rhabdomyosarcoma. By the time of their report (1972), six patients with recurrent orbital rhabdomyosarcoma had been managed by their surgical method. Five of these patients were alive at the time of their report, and detailed protocols were given on 3 living patients without recurrent disease who were followed from 11 to 14 years after surgery. Subsequent pursuits in this field of orbital surgery will be found in the reports of Wilson and Westbury (1973), Sypert and Habal (1978), and Westbury and associates (1975). Sypert and Habal utilized the operation in ten patients with recurrent or extensive squamous cell carcinoma of the orbit.

The aim of the surgical dissection is to encompass the malignancy by a monobloc excision of the eye, all remaining soft parts of the orbital cavity, and most (but not all) of the orbital bones. Clinical or radiographic evidence of bony destruction around the optic foramen and superior orbital fissure, or invasion of the sphenopalatine fossa by the malignant lesion would be considered a relative contraindication to the operation by most surgeons. If there is any question as to the full extent of the malignant process, a preliminary transfrontal exploration of the anterior fossa can be performed to determine its resectability (Sypert and Habal). The technique and extent of the operation are diagrammatically depicted in Figure 360. Superiorly, the roof of the orbit, frontal bone, and frontal sinus are resected. Medially, the lacrimal bone, the ethmoid plate and ethmoid sinus, and the lateral nasal bone with attached turbinates are sacrificed. Inferiorly, the orbital rim, roof of maxillary sinus, and malar bone are removed. Laterally, the orbital portions of the zygomatic bone and sphenoid bone along the posterolateral aspect of the orbit are excised. The exposed dura overlying the anterior and middle cranial fossa is finally covered by a split-thickness skin graft after careful suturing of all rents in the dura.

All who work in this field recommend the advantages of a multidisciplinary approach. The surgical team usually includes surgeons from at least two of the surgical specialties of neurosurgery, maxillofacial surgery, plastic surgery, otorhinologic surgery, ophthalmology, or head and neck oncology. We have had no experience working on a team in this combined surgical specialty effort, but we believe there will be increasing interest in a joint surgical approach to these horizons in oncology among the various medical centers. We are particularly hopeful that these combined surgical procedures involving the orbit may pro-

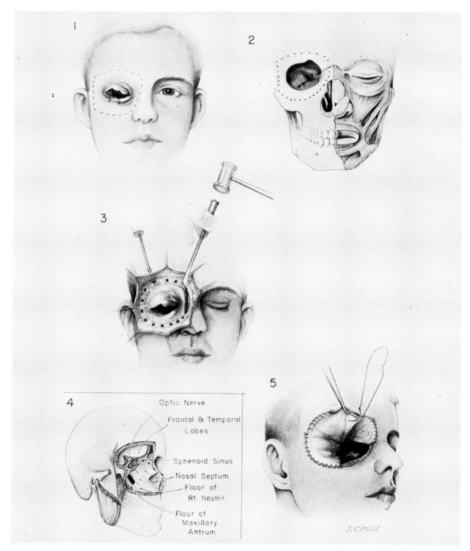

Figure 360.   Cranio-orbital resection (operative technique). 1. A circumorbital skin incision is carried down to periosteum, but the tumor is left untouched during the dissection. 2. The periosteum is elevated and multiple drill holes are made in the frontal, nasal, and maxillary bones. 3. The multiple burr holes are connected by an osteotome. At this point the dura is separated from the bone which encases the tumor. Any dura involved by tumor is resected and replaced by a dural patch graft. 4. Anatomic structure of the defect created by surgical resection. Note that all structures between the frontal lobe and palate are expendable, once the eye has been removed. 5. The defect is resurfaced with a split-thickness skin graft. (From Murray JE, et al: Regional cranio-orbital resection for recurrent tumors with delayed reconstruction. Surg Gynecol Obstet 134:437–447, 1972. By permission of Surgery, Gynecology and Obstetrics.)

long the survival or even improve the cure rate of patients with malignant tumors of the lacrimal gland whose neoplasm is known to have spread beyond the limits of present-day bone resection and soft tissue exenteration. We suspect that Krönlein and other pioneers in the field of orbital bone surgery would applaud these efforts to advance the scope of oncologic surgery in this anatomic area. Truly, the surgery of the orbital cavity and orbital bones has come a long way in its first 100 years.

Bibliography

Combined Lateral and Medial Orbitotomy

McCord CD, Jr: A combined lateral and medial orbitotomy for exposure of the optic nerve and orbital apex. Ophthalmic Surg 9(3):58–66, 1978

Smith JL: Anterolateral approach to the orbit. Trans Am Acad Ophthalmol Otolaryngol 75:1059–1064, 1971

Craniofacial-Orbital Resection

Murray JE, Matson, DM, Habal MB, et al: Regional cranio-orbital resection for recurrent tumors with delayed reconstruction. Surg Gynecol Obstet 134:437–447, 1972

Sypert GW, Habal MB: Combined cranio-orbital surgery for extensive malignant neoplasms of the orbit. Neurosurgery 2:8–14, 1978

Westbury G, Wilson JSP, Richardson A: Combined craniofacial resection for malignant disease. Am J Surg 130:463–469, 1975

Wilson JSP, Westbury G: Combined craniofacial resection for tumor involving the orbital walls. Brit J Plast Surg 26:44–56, 1973

Index

Page numbers followed by t
indicate a table.